TRAVELERS' DIARRHEA

Second Edition

TRAVELERS' DIARRHEA
Second Edition

CHARLES D. ERICSSON, MD
Professor of Medicine
Head, Clinical Infectious Diseases
University of Texas Medical School at Houston
Houston, Texas

HERBERT L. DUPONT, MD
Chief, Internal Medicine
St. Luke's Episcopal Hospital
Director, Center for Infectious Diseases
University of Texas School of Public Health at Houston
Mary W. Kelsey Chair
University of Texas Medical School at Houston
Department of Medicine
Baylor College of Medicine
H. Irving Schweppe Jr. Chair and Vice Chairman
Houston, Texas

PROF ROBERT STEFFEN, MD
Head, Division of Communicable Diseases
Director, World Health Organization Collaborating Centre for
Travellers' Health
Institute of Social and Preventive Medicine
University of Zürich,
Zürich, Switzerland

2008
BC Decker Inc.
Hamilton

BC Decker Inc
P.O. Box 620, L.C.D. 1
Hamilton, Ontario L8N 3K7
Tel: 905-522-7017; 800-568-7281
Fax: 905-522-7839; 888-311-4987
E-mail: info@bcdecker.com
www.bcdecker.com

First Edition 2003.

08/09/10/GP/9 8 7 6 5 4 3 2 1

ISBN 978-1-55009-371-1
Production Editor: Devorah Abrams Farmer Typesetter: Charlesworth; Cover Designer: Lisa Mattinson
Printed in India by Gopsons Papers

Sales and Distribution

United States
BC Decker Inc
P.O. Box 785
Lewiston, NY 14092-0785
Tel: 905-522-7017; 800-568-7281
Fax: 905-522-7839; 888-311-4987
E-mail: info@bcdecker.com
www.bcdecker.com

Canada
BC Decker Inc
50 King St. E.
P.O. Box 620, LCD 1
Hamilton, Ontario L8N 3K7
Tel: 905-522-7017; 800-568-7281
Fax: 905-522-7839; 888-311-4987
E-mail: info@bcdecker.com
www.bcdecker.com

Foreign Rights
John Scott & Company
International Publishers' Agency
P.O. Box 878
Kimberton, PA 19442
Tel: 610-827-1640
Fax: 610-827-1671
E-mail: jsco@voicenet.com

Japan
Igaku-Shoin Ltd.
Foreign Publications Department
1-28-23 Hongo
Bunkyo-ku, Tokyo, Japan 113-8719
Tel: 3 3817 5611
Fax: 3 3815 4114
E-mail: fd@igaku-shoin.co.jp

UK, Europe, Middle East
McGraw-Hill Education
Shoppenhangers Road
Maidenhead
Berkshire, England SL6 2QL
Tel: 44-0-1628-502500
Fax: 44-0-1628-635895
www.mcgraw-hill.co.uk

Singapore, Malaysia, Thailand, Philippines, Indonesia, Vietnam, Pacific Rim, Korea
Elsevier Science Asia
583 Orchard Road
#09/01, Forum
Singapore 238884
Tel: 65-737-3593
Fax: 65-753-2145

Australia, New Zealand
Elsevier Science Australia
Customer Service Department
Locked Bag 16
St. Peters, New South Wales 2044
Australia
Tel: 61 02-9517-8999
Fax: 61 02-9517-2249
E-mail: customerserviceau@elsevier.com
www.elsevier.com.au

Mexico and Central America
ETM SA de CV
Calle de Tula 59
Colonia Condesa
06140 Mexico DF, Mexico
Tel: 52-5-5553-6657
Fax: 52-5-5211-8468
E-mail: editoresdetextosmex@prodigy.net.mx

Brazil
Tecmedd Importadora E Distribuidora De Livros Ltda.
Avenida Maurílio Biagi, 2850
City Ribeirão, Ribeirão Preto – SP – Brasil
CEP: 14021-000
Tel: 0800 992236
Fax: (16) 3993-9000
E-mail: tecmedd@tecmedd.com.br

India, Bangladesh, Pakistan, Sri Lanka
Elsevier Health Sciences Division
Customer Service Department
17A/1, Main Ring Road
Lajpat Nagar IV
New Delhi – 110024, India
Tel: 91 11 2644 7160-64
Fax: 91 11 2644 7156
E-mail: esindia@vsnl.net

Contributors

JAVIER A. ADACHI, MD
Department of Infectious Diseases
University of Texas, MD Anderson Cancer Center
Houston, Texas

ROBERT L. ATMAR, MD
Department of Medicine
Baylor College of Medicine
Houston, Texas

RON H. BEHRENS, BSc, MB ChB, MD
Department of Infectious and Tropical Diseases
University of London, School of Hygiene and Tropical Medicine
London, England

JAIME BELKIND-GERSON, MD, MS
Instituto Nacional de Salud Publica de Mexico
Centro de Investigacion en Salud Poblacional
Cuernavaca, Mexico

ROBERT E. BLACK, MD
Department of International Health
Bloomberg School of Public Health
Johns Hopkins University
Baltimore, Maryland

JEAN-PAUL BUTZLER, MD, PhD
Clinical Microbiology and Epidemiology
Vrije Universiteit Brussel
Brussels, Belgium

SANTIAGO PÉREZ CACHAFEIRO, MD, MSc
Galician Agency for Health Technology Assessment
Santiago de Compostela
A Coruña, Spain

JUAN-PABLO CAEIRO, MD
Department of Medicine
Baylor College of Medicine
Houston, Texas

FRANCESCO CASTELLI, MD
Department of Infectious and Tropical Diseases
University of Brescia
Brescia, Italy

SANTANU CHATTERJEE, MBBS, DTM&H
Travel and Tropical Medicine
Woodlands Medical Centre
Kolkata, India

JOHN D. CLEMENS, MD
International Vaccine Institute
Seoul, Republic of Korea

BRADLEY A. CONNOR, MD
Department of Medicine
Gasterenterology and Hematology
Weill Cornell Medical College
New York, New York

EILIF DAHL, MD, MHA, PHD
Department of Surgery 1
Rikshospitalet – Radiumhospitalet
Oslo, Norway

CHIARA DEBERNARDIS, MD
Division of Communicable Diseases
University of Zürich/ISPM
Zürich, Switzerland

ANDREW W. DUPONT, MD, MSPH
Department of Internal Medicine, Gastroenterology
The University of Texas Medical Branch
Galveston, Texas

HERBERT L. DUPONT, MD
Department of Medicine
Baylor College of Medicine
Houston, Texas

CHARLES D. ERICSSON, MD
Clinical Infectious Diseases
University of Texas Medical School at Houston
Houston, Texas

DAVID O. FREEDMAN, MD
Departments of Medicine and Epidemiology
University of Alabama at Birmingham
Birmingham, Alabama

ROGER I. GLASS, MD, PhD
Fogarty International Center and NIH for International Programs
National Institutes of Health
Bethesda, Maryland

SHERWOOD L. GORBACH, MD
Tufts University School of Medicine
Tufts New England Medical Center
Boston, Massachusetts

WILLIAM B. GREENOUGH III, MD
John Hopkins University
Department of Medicine
Baltimore, Maryland

RICHARD L. GUERRANT, MD
Center for Global Health
Division of Infectious Diseases and International Health
University of Virginia School of Medicine
Charlottesville, Virginia

NIKLAUS GYR, MD, MPH&TM
Department of Internal Medicine
University Hospital Basel
Basel, Switzerland

STEPHEN HANAUER, MD
Section of Gastroenterology and Nutrition
University of Chicago Medical Center
Chicago, Illinois

DAVID R. HILL, MD, DTM&H, FRCP
Department of Tropical and Infectious Diseases
London School of Hygiene and Tropical Medicine
London, England

LYNN L. HORVATH, MD
Army Medical Center, Department of Medicine
Infectious Disease Service
Fort Sam Houston, Texas

DAVID B. HUANG, MD, PhD
Boehringer-Ingelheim Pharmaceuticals
Clinical Operations
Ridgefield, Connecticut

ZHI-DONG JIANG, MD, PhD
Center for Infectious Diseases
University of Texas School of Public Health
Houston, Texas

ERICA N. JOHNSON, MD
Department of Medicine, Infectious Disease Service
Brooke Army Medical Center
Fort Sam Houston, Texas

GILBERT R. KAUFMANN, MD
Department of Internal Medicine
University Hospital Basel
Basel, Switzerland

HERWIG KOLLARITSCH, MD
Institute for Specific Prophylaxis and Tropical Medicine
Medical University of Vienna
Vienna, Austria

PHYLLIS E. KOZARSKY, MD
Department of Medicine
Emory University
Atlanta, Georgia

STEPHANIE A. LEE, MD
Infectious Diseases Associates
Private Practice
Newark, Delaware

MYRON LEVINE, MD, DTPH
Center for Vaccine Development
University of Maryland School of Medicine
Baltimore, Maryland

STUART B. LEVY, MD, FAAM
Department of Molecular Biology and Microbiology and Medicine
Tufts University, School of Medicine
Boston, Massachusetts

LEENA MATILLA, MD, PhD
Faculty of Medicine
University of Helsinki
Helsinki University Central Hospital
Helsinki, Finland

C. KENNETH McALLISTER, MD
Department of Internal Medicine, Infectious Diseases
University of Kentucky School of Medicine
Lexington, Kentucky

PATRICK F. McDERMOTT, PhD
US Food and Administration
Center for Veterinary Medicine
Laurel, Maryland

ROBIN McKENZIE, MD
Department of Medicine
Infectious Diseases
Johns Hopkins University
Baltimore, Maryland

SUSAN L.F. McLELLAN, MD, MPH
Infectious Diseases Section - Medicine
Department of Tropical Medicine, SPHTM
Tulane University Health Sciences Center
New Orleans, Louisiana

JAMES P. NATARO, MD, PhD
Center for Vaccine Development
University of Maryland, School of Medicine
Baltimore, Maryland

DEBORAH J. NICOLLS, MD
Department of Medicine, Infectious Diseases
Emory University, School of Medicine
Atlanta, Georgia

NEBOJŠA NIKOLIĆ, MD, MS
Faculty of Maritime Studies
University of Rijeka
Rijeka, Croatia

RICHARD A. OBERHELMAN, MD
Department of Tropical Medicine and Pediatrics
Tulane University, School of Public Health and Tropical Medicine
New Orleans, Louisiana

PABLO C. OKHUYSEN, MD
Department of Internal Medicine, Infectious Diseases
University of Texas Medical School at Houston
Houston, Texas

PRATIVA PANDEY, MD
Medical Director
The CIWEC Clinic Travel Medicine Center
Kathmandu, Nepal

WILLIAM A. PETRI Jr, MD, PhD
Department of Internal Medicine
University of Virginia
Charlottesville, Virginia

ISRAEL POTASMAN, MD
Faculty of Medicine
B'nai Zion Medical Center
Haifa, Israel

MARK S. RIDDLE, MD, MPH&TM
Naval Medical Research Center
Enteric Diseases Department
Silver Spring, Maryland

ROISIN ROONEY, MS
Department of Public Health and Policy
London School of Hygiene and Tropical Medicine
London, England

EDWARD T. RYAN, MD, DTMH
Associate Professor
Harvard Medical School
Boston, Massachusetts

R. BRADLEY SACK, MS, MD, ScD
Department of International Health
John Hopkins Bloomberg School of Public Health
Baltimore, Maryland

JOHN W. SANDERS, MD, MPH&TM
Uniformed Services University of the Health Sciences
Internal Medicine, Infectious Diseases
Bethesda, Maryland

SUNIL SAZAWAL, MD, MPH, PhD
Department of International Health
Bloomberg School of Public Health
John Hopkins University
Baltimore, Maryland

DAVID R. SHLIM, MD
Jackson Hole Travel and Tropical Medicine
Jackson Hole, Wyoming

CYNTHIA B. SNIDER, MD, MPH
Department of Medicine
University of Virginia School of Medicine
Charlottesville, Virginia

ROBIN C. SPILLER, MD, MSC, FRCP
Wolfson Digestive Diseases Centre
University of Nottingham
Nottingham, England

ROBERT STEFFEN, MD
Division of Communicable Diseases
University of Zürich/ISPM
Zürich, Switzerland

ANN-MARI SVENNERHOLM, MD, PhD
Department of Microbiology & Immunology
Soteborg University
Institute Biomedicin
Göteborg, Sweden

THOMAS D. SZUCS, MD, MPH, MBA, LLM
Institute of Social and Preventive Medicine
University of Zürich
Zürich, Switzerland

CLAUDE THIBEAULT, MD
University of Texas Medical Branch
Preventive and Community Medicine
Galveston, Texas

DAVID R. TRIBBLE, MD, DrPH
Uniformed Services, University of the Health Sciences
Preventive Medicine and Biometrics
Infectious Disease Clinical Research Program
Bethesda, Maryland

JOSEPH TORRESI, MBBS, BMedSci, PhD, FRACP
Department of Medicine
The University of Melbourne
Royal Melbourne Hospital
Parkville, Australia

FRANK VON SONNENBURG, MD, MPH
Division of International Medicine and Public Health
University of Munich
Munich, Germany

JORDI VILA, MD, PhD
Department of Microbiology
University of Barcelona, School of Medicine
Barcelona, Spain

THOMAS WEINKE, MD
Department of Gastroenterology and Infectious Diseases
Klinikum Ernst von Bergmann
Potsdam, Germany

DAVID G. WHITE, BS, MS, PhD
Office of Research
US Food and Drug Administration
Center for Veterinary Medicine
Laurel, Maryland

ANNELIES WILDER-SMITH, MD, PhD, MIH, DTM&H
National University Singapore
Department of Community, Occupational and Family Medicine
Singapore

Contents

PART FOUR: PREVENTION

PREFACE

Although substantial progress has been made in our understanding of the pathogenesis and management of traveler's diarrhea, the hygiene conditions and infrastructure in many developing countries have not significantly improved. Therefore, travelers' diarrhea remains a frequent health problem, with a substantial impact on professional and leisure travelers alike. In this, our second edition of Travelers' Diarrhea, we have chosen many new authors, all thought leaders in their fields, to update the story in comprehensive detail. Some authors are established investigators; some are rising stars. We have once again tried to balance perspectives by insisting on at least two expert authors per chapter. Our aim is to convey an erudite history, a basic understanding of the discipline, state-of-the-art management recommendations, and thoughts for future research.

We have substantial understanding of the risks of acquiring travelers' diarrhea and we continue to learn about differences in host susceptibility. Recent research questions the pivotal role of fluid replacement in the treatment of adults with travelers' diarrhea. An increasing number of medications are available for symptomatic relief, most notably a nonabsorbable antibiotic for specific antimicrobial therapy against causal organisms. Modern molecular and genetic techniques promise to elucidate virulence properties of enteropathogens and protective antibody responses. While vaccine development based on such basic research is at various levels of investigation, hopes remain high for vaccines against some of the pathogens, particularly enterotoxigenic *Escherichia coli*. New production techniques offer the possibility of cheap vaccines, and vaccine delivered in food promises to bypass the cold chain that limits vaccination in some developing countries.

The rate of diarrhea among travelers has not fallen perceptibly over many decades despite improving public health services around the world that have resulted in lowered infant mortality rates in some developing countries. Even at best, vaccines will offer only a partial solution. Continued improvements in public health promise to address the root cause of travelers' diarrhea, namely, fecal-oral contamination. But the world has a long way to go, and until then, traditional approaches of self medication, chemoprophylaxis, and attempts to modify risky behavior will continue to play a central role in our approach to the syndrome.

We hope this book offers something useful to the travel medicine expert, generalist, and researcher alike.

Charles D. Ericsson, MD
Herbert L. DuPont, MD
Robert Steffen, MD

Chapter 1

Historical Perspectives of Travelers' Diarrhea

Herbert L. DuPont, MD

Charles D. Ericsson, MD

Robert Steffen, MD

The early history of the topic of travelers' diarrhea is tied up with military campaigns, where soldiers classically have suffered more losses from diarrhea and dysentery than from war-related injury.[1–3] The later history relates more to international travelers, expatriates, and short-term students spending time in high-risk areas.

With the early recognition of the common occurrence of diarrhea, when individuals traveled to specific tropical and semitropical cities or regions, have emerged popular and colorful terms denoting the disorder: "Delhi Belly," "Turkey Trots," "Montezuma's Revenge," "GIs," "Turista," "Casablanca Crud," "Aztec Two-Step," "Malta Dog," "Singapore Shakes," "Canary Disease," "Gyppy (Egyptian) Tummy," "Aden Gut," "Basra Belly," "Maladie de la Mer Rouge," "Poonah Pooh," "Hongkong Dog," "Ho Chi Minh," "Rangoon Runs," "Tokyo Trot," "San Franciscitis," "Greek Gallop," "Rome Runs," and "Trotsky's."

When considering the syndrome of travelers' diarrhea, historical developments can be divided into at least seven phases:

1. Definitions of populations at risk,
2. Clinical description and epidemiologic features of the syndrome,
3. Specific risk of illness by region and development of immunity,
4. Sources and cause of the disease,
5. Drug prevention,
6. Drug therapy, and
7. Current era of research including refinements in therapy, studies of genetic susceptibility, and immunoprophylaxis.

We will briefly consider the important defining studies of the first six areas.

Definitions of Populations at Risk

In Table 1, the various groups at high risk for developing travelers' diarrhea are outlined along with references dealing with a review of the setting. As stated earlier, military groups have frequently experienced enteric diseases while engaged in campaigns. Kean indicated that the outcome of competition of athletes participating in Olympic Games was often determined by the occurrence of diarrhea.[4] Students to Mexico have served as a setting for the study of travelers' diarrhea for nearly 50 years.[4–9] Persons living for prolonged periods in foreign countries have frequently experienced acute and recurrent diarrhea, whether they be expatriates, missionaries, or Peace Corps volunteers.[10–12] Diarrhea has been an important problem of populations at sea, and an occasional problem among passengers on cruise ships as well as passengers under-

Table 1 Historical Groups at Risk of Acquiring Travelers' Diarrhea

Population	Reference
Military groups	1–3
Olympic competitors	4
Students	4, 8
Expatriates and missionaries	11, 12
Peace Corps volunteers	10
Cruise participants, seafaring populations, and persons taking commercial flights	13–15
Tourists and business persons	16, 17, 20

Table 2 Clinical Description and Epidemiologic Features of the Syndrome

Observation	Reference
Clinical description of the illness	4
Epidemiologic description of the disease	4, 8, 16
Relative risk of various regions of the world	16, 20
Natural immunity occurrence with time in the region	8, 19

taking commercial air travels.[13–15] International travelers on pleasure and business are known to be at high risk for travelers' diarrhea.[16,17] The two key predictive factors for illness occurrence, known for many decades, are place of origin of the travelers and level of hygiene of the country to be visited. International travelers resemble the children of the host country in their intrinsic susceptibility to enteric infection. Invariably, there are high rates of infantile gastroenteritis in those areas at high risk for travelers' diarrhea.

Clinical Description and Epidemiologic Features of the Syndrome

The first good clinical description of travelers' diarrhea was by Kean in his classic article, in which he graphically described the illness and revealed the associated inconvenience (Table 2).[4] From 1963 to 1983, epidemiologic features including timing of occurrence after reaching the high-risk area and risk factors were described.[4,8,16] Illness was generally seen within the first week of arrival to the high-risk area, with nearly all cases occurring within the first 2 weeks. The illness lasted between 2 and 5 days and was self-limiting, the younger travelers were at greatest risk, and recurrences occurred in about 15% of travelers remaining in the area of risk for 5 weeks.[8]

Specific Risk of Illness by Region and Development of Immunity

With the availability of published data describing the occurrence of diarrhea in visitors, it became clear that areas of the world varied in risk of illness acquisition. Based on this information, in 1981, we attempted to divide the world into three categories of risk: high, low, and intermediate.[18] Specific rates of risk were later established by a study of European travelers to various countries.[19] The attack rate of diarrhea occurrence in high-risk regions, including Latin America, Southern Asia, and many parts of Africa, averaged 30 to 50%.[5,8,9,16,17,20] The incidence rate for a 2-week stay often exceeds 60%.[17]

Studies have been carried out with US students in Mexico for nearly five decades and a consistently high rate of diarrhea (33 to 60%) has been seen (Reference details in Table 3). The highest rates were seen when subjects were followed for 4 weeks prospectively by daily visit to the clinic rather than through self-reporting during the first 2 weeks after arrival in Mexico. High rates of illness have remained in US travelers to Mexico despite prevalent knowledge of the cause and reasons for the illness and availability of modern concepts of food and personal hygiene.

Studies of British military troops stationed in Egypt during the years 1939 to 1945 demonstrated that high rates of diarrhea occurred only during the first months after arrival, with very low rates of diarrhea occurring during the second year of observation.[19] Similarly, the rate of illness in Mexico decreased by half as students from the United States remained in the area of risk for one semester.[8] The occurrence of natural immunity by remaining in an area of risk has given hope for the development of a vaccine to prevent the illness.

Sources and Cause of the Disease

The old adage, "don't drink the water" during trips to international settings, was questioned in 1976 and 1977 when diarrhea occurrence was associated with the place at which meals were eaten or by the specific food items consumed (Tables 4, 5).[21,22] Pathogens important as causes of diarrhea were then found in food and it was shown that diarrhea rates were reduced in those careful about the food items selected.[23,24]

The first evidence, albeit indirect, that bacterial agents were the important causes of travelers' diarrhea was seen

Table 3 Risk of Travelers' Diarrhea Seen in US Students to Mexico Attending Summer Classes for at Least 14 Days

Year	Length of Study (wk)	Location in Mexico	Method of Reporting Illness	Rate of Diarrhea (%)	Reference
1958	2	Mexico City	Self-reporting	33	5
1975	4	Cholula	Daily visits to clinic	40	8
1986–7	4	Guadalajara	Daily visits to clinic	50	9
2003	4	Guadalajara	Daily visits to clinic	54	31

Table 4 Food as the Source of Travelers' Diarrhea and Enteric Infection

Observation	Reference
Location of food consumption correlated with development of diarrhea in travelers	21
Observation that consumption of a specific food item could be correlated with occurrence of diarrhea	22
Important pathogens of travelers' diarrhea were found in foods consumed by persons at risk	23
Illness could be prevented by exercising care in foods consumed	24

Table 5 Establishment of the Bacterial Etiology of Travelers' Diarrhea

Observation	Reference
Antibacterial drugs prevented the illness	5, 6, 31
Conventional enteropathogens were not responsible for the illness	7
Enterotoxigenic E. coli (ETEC) found to cause most cases of illness	25
ETEC, enteroaggregative E. coli (EAEC), and a variety of bacterial agents caused most cases of the illness	26, 27
Antibacterial drugs effectively shortened the illness when given therapeutically	26
Antibacterial resistance complicated therapy	32, 33
Immunity to ETEC occurs and ETEC diarrhea may be prevented passively by orally administered antibody or actively by an oral or transcutaneously administered vaccine	38–41

in the effectiveness of antibacterial drugs in reducing the rate of occurrence of illness.

Kean and his colleagues sought to determine the cause of this disease that could be prevented by prophylactic drugs. Early on, his team failed to find conventional bacterial or parasitic agents as causes.[7] In 1973, Gorbach teamed up with Kean in an important study of US students in Mexico, finding that enterotoxigenic *Escherichia coli* (ETEC) was the cause of the illness in a majority of cases.[25] Within the next decade, it became clear that ETEC was the major cause, but it was only one of a number of bacterial agents responsible for travelers' diarrhea.[26] Recently, another *E. coli* strain that shows aggregative adherence to tissue culture cells and is known as *enteroaggregative E. coli* has been shown to rival ETEC as a major cause of travelers' diarrhea.[27] Recently noroviruses have been implicated as important causes of travelers' diarrhea, especially that associated with vomiting.[28]

Drug Prevention

Interestingly, the early drug evaluation of travelers' diarrhea was for prevention, not for therapy. While there had been a number of empiric uncontrolled uses of antibacterial drugs in preventing the disorder, the earliest placebo-controlled trials were carried out by Kean and colleagues in 1958 and 1960.[5,6] The drugs tested were iodochlorhydroxyquin (a halogenated quinoline), neomycin sulfate with kaolin and pectin versus a placebo in one study, and phthalylsulfathiazole and neomycin sulfate versus placebo in the other.[5,6] Moderate protection was seen for neomycin and phthalylsulfathiazole but not for the quinoline. Later, doxycycline was used successfully in preventing diarrhea of international travelers.[29] A Consensus Development Conference held in the US in 1985 concluded that, until we had completely safe drugs not likely to produce antimicrobial resistance, prophylactic drugs should not be employed routinely to prevent this disease.[30] The concern was drug side effects, occurrence of drug resistance, and difficulty in defining who should receive prophylaxis.

Following the development of poorly absorbed (< 0.4%) rifaximin for treatment of travelers' diarrhea, the agent was evaluated as a diarrhea-preventive among US students in Mexico and found to be effective.[31] Further studies with rifaximin prophylaxis are underway.

Drug Therapy

An important and logical observation was that antibacterial drugs would shorten the illness in travelers when used therapeutically.[26] This has become the standard approach to managing the disease. The problem is that antibacterial resistance is becoming a problem worldwide, making it important to search for antibacterial drugs to treat the more severe cases.[32,33] In addition to antibacterial agents, a number of symptom relief drugs emerged once the mechanisms of diarrhea were better appreciated. These include the antimotility agent loperamide, a calmodulin inhibiting drug named zaldaride, and a chloride channel blocker, crofelemer.[34–36] Refinements of therapy have notably included the combination of the symptomatic relief drug, loperamide, and an active antibacterial drug.[37]

Immunoprophylaxis

The natural immunity that occurs as travelers remain at risk appears to be directed to ETEC.[8,38] This observation has encouraged groups to pursue development of immunologic approaches to prevent travelers' diarrhea. While theoretically promising, the approach of using passive protection with colostrum or bovine antibody has not yet been shown to be useful in travelers' diarrhea.[39] Much more successful so far has been the approach of active immunization, specifically with a whole ETEC cell (containing the colonization factors of the organism) and the similar binding subunit of cholera toxin in an oral vaccine that is given twice before travel.[40] A novel approach to ETEC immunization has been through transcutaneous antigen delivery by skin patch.[41] There is every reason to believe that an important proportion of travelers' diarrhea may some day be prevented by an effective ETEC vaccine.

References

1. Davison WC. A bacteriological and clinical consideration of bacillary dysentery in adults and children. Medicine 1922;1:389–510.
2. Butler T, Middleton FG, Earnest DL, Strickland GT. Chronic and recurrent diarrhea in American service-men in Vietnam. An evaluation of etiology and small bowel structure and function. Arch Intern Med 1973;132:373–7.
3. Cook GC. Influence of diarrhoeal disease on military and naval campaigns. J R Soc Med 2001;94:95–7.
4. Kean BH. The diarrhea of travelers to Mexico. Summary of five-year study. Ann Intern Med 1963;59:605–14.
5. Kean BH, Waters SR. The diarrhea of travelers II. Drug prophylaxis in Mexico. N Engl J Med 1959;261:71–4.
6. Kean BH, Schaffner W, Brennan RW, Waters SR. The diarrhea of travelers V. Prophylaxis with phthalylsulfathiazole and neomycin sulphate. J Am Med Assoc 1962;180: 367–71.
7. Varela G, Kean BH, Barrett EL, Keegan CJ. The diarrhea of travelers II. Bacteriologic studies of U.S. students in Mexico. Am J Trop Med 1959;8:353–7.
8. DuPont HL, Haynes GA, Pickering LK, et al. Diarrhea of travelers to Mexico: relative susceptibility of United States and Latin American students attending a Mexican university. Am J Epidemiol 1977;105:37–41.
9. Ericsson CD, DuPont HL, Mathewson JJ III. Epidemiologic observations on diarrhea developing in U.S. and Mexican students living in Guadalajara, Mexico. J Travel Med 1995; 2:6–10.
10. Herwaldt BL, de Arroyave KR, Roberts JM, Juranek DD. A multiyear prospective study of the risk factors for an incidence of diarrheal illness in a cohort of Peace Corps volunteers in Guatemala. Ann Intern Med 2000;132:982–8.
11. Haberberger RL Jr, Lissner CR, Podgore IA, et al. Etiology of acute diarrhea among United States embassy personnel and dependents in Cairo, Egypt. Am J Trop Med Hyg 1994; 51:870–4.
12. Shlim DR, Hoge CW, Rajah R, et al. Persistent high risk of diarrhea among foreigners in Nepal during the first 2 years of residence. Clin Infect Dis 1999;29:613–6.
13. Hershey R. The incidence and effects of travelers' diarrhea in a seafaring population. J Maritime Policy Management 1980;7:147–54.
14. Merson MH, Tenney JH, Meyers JD, et al. Shigellosis at sea: an outbreak aboard a passenger cruise ship., 1975;101:165–75.
15. Tauxe RV, Tormey MP, Mascola L, et al. Salmonellosis outbreak on transatlantic flights; foodborne illness on aircraft: 1947–1984. Am J Epidemiol 1987;125:150–7.
16. Steffen R, Van der Linde F, Gyr K, Schar M. Epidemiology of diarrhea in travelers. J Am Med Assoc 1983;249: 1176–80.
17. von Sonnenburg F, Tornieporth N, Waiyaki P, et al. Risk and aetiology of diarrhea at various tourist destinations. Lancet 2000;356:133–4.
18. DuPont HL, DuPont MW. Travel with health. New York: Appleton-Century-Crofts; 1981.
19. Bulmer E. A survey of tropical diseases as seen in the Middle East. Trans R Soc Trop Med Hyg 1944;37:225–42.
20. Steffen R. Epidemiologic studies of travelers' diarrhea, severe gastrointestinal infections and cholera. Rev Infect Dis 1986;8Suppl 2:S122–30.
21. Tjoa W, DuPont HL, Sullivan P, et al. Location of food consumption and travelers' diarrhea. Am J Epidemiol 1977; 106:61–6.
22. Merson MH, Morris GK, Sack DA, et al. Travelers' diarrhea in Mexico: a prospective study of physicians and family members attending a congress. N Engl J Med 1976;294: 1299–305.
23. Wood LV, Ferguson LE, Hogan P, et al. Incidence of bacterial enteropathogens in foods from Mexico. Appl Environ Microbiol 1983;46:328–32.
24. Kozicki M, Steffen R, Schar M. "Boil it, cook it, peel it or forget it": does this rule prevent travelers' diarrhoea? Int J Epidemiol 1985;14:169–72.
25. Gorbach SL, Kean BH, Evans DG, et al. Travelers' diarrhea and toxigenic Escherichia coli. N Engl J Med 1975;292:933–6.
26. DuPont HL, Reves RR, Galindo E, et al. Treatment of travelers' diarrhea with trimethoprim/sulfamethoxazole and with trimethoprim alone. N Engl J Med 1982;307: 841–4.

27. Adachi JA, Jiang Z-D, Mathewson JJ, et al. Enteroaggregative Escherichia coli as a major etiologic agent in travelers' diarrhea in 3 regions of the world. Clin Infect Dis 2001;32:1706–9.

28. Ko GP, Garcia C, Jiang ZD, et al. Noroviruses as a cause of traveler's diarrhea among students from the United States visiting Mexico. J Clin Microbiol 2005;43:6126–9.

29. Sack DA, Kaminsky DC, Sack RB, et al. Prophylactic doxycycline for travelers' diarrhea: results of a prospective double-blind study of Peace Corps volunteers in Kenya. N Engl J Med 1978;298:758–63.

30. Travelers' Diarrhea—Consensus Conference J Am Med Assoc 1985;253:2700–4.

31. DuPont HL, Jiang ZD, Okhuysen PC, et al. A randomized, double-blind, placebo-controlled trial of rifaximin to prevent travelers' diarrhea. Ann Intern Med 2005;142:805–12.

32. Kuschner RA, Trofa AF, Thomas RJ, et al. Use of azithromycin for the treatment of Campylobacter enteritis in travelers to Thailand, an area where ciprofloxacin resistance is prevalent. Clin Infect Dis 1995;21:536–41.

33. Gomi H, Jiang Z-D, Adachi JA, et al. In vitro antimicrobial susceptibility testing of bacterial enteropathogens causing travelers' diarrhea in four geographic regions. Antimicrob Agents Chemother 2001;45:212–6.

34. Johnson PC, Ericsson CD, DuPont HL, et al. Comparison of loperamide with bismuth subsalicylate for the treatment of acute travelers' diarrhea. J Am Med Assoc 1986;225:757–60.

35. DuPont HL, Ericsson CD, Mathewson JJ, et al. Zaldaride maleate (Zm), an intestinal calmodulin inhibitor, in the therapy of travelers' diarrhea. Gastroenterology 1993;104:709–15.

36. DiCesare D, DuPont HL, Mathewson JJ, et al. A double-blind, randomized, placebo-controlled study of SP-303 (Provir) in the symptomatic treatment of acute diarrhea among travelers to Jamaica and Mexico. Am J Gastroenterol 2002;97:2585–8.

37. Ericsson CD, DuPont HL, Mathewson JJ, et al. Treatment of travelers' diarrhea with sulfamethoxazole and trimethoprim and loperamide. J Am Med Assoc 1990;263:257–61.

38. Brown MR, DuPont HL, Sullivan PS. Effect of duration of exposure on diarrhea due to enterotoxigenic Escherichia coli in travelers from the United States to Mexico. J Infect Dis 1982;145:582.

39. Tacket CO, Losonsky G, Link H, et al. Protection by milk immunoglobulin concentrate against oral challenge with enterotoxigenic Escherichia coli. N Engl J Med 1988;318:1240–3.

40. Peltola H, Siitonen A, Kyronseppa H, et al. Prevention of travelers' diarrhoea by oral B-subunit/whole-cell cholera vaccine. Lancet 1991;338:1285–9.

41. Glenn GM, Villar CP, Flyer DC, et al. Safety and Immunogenicity of an Enterotoxigenic Escherichia coli Vaccine Path Containing Heat-Labile Toxin: Use of Skin Pretreatment to Discrupt the Stratum Corneum. Infect Immun 2007;75(5):2163–70.

PART ONE

ETIOLOGY AND PATHOGENESIS

CHAPTER 2

THE BACTERIAL PATHOGENS

ZHI-DONG JIANG, MD, PhD

JEAN-PAUL BUTZLER, MD, PhD

An infectious etiology for travelers' diarrhea was finally confirmed in the 1970s.[1] A number of surveys carried out in different geographical areas have identified a range of bacterial, viral, and parasitic agents as being responsible for travelers' diarrhea. Bacterial pathogens are responsible for fewer than 5% of cases of diarrhea illness in the United States.[2] In contrast, however, bacteria are the etiologic agents in 50 to 80% of cases of diarrheal illness in developing countries.[3] The bacterial etiology of traveler's diarrhea, based on the results of studies in a variety of geographic areas, is outlined in Table 1.[4–10]

In their studies carried out in the early 1960s, when they demonstrated that antimicrobial agents were useful to prevent diarrhea, Kean and colleagues[11] provided the first clues that the majority of diarrhea of travelers was caused by bacterial agents. Later, in 1975, Kean teamed up with Gorbach and colleagues,[12] making the important discovery that enterotoxigenic *Escherichia coli* (ETEC) was a major cause of travelers' diarrhea. Current studies have shown that infectious microorganisms are the primary causes of travelers' diarrhea, and among them, bacterial enteric pathogens are the most important etiologic agents isolated. ETEC, enteroaggregative *E. coli* (EAEC), *Shigella* species, *Campylobacter jejuni*, *Salmonella* species, *Aeromonas* species, *Plesiomonas* species, and non-*cholerae Vibrio* species are the agents most commonly identified.[13,14] As a group, the diarrheagenic *E. coli* are responsible for the vast majority of travelers' diarrhea cases. Based on clinical associations, serotyping, and phenotypic assays of different virulence characteristics, the diarrheagenic *E. coli* have been loosely classified into five major categories. These are ETEC, enteropathogenic *E. coli* (EPEC), enterohemorrhagic *E. coli*, EAEC, and enteroinvasive *E. coli*. In recent years a number of isolates not conforming to this classification have been reported. These nonclassified isolates and the enteropathogenic, enterohemorrhagic, and enteroinvasive forms are rarely causes of diarrhea in adults, and their role as agents of travelers' diarrhea has not been determined.

Enterotoxigenic *E. coli*

ETEC are those strains of *E. coli* that elaborate at least one member of two defined groups of enterotoxins: heat-stable (ST) and heat-labile (LT) enterotoxins.[15] ETEC has a worldwide distribution and is an important cause of diarrhea in children in developing countries and of diarrhea in travelers visiting these areas.[16,17]

EPIDEMIOLOGY

In the 1970s and early 1980s, ETEC was found to be the most important cause of diarrhea among US students to Mexico.[12,18] Later it was shown that ETEC was an important cause of travelers' diarrhea worldwide[13,19,20] accounting for 5 to 60% of cases in all developing

Table 1. Geographic Distribution of Bacterial Etiology of Travelers' Diarrhea

Pathogen	Mexico (%)	Jamaica (%)	India (%)	Kenya (%)	Thailand (%)	Total (%)
Enterotoxigenic *E. coli*	15–60	15–40	5–40	5–40	10–20	5–60
Enteroaggregative *E. coli*	0–40	0–30	0–20	0–15	5–10	0–40
Campylobacter spp.	0–5	0–5	0–10	0–30	10–40	0–40
Salmonella spp.	0–15	0–15	0–30	5–25	0–10	0–30
Shigella spp.	0–30	0–15	0–15	0–10	0–15	0–30
No Pathogen	20–60	20–70	10–55	10–55	20–60	10–70

tropical and semitropical regions. It also causes high frequency of gastroenteritis in local pediatric populations of developing countries[21–23] where these children and travelers are exposed to ETEC-contaminated food.[24–26]

The prevalence of ETEC is common in most regions of Latin America, the Caribbean, and many parts than in Asia and Africa (see Table 1). In some parts of Asia, such as Thailand, ETEC rates are lower than *Campylobacter*[27–29] Steffen and colleagues[30] did not find a seasonal pattern for ETEC diarrhea in travelers to Jamaica, while Mattila and colleagues described a higher prevalence in summer and fall (> 50% of cases) than in winter (15%)[31] and a similarly in Mexico there appears to be a season association, where ETEC is the most common pathogen in travelers with diarrhea in the rainy summer, nearly disappearing in the dry winter.[32]

MICROBIOLOGY AND IDENTIFICATION

E. coli is the type species of the genus *Escherichia*, which contains mostly motile gram-negative bacilli within the family *Enterobacteriaceae*.[33] *E. coli* can easily be isolated from clinical specimens on general or selective media incubated at 37°C under aerobic conditions. *E. coli* in stool are most often recovered on MacConkey or eosin methylene-blue agar. These media contain chemicals that inhibit gram-positive organisms and contain lactose, a disaccharide that permits a presumptive differentiation of lactose fermenters from nonlactose fermenters. They selectively grow members of the *Enterobacteriaceae* and permit differentiation of enteric organisms on the basis of morphology.[33]

Confirmation that the *E. coli* are ETEC relies on detection of the enterotoxins LT and/or ST. ST was initially detected in a rabbit ligated ileal loop assay,[34] then subsequently superceded due to expense of the technique and lack of standardization, by the suckling mouse assay.[35] The traditional bioassay for detection of LT employs cell culture, either the Y1 adrenal cell assay or the Chinese hamster ovary (CHO) cell assay. In the Y1 assay, ETEC culture supernatants are added to Y1 cells, and the cells are examined for rounding.[36] In the CHO cell assay, LT will cause elongation of the CHO cells.[37] ETEC were among the first pathogenic microorganisms for which molecular diagnostic techniques were developed. As early as 1982,[38] deoxyribonucleic acid (DNA) probes were utilized for the detection of LT and ST encoding genes isolated from stool and environmental samples. Although the LT polynucleotide probe provides good sensitivity and specificity when labeled with radioisotopes,[39] ST polynucleotide probes have had problems of poor sensitivity and specificity due to the small size of the gene. For this reason, oligonucleotide probes, which are generally more sensitive and specific for ST detection, have been developed.[40]

For the detection of ST and LT by hybridization after incubation, lactose fermenting *E. coli* are transferred to a Whatman filter paper (#541). The bacteria transferred on the paper can be lysed, denatured, and hybridized with the probe in situ, and then a radiographic image is generated by exposure to X-ray film. Recommended oligonucleotide probes consist of the following sequences: ST-h, 5'-GCTGTGAATTGTGTTGTAATCC-3'; ST-p, 5'-GCTGTGAACTTTGTTGTAATCC-3' ;[33] and LT, 5'-GCGAGAGGAACACAAACCGG-3'.

PATHOGENESIS AND VIRULENCE FACTORS

Like most mucosal pathogens, *E. coli* can be said to follow a requisite strategy of infection: (1) colonization of the mucosal site, (2) elaboration of enterotoxins, (3) development of a net secretory state.

The LT is closely related in structure and function to the cholera enterotoxin (CT) expressed by *Vibrio cholerae*.[41] The LT activates adenylate cyclase,[42] which is located on the basolateral membrane of polarized intestinal epithelial cells and leads to an increase in levels of intracellular cyclic AMP (cAMP).[43] Although the stimulation of chloride (Cl), as a result of increased intracellular levels of cAMP, is the classical explanation for the mechanism by which LT or CT cause diarrhea, there is increasing evidence that LT or CT could evoke an intestinal inflammatory response.[44] CT has been reported to stimulate production of the proinflammatory cytokine interleukin (IL)-6, activating the enteric immune system.[45]

In contrast to the large, oligomeric LTs, the STs are small, monomeric toxins. There are two unrelated classes of STs that differ in structure and mechanism of action. Genes for both classes are found predominantly on plasmids, and some ST-encoding genes have been found on transposons. ST-I toxin is produced by ETEC and several other gram-negative bacteria including *Yersinia enterocolitica* and *V. cholerae* non-01. ST-II has been found only in ETEC. The major receptor for ST-I is guanylate cyclase C (GC-C). GC-C is located in the apical membrane of intestinal epithelial cells, and binding of ligands to the extracellular domain stimulates the intracellular enzymatic activity. Binding of ST-I to GC-C stimulates GC activity, leading to an increase in intracellular cyclic quanosine monophosphate (cGMP) levels.[46] This activity leads ultimately to stimulation of chloride secretion and/or inhibition of sodium chloride absorption, resulting in net intestinal fluid secretion. Unlike ST-I, ST-II induces histologic damage of the intestinal epithelium. The receptor for ST-II is unknown. Unlike the chloride secretion elicited by ST-I, ST-II stimulates the secretion of bicarbonate from intestinal cells.[44]

In order to colonize the intestine, ETEC isolates express fimbrial antigens on their surfaces called colonization factor antigens (CFAs).[47] Initially two colonization factors antigens, CFA/I and CFA/II, were described in ETEC isolated from humans,[48] but others have since been identified.[49] CFA/I is a rigid, rod-like fimbria, while CFA/II and CFA/IV may contain a mixture of rigid fimbriae and nonfimbrial antigens. The CFA/II antigen was later shown to consist of three subcomponents, coli surface (CS)-associated antigens, CS1, CS2, and CS3.[50] CS3 is present in all strains of the CFA/II group, either alone or in combination with CS1 or CS2. The best characterized colonization factors of ETEC are CFA/I, CFA/II, and CFA/IV. CFA/IV consists of three distinct antigens, CS4, CS5, and CS6.[51] Similarly to CFA/II, CS6 can be produced alone or together with CS4 and CS5. The role of CFA/III in colonization has also been demonstrated recently.[52]

ETEC VACCINE DEVELOPMENT

Natural ETEC immunity develops and persists as people remain at risk of infection.[53] This observation has given researchers encouragement that a protective ETEC vaccine may be produced to prevent the disease, with a number of vaccine candidates currently under development. Some of the most promising vaccine candidates use the cholera toxin B-subunit,[54] which is immunologically and physiologically related to the LT of ETEC. The Anti-LT immunity elicited is specific and does not appear to offer any cross protection against ST-only producing ETEC. ST is not immunogenic unless coupled to a carrier[55] and it has proven impossible to synthesize ST toxoids that induce a good neutralizing antibody response without residual toxicity.[55] Approximately half of the ETEC isolated in one of the studies[13] produced ST-only and would not be expected to be prevented by an anti-LT vaccine. To be effective, vaccine candidates should probably contain a number of ETEC CFAs, which is the approach employed by the developers of the oral cholera toxin B-subunit vaccine previously mentioned.

Defined CFAs are produced in over 50% of ETEC.[13] CFA/II was found to be the principal adhesin type among ETEC studied in two South American countries,[56,57] while a study carried out in Peru demonstrated the importance of CFA/IV.[58] For a vaccine designed for Mombasa (Kenya), Goa (India), and Montego Bay (Jamaica), the preparation should optimally include CFA/II (CS3 is the most important) and CFA/IV (in particular CS6) components.[13] It is recommended therefore that an ETEC vaccine for widespread use in the developing countries should contain CS6 and probably CS3 as part of multivalent combination.

Enteroaggregative *E. coli*

EAEC is an emerging enteric pathogen of worldwide distribution that probably accounts for as many cases of travelers' diarrhea as ETEC. This *E. coli* pathotype is defined by its ability to produce a unique pattern of adhesion when added to HEp-2 cells in culture, resembling a pile of bricks that have been stacked. EAEC has been isolated in 19 to 33% of patients with travelers' diarrhea.[59]

EPIDEMIOLOGY

EAEC was first implicated as a cause of travelers' diarrhea in 1985 by Mathewson and colleagues.[60] Subsequent studies have further substantiated the pathogenic role of EAEC strains as etiologic agents in acute travelers' diarrhea,[59,61] in persistent diarrhea in children in developing regions[62,63] and in AIDS-associated chronic diarrhea.[64,65] Adachi and colleagues demonstrated that up to 26% of travelers' diarrhea from multiple regions of the world may be attributable to EAEC[59] which thus a major cause of this illness. A recent study demonstrated that co-infection of EAEC with ETEC and occurrence of asymptomatic EAEC infection were common to travelers in developing regions.[66] It was not possible to define whether the EAEC was the true pathogen in these cases. However, 56% (90 of 162) of the diarrheal cases where EAEC was the sole pathogen explains the etiology of approximately 30% of the otherwise undiagnosed cases. EAEC as the causative agent is further substantiated by a previous observation that diarrhea, in subjects whom no other pathogen was isolated, improved with antimicrobial therapy.[67,68]

MICROBIOLOGY AND IDENTIFICATION

The term enteroaggregative *E. coli* describes those strains of *E. coli* that attach to HEp-2 cells in a solely adhesion pattern (stacked brick arrangement) but do not belong to serotypes often associated with EPEC.

The HEp-2 adherence assay was originally reported by Cravioto and colleagues.[69] The adhesion assay is performed by incubating fresh bacterial cultures with a monolayer of HEp-2 cells (ATCC, Rockville, MD), then fixing and staining the monolayer and observing the pattern of bacterial adhesion. A sample is interpreted as positive for EAEC if it shows the characteristic "stacked-brick" aggregative appearance as described by Nataro and colleagues.[70]

PATHOGENESIS & VIRULENCE FACTORS

Strains of EAEC differ in their pathogenicity,[70] though the mechanisms of pathophysiology and the virulence traits that enable the organism to cause diarrhea are not well understood. Host and environmental factors may influence the occurrence of EAEC diarrhea (eg, diet, inoculum size, genetic makeup, stress, relocation, etc), and the specific role of defined EAEC virulence determinants in the pathogenicity of diarrhea in humans is currently under investigation.[71] EAEC strains have been found in food in endemic areas[26] although as stated earlier, asymptomatic infection is commonly observed in these areas.[66] The frequent occurrence of asymptomatic EAEC infection in travelers to Mexico and lack of intestinal inflammatory markers have raised questions about pathogenicity in these cases.

EAEC typically do not secrete LT or ST enterotoxins but can produce other enterotoxins such as Pet (plasmid encoded toxin), EAST-1 (heat stable enterotoxin), Shet1 and Shet2 (*Shigella* enterotoxins), the cryptic secreted protein AspU and flagellin (fliC). EAEC also produce a mucus biofilm in the intestinal mucosa. The characteristic adherence pattern is encoded in genes that are carried in a large 60 MDa plasmid (pAA). EAEC attach to intestinal epithelia via the aggregative adherence fimbriae AAF/I, AAF/II, which are encoded in this large plasmid by *aggA* and *aafA* and regulated by the transcriptional activator of fimbrial expression *aggR* as well as recently described AAF/III fimbriae. Volunteer challenge studies have demonstrated heterogeneity in the ability of EAEC isolates to cause disease, and several studies have been unable to make clear associations with EAEC and diarrhea. It was recently shown that EAEC carrying the *aggR* regulated virulence factors are more likely to be associated with illness and that these strains should be referred to as "typical" EAEC.

IMMUNITY AND CYTOKINE PRODUCTION

It has been shown that strains of EAEC commonly induce an immune response in patients with travelers' diarrhea (50%).[72]

In a separate study of US adult tourists visiting Mexico it was observed that the number of subjects with EAEC colonization increased over time, while the number of EAEC diarrhea cases decreased with the time of stay.[66] During the first 2-weeks stay, subjects with EAEC diarrhea and EAEC colonization were more frequently identified than those with ETEC infection. However, the ratio of diarrhea cases to asymptomatic subjects by week was found to be similar for both pathogens (0.8 to 0.9 for EAEC versus 0.7 to 1.1 for ETEC).[66] During the third and fourth weeks, the diarrhea to asymptomatic infection ratio for EAEC dropped eightfold compared with the first week of study, yet the absolute number of subjects with EAEC colonization increased. This implies that immunity to symptomatic disease occurs quite early, though it is unable to block actual enteric infection.[66] These observations suggest that although travelers are commonly colonized by EAEC, as reported previously,[73] there may be other factors involved in the development of EAEC diarrheal disease. Possible explanations for the relatively high prevalence of asymptomatic infections are: a) the development of an acquired partial immunity to EAEC by the host; b) the presence of a heterogeneous group of EAEC strains with different capacity to colonize the intestinal lumen, or c) difference in virulence properties between strains of EAEC. These hypotheses could explain the following observations: prolonged EAEC colonization with increasing frequency as persons remain in Mexico, the dichotomy in the trends of EAEC infection and colonization, the presence of some cases with EAEC diarrhea preceded by EAEC colonization, and the lack of any repeated EAEC diarrhea episode in the same patient.

Steiner and Sutijia have presented two possible mechanisms of anti-EAEC immunity, the development of anti-EAEC secretory immunoglobulin A,[72] and the activation of cytokines and interleukins,[74] though the actual protective role these mechanisms may play remain unclear. One further hypothesis is that EAEC strains represent a group of heterogeneous diarrheagenic *E. coli* that share the distinctive aggregative adherence pattern to HEp-2 cells. A number of observations support this: 1) different EAEC strains have been shown to have variable virulence in volunteers,[70] 2) the organisms have a variety of possible pathogenic factors, identified in a selected group of EAEC isolates,[75,76] and 3) strains of EAEC infecting persons in a common geographic area are quite genotypically diverse as determined by pulse field gel electrophoresis[59] and plasmid analysis.[66]

Recent studies have documented in vitro production of IL-8 by EAEC infected epithelial cells.[74] These findings are reminiscent of inflammatory bowel disease, in which increased level of fecal cytokines IL-1β,[77] tumor necrosis factor-α (TNF-α)[78] and IL-8[78] have been demonstrated. Elevated TNF-α and IL-6 levels in stool and in serum of children with shigellosis have also been associated with disease complications.[79]

Evidence also exists to indicate that EAEC may produce inflammatory enteritis with secretion of IL-8.[80] Diarrhea caused by a variety of inflammatory bacterial enteropathogens including EAEC, *Shigella*, and *Salmonella* in adults was associated with production of cytokines in diarrheal stools.[81] In addition, Bouckenooghe and colleagues demonstrated that naturally occurring EAEC diarrhea in travelers was associated with another marker of intestinal inflammation, fecal lactoferrin,[82] whilst IL-8 was detected at ~ 200-fold higher concentrations in fecal samples from patients with diarrhea in whom the infecting strains of EAEC were positive for *aggR*, *aafA*, or any combination of virulence factors when compared with patients with diarrhea from whom nonadherent *E. coli* were identified.[71] When infecting EAEC isolates in the patients with diarrhea were positive for *aggR* or *aafA* factors, they were more likely to be associated with increased level of IFN-γ when compared with patients infected with EAEC without those virulence factors.[71] Detection of high concentrations of fecal cytokines in patients with EAEC diarrhea suggests increased production and secretion from an inflamed bowel, though studies show that diarrhea in international travelers with EAEC infection may or may not be associated with intestinal release of markers of inflammation. Steiner and colleagues[80] demonstrated that concentrations of IL-1β were elevated in EAEC infection either in the presence or absence of symptoms. In the study by Nataro and colleagues[83] patients with EAEC had higher rates of IL-1β:IL-1ra ratios compared with uninfected controls. Jiang and colleagues showed that there was no significant elevation in fecal IL-1β for patients with diarrhea and infection with EAEC positive or negative for virulence factors.[71] One possible explanation for variation in intestinal markers of inflammation with EAEC-associated diarrhea may well be because not all strains are pathogenic.

Shigella spp.

The *Shigellae* are an important cause of bacillary dysentery. Clinical features of shigellosis classically include watery or bloody diarrhea, abdominal pain, fever, and malaise. There are four species of *Shigella: boydii, dysenteriae, flexneri*, and *sonnei*.

EPIDEMIOLOGY

In endemic areas, *Shigella* infection occurs predominantly in young children, though the peak incidence occurs in preschool children rather than in infants.[84] The lower incidence rates in older children and adults suggest the presence of an exposure-dependent immunity. This is highlighted in the fact that adult travelers to such endemic areas commonly acquire *Shigella* infection because they are likely to be immunologically naive. Furthermore, the immunity-acquired appears to be strain specific. This is supported by the observation that when a new *Shigella* serotype is introduced that is serologically distinct from strains previously encountered, diarrheal diseases occurs equally in all age groups.[84]

The *Shigellae* spp. are the cause of travelers' diarrhea in up to 10% of travelers to developing countries.[13] Approximately 14,000 laboratory confirmed cases of shigellosis and an estimated 448,000 total cases (mostly due to *S. sonnei*) occur in the United States each year.[85] In the developing world, *S. flexneri* tends to predominate.[86] Epidemics of *S. dysenteriae* type 1 have occurred in Africa and Central America with case fatality rates of 5 to 15%.[86]

Infection with *Shigellae* readily spreads among individuals living in cramped over-crowded conditions.[86] Transmission is via the fecal-oral route and the inoculum size needed to initiate infection can be as few as 200 or less organisms.[86,87] It may be transmitted through contaminated food and water; however, person-to-person spread and transmission by flies may also occur because so few organisms are necessary to cause disease.[86] Clinical cases may excrete 10^5 to 10^8 organisms/g of feces, and even convalescent carriers have in excess of 10^2 *Shigella* per gram of feces.[88]

The enteritis caused by *Shigella* spp. varies in severity, with the diarrhea ranging from watery to dysenteric. Dysentery more commonly results from *S. dysenteriae* and *S. flexneri* infections, while *S. boydii* and *S. sonnei* usually produce a watery diarrhea. Patients *with Shigella dysentery* tend to cause have severe symptoms, usually with high fever, severe abdominal pain and fractionated stools.

MICROBIOLOGY AND IDENTIFICATION

Shigella are gram-negative, rod-shaped bacilli that lack flagellae. While they share many biochemical properties with *E. coli*, major phenotypic differences include their failure to ferment lactose within 24 hours, their inability to produce gas, and their lack of motility.

In order of decreasing bacterial recovery, rectal swab, stool, and anal swab are the specimens of choice.[89] Blood, mucus, or pus, if present in the stool, are extremely productive and should be cultured. For optimal chances of isolating *Shigella* spp., a differential enteric agar medium and a moderately selective agar medium should be used.[90]

The four *Shigella* species are also biochemically similar to each other, except for the inability of *S. dysenteriae* to ferment mannitol, positive ornithine utilization by *S. sonnei*, and ability of most *S. sonnei* to ferment lactose after several days in culture. Final identification to species and group level is usually accomplished by serology.

Shigella spp. is susceptible to changes in stool pH that occurs during prolonged transport, and a number of organisms may die under such conditions. If shigellosis is suspected, the stool specimen should be transported promptly to the laboratory or a suitable transport media should be used, eg, Enteric Plus (Meridian Diagnostics, Cincinnati, OH).

PATHOGENESIS AND VIRULENCE FACTORS

Shigella possess specialized adaptive processes that enable them to coopt epithelial cell functions to augment their penetration of the host intestinal epithelium. A necessary step in the successful colonization and ultimate production of disease is the ability of *Shigella* to adhere to host surfaces, which is an important determinant of virulence.[91] Generally, binding to intestinal host cells is essential for *Shigella* to resist both the fluid flow of the luminal contents and the peristalsis of intestinal contraction. Once bound to the epithelial surface, *Shigella* may colonize and establish a permanent residence in the gut. Adhesion of the bacteria to host cells or surfaces is essential for the successful development of infection. A wide range of mammalian cell surface constituents, including glycoproteins and glycolipids, can serve as receptors for bacterial attachment.[92] This process allows *Shigella* to invade epithelial cells via their basolateral pole and subsequently to spread laterally from one enterocyte to another. The accompanying inflammatory response this elicits is characterized by IL-8 production and polymorphonuclear leukocyte transmigration.[93] The host cell is often an active participant in the adhesion process and does not function simply as an inert surface for attachment. The host has specialized strategies to resist such infections, often in response to these virulence factors or the damage caused by them. This interaction defines the disease process.[94]

Evidence for an essential role of a plasmid in entry came from the observation that a plasmid of 200 kb was present in invasive isolates of *Shigella*, and loss of this plasmid eliminated entry.[95] The nucleotide sequence of the 30.5 kb region that is necessary for entry of *Shigella* into epithelial cells has been determined.[96] The plasmid encodes the invasion plasmid antigens (*ipa*) operon, which includes IpaB, C, and D—three proteins essential for invasion.[97]

In contrast to the pathogenic *E. coli*, flagellae and pili are not recognized to be the virulence factors for *Shigella*. It has been demonstrated that *Shigella* of all serogroups elaborate an exotoxin that exhibits cytotoxic, neurotoxic, and enterotoxic activity.[98,99] There is sufficient evidence that Shiga toxin uses cytotoxic effects on intestinal epithelial cells, including human colonic cells in primary culture.[100] However, the in vivo situation is much more complicated because not only is there free toxin in the lumen, but *Shigella* also invades and multiplies with epithelial cells.[101] making it difficult to distinguish invasion and an elicited inflammatory response from the specific direct effects of toxin.

Salmonella spp. (Nontyphoidal Salmonella Infection)

Nontyphoidal salmonellosis refers to disease caused by any serotype of organism in the genus *Salmonella*, other than *Salmonella typhi*, the causative agent of typhoid fever. The most common manifestation of nontyphoidal salmonellosis is acute enterocolitis, though the organism can produce invasive infections leading to septicaemia, meningitis, and fever that may be clinically indistinguishable from that caused by *S. typhi*.

EPIDEMIOLOGY

Human salmonellosis is initiated by the ingestion of food or water that is contaminated with one or another *Salmonella* spp. Nontyphoidal *Salmonella* infection is widely distributed among different animal species but is particularly prevalent in animals raised for food. For example, *Salmonella* spp. have previously been isolated from approximately 50% of commercially available chickens, from 20% of frozen egg whites, from a varying percentage of raw milk sources, and from ground beef used to make hamburgers.[102,103] Food products also become contaminated during collection and processing via the food handlers.

The *Salmonella* spp. are the cause of travelers' diarrhea in up to 10% of travelers to developing countries.[13] *Salmonella* enterocolitis remains an important cause of infectious enterocolitis in developing countries despite the public health measures that have decreased endemic fever and cholera. One of the major contributors to the persistence of the salmonellae, as a major cause of diarrheal and invasive disease, is the variety and abundance of animal reservoirs they are able to infect.

Salmonella enterocolitis usually occurs after an incubation period of between 6 to 48 hours. There is a marked seasonal variation in the occurrence of *Salmonella* infection: in the US, peak incidences in summer and fall are due to many small outbreaks of food poisoning (*Salmonella* infection accounts for 10 to 15% of food poisoning cases). Inadequate cooking practices that affect relatively large numbers of people are most common at these times (for example, at picnics and barbecues). The highest rates of *Salmonella* infection are observed in children under the age of 5 years, particular infants, and in elderly individuals.

The colossal scale of contamination of animals and associated food products cannot be overstated and, despite at times heroic public health efforts to limit human encounters with salmonella in food, the major defense against human infection is appropriate food handling and cooking practices. Person to person spread via the fecal-oral route is also a major source of infection.[104]

MICROBIOLOGY AND IDENTIFICATION

Salmonellae are gram-negative, flagellated, nonsporulating, aerobic bacilli. Isolation of salmonellae from stool is best performed on selective and differential media. *Salmonella-Shigella*, and Hektoen enteric agars are widely used to screen for *Salmonella* because they support the growth of the organism and are considered moderately selective media. The purpose of these selective media is to suppress the growth of other *Enterobacteriaceae* and differentiate among gram-negative bacteria based on their ability to ferment lactose. Hektoen enteric agar is a useful medium for stool cultures because it demonstrates the production of hydrogen sulfide-producing organisms. Most *Salmonellae* produce abundant hydrogen sulfide, form gas in glucose media, and do not ferment sucrose. *Salmonellae* are distinguished from several *Proteus* species by their inability to metabolize urea.

PATHOGENESIS AND VIRULENCE FACTORS

The pathogenesis of *Salmonella* infection is not fully understood. The bacteria penetrate and damage the intestinal mucosa, are ingested by macrophages, and may multiply in a limited fashion in mesenteric lymphoid tissues. In severe invasive infection, bacteremia and focal infections in distant tissues occur.

The process includes several distinct steps, no single one of which explains the entire pathogenic spectrum: (1) Attachment and penetration. Adhesins facilitate the attachment of *Salmonellae* to intestinal mucosal cells, and may be necessary for mucosal invasion.[105] (2) Secretory response. The diarrhea associated with salmonellosis may reflect bacterial properties that cause fluid loss. Some invasive strains of *Salmonella* can cause fluid to accumulate in the rabbit ileal loop model, and the characteristics of the fluid suggest active secretion rather than just passive leaking through a damaged mucosa.[106] This fluid accumulation is accompanied by high levels of tissue cyclic AMP, is abolished by indomethacin, and suggests the presence of an enterotoxin.[107] (3) Inflammation and tissue destruction. The fever, bloody diarrhea, and evidence of colitis that often accompany *Salmonella* may be the result of local inflammation, effects of bacterial endotoxin, or of specific cytotoxins that cause mucosal cell death.[108] A cytotoxin has been identified in *Salmonella* that inhibits protein synthesis in cultured vero cells, in a manner analogous to the cytotoxins present in *Shigella dysenteriae* 1 and verotoxigenic *Escherichia coli.*[109]

A great deal of progress has been made in the understanding of the molecular bases of *Salmonella* entry into host cells. It is now evident that *Salmonella* entry is encoded on a 35 to 40 kb region of the *Salmonella* chromosome located at centisome.[63,110] It has been demonstrated the similarity between the genetic bases of *Salmonella* and *Shigella* proteins that mediate the entry of these organisms into cultured epithelial cells.[111]

Campylobacter spp.

Campylobacter jejuni has emerged as one of the most commonly identified bacterial causes of acute gastroenteritis worldwide.[112–114] Although several other *Campylobacter* species (*C. upsaliensis, C. lari, C. concisus, C. jejuni, C. fetus subsp. fetus, C. jejuni subsp doylei, C.hyointestinalis, and Arcobacter butzleri*) have been shown to cause diarrhea, *C. jejuni* is by far the most frequently isolated species from humans.

EPIDEMIOLOGY

The reported incidence of campylobacteriosis in most developed countries has risen substantially during the past 20 years. In these countries *Campylobacter* enteritis affects people of all ages and is prominent in infants and young adults. In developing countries, campylobacteriosis is widespread and causes significant morbidity and even mortality. In these countries the disease is confined to young children who develop immunity early in life through repeated exposure to infection.[113] The high prevalence of the organism in the tropics and its short incubation period are reflected in its frequency as a cause of traveler's diarrhea. A 1998 study from Austria found that *C. jejuni* was the most frequent bacterial cause of diarrhea among 322 travelers returning from destinations in Asia, Africa, and Latin America.[115] During the last 10 years, *Campylobacter* has consistently been the leading cause of traveler's diarrhea among US troops participating in military exercises in Thailand with isolation rates as high as 39%.[29] In Sweden, over 70% of cases of *Campylobacter* enteritis were acquired outside the country.[116] The infection is seasonal in temperate climates. About twice as many infections occur in summer than in winter. Campylobacteriosis is a zoonosis. The reservoir of infection is in wild and domestic animals, particularly birds. Chickens constitute by far the largest potential source of human infection.[112–114] Many cases of campylobacteriosis are associated with foreign travel, from 10 to 50% or more of all cases depending on the country, and usually result from the consumption of contaminated food or water in the countries visited. Many risk factors for *Campylobacter* transmission have been identified. In developed countries, for example, handling and consumption of poultry meat are primary sources of infection and are likely to account for much of the increased incidence of campylobacteriosis. Other risk factors in developed countries include foods of animal origin, including raw milk, inadequately treated water, contact with farm animals and pets, and foreign travel. In developing countries, inadequately treated water and contact with farm animals are assumed to be the most important risk factors. The significance of different transmission pathways varies with time and location.[116]

MICROBIOLOGY

Campylobacter species are small, curved, or spiral-shaped gram-negative bacilli that exhibit rapid darting and spinning motions. The isolation of *Campylobacters* requires special selective techniques that depend either on differential filtration or direct plating on agar-containing antibiotics.

The plates must be incubated under conditions of reduced oxygen tension. *C. jejuni* and *C. coli* grow best at 42°C. Seventy-two to ninety-six hours are required for primary isolation from stool samples and isolation from blood takes even longer. Because some non-*jejuni-coli Campylobacter* species are susceptible to cephalotin (an antibiotic used in most selective media) the filter method and antibiotic-free media are recommended in addition of the selective medium.

The minimal standards for identifying *Campylobacter* after primary isolation are: colony morphology, gram stain response, motility, and an oxidase test. The hippurate hydrolysis test differentiates most *C. jejuni* strains from other *Campylobacter* species. For organisms other than *C. jejuni* and *C. coli*, including atypical *C. jejuni* strains, additional biochemical tests are required. Several molecular tests can further characterize the strains.

PATHOGENESIS

The mechanisms by which *C. jejuni* causes disease are not well known. *C. jejuni* depends on flagellum-mediated motility to display full virulence. At least three mechanisms by which *Campylobacter* may induce illness can be postulated on the basis of clinical syndromes[113,114,116]:

1. *C. jejuni* may cause an enterotoxigenic-like illness with watery diarrhea, as seen in patients in developing countries.
2. The frequent finding of dysenteric stools suggests that mucosal damage due to an invasive process analogous to that seen in Shigellosis is also important in the pathogenesis. Indeed, the fact that many patients have erythrocytes and leukocytes in their stools suggest colonic involvement.
3. Extraintestinal translocation is where the organisms cross the intestinal mucosa and migrate via the lymphatic system to various extraintestinal sites, leading to sepsis, meningitis, cholecystitis, endocarditis, osteomyelitis and septic arthritis.

References

1. Rowe B, Taylor J, Bettelheim KA. An investigation of traveler's diarrhea. Lancet 1970;1:1–5.
2. MacDonald KL, Cohen ML. Epidemiology of travelers' diarrhea: current perspectives. Rev Infect Dis 1986;8(suppl 2):S117–21.
3. Layton M, Bia FJ. Emerging issues in travel medicine. Curr Opin Infect Dis 1992;5:338–44.
4. MacDonald KL, Cohen ML. Epidemiology of travelers' diarrhea: current perspectives. Rev Infect Dis 1986;8(suppl 2):S117–21.
5. Taylor DN, Echeverria P. Etiology and epidemiology of travelers' diarrhea in Asia. Rev Infect Dis 1986;8(suppl 2): S136–41.
6. Black RE. Pathogens that cause travelers' diarrhea in Latin America and Africa. Rev Infect Dis 1986;8(suppl2):S131–5.
7. Hyams KC, Bourgeois Al, Merrell BR, et al. Diarrhea disease during Operation Desert Shield. N Engl J Med 1991;325:1423–8.
8. Heck JE, Staneck JL, Cohen MB, et al. Prospective, controlled, double-blind randomized comparison of ciprofloxacin vs trimethoprim/sulfamethoxazole vs placebo for prevention of traveler's diarrhea [Abstract]. Interscience Conference on Antimicrobial Agents and Chemotherapy; Anaheim, California, October 1992.
9. Steffen R, van der Linde F, Gyr K, Schar M. Epidemiology of diarrhea in travelers. JAMA 1983;249:1176–80.
10. Sanders JW, Isenbarger DW, Walz SE, et al. An observational clinic-based study of diarrheal illness in deployed United States military personnel in Thailand: presentation and outcome of *Campylobacter* infection. Am J Trop Med Hyg 2002;67:533–8.
11. Kean BH, Schaffner W, Brennan RW, Waters SR. The diarrhea of travelers V. Prophylaxis with phthalylsufathiazole and neomycin sulphate. JAMA 1962;180:367–71.

12. Gorbach SL, Kean BH, Evans DG, et al. Travelers' diarrhea and toxigenic *Escherichia coli.* N Engl J Med 1975;292: 933–6.

13. Jiang Z-D, Lowe B, Verenkar MP, et al. Prevalence of enteric pathogens among international travelers with diarrhea acquired in Kenya (Mombasa), India (Goa) and Jamaica (Montego Bay). J Infect Dis 2002;185:497–502.

14. Black RE. Epidemiology of travelers' diarrhea and relative importance of various pathogens. Rev Infect Dis 1990;12 (suppl 1):S73–9.

15. Levine MM. *Escherichia coli* that cause diarrhea: enterotoxigenic, enteropathogenic, enteroinvasive, enterohemorrhagic, and enteroadherent. J Infect Dis 1987;155: 377–9.

16. von Sonnenburg F, Tornieporth N, Collard F, et al. Risk and etiology of diarrhoea at various tourist destinations. Lancet 2000;356:133–4.

17. Ericsson CD. Travelers' diarrhea: epidemiology, prevention and self-treatment. Infect Dis Clin North Am 1998; 12:285–302.

18. DuPont HL, Reves RR, Galindo E, et al. Treatment of travelers' diarrhea with trimethoprim/sulfamethoxazole and with trimethoprim alone. N Engl J Med 1982;307: 841–4.

19. Echeverria P, Blacklow NR, Sanford LB, et al. Travelers' diarrhea among American Peace Corps volunteers in rural Thailand. J infect Dis 1981;143:767–71.

20. Steffen R, Mathewson JJ, Ericsson CD, et al. Travelers' diarrhea in West Africa and in Mexico: fecal transport systems and liquid bismuth subsalicylate for self-therapy. J Infect Dis 1988;157:1008–13.

21. Evans Dg, Olarte J, DuPont HL, et al. Enteropathogens associated with pediatric diarrhea in Mexico City. J Pediatr 1977;91:65–8.

22. Pickering LK, Evans DJ Jr, Munoz O, et al. Prospective study of enteropathogens in children with diarrhea in Houston and Mexico. J Pediatr 1978;93:383–8.

23. Long KZ, Wood JW, Garibay EV, et al. Proportional hazards analysis of diarrhea due to enterotoxigenic *Escherichia coli* and breast feeding in a cohort of urban Mexican children. Am J Epidemiol 1994;139:193–205.

24. Tjoa WS, DuPont HL, Sullivan P, et al. Location of food consumption and travelers' diarrhea. Am J Epidemiol 1977;106:61–6.

25. Wood LV, Ferguson LE, Hogan P, et al. Incidence of bacterial enteropathogens in foods from Mexico. Appl Environ Microbiol 1983;46:328–32.

26. Adachi JA, Mathewson JJ, Jiang ZD, et al. Enteric pathogens in Mexican sauces of popular restaurants in Guadalajara, Mexico, and Houston, Texas. Ann Intern Med 2002;136:884–7.

27. Kuschner R, Trofa AF, Thomas RJ, et al. Use of azithromycin for the treatment of *Campylobacter* enteritis in travelers to Thailand, an area where ciprofloxacin resistance is prevalent. Clin Infect Dis 1995;21: 536–41.

28. Echeverria P, Jackson LR, Hoge CW, et al. Diarrhea in U.S. troops deployed to Thailand. J Clin Microbiol 1993; 31:3351–2.

29. Hoge CW, Gambet JM, Srijan A, et al. Trends in antibiotics resistance among diarrhea pathogens isolated in Thailand over 15 years. Clin Infect Dis 1998;26: 341–5.

30. Steffen R, Colland F, Tornieporth N, et al. Epidemiology, etiology, and impact of traveler's diarrhea in Jamaica. JAMA 1999;281:811–7.

31. Mattila L, Siitonen A, Kyronseppa H, et al. Seasonal variation in etiology of travelers' diarrhea. Finninsh-Moroccan Study Group. J Infect Dis 1992;165:385–8.

32. Ericsson CD, DuPont HL. Travelers' diarrhea: approaches to prevention and treatment. Clin Infect Dis 1993;16:616–26.

33. Larry Gray. *Escherichia, Salmonella, Shigella,* and *Yersinia.* In: Murray PR, Baron EJ, Pfaller MA, et al, editors. Manual of clinical microbiology, 6th ed. American Society for Microbiology, Washington, D.C. 1996. p. 450–6.

34. Evans DG, Evans DJ, Pierce NF. Differences in the response of rabbit small intestinal to heat-labile and heat-stable enterotoxins of *Escherichia coli.* Infect Immun 1973; 7:873–80.

35. Gianella RA. Suckling mouse model for detection of heat-stable *Escherichia coli* enterotoxin: characteristics of the model. Infect Immun 1976;14:95–9.

36. Donta ST, Moon HW, Whipp SC. Detection of heat-labile *Escherichia coli* enterotoxin with the use of adrenal cells in tissue culture. Science 1974;183:334–6.

37. Guerrant RL, Brunton LL, Schnaitman TC, et al. Cyclic adenosine monophosphate and alteration of Chinese hamster ovary cell morphology: a rapid, sensitive in vitro assay for the enterotoxins of *Vibrio cholerae* and *Escherichia coli.* Infect Immun 1974;10:320–7.

38. Moseley SL, Echeverria P, Seriwatana J, et al. Identification of enterotoxigenic *Escherichia coli* by colony hybridization using three enterotoxin gene probes. J Infect Dis 1982;145:863–9.

39. Lanata CF, Kaper JB, Baldini MM, et al. Sensitivity and specificity of DNA probes with the stool blot technique detection of *Escherichia coli* enterotoxins. J Infect Dis 1985;152:1087–90.

40. Schultsz C. Detection of enterotoxigenic *Escherichia coli* in stool samples by using nonradioactively labeled oligonucleotide DNA probes and PCR. J Clin Microbiol 1994;32: 2393–7.

41. Sixma TK, Kalk KH, van zanten BA, et al. Refined structure of *Escherichia coli* heat-labile enterotoxin, a close relative of cholera toxin. J Mol Biol 1993;230:890–918.

42. Evans DJ Jr, Chen LC, Curlin GT, Evans DG. Stimulation of adenylate cyclase by *Escherichia coli enterotoxin.* Nature 1972;236:137–8.

43. Lencer WI, Constable IC, Moe S, et al. Targeting of choleratoxin and *Escherichia coli* heat labile toxin in polarized epithelia: role of COOH-terminal KDEL. J Cell Biol 1995;131:951–62.

44. Sears CL, Kaper JB. Enteric bacterial toxins: mechanisms of action and linkage to intestinal secretion. Microbiol Rev 1996;60:167–215.

45. McGee DW, Elson CO, McGhee JR. Enhancing effect of cholera toxin on interleukin-6 intestinal epithelial cells: mode of action and augmenting effect of inflammatory cytokines. Infect Immun 1993;61:4637–44.

46. Mezoff AG, Giannella RA, Eade MN, Cohen MB. *Escherichia coli* enterotoxin (Sta) binds to receptors, stimulates guanyl cyclase, and impairs absorption in rat colon. Gastroenterology 1992;102:816–22.

47. Radin A, Svennerhdm AM. Colonization factor antigens (CFAs) of enterotoxigenic *Escherichia coli* can prime and boost immune responses against heterologous CFAs. Microbial Pathog 1994;16:131–9.

48. Evans DG, Evans DJ Jr. New surface associated heat-labile colonization factor antigen (CFA/II) produced by enterotoxigenic *Escherichia coli* of serogroups O6 and O8. Infect Immun 1978;21:638–47.

49. McConnell M. Newly characterized putative colonization factors of human enterotoxigenic *Escherichia coli.* FEMS Symp 1991;58:79–82.

50. Smyth CJ. Two mannose-resistant haemagglutinins on enterotoxigenic *Escherichia coli* of serotype O6:K15:H16 or H-isolated from travelers and infantile diarrhea. J Gen Microbiol 1982;128:2081–96.

51. Thomas LV, McConnell MM, Rowe B, Field AM. The possession of three novel *coli* surface antigens by enterotoxigenic *Escherichia coli* strains positive for the new putative colonization factor PCF8775. J Gen Microbiol 1985;131:2319–26.

52. Svennerholm AM, McConnell MM, Wilklund G. Roles of different putative colonization factors antigens in colonization of human enterotoxigenic *Escherichia coli* in rabbits. Microb Path 1993;13:381–9.

53. Rudin A, Wiklund G, Wenneras C, Qadri F. Infection with colonization factor antigen I-expressing enterotoxigenic *Escherichia coli* boosts antibody responses against heterologous colonization factors in primed subjects. Epidemiol Infect 1997;119:391–3.

54. Peltola H, Siitonen A, Kyronseppa H, et al. Prevention of travelers' diarrhea by oral B-subunit/whole-cell cholera vaccine. Lancet 1991;338:1285–9.

55. Svennerholm AM, Holmgren J. Oral B subunit whole cell vaccines against cholera and enterotoxigenic *Escherichia coli* diarrhea. In: Ala' Aldeen DA, Hormaeche CE, editors. Molecular and clinical aspects of bacterial vaccine development. New York: John Wiley & Sons Ltd.; 1995. p. 205–32.

56. Aguero M, Reyes L, Prado V, et al. Enterotoxigenic *Escherichia coli* in a population of infants with diarrhea in Chile. J Clin Microbiol 1985;22:576–81.

57. Binsztein N, Jouve M, Viboud G, et al. Colonization factors of enterotoxigenic *Escherichia coli* isolated from children with diarrhea in Argentina. J Clin Microbiol 1991;29:1893–8.

58. McConnell M, Hibberd M, Penny M, et al. Surveys of human enterotoxigenic *Escherichia coli* from three different geographical areas for possible colonization factors. Epidemiol Infect 1991;106:477–84.

59. Adachi JA, Jiang ZD, Mathewson JJ, et al. Enteroaggregative *Escherichia coli* as a major etiologic agent in travelers' diarrhea in 3 regions of the world. Clin Infect Dis 2001;32:1706–9.

60. Mathewson JJ, Johnson PC, DuPont HL, et al. A newly recognized cause of travelers' diarrhea: Enteroadherent *Escherichia coli.* J Infect Dis 1985;151:471–5.

61. Gascon J, Vargas M, Quinto L, et al. Enteroaggregative *Escherichia coli* strains as a cause of traveler's diarrhea: a case-control study. J Infect Dis 1998;177:1409–12.

62. DuPont HL, Ericsson CD. Prevention and treatment of travelers' diarrhea. N Engl J Med 1993;328:1821–7.

63. Lima AA, Fang G, Schorling JB, et al. Persistent diarrhea in Northeast Brazil: etiologies and interactions with malnutrition. Acta Paediatr Suppl 1992;381:39–44.

64. Mathewson JJ, Jiang ZD, Zumla A, et al. HEp2 cell adherent *Escherichia coli* in patients with human immunodeficiency virus-associated diarrhea. J Infect Dis 1995; 171:1636–9.

65. Wanke CA, Gerrior J, Blais V, et al. Successful treatment of diarrhea disease associated with enteroaggregative *Escherichia coli* in adults with human immunodeficiency virus. J Infect Dis 1998;178:1369–72.

66. Adachi JA, Jiang ZD, Pulido C, et al. Natural history of enteroaggregative *Escherichia coli* infection among American travelers to Mexico. J Infect Dis 2002;136: 884–7.

67. Ericsson CD, Johnson PC, DuPont HL, et al. Ciprofloxacin or trimethoprim-sulfamethoxazole as initial therapy for travelers' diarrhea: a placebo-controlled trial. Ann Intern Med 1987;106:216–20.

68. DuPont HL, Ericsson CD, Mathewson JJ, et al. Oral aztreonam, a poorly absorbed yet effective therapy for bacterial diarrhea in US travelers to Mexico. JAMA 1992; 267:1932–5.

69. Cravioto A, Gross RJ, Scotland SM, Rowe B. An adhesive factor found in strains of *Escherichia coli* belonging to the traditional infantile enteropathogenic serotypes. Curr Microbiol 1979;3:95–9.

70. Nataro JP, Deng Y, Cookson S, et al. Heterogeneity of enteroaggregative *Escherichia coli* virulence demonstrated in volunteers. J Infect Dis 1995;171:465–8.

71. Jiang ZD, Greenberg D, Nataro JP, et al. Occurrence and pathogenic effect of enteroaggregative *E. coli* virulence factors in international travelers. J Clin Microbiol 2002;40: 4185–90.

72. Sutijia M, Bouckenooghe AR, Adachi JA, et al. Intestinal secretory immunoglobulin A response to enteroaggregative *Escherichia coli* in travelers with diarrhea. Clin Diagn Lab Immun 2000;7:501–3.

73. Cohen MB, Hawkins JA, Weckbach LS, et al. Colonization by enteroaggregative *Escherichia coli* in travelers with and without diarrhea. J Clin Microbiol 1993;31:351–3.

74. Steiner TS, Nataro JP, Poteet-Smith CE, et al. Enteroaggregative *Escherichia coli* expresses a novel flagellin that causes IL-8 release from intestinal epithelial cells. J Clin Investig 2000;105:1769–77.

75. Czeczulin JR, Balepur S, Hicks S, et al. Aggregative adherence fimbria II, a second fimbrial antigen mediating aggregative adherence in enteroaggregative *Escherichia coli*. Infect Immun 1997;65:4135–45.

76. Czeczulin JR, Whittam TS, Henderson IR, et al. Phylogenetic analysis of enteroaggregative and diffusely adherent *Escherichia coli*. Infect Immun 1999;67:2693–9.

77. Brynskov J, Tvede N, Anderson CB, Vilien M. Increased concentrations of interleukin-1β, interleukin-2, and soluble interleukin-2 receptors in endoscopical mucosal biopsy specimens with active inflammatory bowel disease. Gut 1992;33:55–8.

78. Izzo RS, Witkon K, Chen AI, et al. Interleukin-8 and neutrophil markers in colonic mucosa from patients with ulcerative colitis. Am J Gastroenterol 1992;87:1447–52.

79. Harenda de Silva DG, Mendis LN, Sheron N, et al. Concentrations of interleukin-6 and tumor necrosis factor in serum and stools of children with *Shigella dysenteriae* 1 infection. Gut 1993;34:194–8.

80. Steiner TS, Lima AAM, Nataro JP, Guerrant RL. Enteroaggregative *Escherichia coli* produce intestinal inflammation and growth impairment and cause interleukin-8 release from intestinal epithelial cells. J Infect Dis 1998;177:88–96.

81. Greenberg D, Jiang ZD, Steffen R, Verenkar MP, DuPont HL. Enteroaggregative *Escherichia coli* produce markers of inflammation among travelers who develop acute diarrhea. J Infect Dis 2002;185:944–9.

82. Bouckenooghe AR, Dupont HL, Jiang ZD, et al. Markers of enteric inflammation in enteroaggregative *Escherichia coli* diarrhea in travelers. Am J Trop Med Hyg 2000;62: 711–3.

83. Nataro J, Kaper J, Robins-Browne R, et al. Patterns of adherence of diarrheagenic *Escherichia coli* to HEp-2 cells. Pediatr Infect Dis J 1987;6:829–31.

84. Keusch GT, Bennish ML. Shigellosis: recent progress, persisting problems and research issues. Pediatr Infect Dis J 1989;8:713–9.

85. Blaser MJ, Pollard RA, Feldman RA. Shigella infections in the United States, 1974–1980. J Infect Dis 1983;147: 771–5.

86. Keusch GT, Bennish ML. Shigellosis. In: Evans AS, Brachman P, editors. Bacterial infections of humans. 3rd ed. New York: Plenum; 1998.

87. DuPont HL, Hornick RB, Dawkins AT, et al. The response of man to virulent *Shigella flexneri* 2a. J Infect Dis 1969; 119:296–9.

88. Dale DC, Mata LJ. Studies of diarrheal disease in Central America. XI. Intestinal bacterial flora in malnourished children with shigellosis. Am J Trop Med Hyg 1968;17: 397–403.

89. Escheverria P, Sethabuts O, Pitarangsi C. Microbiology and diagnosis of infections with *Shigella* and enteroinvasive *Escherichia coli*. Rev Infect Dis 1991;13(suppl 4):S220–5.

90. Grasmick A. Processing and interpretation of bacterial fecal cultures. In: Isenberg HD, editor. Clinical microbiology procedures handbook American Society for Microbiology, Washington, DC; 1996. p. 1.10.1–1.10.25.

91. Sansonetiti PJ. Molecular mechanisms of cell and tissue invasion by *Shigella flexneri*. Infect Agents Dis 1993;2:201–6.

92. Schauer D. Indigenous microflora: paving the way for pathogens? Curr Biol 1997;7:775–7.

93. Sansonetti P, Phalipon A. M cells as ports of entry for enteroinvasive pathogens: mechanisms of interaction, consequences for the disease process. Semin Immunol 1999;11:193–203.

94. Finlay B. Bacterial disease in diverse hosts. Cell 1999;96: 315–8.

95. Sansonetti PJ, d'Hauteville H, Ecobichon C, Pourcel C. Molecular comparison of virulence plasmids in *Shigella* and enteroinvasive *Escherichia coli*. Ann Microbiol 1983; 134A:295–318.

96. Allaoui A, Sansonetti PJ, Menard R, et al. MxiG, a membrane protein required for secretion of *Shigella* spp. Ipa invasins: involvement in entry into epithelial cells and in intercellular dissemination. Mol Microbiol 1995;17: 461–70.

97. Menard R. Sansonetti PJ. Parsot C. Nonpolar mutagenesis of the *ipa* genes defines IpaB, IpaC, and IpaD as effectors

of *Shigella flexneri* entry into epithelial cells. J Bacteriol 1993;175:5899–906.

98. Keusch GT, Grady GF, Mata LJ, Mclver J. The pathogenesis of *Shigella* diarrhea. I. Enterotoxin production by *Shigella dysenteriae* I. J Clin Invest 1972;5:1212–8.

99. O'Brien AD, Thompson MR, Gemski P, et al. Biological properties *of Shigella flexneri* 2A toxin and its serological relationship to *Shigella dysenteriae* 1 toxin. Infect Immun 1977;15:796–8.

100. Moyer MP, Dixon PS, Rothman SW, Brown JE. Cytotoxicity of Shiga toxin for primary cultures of human colonic and ileal epithelial cells. Infect Immun 1987;55:1533–5.

101. Sansonetti PJ. Genetic and molecular basis of epithelial cell invasion by *Shigella* species. Rev Infect Dis 1991; 13Suppl 4:S285–92.

102. Wilder AN, MacCready RA. Isolation of *Salmonella* from poultry. N Engl J Med 1966;274:1453.

103. Hargrett-Bean NT, Pavia AT, Tauxe RV. *Salmonella* isolates from humans in the United States, 1984–1986. MMWR CDC Surveill Summ 1988;2:25.

104. Goldberg MB, Rubin RH. The spectrum of *Salmonella* infection. Infect Dia Clin North Am 1988;2:571.

105. Jones GW, Richardson LA. The attachment to and invasion of HeLa cells by *Salmonella typhimurium*: the contribution of mannose-sensitive and monnose-resistant haemagglutinating activities. J Gen Microbiol 1981;127: 361–70.

106. Giannella RA, Formal SB, Collins H. Role of plasma filtration in the intestinal fluid secretion mediated by infection with *Salmonella typhimurium.* Infect Immun 1976;13:470–4.

107. Baloda SB, Faris A, Krovacek K, Wadstrom T. Cytotonic enterotoxins and cytotoxic factors produced by *Salmonella enteritidis* and *Salmonella typhimurium.* Toxixon 1983;21:785–96.

108. Giannelia RA. Importance of intestinal inflammatory reaction in *Salmonella*-mediated intestinal secretion. Infect Immun 1979;23:140–5.

109. Koo FCW, Peterson JW, Houston CW, Molina NC. Pathogenesis of experimental salmonellosis: inhibition of protein synthesis by cytotoxin. Infect Immun 1984;43:93–100.

110. Mills DB, Bajaj V, Lee CA. A 40 kilobase chromosomal fragment encoding *Salmonella typhimurium* invasion genes is absent from the corresponding region of the *Escherichia coli* K-12 chromosome. Mol Microbiol 1995; 15:749–59.

111. Groisman EA, Ochman H. Cognate gene clusters govern invasion of host epithelial cells by *Salmonella typhimurium* and *Shigella flexneri.* EMBO J 1993;12:3779–87.

112. Butzler JP, Mégreaud F. *Campylobacter* and Helicobacter pylori. In: Zinner S, Young LS, Acar JF, et al, editors. Expanding indications for the new macrolides, azalides and streptogramins, New York: 1997. p. 237–49.

113. Butzler JP. Campylobacteriosis in humans in the increasing incidence of human WHO/CDS/CSR/APH 2001;7:38–41.

114. Allos BM. *Campylobacter jejuni* infections: update on emerging issues and trends CID 2001;32:1201–6.

115. Reinthaler FF, Feierl G, Stunzner D, Marth E. Diarrhea in returning Austrian tourists: epidemiology, etiology and cost-analysis. J Travel Med 1998;5:65–72.

116. Tauxe R. Incidence, trends and sources in developed countries: an overview in the increasing incidence of human campylobacteriosis. WHO/CDS/CSR/APH 2001;7: 42–3.

CHAPTER 3

THE VIRAL PATHOGENS

ROBERT L. ATMAR, MD

ROGER I. GLASS, MD, PhD

Gastroenteritis is one of the most common afflictions of humanity.[1] Enteric viruses are being increasingly recognized as important causes of this disease, but the true burden of viral origins is not known.[2] Diarrhea also can be a common symptom of a number of viral infections (eg, influenza, hepatitis, dengue, severe acute respiratory syndrome [SARS]); however, other clinical signs and symptoms usually suggest the presence of an extra-intestinal infection. This chapter will focus upon the enteric viruses that contribute to the worldwide burden of gastroenteritis.

Historical Background

Viruses have been suspected to be a cause of gastroenteritis for more than 50 years. In 1929, Zahorsky described an outbreak of epidemic nonbacterial gastroenteritis and proposed the name "winter vomiting disease."[3] During the 1930s and 1940s, no bacterial pathogen could be identified in the majority of outbreaks of gastroenteritis that were investigated by the New York State Department of Health. In 1947, Gordon and colleagues pooled stool filtrates collected from two subjects in an outbreak of nonbacterial gastroenteritis and produced an experimental challenge inoculum to infect volunteers.[4] Subjects developed gastroenteritis within 1 to 5 days of inoculation. The agent could be passed serially through humans, suggesting that it was not a preformed toxin, and its ability to cause illness was lost following heat inactivation by autoclaving. No bacteria were isolated from the inocula, but attempts to grow a viral pathogen in embryonated chicken eggs failed.

Outbreaks of nonbacterial gastroenteritis continued to occur without an etiologic agent being identified. One such outbreak occurred in an elementary school in Norwalk, Ohio during October 1968.[5] This outbreak was associated with a 50% attack rate involving both students and teachers and a secondary attack rate of 32% among family contacts. Challenge inocula to infect human subjects were produced from stools collected during the outbreak.[6] In 1972, Kapikian and colleagues were able to exploit a new diagnostic method, immunoelectron microscopy (IEM), to identify viral particles in the stools of volunteers infected with a passage of the Norwalk inoculum.[7] This became the first clear evidence documenting a specific virus as the cause of gastroenteritis.

Over the next 4 years, all of the other recognized viral causes of gastroenteritis (Table 1) were identified by electron microscopy; ie, rotavirus, enteric adenovirus, astrovirus, and "classical" calicivirus.[8–12] Other viruses have also been detected in stool samples of persons with diarrhea. Some of these are recognized to cause diarrhea in animals (eg, toroviruses, pestiviruses, coronaviruses, picobirnaviruses), while others from some of these families as well as the recently described picornavirus, Aichi virus, are more prevalent in stool samples from persons with diarrhea than in samples from asymptomatic individuals. However, the role of these viruses as causes of gastroenteritis in humans remains to be determined.[13] The remainder of this chapter will focus upon the four virus families that have clearly been established to cause gastroenteritis (Table 2).

Table 1 Established and Candidate Viral Agents as Causes of Gastroenteritis in Humans

Established Agents	Candidate Agents
Adenoviruses (Group F – enteric)	Aichi virus (a picornavirus)
Astroviruses	Coronaviruses
Caliciviruses	Pestiviruses
Noroviruses	Picobirnaviruses
Sapoviruses	Toroviruses
Rotaviruses	
Group A	
Groups B and C	

Table 2 Characteristics, Epidemiology, and Diagnosis of Enteric Viruses Recognized to Cause Diarrhea

	Norovirus	Sapovirus	Rotavirus	Astrovirus	Enteric Adenovirus
Family	Caliciviridae	Caliciviridae	Reoviridae	Astroviridae	Adenoviridae
genome	ssRNA, positive sense, polyadenylated	ssRNA, positive sense, polyadenylated	dsRNA, segmented (11 segments)	ssRNA, positive sense, polyadenylated	dsDNA
Viral Particle Size	28–35 nm	28–35 nm	75 nm	28–30 nm	65–80 nm
Age Groups Affected	All age groups	Predominantly children; occasionally adults	Predominantly children; also elderly and adults	Predominantly children; occasionally adults	Young children; other age groups uncommon
Diagnostic Assays	RT-PCR, EM, EIA	RT-PCR, EM, EIA	EIA, Latex agglutination, RT-PCR, EM, culture	RT-PCR, EIA, EM, culture	EIA, PCR, EM, culture
Likely to Cause Travelers Diarrhea?	Yes	No	Yes	No	No

dsDNA = double-stranded deoxyribonucleic acid; dsRNA = double-stranded ribonucleic acid; EIA = enzyme immunoassay; EM = electron microscopy; PCR = polymerase chain reaction; RT-PCR = reverse transcription-polymerase chain reaction; ssRNA = single-stranded ribonucleic acid.

Caliciviruses

VIRAL CHARACTERISTICS AND BIOLOGY

Caliciviruses are nonenveloped, icosahedral viruses that have a single-stranded, positive-sense ribonucleic acid (RNA) genome.[14] There are four recognized genera within the family *Caliciviridae*: *Norovirus*, *Sapovirus*, *Lagovirus*, and *Vesivirus*. Currently, only animal strains are recognized to be members of the latter two genera, while noroviruses and sapoviruses contain both human and animal strains. A fifth genus that currently only contains bovine strains has been proposed.[15]

The name "calicivirus" is derived from the Latin word calix, meaning "cup" or "goblet," a reference to the cup-like depressions that can be seen by electron microscopy (EM) on the surface of viral particles. Sapoviruses have the traditional calicivirus morphology. In contrast, noroviruses are less likely to have visible cup-like depressions, and many were previously identified morphologically as small round structured viruses (SRSVs). However, some noroviruses have the distinctive calicivirus EM appearance, so definitive classification of an individual virus strain is dependent upon sequencing data and phylogenetic analysis.

Noroviruses have a genome that ranges in size from 7.5 to 7.7 kb with three open reading frames (ORFs).[16] The first ORF encodes a large polyprotein that is thought to be cleaved post-translationally into several nonstructural proteins, including a viral protease, polymerase, and nucleoside triphosphate hydrolase (NTPase). The second ORF encodes the major structural protein (VP1), while the third ORF encodes a basic protein that is also a minor structural protein (VP2). The VP1 protein spontaneously assembles into virus-like particles (VLPs) when expressed in a baculovirus expression system.[17] These VLPs are antigenically and morphologically similar to native virions and have been useful reagents because human caliciviruses cannot be propagated in vitro.[18] Sapoviruses have a genomic organization similar to that of the noroviruses, with the exception that the VP1 gene is in the same ORF as those for the nonstructural proteins.[19]

The lack of a cell culture system has led to the application of other classification systems for characterization of norovirus and sapovirus strains. Both antigenic and genetic classification schemes have been employed. Early studies relied on reactivity with human convalescent sera (eg, solid phase immune electron microscopy), but more recent methods have utilized hyperimmune animal sera generated against recombinant VLPs.[20] However, sequence-based strain characterization is currently the most common means of strain classification. The norovirus and sapovirus genera each can be subdivided into five genogroups based upon phylogenetic analyses.[21,22] The genogroups can be further subdivided into genetic clusters, or genotypes, based upon pairwise comparisons of the VP1 amino acid sequences of viral strains. How well the genetic classification scheme reflects biologic (ie, serotypic) differences between groups has not yet been determined.

EPIDEMIOLOGY

Human caliciviruses infect persons of all ages. These viruses cause infection throughout the year, although there is a peak incidence during the cold-weather months.[23] Noroviruses were previously referred to as "Norwalk-like" viruses and Norwalk virus is the prototype strain. In the United States, there are an estimated 23 million cases of norovirus-associated gastroenteritis per year.[2] Worldwide, noroviruses are the major cause of epidemic nonbacterial gastroenteritis, being identified in 70 to > 95% of outbreaks.[24–26] Noroviruses are also the most common viral cause of gastroenteritis identified in recent community-based studies.[24,27,28] Seroprevalence rates in developed countries increase during the first several years of life, reaching levels of 80 to 90% by young adulthood.[29] In contrast, sapoviruses are only occasionally identified in outbreaks and are instead more commonly recognized as to cause diarrhea among young children.[30,31]

Human caliciviruses are principally spread by the fecal–oral route, but airborne transmission (following exposure to a vomiting person) may also occur.[32] Spread from person-to-person and by consumption of contaminated foods or water are common mechanisms by which infection is established, although fomites may also serve as the source of infection. Some foods more commonly associated with norovirus infection include uncooked shellfish, salads, and cold foods.[33] Recreational activities, including canoeing, rafting, and football, are another means by which viral transmission has occurred, either through consumption of contaminated water or by more direct exposure to ill participants.[34,35] These viruses are relatively resistant to many disinfectants, making it difficult to eradicate them from the environment. This characteristic has led to continued virus transmission from contaminated environmental surfaces to guests and has necessitated the closure of hotels and cruise ships in order to decontaminate potentially contaminated areas.[36,37] Features that favor transmission of noroviruses include low infectious dose, stability in the environment and infectivity even in presence of 10 ppm chlorine.[38]

CLINICAL MANIFESTATIONS AND IMMUNITY

The acute onset of vomiting, nonbloody diarrhea, or both, is characteristic of human calicivirus infection. From human experimental infection studies, vomiting may be the predominant symptom in one person, while diarrhea without vomiting may occur in another individual infected with the same virus.[6,39] Other associated symptoms may include nausea, anorexia, abdominal cramps, malaise, and low-grade fever. Up to one-third of individuals infected during experimental challenge studies are asymptomatic, while other individuals are not infected, even upon repeated challenge.[39,40] The incubation period ranges from 1 to 2 days, and symptoms generally persist for 12 to 60 hours.

In persons who are infected following exposure to virus, short-term, homologous immunity (6 to 14 weeks) is induced following infection.[40] In some studies, higher levels of serum antibody have correlated with protection from illness.[41,42] Natural resistance to infection, based upon expression of histoblood-group antigens (ABH, secretor status) that may serve as virus receptors, also influence the likelihood of symptomatic illness following exposure to virus.[43–45]

DIAGNOSIS

Human calicivirus infection can be diagnosed by a number of different methods, but few are readily available to the clinician. Electron microscopy, the first method for detection of these viruses, is still employed by many laboratories to screen stools for potential viral pathogens, but the low number of noroviruses shed in stool makes this method relatively insensitive. The sensitivity can be increased somewhat with IEM, in which specific antisera aggregate viruses to make them easier to detect, but the antisera used in this assay are not widely available.

Currently, the most common assay for human calicivirus diagnosis is the reverse transcription-polymerase chain reaction (RT-PCR).[20] In this assay virus-specific primers that target conserved regions of the genome (usually in the polymerase or VP1 genes) prime complementary deoxyribonucleic acid (DNA) synthesis and then amplify portions of the virus genome. The specificity of the amplification is confirmed using probe hybridization or sequencing of the amplicons. Unfortunately, the sequence diversity of the human caliciviruses is such that no single primer pair can detect all viruses, and most laboratories use separate primer pairs for genogroups I and II noroviruses and a third pair for sapoviruses.[20]

Antigen and antibody detection assays have also been investigated, but their application is largely restricted to research laboratories. Early generation antigen detection enzyme-linked immunosorbent assays (ELISA) were too specific, only detecting viruses closely related to the antigen from which the hyperimmune sera were made. The description of more broadly reactive monoclonal antibodies suggests that a more broadly reactive antigen detection assay can be developed.[46,47] However, commercial antigen detection assays developed with these antibodies have had poor sensitivity or specificity.[48–50] Antibody assays have relied largely on the analysis of paired sera, making the assay of more value for epidemiologic studies than for evaluation of the individual patient.

TREATMENT AND PREVENTION

The illness caused by human caliciviruses is generally mild and self-limited, and treatment is supportive (eg, rehydration, analgesics, antiemetics). Recovery is the rule, although some patients become ill enough to require hospitalization for fluid replacement. Mortality is rare, but it has occurred as a result of aspiration and in the elderly due to dehydration and electrolyte disturbances. Currently, the principal means of prevention is avoidance of contaminated foodstuffs and water. The potential value of VLPs as a vaccine is being explored.[51]

Rotaviruses

VIRAL CHARACTERISTICS AND BIOLOGY

Rotaviruses are nonenveloped, icosahedral viruses that have a double-stranded, segmented RNA genome. Rotavirus is a genus within the family *Reoviridae*, and there are both animal and human strains within the genus.[52] The name "rotavirus" is derived from the Latin word, *rota*, meaning "wheel," and refers to the morphologic appearance of the virus particle. The virus particle is made up of three layers of structural protein: VP1, VP2, and VP3 form the inner core; VP6, which makes up 50% of the total weight of the viral particle, forms the second layer; and VP4 and VP7 form the outer layer. The inner core layer encloses the 11 segments of the RNA genome. The segmented genome allows reassortment of virus genes to occur in cells that are co-infected with more than one virus strain.

Rotaviruses are classified into different groups based upon the presence of cross-reactive antigenic epitopes on the VP6 protein. Group A rotaviruses are the major cause of human disease. Groups B and C rotaviruses are primarily animal pathogens but are also a cause of disease in humans, including a few large outbreaks, while other groups (D to F) infect only animals.[53–55] The group A rotaviruses are further subdivided into serotypes based upon antigenic characteristics of the VP7 (G type) and VP4 (P type) proteins. Fourteen different G types and 20 P types have been identified, with at least 10 G types and 11 P types being found in humans.[53]

One of the viral proteins, nonstructural protein 4 (NSP4), has been found to be a viral enterotoxin.[56] Its toxigenic effect is mediated through a calcium-dependent signaling pathway that leads to excess chloride secretion. The toxigenic properties of this protein are not the only means by which rotavirus causes diarrhea; villous shortening with malabsorption and activation of the enteric nervous system are also likely to have a role in the pathogenesis of disease.[57–59]

EPIDEMIOLOGY

Rotavirus infection is the principal cause of dehydrating diarrhea of young children in the world. In the developing world, it is a major cause of mortality in the first years of life and is estimated to cause 600,000 deaths per year.[60] In contrast, in the United States there is little mortality associated with rotavirus infection (20 to 60 deaths per year); nevertheless, primary infection leads to a significant use of medical resources due to doctor visits (~ 600,000 per year) and hospitalizations (55,000 to 70,000 per year).[60,61] Almost all children are infected at least once by the age of 3 years, with the peak incidence occurring between ages 6 and 24 months.

Infection in adults is recognized less frequently. It occurs following contact with a pediatric case, in foodborne or waterborne outbreaks, in travelers, in epidemics in closed populations (ie, institutionalized individuals), and as a sporadic cause of endemic disease.[62,63] It was identified in 1% of 263 nonbacterial gastroenteritis outbreaks investigated by the Centers for Disease Control and Prevention between 1998 and 2000.[64] All three of the rotavirus-associated outbreaks in the United States and several recent outbreaks in Japan were caused by viruses with a G2 serotype.[64] In children, the most common infecting serotypes are G1 to G4 and G9.[65,66] The reasons for the predominance of G2 serotypes among outbreaks in adults are not clear, but possibilities include increased virulence of G2 viruses and lack of protective heterotypic immunity in affected individuals.[64,67] Group C rotaviruses have been identified as causes of both sporadic disease and outbreaks of gastroenteritis in pediatric and adult patients when appropriate diagnostics have been utilized.[55,68,69]

Transmission of rotavirus infection is by the fecal–oral route. Fomites and contaminated foods and water all serve as vehicles for virus transmission. Rotaviruses survive less well in the environment than do caliciviruses, based on the observations that they are commonly found in shellfish and in sewage, but they are uncommonly identified as causes of foodborne or waterborne outbreaks.[26,64,70,71] In the United States, there is a distinct winter seasonality, but in other parts of the world, autumn and spring peaks of infection occur, and in the tropics (within 10° of the equator), a seasonal trend often is not apparent.[70]

CLINICAL MANIFESTATIONS AND IMMUNITY

Diarrhea, vomiting, and fever are all common symptoms of rotavirus-associated gastroenteritis.[64,72] Diarrhea is usually watery and is typically of longer duration (4 days or more) than that seen with norovirus-associated illness. Vomiting occurs in the first 1 to 2 days of illness, and fever may be as high as 39° to 40°C in young children.[73,74] Volume depletion occurs frequently and is a reason that patients seek medical care. The overall illness tends to be somewhat more severe than that associated with norovirus infection, which may explain the relatively greater frequency of identification of rotavirus infection in persons seeking medical attention.[28,73,75,76] Asymptomatic infection also occurs commonly, particularly in older children and adults. The incubation period is estimated to be 1 to 3 days.[74]

Repeated infection leads to protection from more severe disease.[77] Serum antibody levels have been the best correlate of protection from disease based upon a variety of studies in humans.[78] Additional host factors, such as nutritional status, and virus factors also likely contribute to the development of symptomatic infection.[64,74]

DIAGNOSIS

Antigen detection assays are currently the principal means of diagnosis of rotavirus infections. Both ELISA and latex agglutination assays detect shared epitopes on the VP6 protein of group A rotaviruses.[74] In some laboratories, stools that are negative in group A rotavirus antigen assays are screened by EM. Such a strategy allows the detection of groups B and C viruses that are missed by the group A-specific antigen detection assays. RT-PCR assays are also employed for diagnosis of rotavirus infection, and group A rotaviruses may be isolated with cell culture. Serologic assays (eg, ELISA, neutralization assay) rely on the identification of fourfold or greater rises in serum antibody, restricting the utility of these assays to epidemiologic studies.

Rotaviruses identified in stool specimens or isolated in cell culture may be further characterized with a variety of methods. The differential mobility of the RNA genome segments by polyacrylamide gel electrophoresis (PAGE) may allow differentiation of rotavirus strains.[79] G and P types can be characterized based upon the reactivity of the virus with a panel of monoclonal antibodies.[79,80] Sequencing of the VP4 and VP7 genes is also employed to characterize the genetic variability of strains within a region and over time.[79,81]

TREATMENT AND PREVENTION

Treatment of rotavirus infection is supportive; no specific effective antiviral therapy is available. Therapy is targeted at maintaining volume status, and this is accomplished with either oral or intravenous rehydration.[82] Early reinstitution of feeding during the illness (~24 hours after onset) does not prolong diarrhea and may shorten it. There are insufficient data available to show a clinical benefit from the prescription of antimotility agents, such as loperamide, and these agents are not recommended for children.[82] Chronic rotavirus diarrhea in immunocompromised children has been successfully treated by passive immunotherapy with oral immunoglobulins, but this approach is not recommended for general use.[83]

Active immunization can prevent or ameliorate the severity of rotavirus-induced illness.[60] The first licensed rotavirus vaccine was a quadrivalent, live, attenuated vaccine that was withdrawn from the market due to its association with the occurrence of intussusception within the first 2 weeks of the first dose of the vaccine.[84] Two additional live attenuated rotavirus vaccines have recently been licensed after clinical evaluations demonstrated efficacy without an increased risk of intussusception.[60] Additional nonspecific control measures include hand-washing, cohorting of ill individuals, and disinfection of potential fomites.

Astroviruses

VIRAL CHARACTERISTICS AND BIOLOGY

Astroviruses are nonenveloped, icosahedral viruses that have a single-stranded, positive-sense genome. *Astrovirus* is a genus within the family *Astroviridae*, and there are both animal and humans strains that tend to cause species-specific disease. The name "astrovirus" is derived from the Greek word, *astron*, meaning "star," and refers to the five- or six-point star-like appearance of the viruses as seen by EM.[85]

The 6.8 kb astrovirus genome has three large ORFs: ORF1a, ORF1b, and ORF2. ORF1a encodes several nonstructural proteins, including a 3C-like serine protease, while ORF1b contains the RNA-dependent RNA polymerase gene and is translated by ribosomal frameshifting. ORF2 is contained in both genomic and a subgenomic RNA, and it is translated into a precursor that is proteolytically cleaved into at least three capsid proteins.[85,86]

Eight different human astrovirus antigenic types have been identified.[87] Phylogenetic analysis of the capsid gene also yields the eight groups that correspond to the serologic classification.[88,89] Although the different astrovirus types can be distinguished serologically, they also share a shared group antigen that makes their identification possible with monoclonal antibodies in an enzyme immunoassay.[90]

EPIDEMIOLOGY

Astroviruses are recognized to cause disease in four different groups of individuals: 1) infants and young children; 2) the immunocompromised; 3) the institutionalized elderly; and 4) otherwise healthy persons exposed to contaminated food or water.[85,87] These viruses are one of the most common causes of viral diarrhea among infants and children. For example, in China, astroviruses were the second most common virus identified, after rotavirus, in children hospitalized for acute diarrhea.[91] In several other studies, astroviruses have been identified in 2 to 6% of persons with acute gastroenteritis.[27,28,76,92–94]

Astroviruses have been associated with gastroenteritis in a number of groups with immunodeficiencies. These viruses have caused an outbreak of gastroenteritis in a bone marrow transplant unit and were one of the more commonly identified viruses in human immunodeficiency virus (HIV)-infected patients with diarrhea.[95,96] The severely immunocompromised (eg, bone marrow transplant, fludarabine-treated) patient may have protracted courses of diarrhea.[97–99] Several outbreaks of astrovirus infection among the institutionalized elderly have been reported, with attack rates ranging from 12 to 100%.[85,100]

Outbreaks of astrovirus infection among otherwise healthy persons have been reported.[101–103] At least some of these outbreaks are thought to have been caused by contaminated food or water. However, none of the outbreaks of epidemic gastroenteritis investigated by the Centers for Disease Control and Prevention from 1996 to 1997 were attributed to astrovirus infection, and these viruses have only rarely been identified as causes of foodborne disease.[104,105] Furthermore, although astroviruses can be demonstrated to be common contaminants in uncooked shellfish, this foodstuff has rarely been documented to be a source of astrovirus infection.[71,106] Thus, although astroviruses can cause either foodborne or waterborne disease, epidemic gastroenteritis caused by these viruses via this route of transmission appears to be uncommon.

Astroviruses are spread by the fecal–oral route. Transmission is from person-to-person, spread by food or water and possibly by fomites. Infection occurs most commonly during the winter months in temperate climates and during the rainy season in the tropics.[85,97] Type 1 astroviruses are the most prevalent worldwide, although in a given location, the predominant circulating serotype may vary over time.

CLINICAL MANIFESTATIONS AND IMMUNITY

Astrovirus causes a mild gastroenteritis, with diarrhea lasting approximately 4 days and vomiting occurring in up to 60% of cases.[87] Low-grade fever may also occur in up to one-quarter of patients. Dehydration is much less common than is seen with rotavirus infections in the same age group, and the overall illness associated with astrovirus infection is milder than with rotavirus.[107,108] The incubation period is estimated to be approximately 3 to 4 days, based upon experimental challenge studies, and to be as little as 24 to 36 hours, based upon epidemiologic investigations of epidemic disease.[85]

The epidemiologic pattern of disease, occurring primarily in young children and in the elderly, suggests that immunity, which protects older children and adults from symptomatic infection, develops. In studies of experimental challenge of adults, the presence of serum antibody correlated with protection from infection.[106] Clearance of infection in an immunocompromised patient following administration of intravenous gamma globulin also suggests a possible role of antibody in disease resolution.[98]

DIAGNOSIS

RT-PCR is the most sensitive assay for the diagnosis of astrovirus infection. Primer pairs have been developed that target conserved areas of the genome, including a region in ORF1a just upstream of the putative protease domain, a region in ORF1b (the RNA-dependent RNA polymerase gene) and the 3' untranslated region.[89,101,109] Sequencing of the RT-PCR products has been performed to further characterize detected strains. Antigen detection enzyme immunoassays (EIAs) are also employed to diagnose astrovirus infection.[85,87,88,90] The EIA is not generally available in the United States, but an astrovirus-specific EIA is commercially available in Europe. Astroviruses can also be typed with type-specific EIAs.[88] Electron microscopy is the least sensitive, but one of the most commonly available techniques for diagnosing astrovirus infection.[96]

Astroviruses can be isolated in cell culture. A number of different cell lines have been evaluated, but the intestinally derived cell lines, CaCo-2 and T84, are among the most sensitive.[110,111] A rapid shell vial assay, which relies on detection of viral replication by immunofluorescent staining 18 hours after inoculation, has also been described.[110] Amplification of virus in cell culture prior to detection with RT-PCR assays is another strategy to diagnose astrovirus infection.[112]

TREATMENT AND PREVENTION

Treatment is supportive, and no specific therapy is available. If volume depletion occurs, oral or intravenous volume rehydration should be provided. An anecdotal report describing the administration of gamma globulin to resolve protracted illness in an immunocompromised patient requires confirmation in additional patients.[98] Prevention is targeted toward maintenance of hygienic standards and disinfection of potential fomites. No vaccine is currently available.

Enteric Adenoviruses

VIRAL CHARACTERISTICS AND BIOLOGY

Enteric adenoviruses are nonenveloped, icosahedral viruses that have a double-stranded DNA genome. They are members of the family *Adenoviridae*, which contains six subgroups (or subgenera), A through F, that cause human disease. The subgroup F adenoviruses are the enteric adenoviruses. Adenovirus types 40 and 41 are the two members of the subgroup F adenoviruses, and variants among each of these types have been described.[113,114]

The adenovirus genome is approximately 32 kb in size and encodes a number of structural and nonstructural proteins. The relationships between viruses in the different subgroups have been determined and characterized by analysis of genomic DNA restriction patterns.[115] Subgroups have also been characterized by their abilities to hemagglutinate rat or monkey red blood cells. Group F adenoviruses partially hemagglutinate rat red blood cells.[116]

The adenovirus capsid is made up of 240 hexons and 12 pentons, with the latter present at the vertices of the virus particle. A protein fiber extends from the penton base. A knob region at the tip of the fiber interacts with cellular receptors as the initial event in infection. The hexon protein has a group-specific antigen that is shared by all of the human adenoviruses.[116]

EPIDEMIOLOGY

Seroepidemiologic studies indicate that enteric adenoviruses cause disease in both developed and developing countries.[113] These viruses have been identified in 1 to 2% of cases of gastroenteritis in most studies, although higher frequencies have been reported.[27,28,76,92,93,117,118] Children under 2 years of age are the most likely to have infection and disease. Some HIV-infected patients with chronic diarrhea have adenoviruses present in their feces, but it is not clear whether the enteric adenoviruses have a specific role in causing diarrhea in this patient population.[119,120] Such a role is suggested by a single case report that noted the prolonged excretion of adenovirus type 40 in the absence of other enteric pathogens in an acquired Immune Deficiency Syndrome (AIDS) patient with chronic diarrhea.[121]

Transmission is by person-to-person spread. Foodborne or waterborne transmission has not been demonstrated, and transmission to adults is uncommon. Unlike the other viral causes of gastroenteritis, there is no seasonal pattern of enteric adenovirus disease.[113]

CLINICAL MANIFESTATIONS AND IMMUNITY

Diarrhea and vomiting are the principal manifestations of enteric adenovirus infection. Adenovirus-infected patients are less likely to have high fever (over 39°C) than rotavirus-infected children (3% versus 42%, respectively), but their diarrhea tends to last longer (mean duration 10.8 days versus 5.8 days in rotavirus-infected patients).[122] The incubation period is approximately 1 week.[113]

DIAGNOSIS

Enzyme immunoassays to detect enteric adenoviruses are commercially available.[113] These assays utilize a group-specific polyclonal antiserum to capture and monoclonal subgroup F-specific antibodies as the detector. Sensitivity and specificity of the assay are high.[123] Electron microscopy is another common means for detection of adenoviruses in the stool. To confirm that the adenovirus is an enteric adenovirus, IEM must be performed with type- or subgroup-specific antisera.

A number of nucleic acid detection methods for the enteric adenoviruses have been described. Dot blot hybridization was one of the initial assays, but more recently, PCR assays have been developed.[113,124,125] A multiplex PCR assay allows the distinction of subgroup F adenoviruses from those of other subgroups based on amplicon size.[125] Although fastidious, the enteric adenoviruses can be isolated in cell culture and classified by type or subgroup with monoclonal antibodies or by restriction analysis.[113,126,127]

TREATMENT AND PREVENTION

Similar to the other enteric viruses, treatment of enteric adenovirus infection is supportive. No specific antiviral therapy is available. Because of their relatively low impact as a cause of diarrhea, compared to other enteric pathogens, vaccine development for adenoviruses has not been a priority. Additional studies are needed to clarify the correlates and duration of immunity.

Relative Importance of the Viral Pathogens as Causes of Diarrhea

The importance of viruses, other than rotavirus, as causes of diarrhea has been underappreciated due to the lack of readily available, sensitive diagnostics for these agents. Community and outpatient studies of gastroenteritis show that each of the enteric viruses have been found to be causes of diarrhea in different settings (in the community, presenting for outpatient care, admitted to the hospital) in several countries, and the prevalence of

Table 3 Frequency of Identification of Enteric Viruses in Persons with Gastroenteritis in Different Settings

Country	United Kingdom[28]		The Netherlands[27,92]		Finland[75]	Peru[128,130]	France[76]	Sweden[93]	
Setting	Community (%)	General Practice (%)	Community (%)	General Practice (%)	Clinical Study Cohort (%)	Inpatient (%)	Outpatient (%)	Outpatient (%)	Inpatient (%)
Age groups	All ages		All ages		0–2 years	0–2 years	0–13 years	≥ 15 years	
Calicivirus	7.5	7.3	22.4	7.5	29.5	55	14	2.8	2.7
Rotavirus	3.7	6.9	7.3	5.3	31	52	61	2.1	4.5
Astrovirus	2.0	2.6	2.0	1.5	8.8	4	6.3	1.8	1.9
Adenovirus	1.5	2.7	3.8	2.2	6.3	4	3.1	1.3	0.5

Table 4 Number (Frequency) of Enteric Viruses Identified* in Association with Travelers' Diarrhea in Selected Studies Reported Since 1990

Author	Traveler (Number)	Travel Location	Norovirus	Rotavirus	No Pathogen
Haberberger et al.[131]	Military (183)	Egypt	NT†	NT	93 (51%)
Mattila et al.[132]	Adult tourists (171)	Morocco	NT	5 (3%)	70 (41%)
Petruccelli et al.[133]	Military (137)	Thailand	NT	2 (1%)	57 (42%)
Bourgeois et al.[134]	Military (289)	South America, West Africa	26 (9%)‡	31 (11%)	143 (49%)
Sharp et al.[135]	Military (113)	Somalia	NT	1 (1%)	39 (35%)
Oyofo et al.[136]	Military (49)	Southeast Asia	21 (43%)**	0	14 (29%)
Steffen et al.[137]	Adult tourists (322)	Jamaica	NT	26 (9%)	220 (68%)
Chapin et al.[138]	Adult tourists (34)	Mexico Guatemala	22 (65%)**	1 (3%)	5 (15%)
Ko et al.[139]	Adult tourists (124)	Mexico	21 (17%)**	NT	39 (31%)

*Identification of viral pathogen performed using antigen detection assay, unless noted otherwise; few studies tested for astroviruses, adenoviruses, or sapoviruses.
†NT = not tested (for this viral pathogen).
‡Antigen and antibody detection assays using human-based reagents.
**Reverse transcription--polymerase chain reaction (RT-PCR) used as the diagnostic test.

each virus varies by age, severity, and setting studied (Table 3). The prevalence of rotaviruses and human caliciviruses increases significantly when only severe cases of gastroenteritis are considered; rotaviruses cause more than 25 to > 50% of cases of gastroenteritis requiring hospitalization in children < 5 years of age and human caliciviruses (noroviruses and sapoviruses combined) are found in 20% or more of cases.[75,128–130] Although all of the enteric viruses were found in each of the countries studied, they are not all likely to be a burden to the traveler. This is because astroviruses and enteric adenoviruses cause the greatest disease burden in young children. Thus, the most likely viral agents to cause diarrhea in the traveler are the human caliciviruses (particularly noroviruses) and rotaviruses. This conclusion is borne out by observational studies of travelers' diarrhea (Table 4).[131–139] However, the relative importance of enteric viruses as causes of travelers' diarrhea is likely to be underestimated because few studies have employed molecular methods for diagnosis of virus infections. When the best diagnostic assay available (RT-PCR) has been applied for identification of norovirus infection, these viruses have been identified in 16 to 65% of samples.[136,138,139] Furthermore, noroviruses are a major cause of gastroenteritis in deployed military populations and among travelers on cruise ships.[37,38,140–142] Additional studies using newer diagnostic methods are warranted for the identification of potential viral etiologies of travelers' diarrhea, especially given the large number of cases for which no enteric pathogen is identified (see Table 4). Furthermore, improved strategies to prevent or ameliorate disease caused by the human caliciviruses and rotaviruses are needed for travelers.

Acknowledgments

This work was supported by Public Health Service grants AI25465 and AI57788 from the National Institute of Allergy and Infectious Diseases.

References

1. Guerrant RL, Hughes JM, Lima NL, Crane J. Diarrhea in developed and developing countries: magnitude, special settings, and etiologies. Rev Infect Dis 1990;12 Suppl 1: S41–50.

2. Mead PS, Slutsker L, Dietz V, et al. Food-related illness and death in the United States. Emerg Infect Dis 1999;5: 607–25.

3. Zahorsky J. Hyperemesis hiemis or the winter vomiting disease. Arch Pediatr 1929;46:391–5.

4. Gordon I, Ingraham HS, Korns RF. Transmission of epidemic gastroenteritis to human volunteers by oral administration of fecal filtrates. J Exp Med 1947;86:409–22.

5. Adler JL, Zickl R. Winter vomiting disease. J Infect Dis 1969;119:668–73.

6. Dolin R, Blacklow NR, DuPont H, et al. Transmission of acute infectious nonbacterial gastroenteritis to volunteers by oral administration of stool filtrates. J Infect Dis 1971; 123:307–12.

7. Kapikian AZ, Wyatt RG, Dolin R, et al. Visualization by immune electron microscopy of a 27-nm particle associated with acute infectious nonbacterial gastroenteritis. J Virol 1972;10:1075–81.

8. Bishop RF, Davidson GP, Holmes IH, Ruck BJ. Virus particles in epithelial cells of duodenal mucosa from children with acute non-bacterial gastroenteritis. Lancet 1973;2:1281–3.

9. Appleton H, Higgins PG. Letter: viruses and gastroenteritis in infants. Lancet 1975;1:1297.

10. Madeley CR, Cosgrove BP. Letter: 28 nm particles in faeces in infantile gastroenteritis. Lancet 1975;2:451–2.

11. Flewett TH, Bryden AS, Davies H, Morris CA. Epidemic viral enteritis in a long-stay children's ward. Lancet 1975; 1:4–5.

12. Madeley CR, Cosgrove BP. Letter: caliciviruses in man. Lancet 1976;1:199–200.

13. Kilgore PE, Glass RI. Viral gastroenteritis. In: Richman DD, Whitley RJ, Hayden FG, editors. Clinical virology. Washington: ASM Press; 2002. p. 45–57.

14. Koopmans MP, Green KY, Ando T, et al. *Caliciviridae.* In: Fauquet CM, Mayo MA, Maniloff J, et al, editors. Virus taxonomy: classification and nomenclature of viruses; eighth report of the International Committee on Taxonomy of Viruses. San Diego: Elsevier Academic Press; 2005. p. 843–51.

15. Oliver SL, Asobayire E, Dastjerdi AM, Bridger JC. Genomic characterization of the unclassified bovine enteric virus Newbury agent-1 (Newbury1) endorses a new genus in the family *Caliciviridae.* Virology 2006;350: 240–50.

16. Katayama K, Shirato-Horikoshi H, Kojima S, et al. Phylogenetic analysis of the complete genome of 18 Norwalk-like viruses. Virology 2002;299:225–39.

17. Jiang X, Wang M, Graham DY, Estes MK. Expression, self-assembly, and antigenicity of the Norwalk virus capsid protein. J Virol 1992;66:6527–32.

18. Green KY, Lew JF, Jiang X, et al. Comparison of the reactivities of baculovirus-expressed recombinant Norwalk virus capsid antigen with those of the native Norwalk virus antigen in serologic assays and some epidemiologic observations. J Clin Microbiol 1993;31: 2185–91.

19. Liu BL, Clarke IN, Caul EO, Lambden PR. Human enteric caliciviruses have a unique genome structure and are distinct from the Norwalk-like viruses. Arch Virol 1995; 140:1345–56.

20. Atmar RL, Estes MK. Diagnosis of noncultivatable gastroenteritis viruses, the human caliciviruses. Clin Microbiol Rev 2001;14:15–37.

21. Zheng DP, Ando T, Fankhauser RL, et al. Norovirus classification and proposed strain nomenclature. Virology 2006;346:312–23.

22. Farkas T, Zhong WM, Jing Y, et al. Genetic diversity among sapoviruses. Arch Virol 2004;149:1309–23.

23. Mounts AW, Ando T, Koopmans M, et al. Cold weather seasonality of gastroenteritis associated with Norwalk-like viruses. J Infect Dis 2000;181 Suppl 2:S284–7.

24. Atmar RL, Estes MK. The epidemiologic and clinical importance of norovirus infection. Gastroenterol Clin N Am 2006;35:275–90.

25. Blanton LH, Adams SM, Beard RS, et al. Molecular and epidemiologic trends of caliciviruses associated with outbreaks of acute gastroenteritis in the United States, 2000–2004. J Infect Dis 2006;193:413–21.

26. Lopman BA, Reacher MH, van Duijnhoven Y, et al. Viral gastroenteritis outbreaks in Europe, 1995–2000. Emerg Infect Dis 2003;9:90–6.

27. de Wit MA, Koopmans MP, Kortbeek LM, et al. Sensor, a population-based cohort study on gastroenteritis in the Netherlands: incidence and etiology. Am J Epidemiol 2001;154:666–74.

28. Wheeler JG, Sethi D, Cowden JM, et al. Study of infectious intestinal disease in England: rates in the community, presenting to general practice, and reported to national surveillance. The Infectious Intestinal Disease Study Executive. BMJ 1999;318:1046–50.

29. Lopman BA, Brown DW, Koopmans M. Human caliciviruses in Europe. J Clin Virol 2002;24:137–60.

30. Chiba S, Nakata S, Numata-Kinoshita K, Honma S. Sapporo virus: history and recent findings. J Infect Dis 2000;181 Suppl 2:S303–8.

31. Gallimore CI, Iturriza-Gomara M, Lewis D, et al. Characterization of sapoviruses collected in the United Kingdom from 1989 to 2004. J Med Virol 2006;78:673–82.

32. Chadwick PR, McCann R. Transmission of a small round structured virus by vomiting during a hospital outbreak of gastroenteritis. J Hosp Infect 1994;26:251–9.

33. Schwab KJ, Estes MK, Atmar RL. Norwalk and other human caliciviruses: molecular characterization, epidemiology, and pathogenesis. In: Cary JW, Linz JE, Bhatnagar D, editors. Microbial foodborne diseases: mechanisms of pathogenicity and toxin-synthesis. Lancaster: Technomic Publishing Co., Inc.; 2000. p. 460–93.

34. Gray JJ, Green J, Cunliffe C, et al. Mixed genogroup SRSV infections among a party of canoeists exposed to contaminated recreational water. J Med Virol 1997;52: 425–9.

35. Becker KM, Moe CL, Southwick KL, MacCormack JN. Transmission of Norwalk virus during football game. N Engl J Med 2000;343:1223–7.

36. Cheesbrough JS, Green J, Gallimore CI, et al. Widespread environmental contamination with Norwalk-like viruses (NLV) detected in a prolonged hotel outbreak of gastroenteritis. Epidemiol Infect 2000;125:93–8.

37. Widdowson MA, Cramer EH, Hadley L, et al. Outbreaks of acute gastroenteritis on cruise ships and on land: identification of a predominant circulating strain of norovirus—United States, 2002. J Infect Dis 2004;190: 27–36.

38. Isakbaeva ET, Widdowson MA, Beard RS, et al. Norovirus transmission on cruise ship. Emerg Infect Dis 2005;11: 154–8.

39. Graham DY, Jiang X, Tanaka T, et al. Norwalk virus infection of volunteers: new insights based on improved assays. J Infect Dis 1994;170:34–43.

40. Parrino TA, Schreiber DS, Trier JS, et al. Clinical immunity in acute gastroenteritis caused by Norwalk agent. N Engl J Med 1977;297:86–9.

41. Nakata S, Chiba S, Terashima H, et al. Humoral immunity in infants with gastroenteritis caused by human calicivirus. J Infect Dis 1985;152:274–9.

42. Ryder RW, Singh N, Reeves WC, et al. Evidence of immunity induced by naturally acquired rotavirus and Norwalk virus infection on two remote Panamanian islands. J Infect Dis 1985;151:99–105.

43. Lindesmith L, Moe C, Marionneau S, et al. Human susceptibility and resistance to Norwalk virus infection. Nat Med 2003;9:548–53.

44. Hutson AM, Airaud F, LePendu J, et al. Norwalk virus infection associates with secretor status genotyped from sera. J Med Virol 2005;77:116–20.

45. Thorven M, Grahn A, Hedlund KO, et al. A homozygous nonsense mutation (428G-->A) in the human secretor (FUT2) gene provides resistance to symptomatic norovirus (GGII) infections. J Virol 2005;79:15351–5.

46. Kitamoto N, Tanaka T, Natori K, et al. Cross-reactivity among several recombinant calicivirus virus-like particles (VLPs) with monoclonal antibodies obtained from mice immunized orally with one type of VLP. J Clin Microbiol 2002;40:2459–65.

47. Parker TD, Kitamoto N, Tanaka T, et al. Identification of Genogroup I and Genogroup II broadly reactive epitopes on the norovirus capsid. J Virol 2005;79:7402–9.

48. Burton-MacLeod JA, Kane EM, Beard RS, et al. Evaluation and comparison of two commercial enzyme-linked immunosorbent assay kits for detection of antigenically diverse human noroviruses in stool samples. J Clin Microbiol 2004;42:2587–95.

49. Richards AF, Lopman B, Gunn A, et al. Evaluation of a commercial ELISA for detecting Norwalk-like virus antigen in faeces. J Clin Virol 2003;26:109–15.

50. Gonzalez GG, Liprandi F, Ludert JE. Evaluation of a commercial enzyme immunoassay for the detection of norovirus antigen in fecal samples from children with sporadic acute gastroenteritis. J Virol Methods 2006;136: 289–91.

51. Estes MK, Ball JM, Guerrero RA, et al. Norwalk virus vaccines: challenges and progress. J Infect Dis 2000;181 Suppl 2:S367–73.

52. Estes MK. Rotaviruses and their replication. In: Knipe DM, Howley PM, editors. Fields virology, Vol 2. Philadelphia: Lippincott Williams & Wilkins; 2001. p. 1747–85.

53. Desselberger U, Iturriza-Gomara M, Gray JJ. Rotavirus epidemiology and surveillance. In: Chadwick D, Goode JA, editors. Novartis Foundation Symposium 238. Gastroenteritis viruses. New York: John Wiley & Sons, Inc.; 2001. p. 125–47.

54. Fang ZY, Ye Q, Ho MS, et al. Investigation of an outbreak of adult diarrhea rotavirus in China. J Infect Dis 1989;160: 948–53.

55. Nilsson M, Svenungsson B, Hedlund KO, et al. Incidence and genetic diversity of group C rotavirus among adults. J Infect Dis 2000;182:678–84.

56. Ball JM, Tian P, Zeng CQ, et al. Age-dependent diarrhea induced by a rotaviral nonstructural glycoprotein. Science 1996;272:101–4.

57. Mavromichalis J, Evans N, McNeish AS, et al. Intestinal damage in rotavirus and adenovirus gastroenteritis assessed by d-xylose malabsorption. Arch Dis Child 1977;52:589–91.

58. Hyams JS, Krause PJ, Gleason PA. Lactose malabsorption following rotavirus infection in young children. J Pediatr 1981;99:916–8.

59. Lundgren O, Peregrin AT, Persson K, et al. Role of the enteric nervous system in the fluid and electrolyte secretion of rotavirus diarrhea. Science 2000;287:491–5.

60. Glass RI, Parashar UD, Bresee JS, et al. Rotavirus vaccines: current prospects and future challenges. Lancet 2006;368: 323–32.

61. Malek MA, Curns AT, Holman RC, et al. Diarrhea- and rotavirus-associated hospitalizations among children less than 5 years of age: United States, 1997 and 2000. Pediatrics 2006;117:1887–92.

62. Hrdy DB. Epidemiology of rotaviral infection in adults. Rev Infect Dis 1987;9:461–9.

63. Marshall J, Botes J, Gorrie G, et al. Rotavirus detection and characterisation in outbreaks of gastroenteritis in aged-care facilities. J Clin Virol 2003;28:331–40.

64. Griffin DD, Fletcher M, Levy ME, et al. Outbreaks of adult gastroenteritis traced to a single genotype of rotavirus. J Infect Dis 2002;185:1502–5.

65. Matson DO, Estes MK. Impact of rotavirus infection at a large pediatric hospital. J Infect Dis 1990;162:598–604.

66. Griffin DD, Kirkwood CD, Parashar UD, et al. Surveillance of rotavirus strains in the United States: identification of unusual strains. The National Rotavirus Strain Surveillance System collaborating laboratories. J Clin Microbiol 2000;38:2784–7.

67. Cascio A, Vizzi E, Alaimo C, Arista S. Rotavirus gastroenteritis in Italian children: can severity of symptoms be related to the infecting virus? Clin Infect Dis 2001;32:1126–32.

68. Jiang B, Dennehy PH, Spangenberger S, et al. First detection of group C rotavirus in fecal specimens of children with diarrhea in the United States. J Infect Dis 1995;172:45–50.

69. Sanchez-Fauquier A, Roman E, Colomina J, et al. First detection of group C rotavirus in children with acute diarrhea in Spain. Arch Virol 2003;148:399–404.

70. Cook SM, Glass RI, Lebaron CW, Ho MS. Global seasonality of rotavirus infections. Bull World Health Organ 1990;68:171–7.

71. Le Guyader F, Haugarreau L, Miossec L, et al. Three-year study to assess human enteric viruses in shellfish. Appl Environ Microbiol 2000;66:3241–8.

72. Ruuska T, Vesikari T. Rotavirus disease in Finnish children: use of numerical scores for clinical severity of diarrhoeal episodes. Scand J Infect Dis 1990;22:259–67.

73. Pang XL, Joensuu J, Vesikari T. Human calicivirus-associated sporadic gastroenteritis in Finnish children less than two years of age followed prospectively during a rotavirus vaccine trial. Pediatr Infect Dis J 1999;18:420–6.

74. Bass DM Greenberg HB. Group A rotaviruses. In: Blaser MJ, Smith PD, Ravdin JI, et al, editors. Infections of the gastrointestinal tract. Philadelphia: Lippincott, Williams and Wilkins; 2002. p. 859–77.

75. Pang XL, Honma S, Nakata S, Vesikari T. Human caliciviruses in acute gastroenteritis of young children in the community. J Infect Dis 2000;181 Suppl 2:S288–94.

76. Bon F, Fascia P, Dauvergne M, et al. Prevalence of group A rotavirus, human calicivirus, astrovirus, and adenovirus type 40 and 41 infections among children with acute gastroenteritis in Dijon, France. J Clin Microbiol 1999;37:3055–8.

77. Velazquez FR, Matson DO, Calva JJ, et al. Rotavirus infections in infants as protection against subsequent infections. N Engl J Med 1996;335:1022–8.

78. Jiang B, Gentsch JR, Glass RI. The role of serum antibodies in the protection against rotavirus disease: an overview. Clin Infect Dis 2002;34:1351–61.

79. Ramachandran M, Gentsch JR, Parashar UD, et al. Detection and characterization of novel rotavirus strains in the United States. J Clin Microbiol 1998;36:3223–9.

80. Taniguchi K, Urasawa T, Morita Y, et al. Direct serotyping of human rotavirus in stools by an enzyme-linked immunosorbent assay using serotype 1-, 2-, 3-, and 4-specific monoclonal antibodies to VP7. J Infect Dis 1987;155:1159–66.

81. Mascarenhas JD, Linhares AC, Bayma AP, et al. Molecular analysis of VP4, VP7, and NSP4 genes of P[6]G2 rotavirus genotype strains recovered from neonates admitted to hospital in Belem, Brazil. J Med Virol 2006;78:281–9.

82. American Academy of Pediatrics. Practice parameter: the management of acute gastroenteritis in young children. Pediatrics 1996;97:424–35.

83. Guarino A, Guandalini S, Albano F, et al. Enteral immunoglobulins for treatment of protracted rotaviral diarrhea. Pediatr Infect Dis J 1991;10:612–4.

84. Murphy TV, Gargiullo PM, Massoudi MS, et al. Intussusception among infants given an oral rotavirus vaccine. N Engl J Med 2001;344:564–72.

85. Matsui SM. Astroviruses. In: Richman DD, Whitley RJ, Hayden FG, editors. Clinical virology. Washington: ASM Press; 2002. p. 1075–86.

86. Bass DM, Qiu S. Proteolytic processing of the astrovirus capsid. J Virol 2000;74:1810–4.

87. Mitchell DK. Astrovirus gastroenteritis. Pediatr Infect Dis J 2002;21:1067–9.

88. Monroe SS, Holmes JL, Belliot GL. Molecular epidemiology of human astroviruses. In: Chadwick D, Goode JA, editors. Novartis Foundation Symposium 238. Gastroenteritis viruses. New York: John Wiley & Sons, Inc.; 2001. p. 237–45.

89. Guix S, Bosch A, Pinto RM. Human astrovirus diagnosis and typing: current and future prospects. Lett Appl Microbiol 2005;41:103–5.

90. Herrmann JE, Hudson RW, Perron-Henry DM, et al. Antigenic characterization of cell-cultivated astrovirus serotypes and development of astrovirus-specific monoclonal antibodies. J Infect Dis 1988;158:182–5.

91. Qiao H, Nilsson M, Abreu ER, et al. Viral diarrhea in children in Beijing, China. J Med Virol 1999;57:390–6.

92. de Wit MA, Koopmans MP, Kortbeek LM, et al. Etiology of gastroenteritis in sentinel general practices in the Netherlands. Clin Infect Dis 2001;33:280–8.

93. Svenungsson B, Lagergren A, Ekwall E, et al. Enteropathogens in adult patients with diarrhea and healthy control subjects: a 1-year prospective study in a Swedish clinic for infectious diseases. Clin Infect Dis 2000; 30:770–8.

94. Espul C, Martinez N, Noel JS, et al. Prevalence and characterization of astroviruses in Argentinean children with acute gastroenteritis. J Med Virol 2004;72:75–82.

95. Grohmann GS, Glass RI, Pereira HG, et al. Enteric viruses and diarrhea in HIV-infected patients. Enteric Opportunistic Infections Working Group. N Engl J Med 1993;329:14–20.

96. Cubitt WD, Mitchell DK, Carter MJ, et al. Application of electronmicroscopy, enzyme immunoassay, and RT-PCR to monitor an outbreak of astrovirus type 1 in a paediatric bone marrow transplant unit. J Med Virol 1999;57:313–21.

97. Kurtz JB, Lee TW. Astroviruses: human and animal. Ciba Found Symp 1987;128:92–107.

98. Bjorkholm M, Celsing F, Runarsson G, Waldenstrom J. Successful intravenous immunoglobulin therapy for severe and persistent astrovirus gastroenteritis after fludarabine treatment in a patient with Waldenstrom's macroglobulinemia. Int J Hematol 1995;62:117–20.

99. Coppo P, Scieux C, Ferchal F, et al. Astrovirus enteritis in a chronic lymphocytic leukemia patient treated with fludarabine monophosphate. Ann Hematol 2000;79:43–5.

100. Lewis DC, Lightfoot NF, Cubitt WD, Wilson SA. Outbreaks of astrovirus type 1 and rotavirus gastroenteritis in a geriatric in-patient population. J Hosp Infect 1989;14:9–14.

101. Belliot G, Laveran H, Monroe SS. Outbreak of gastroenteritis in military recruits associated with serotype 3 astrovirus infection. J Med Virol 1997;51:101–6.

102. Utagawa ET, Nishizawa S, Sekine S, et al. Astrovirus as a cause of gastroenteritis in Japan. J Clin Microbiol 1994;32: 1841–5.

103. Oishi I, Yamazaki K, Kimoto T, et al. A large outbreak of acute gastroenteritis associated with astrovirus among students and teachers in Osaka, Japan. J Infect Dis 1994; 170:439–43.

104. Fankhauser RL, Noel JS, Monroe SS, et al. Molecular epidemiology of "Norwalk-like viruses" in outbreaks of gastroenteritis in the United States. J Infect Dis 1998;178: 1571–8.

105. Bresee JS, Widdowson MA, Monroe SS, Glass RI. Foodborne viral gastroenteritis: challenges and opportunities. Clin Infect Dis 2002;35:748–53.

106. Kurtz JB, Lee TW, Craig JW, Reed SE. Astrovirus infection in volunteers. J Med Virol 1979;3:221–30.

107. Guerrero ML, Noel JS, Mitchell DK, et al. A prospective study of astrovirus diarrhea of infancy in Mexico City. Pediatr Infect Dis J 1998;17:723–7.

108. Jakab F, Peterfai J, Meleg E, et al. Comparison of clinical characteristics between astrovirus and rotavirus infections diagnosed in 1997 to 2002 in Hungary. Acta Paediatr 2005;94:667–71.

109. Jonassen TO, Monceyron C, Lee TW, et al. Detection of all serotypes of human astrovirus by the polymerase chain reaction. J Virol Methods 1995;52:327–34.

110. Brinker JP, Blacklow NR, Herrmann JE. Human astrovirus isolation and propagation in multiple cell lines. Arch Virol 2000;145:1847–56.

111. Willcocks MM, Carter MJ, Laidler FR, Madeley CR. Growth and characterisation of human faecal astrovirus in a continuous cell line. Arch Virol 1990;113:73–81.

112. Mustafa H, Palombo EA, Bishop RF. Improved sensitivity of astrovirus-specific RT-PCR following culture of stool samples in CaCo-2 cells. J Clin Virol 1998;11:103–7.

113. Herrmann JE, Blacklow NR. Enteric adenoviruses. In: Blaser MJ, Smith PD, Ravdin JI, et al, editors. Infections of the gastrointestinal tract. Philadelphia: Lippincott, Williams and Wilkins; 2002. p. 941–8.

114. van der Avoort HG, Wermenbol AG, Zomerdijk TP, et al. Characterization of fastidious adenovirus types 40 and 41 by DNA restriction enzyme analysis and by neutralizing monoclonal antibodies. Virus Res 1989;12:139–57.

115. Adrian T, Wadell G, Hierholzer JC, Wigand R. DNA restriction analysis of adenovirus prototypes 1 to 41. Arch Virol 1986;91:277–90.

116. Ruuskanen O, Meruman O, Akusjarvi G. Adenoviruses. In: Richman DD, Whitley RJ, Hayden FG, editors. Clinical virology. Washington: ASM Press; 2002. p. 515–35.

117. Basu G, Rossouw J, Sebunya TK, et al. Prevalence of rotavirus, adenovirus and astrovirus infection in young children with gastroenteritis in Gaborone, Botswana. East Afr Med J 2003;80:652–5.

118. Liu C, Grillner L, Jonsson K, et al. Identification of viral agents associated with diarrhea in young children during a winter season in Beijing, China. J Clin Virol 2006;35:69–72.

119. Janoff EN, Orenstein JM, Manischewitz JF, Smith PD. Adenovirus colitis in the acquired immunodeficiency syndrome. Gastroenterology 1991;100:976–9.

120. Smith PD, Quinn TC, Strober W, et al. NIH conference. Gastrointestinal infections in AIDS. Ann Intern Med 1992; 116:63–77.

121. Dionisio D, Arista S, Vizzi E, et al. Chronic intestinal infection due to subgenus F type 40 adenovirus in a patient with AIDS. Scand J Infect Dis 1997;29:305–7.

122. Uhnoo I, Olding-Stenkvist E, Kreuger A. Clinical features of acute gastroenteritis associated with rotavirus, enteric adenoviruses, and bacteria. Arch Dis Child 1986;61:732–8.

123. De Jong JC, Bijlsma K, Wermenbol AG, et al. Detection, typing, and subtyping of enteric adenoviruses 40 and 41 from fecal samples and observation of changing incidences of infections with these types and subtypes. J Clin Microbiol 1993;31:1562–9.

124. Takiff HE, Seidlin M, Krause P, et al. Detection of enteric adenoviruses by dot-blot hybridization using a molecularly cloned viral DNA probe. J Med Virol 1985;16:107–18.

125. Xu W, McDonough MC, Erdman DD. Species-specific identification of human adenoviruses by a multiplex PCR assay. J Clin Microbiol 2000;38:4114–20.

126. Kidd AH, Madeley CR. In vitro growth of some fastidious adenoviruses from stool specimens. J Clin Pathol 1981;34:213–6.

127. Wigand R, Baumeister HG, Maass G, et al. Isolation and identification of enteric adenoviruses. J Med Virol 1983;11:233–40.

128. Parashar UD, Li JF, Cama R, et al. Human caliciviruses as a cause of severe gastroenteritis in Peruvian children. J Infect Dis 2004;190:1088–92.

129. Colomba C, De Grazia S, Giammanco GM, et al. Viral gastroenteritis in children hospitalised in Sicily, Italy. Eur J Clin Microbiol Infect Dis 2006;25:570–5.

130. Cama RI, Parashar UD, Taylor DN, et al. Enteropathogens and other factors associated with severe disease in children with acute watery diarrhea in Lima, Peru. J Infect Dis 1999;179:1139–44.

131. Haberberger RL Jr, Mikhail IA, Burans JP, et al. Travelers' diarrhea among United States military personnel during joint American-Egyptian armed forces exercises in Cairo, Egypt. Mil Med 1991;156:27–30.

132. Mattila L, Siitonen A, Kyronseppa H, et al. Seasonal variation in etiology of travelers' diarrhea. Finnish-Moroccan Study Group. J Infect Dis 1992;165:385–8.

133. Petruccelli BP, Murphy GS, Sanchez JL, et al. Treatment of traveler's diarrhea with ciprofloxacin and loperamide. J Infect Dis 1992;165:557–60.

134. Bourgeois AL, Gardiner CH, Thornton SA, et al. Etiology of acute diarrhea among United States military personnel deployed to South America and west Africa. Am J Trop Med Hyg 1993;48:243–8.

135. Sharp TW, Thornton SA, Wallace MR, et al. Diarrheal disease among military personnel during Operation Restore Hope, Somalia, 1992–1993. Am J Trop Med Hyg 1995;52:188–93.

136. Oyofo BA, Soderquist R, Lesmana M, et al. Norwalk-like virus and bacterial pathogens associated with cases of gastroenteritis onboard a US Navy ship. Am J Trop Med Hyg 1999;61:904–8.

137. Steffen R, Collard F, Tornieporth N, et al. Epidemiology, etiology, and impact of traveler's diarrhea in Jamaica. JAMA 1999;281:811–7.

138. Chapin AR, Carpenter CM, Dudley WC, et al. Prevalence of norovirus among visitors from the United States to Mexico and Guatemala who experience traveler's diarrhea. J Clin Microbiol 2005;43:1112–7.

139. Ko G, Garcia C, Jiang ZD, et al. Noroviruses as a cause of traveler's diarrhea among students from the United States visiting Mexico. J Clin Microbiol 2005;43:6126–9.

140. Thornton SA, Sherman SS, Farkas T, et al. Gastroenteritis in US Marines during Operation Iraqi Freedom. Clin Infect Dis 2005;40:519–25.

141. Halperin T, Yavzori M, Amitai A, et al. Molecular analysis of noroviruses involved in acute gastroenteritis outbreaks in military units in Israel, 1999–2004. Eur J Clin Microbiol Infect Dis 2005;24:697–700.

142. Bailey MS, Boos CJ, Vautier G, et al. Gastroenteritis outbreak in British troops, Iraq. Emerg Infect Dis 2005;11:1625–8.

CHAPTER 4

THE PARASITIC PATHOGENS

WILLIAM A. PETRI JR, MD, PhD

CYNTHIA SNIDER, MD, MPH

PABLO C. OKHUYSEN, MD

Diarrhea caused by protozoan parasites is the most common reason for a returning traveler to seek medical attention, accounting for nearly one-third of all physician visits (Figure 1).[1,2] The longer incubation period for parasitic agents and the use of antibiotics for self treatment of diarrhea while traveling are probably responsible for their predominance as a cause of diarrhea in the returning traveler.

The most common enteric protozoa identified in returning travelers are *Giardia lamblia* and *Entamoeba histolytica*. Much less frequent are infections due to Cryptosporidia, Cyclospora, Microsporidiae, and Isospora. The risk factors for acquisition of intestinal parasites have not been well defined. In general, length of stay, hygiene, and level of development in the host country have been thought to be associated with the acquisition of intestinal protozoa.[3] For example, in studies done in Nepal, giardiasis was most commonly diagnosed in travelers with diarrhea lasting more than 2 weeks than in those with diarrhea of less than 2 weeks duration.[4] Of course travel is not required to acquire infection because the enteric protozoa are endemic to the US: the three most common intestinal parasites identified as causes of diarrhea in the United States are *Giardia lamblia* (9.5 cases per 100,000 population), *Cryptosporidium parvum* (1.4 cases/100,000 population), and *Entamoeba histolytica* (1.2 cases/100,000 population). The individual parasites are discussed below, in order from the most to least frequent causes of travelers' diarrhea.

Etiology of Acute Diarrhea in Returned Travelers

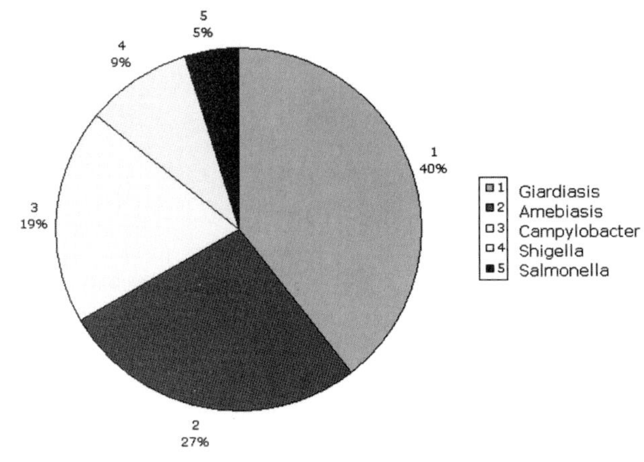

Figure 1 Etiology of acute diarrhea in returned travelers. Data reported by the GeoSentinel Surveillance Network of 30 travel or tropical-medicine clinics on six continents.[1]

Giardia

Giardia lamblia is in the Sarcomastigophora phylum. It is also known as *G. intestinalis* or *G. duodenalis* and can produce infection in humans and a number of animal hosts. In most series, it is the most common parasitic cause of diarrhea in travelers. Molecular analysis of Giardia isolates has shown that these parasites belong to distinct genotypes called assemblages A and B.[5–8] the genome is nearly complete for A1 and is estimated to be 12 Mb with 9,600 genes. A large case-control study in Dhaka Bangladesh demonstrated that assemblage A was more commonly associated with diarrhea.[8]

Giardiasis is highly infectious: ingestion of as few as 10 to 25 cysts produces disease in human volunteers. Giardiasis occurs in all parts of the world and is a common cause of water borne outbreaks of diarrhea in the United States. In some urban slums in developing countries rates of giardia infection approach 100%.[9] Modes of transmission include fecal-oral, waterborne, and foodborne.[10] Person to person spread of giardia infection is documented in children and employees in day care centers, in men who have sex with men, and in residents of institutions for the mentally handicapped. Water borne outbreaks have occurred in the Rocky Mountain areas of the United States and Canada and the Northwestern and Northeastern United States. Proper filtration of surface water supplies is the most important factor in prevention of these outbreaks because the cysts of giardia are not completely inactivated by the flocculation, sedimentation, and chlorination steps of water purification. The risk of acquiring giardia may vary based on the region visited: a study done on German travelers demonstrated it to be more likely acquired during travel to the Indian subcontinent and Africa than to Asia or Latin America.[11]

After ingestion of the cyst, excystation follows ingestion, with the trophozoites multiplying in the small bowel (Figure 2). Giardia trophozoites adhere to the intestinal mucosal via the ventral disk as well as parasite lectins.[10,12] While Giardia is not invasive, it causes damage to the microvillus layer and results in a lymphocytic infiltration of the lamina propria. Also, there is an association of Giardia infection with overgrowth of bacteria in the small intestines. Malabsorption of protein, D-xylose, and fat-soluble vitamins as well as disaccharidase deficiency occurs in some patients with giardiasis. Trophozoites encyst in the bowel lumen, with an encystation-specific secretory vesicle system implicated in synthesis of the cyst wall.

Worldwide, most patients infected with Giardia are asymptomatic.[10,12] When present, clinical symptoms follow an incubation period of 1 to 3 weeks (Table 1).

Table 1. Symptoms and Signs of Giardiasis

Prolonged diarrhea	100%
Fatigue	97%
Abdominal cramps	83%
Bloating	79%
Malodorous stool	79%
Flatulence	76%
Weight loss	59%
Fever	21%
Vomiting	17%

The most notable feature of the illness is the prolonged nature of the diarrhea and the malabsorption that may be present. In most cases, the stools are described as foul smelling and greasy. Accompanying symptoms may include malaise, flatulence, cramping, bloating, nausea, anorexia, and weight loss. Less common symptoms include vomiting, fever, and urticaria. Symptoms often last for over 10 days and may continue beyond 1 month.

Diagnosis of giardiasis is best accomplished by antigen detection or real-time polymerage chain reaction (PCR) testing of stool samples. The classical ova and parasite microscopic exam is both insensitive and nonspecific.[10,13] Immunofluorescent and enzyme-linked immunosorbent assay (ELISA) techniques are commercially available.[14] Real-time PCR offers the advantage of being able to distinguish between giardia genotyopes.[8]

Nitroimidazoles such as multiple doses of metronidazole or a single dose of tinidazole are the main treatments of choice for giardiasis (Table 2).[10,12,13] Isolates with decreased susceptibility to metronidazole

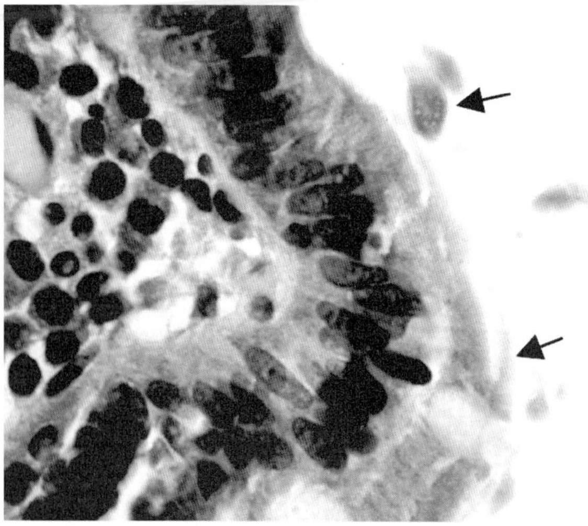

Figure 2 *Giardia lamblia* trophozoites in the human small intestine. These trophozoites (arrows) are adherent to human small intestinal epithelial cells and in the intestinal lumen. Reprinted with permission from Petri WA Jr.[20]

Table 2. Treatment of Intestinal Enteric Protozoa Infections

Infection	Drug of Choice	Alternatives
Amebiasis		
Asymptomatic	Paromomycin	Iodoquinol or Diloxanide furoate
Invasive Disease[1]	Tinidazole	Metronidazole
Cryptosporidiosis	Nitazoxanide[2]	
Cyclosporiasis	Trimethoprim-sulfamethoxazole	
Giardiasis	Tinidazole	Metronidazole, nitazoxanide, paromomycin, furazolidone, quinacrine
Isosporiasis	Trimethoprim-sulfamethoxazole	Pyrimethamine
Microsporidiosis		
E. intestinalis	Albendazole	
E. bieneusi	Fumagillin	

[1]After completion of therapy, the patient should be additionally treated with paromomycin to eradicate intestinal lumen infection to prevent relapse.
[2]Not shown to be effective in HIV-infected patients.

have been described: in 5 out of 6 patients with metronidazole-resistant giardiasis, a combination regimen of quinacrine and metronidazole was effective.[12,15] Quinacrine is another effective treatment; however, it is no longer marketed in much of the world and may not be manufactured.[12] Nitazoxanide is a broad-spectrum antiparasitic agent that is currently licensed in many parts of the world, including the US. In controlled trials, it was as effective as metronidazole in the treatment of giardiasis.[16,17] It may also be effective in metronidazole-resistant cases.[18,19] Albendazole, furazolidone, and paromomycin are alternative agents.[19,20] New targets may be identified as the parasite's genome is analyzed.[21]

Prevention of water borne outbreaks requires proper flocculation, sedimentation, filtration, and chlorination of water supplies. Filtration is the single most important step for removal of the chlorine-resistant giardia cysts from community water supplies. Good personal hygiene is required to prevent transmission by food handlers and in day care centers. For backpackers and campers, all surface water should be considered to be contaminated with giardia. Approaches to field water purification include bringing the water to a boil for 1 minute, filtration through a 2 µm filter, or treatment for 30 minutes with halazone (5 tablets/liter for 30 minutes), Globaline (tetraglycine hydroperiodide, 1 tablet per quart), or saturated crystalline iodine (12.5 mL/liter for 30 minutes). Halazone or iodine treatment of water is less effective at 3°C than at 20°C.

Entamoeba

Entamoeba histolytica is in the Sarcomastigophora phylum. It was responsible for one-third of cases of diarrhea seen in returning travelers in the GeoSentinel Surveillance Nework.[1] *Entamoeba histolytica* has been reclassified into three species that are morphologically identical: *E. histolytica*, which is the cause of amebic diarrhea, colitis, and liver abscess, and E. dispar and E. moshkovskii, which are common colonizers of humans but do not cause disease.[22–24] A prototype strain of *E. histolytica* has been sequenced with a genome size of 23.7 Mb and approximately 7,000 genes. The partial sequence of *E. dispar* shows it to be 95% identical to *E. histolytica*. The species can be differentiated by monoclonal antibodies and PCR.[25,26] The infectious cyst form of the parasite is resistant to chlorine, and outbreaks due to contaminated municipal water supplies have occurred.[27] Major routes of transmission are through contaminated water and food or by direct fecal–oral contact. Individuals at highest risk for infection include children in, and travelers to the developing world, immigrants or migrant workers, and individuals housed in mental institutions.[22]

Infection is initiated by ingestion of the cyst form of the parasite. In the intestine, the invasive trophozoite emerges from the cyst and can then either colonize the intestine and form new cysts, or invade and cause amebic diarrhea and/or colitis (Table 3). Invasive infection of the colon can then spread hematogenously to other organs such as the liver and brain. The parasite has a unique transcriptional profile when residing in the intestine.[28] The determinants of whether infection results in colonization or disease include the parasite (not every genotype is equally invasive), host (certain human leukogite antigen (HLA) class II alleles influence resistance), and environment (malnutrition is associated with susceptibility).[29–32] Invasion into the intestine requires contact-dependent killing of host cells by the parasite, a process that is initiated by the *E. histolytica* Gal/GalNAc adherence lectin.[33] Ingestion of the host cell corpse follows killing and is mediated in part by a family of transmembrane kinases discovered by the genome project.[34–37] Host leukocytes, neutrophils, and macrophages may also play a role in cell damage when they are lysed by the amebae and release their toxic products. Ulcerative lesions in the intestinal mucosa and liver abscesses are characterized by a moderate inflammatory response. Advanced lesions have necrotic centers with amebae concentrated at the outer zone of normal tissue.[22]

The immune response to intestinal infection in the mouse model is an IL-10 mediated and neutrophil-dependent innate immune response, likely acting at the level of the intestinal epithelium and resulting in rapid expulsion of the parasite.[38,39] Chronic amebic colitis in the murine model is characterized by a CD4+ T cell response that is disease-exacerbating and associated with the production of Th2-phenoytpe cytokines.[40] Immune responses associated with protection from re-infection in children include mucosal immunoglobalin A (IgA)

Table 3. Clinical Manifestations of Entamoeba Histolytica Infection

Asymptomatic colonization Intestinal amebiasis and its complications
Amebic colitis
Ameboma
Toxic megacolon
Peritonitis
Cutaneous amebiasis
Extraintestinal amebiasis
Amebic liver abscess
Splenic abscess
Brain abscess
Empyema
Pericarditis

against the Gal/GalNAc lectin[32,41] and systemic interferon gamma production by peripheral blood mononuclear cells.[42] The presence of protective immunity and promise for a vaccine is borne out in the mouse model, where immunization with the Gal/GalNAc lectin prevents amebic intestinal infection and invasion.[43]

The manifestations of human infection by *E. histolytica* include colonization and intestinal and extraintestinal disease. Prospective observation of a cohort of Bangladeshi children has shown that amebic diarrhea without blood or mucus is three times more common than overt amebic dysentery, with an incidence of 6% per child per year (Table 4).[32] One therefore must consider amebiasis as part of the differential diagnosis of diarrhea and not just dysentery. Amebic colitis is characterized by ulcerations of the colonic mucosa with pathognomonic (but not always observed) flask-shaped abscesses (Figures 3 and 4). Another form of colonic amebiasis is an ameboma, which is a granulomatous inflammatory mass in the colon lumen that can mimic colonic adenocarcinoma by radiologic appearance.[22] Children and adults can be intestinally infected for months to years.[32,44] Some forms of chronic amebic colitis are difficult to distinguish from inflammatory bowel disease (IBD); thus, it is important to obtain amebic serology and fecal antigen detection prior to initiating therapy for IBD, especially in an individual with a history of travel or residence in the developing world.

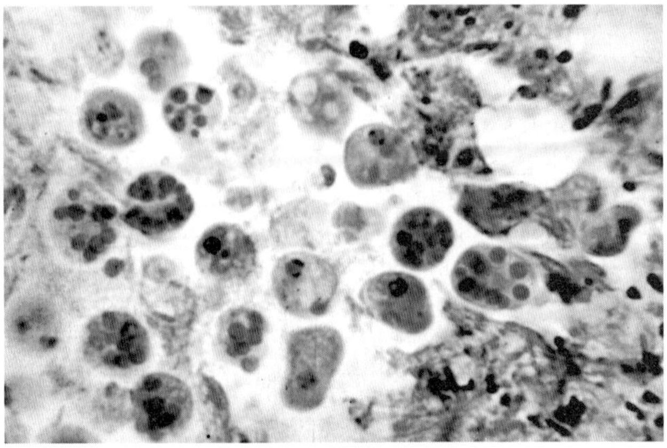

Figure 4 *Entamoeba histolytica* trophozoites in a human colonic ulcer. Note the numerous amebae, some containing phagocytosed erythrocytes, surrounded by extensive tissue destruction. Reprinted with permission from Petri WA Jr.[20]

Table 4 Amebic Diarrhea or Dysentery: Symptoms, Signs and Diagnosis

Finding	Proportion of patients
History of immigration from or travel to area of endemicity	Most
Gradual onset, symptoms >1 week	Most
Diarrhea	94%–100%
Heme-positive stools	25%
Abdominal pain	12%–80%
Weight loss	44%
Fever > 38°C	10%
Positive Entamoeba histolytica–specific stool antigen test	87%
Positive amebic serology	70%
Positive colonoscopic biopsies	80%

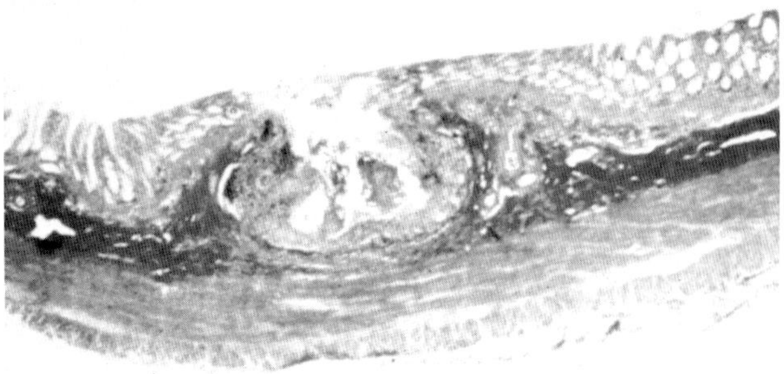

Figure 3 Flask shaped colonic ulcer due to *Entamoeba histolytica*. From the collection of the late Harrison Juniper.

Amebic liver abscess can present months after travel to an endemic area, likely due to the long latency of the parasite in the intestine (Table 5).[45,46] Liver abscess is in 90% of cases a disease of young men, with children or women uncommonly affected. Diarrhea or dysentery is not present in two-thirds of patients at the time of diagnosis of liver abscess.[46] Most patients complain of 2 to 4 weeks of fever, cough, and constant dull right upper quadrant or epigastric abdominal pain. Involvement of the diaphragm may lead to right-sided pleurisy or referred shoulder pain. On physical exam hepatomegaly and tenderness over the liver is a typical finding. Infective trophozoites can migrate hematogenously to either lobe of the liver, causing abscess formation, abdominal pain, jaundice, and fever (Figures 5 and 6). Adjacent anatomical structures, such as the pulmonary parenchyma, peritoneum, and pericardium can become involved.[46–48] Amebae can also rarely disseminate to the brain, with amebic brain abscess seen mostly in patients with coexisting amebic liver abscess.[49] Indications for surgical drainage of an amebic abscess include large dimensions, impending rupture, left lobe location, or lack of therapeutic response.

The diagnosis of intestinal amebic infection is best accomplished with a combination of amebic serology plus antigen or real-time PCR fecal detection of *E.*

Table 5 Pyogenic versus Amebic Liver Abscess

	Pyogenic Abscess	Amebic Abscess
Male/female ratio	1/1	10/1
Age, years	> 50	20–40
Aspirate or blood cultures (+) bacteria	Positive	Negative[1]
Biliary disease	Yes	No
Diabetes mellitus	Yes	No
Immigrant from or traveler to developing world[2]	No	Yes

[1]In some cases an amebic liver abscess can be co-infected with bacteria, potentially leading to diagnostic confusion.
[2]The incubation period can be protracted (months or even years) due to prolonged latent infection.

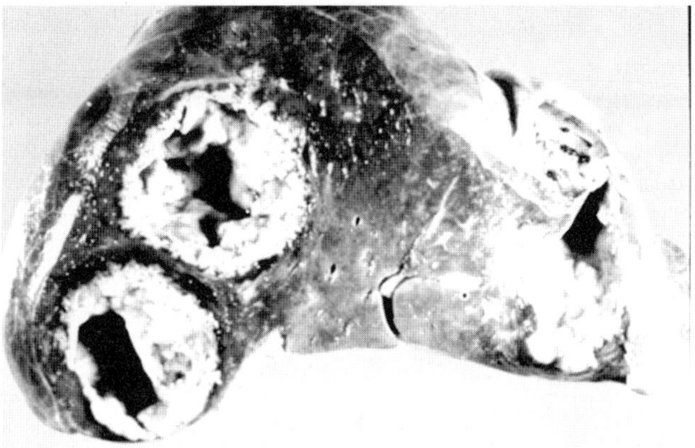

Figure 5 Amebic liver abscess. There are two abscesses in the right lobe and one abscess in the left lobe. Reprinted with permission from Haque R et al.[22]

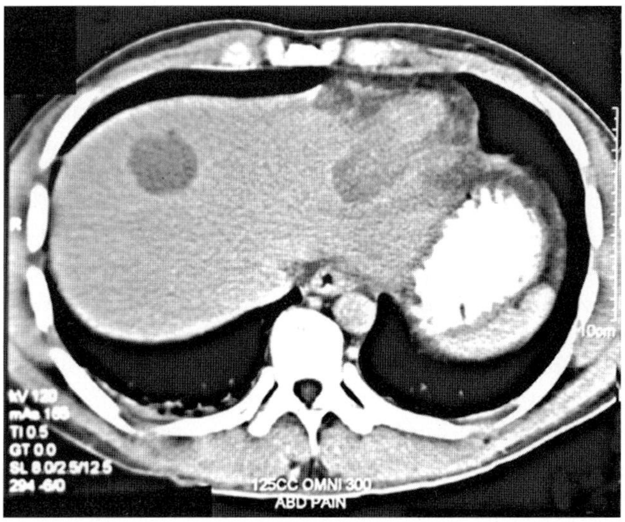

Figure 6 Abdominal computed tomography in a patient with amebic liver abscess. There is one abscess in the right lobe and one abscess in the left lobe. Reprinted with permission from Haque R et al.[22]

histolytica.[25,26] This combination approach gives close to 100% sensitivity. The traditional stool ova and parasite exam should not be used for diagnosis because it is notoriously nonspecific, insensitive, and incapable of distinguishing *E. histolytica* from *E. dispar* or *E. moshkovskii.*[50] Colonoscopy can be helpful in difficult cases, with the rare amebae in intestinal ulcers best visualized with immunoperoxidase or Periodic acid–Schiff (PAS) stains (Figure 7).[51]

Ultrasound, computer tomography, and magnetic resonance imaging are all sensitive tests for hepatic abscess, but none are capable of distinguishing an amebic from a bacterial abscess (see Figure 6). The diagnosis of amebic liver abscess in a patient with a space-occupying lesion of the liver is best accomplished by a combination of amebic serology and antigen detection because neither test alone is completely sensitive. For example serum antiamebic antibodies were detected in only half of amebic liver abscess patients at first presentation.[25] Amebic antigen should be searched for in stool, abscess pus, and serum: amebic antigen was detected in 96% (22/23) of sera, 42% (3/7) stools, and 100% (3/3) of liver abscess aspirates tested in one study prior to patient treatment with metronidazole.[25] Metronidazole treatment quickly rendered these specimens negative.

Treatment of luminal noninvasive amebiasis should be with paromomycin, or with the alternative agents diloxanide or iodoquinol (see Table 2).[19,52] Invasive disease, such as amebic dysentery and liver abscess, should be treated with metronidazole or tinidazole, followed by a luminal agent such as diloxanide or paromomycin to prevent future invasion with any remaining cysts. A stool *E. histolytica* antigen or PCR test at the completion of therapy as a test of cure is advisable.

Cryptosporidium

Cryptosporidia is in the Apicomplexa phylum. They are protozoan parasites that preferentially infect the small bowel of many animal species including humans (Figure 8).[53,54]

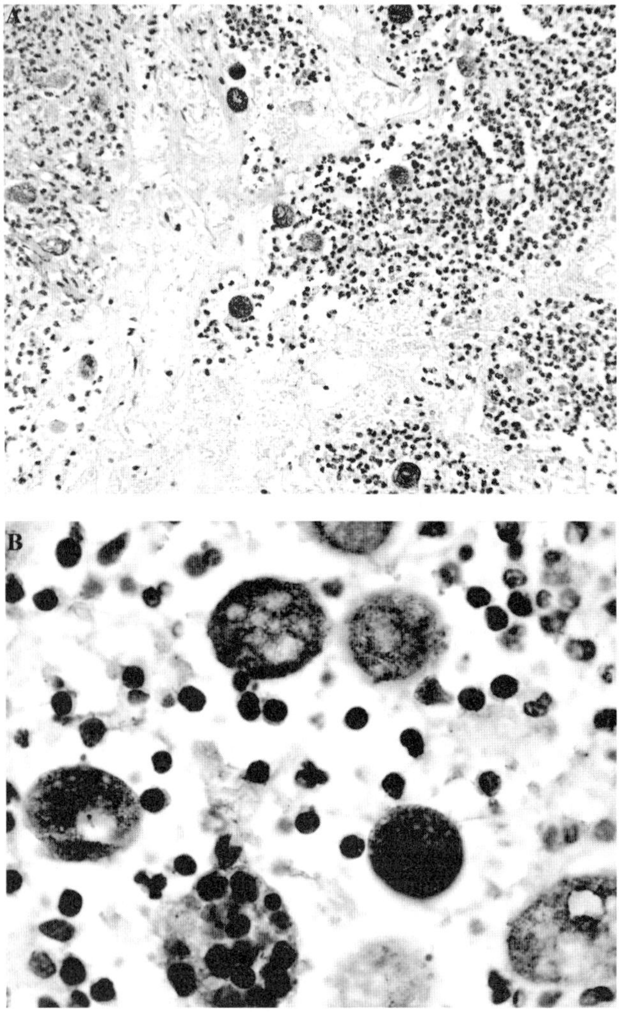

Figure 7 Immunoperoxidase stain for *Entamoeba histolytica* trophozoites in human intestine. *A*, Low power; *B*, high power. Note in (B) ameba with multiple ingested host cells. Tissue sections stained with a monoclonal antibody against the *E. histolytica* Gal/GalNAc lectin. Courtesy of Dr. James S. McCarthy.

Oocysts are resistant to water chlorination and can survive in aquatic environments for prolonged periods of time,[55] At least two distinct transmission cycles occur in nature and are related to specific species. Infections with *C. hominis* demonstrate preference for causing infection in humans while *C. parvum* favors a zoonotic transmission.[56–58] In addition, human infection can be caused by C. meleagridis and rarely other species of Cryptosporidia. C. hominis and C. parvum have completed genome sequences, with essentially every gene present in both. Genome size is 9.1 Mb with approximately 3,800 genes. Energy metabolism is from glycolysis and few biosynthetic pathways are present, with most metabolites acquired via a series of transporters, perhaps explaining the current difficulties in finding effective therapies for cryptosporidia.[59,60]

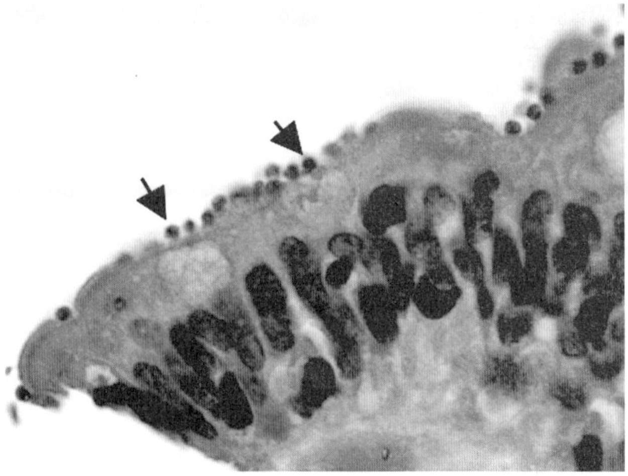

Figure 8 *Cryptosporidium parvum* intracellular replication within human small intestinal epithelial cells (arrows). Reprinted with permission from Petri WA Jr.[20]

Cryptosporidia are transmitted via the fecal–oral route.[61] Risk factors for transmission include contact with farm animals or pets, drinking untreated water, ingestion of contaminated food, and contact with patients or day care centers.[62–64] As few as 10 oocysts can cause infection in healthy volunteers and perhaps even fewer in immunocompromised individuals.[65] Healthy individuals can develop specific antibody responses after infection, and those with preexisting antibodies to *C. parvum* are less susceptible to lower innocula.[66,67] However, healthy adults may experience repeated infections.[68]

Few studies have been performed to assess the prevalence of cryptosporidiosis in long-term travelers. Cohort studies have documented extremely high infection rates among children in developing countries, with seroconversion in virtually all children by age 5.[69–71] There are fewer data on the epidemiology in travelers, but cryptosporidiosis may occur in long-term travelers. For example, a survey of Peace Corps volunteers residing in West Africa demonstrated 13.6% increases in seroprevalence over a 2-year period of time.[72]

Cryptosporidium multiplies in the intestinal microvillus layer. Infection causes villous atrophy, crypt hyperplasia, and infiltration of lymphocytes, neutrophils, plasma cells, and macrophages into the lamina propria.[73] In immunocompromised patients, Cryptosporidium may be found in the entire gastrointestinal tract and within the epithelial cells of the biliary tree, the pancreatic duct, and the airways.[74] Infection causes increases in intestinal permeability and chloride secretion, which are thought to result from the host inflammatory response.[75,76] Control of infection depends on the host cellular immune response and the production of cytokines such as interferon gamma. Individuals with immunoglobulin A (IgA) deficiencies can develop chronic disease.[77]

Symptoms of cryptosporidial infection include watery stools, fatigue, abdominal pain, general malaise, and in 20% of cases, nausea and vomiting. Low-grade fever can also occur. Many patients will have a relapsing course. In human immunodeficiency virus (HIV)-infected individuals, when CD4 (T cells) counts are > 200/mL3, *C. parvum* infection resolves spontaneously. In the later stages of HIV disease (CD4 counts < 100/mL3), chronic infection can lead to dehydration, malnutrition, wasting, and death.[78] Patients with HIV should exert particular caution when traveling abroad to prevent cryptosporidiosis. Specifically, they should avoid drinking water that has not been boiled or purified and that is not available in sealed containers.

Diagnosis depends on the identification of oocysts in stool. The organisms are 4 to 6 μm in diameter, approximately the size of yeast found in normal stool. Staining of a fresh fecal specimen with a modified acid-fast stain aids in the diagnosis but the level of sensitivity is low. Commercially available ELISAs to detect Cryptosporidia antigens in stool are sensitive and specific.[79] The newest advance in diagnosis is real-time PCR to detect parasite deoxyribonucleic acid (DNA) in stool; this approach offers sensitive Cryptosporidia species-specific diagnosis and the capability of multiplex formats to detect multiple parasites simultaneously from a single sample (Figure 9).[80,81]

Treatment in the immunocompetent host is primarily supportive because cryptosporidiosis is self limited. In one randomized, placebo-controlled trial of normal children and adults, nitazoxanide decreased the duration of diarrhea and oocysts shedding (see Table 2).[82] The dose used in the trial was 500 mg twice a day for 3 days, with doses of 200 mg and 100 mg twice a day in children. A randomized trial in HIV patients with cryptosporidiosis, conducted in Mexico, showed improvement with treatment of patients having CD4 cell counts above (but not in those with below) 50/mL.[83] Nitazoxanide is approved for use in some countries and has recently been licensed in the United States by the manufacturer, Romark Laboratories.

A small study using bovine anti-Cryptosporidium immunoglobulin in healthy adults exposed to *C. parvum* demonstrated a decrease in parasite excretion but no significant decrease in diarrhea.[84] Few options exist for acquired immune deficiency syndrome (AIDS) patients that fail highly active antiretroviral therapy. Paromomycin was not shown to be more effective than placebo for the treatment of symptomatic cryptosporidial enteritis.[85]

Treatment of water and avoiding contaminated food are the main methods for prevention of cryptosporidiosis. Specifically, travelers should avoid drinking water that has not been boiled or filtered. Personal-use water filters should be capable of removing particles of 1 mm in diameter.[86] Patients with HIV should exert particular caution when traveling abroad to prevent contracting the disease.

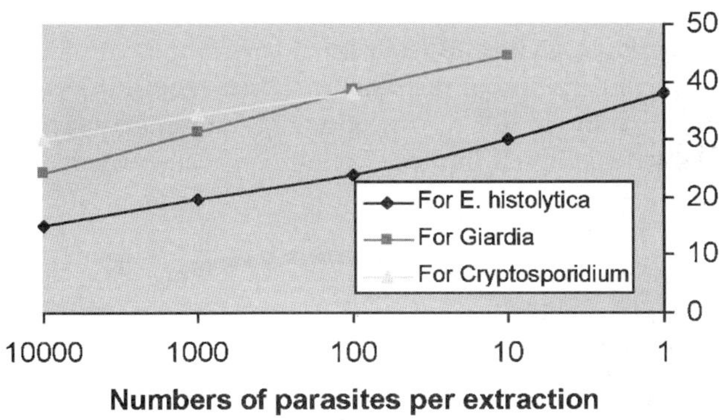

Figure 9 Analytical sensitivity of the multiplex real-time PCR assay for detection of *E. histolytica, G. intestinalis,* and *Cryptosporidium* spp. Reprinted with permission from Haque R et al.[81]

Cyclospora

Cyclospora is in the Apicomplexa phylum. Unlike Cryptosporidium, which is readily infectious after excretion, *Cyclospora cayetanensis* requires sporulation in the environment before becoming infectious. This coccidian parasite has been found in developing countries, particularly in Nepal and Peru, and was previously referred to as a cyanobacteria-like body. It appears that humans are the only reservoir for infection because extensive evaluation of domestic animals has failed to reveal carriage in endemic regions.[87] However, it is genetically related to Eimeria species (a common cause of infection in avian species), and it is possible that a yet unidentified avian reservoir exists. The vehicles of transmission are most likely contaminated water and food.[88] Cases in developed countries have been acquired mostly during outbreaks that have been related to imported raspberries, or diagnosed in travelers returning from developing nations.[89,90]

Studies in developing countries like Peru and Haiti have demonstrated a high frequency of asymptomatic excretion in indigenous populations. After an incubation period of approximately 7 days (range 2 to 11 days), diarrhea occurs accompanied by cramping, abdominal pain, nausea, vomiting, fatigue, and occasionally, fever. In general, infection is self limited in otherwise healthy adults, but diarrhea can be prolonged and appears to be more severe than that experienced with Cryptosporidium if untreated. In the immunocompromised host, infection with Cyclospora may also result in chronic diarrhea if left untreated and requires chronic suppressive therapy in some cases, such as AIDS.

Cyclospora should be considered the likely cause of persistent or recurrent diarrhea among international travelers to Nepal in the spring or summer months. It is also endemic and of potential importance to travelers to other areas of the world and should be considered because of the chronicity of symptoms.

Cyclospora and Cryptosporidium show staining similarity, but Cyclospora oocysts are twice as large (8 to 10 μm versus 3 to 5 μm). It can be identified in fecal samples by autofluorescence at 330 to 380 nm under ultraviolet microscopy.[91] A 10-day course of therapy with combined trimethoprim (TMP) and sulfamethoxazole (SMX) results in clinical improvement and eradication of this parasite (see Table 2).

Isospora

Isospora belli is in the Apicomplexa phylum. It produces large, oval-shaped oocysts that sporulate outside the body. This process takes 2 to 3 days before the oocysts become infectious. The organism is endemic in tropical and subtropical environments, is associated with outbreaks of diarrheal disease, and has also been implicated in travelers' diarrhea. I. belli infection is confined to humans and perhaps to dogs. No other animal reservoir has been identified. Transmission is postulated to be associated with contaminated water; however, this has not been proven. The watery diarrhea caused by this organism suggests an enterotoxin, but no evidence for this molecule exists to date. The clinical features of I. belli infection in immunocompetent hosts are abdominal pain, cramping, nausea, and watery diarrhea, occasionally with eosinophilia. In immunodeficient hosts, prolonged diarrhea with malnutrition may occur. Several case reports have documented dissemination to the mesenteric lymph nodes or acalculous cholecystitis in advanced HIV infection.

Oocysts can be visualized with an acid-fast stain. Symptomatic infection responds to treatment with combined TMP–SMX. In AIDS patients with recurrent disease, secondary prophylaxis with TMP–SMX and pyrimethamine–sulfadoxine prevents relapses (see Table 2).

Microsporidia

Microsporidia are a phylum of species that are small obligate intracellular parasites that infect vertebrate and invertebrate hosts. Only a few of the over 1,000 species known to belong in this phylum have been identified as pathogenic agents for humans. Microsporidia species have been sporadically reported as a cause of chronic diarrhea in both otherwise healthy adults and HIV-infected patients after travel and should be a consideration in cases of chronic diarrhea. Members of the microsporidia include *Enterocytozoon bieneusi, Encephalitozoon cuniculi, Brachiola algerae, Encephalitozoon hellem,* and *Encephalitozoon intestinalis.* The *Encephalitozoon cuniculi* genome has been sequenced and is extraordinarily small, containing 2.5 mb and approximately 2,000 genes. The lack of many metabolic pathways in the organism may explain the current paucity of therapies for microsporidia.

Microsporidia share several common characteristics, including specialized polar tubes that mediate parasite invasion into the epithelium, intracellular asexual reproduction, and the formation of thick-walled spores that are able to survive for months in the environment (Figure 10).[92,93] *E. bieneusi* and *E. intestinalis* can be distinguished morphologically by electron microscopy of small bowel biopsies or by PCR techniques.

Microsporidia may rarely cause travelers' diarrhea in healthy, nonimmunocompromised hosts. The epidemiology and pathogenesis in these cases are uncertain. Both *E. bieneusi* and *E. intestinalis* infections are identified by diarrhea in individuals with CD4 counts less than 100/mL3, and frequently also in asymptomatic carriers. *E. bieneusi* infects the enterocytes of the proximal jejunum and occasionally spreads to the biliary tract. In comparison, *E. intestinalis* is found in enterocytes, macrophages, and fibroblasts and may also disseminate to the mesenteric nodes and kidney.

Free and intracytoplasmic spores can be stained with Giemsa stain, Weber's trichrome stain, or fluorochrome (calcofluor, Uvitex 2B) stains that have affinity for chitin, but identification of the specific species requires electron microscopy or PCR. Infection of immunocompetent individuals is self limited. Preliminary data suggest that

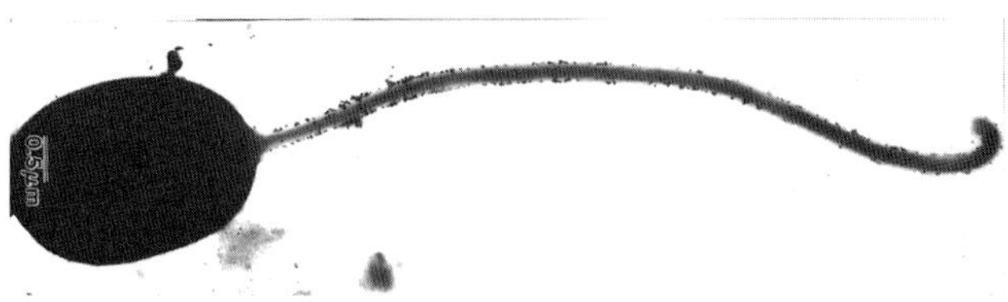

Figure 10 Electron micrographs of the reaction of extruded microsporidian polar tubes of *B. algerae* with colloidal gold-labeled ConA. Reprinted with permission from Xu Y et al.[93]

albendazole may be of use in the treatment of *E. intestinalis* and in Encephalitozoon infections. Fumagillin has been shown to be of potential use in AIDS-associated microsporidiosis (see Table 2).[92]

Other Protozoa

The roles of *Dientamoeba fragilis* and *Blastocystis hominis* as a causal agent of travelers' diarrhea remains a subject of debate; some authorities suggest treatment of symptomatic infections.[94] A number of nonpathogenic protozoa are commonly identified in travelers with acute or chronic diarrhea; however, their role as causative agents of diarrhea has not been established. Patients in whom parasites such as *Entamoeba coli*, *Endolimax nana*, and other species of Entamoeba are identified do not require specific treatment.

Helminths and Diarrhea in Travelers

Numerous helminths infect the human intestinal tract, and in many developing countries, the majority of the population is infected with one or more intestinal helminths. However, intestinal helminths are rarely identified as causes of diarrhea. Trichinosis can present with a diarrheal illness, typically associated with eosinophilia. This is particularly true in cases acquired in Arctic regions.[95] Illness can last for up to 14 weeks. Strongyloidiasis can be associated with diarrhea.[96,97] In most patients with intact host defenses, gastrointestinal illness is mild. However, patients can develop hyperinfection, which can be associated with watery or bloody diarrhea and prominent gastrointestinal complaints. Hyperinfection primarily develops in patients with compromised host defenses, particularly due to corticosteroid therapy. There is no sensitive diagnostic test for chronic strongyloidiasis.[98] Capillariasis may present with abdominal pain, diarrhea, and malabsorption.[99] Heavy infection with Trichuris may present with bloody diarrhea. Acute schistosomiasis is characterized by a systemic febrile illness termed Katayama fever. Travelers typically present at between 2 and 8 weeks after exposure with a systemic illness. Prominent features can include urticaria, hematospermia, or spinal cord involvements.[100] Gastrointestinal complaints are common and, in some cases, diarrhea may be the most prominent symptom. Chronic intestinal schistosomiasis is associated with a granulomatous inflammation, polyps in the intestine, and bloody diarrhea.[101] Heavy infection with Hymenolepis tapeworms can be associated with diarrhea.

Other Considerations

The evaluation of diarrhea in travelers who do not respond to antimicrobial therapy or who experience prolonged illness requires a careful parasitologic examination of repeated stool specimens. In cases where a specific agent cannot be identified, other considerations should be entertained, such as Clostridium difficile antibiotic associated colitis, tropical sprue, celiac disease, postinfective irritable bowel syndrome, HIV infection, or inflammatory bowel disease, among others.

References

1. Freedman DO, Weld LH, Kozarsky PE, et al. The GeoSentinel Surveillance Network. Spectrum of disease and relation to place of exposure among ill returned travelers. N Engl J Med 2006;354:119–30.
2. Reinthaler FF, Feierl G, Stunzner D, Marth E. Diarrhea in returning Austrian tourists: epidemiology, etiology, and cost-analyses. J Travel Med 1998;5:65–72.
3. Shlim DR, Hoge CW, Rajah R, et al. Persistent high risk of diarrhea among foreigners in Nepal during the first 2 years of residence. Clin Infect Dis 1999;29:613–6.
4. Taylor DN, Houston R, Shlim DR, et al. Etiology of diarrhea among travelers and foreign residents in Nepal. J Am Med Assoc 1988;260:1245–8.
5. Monis PT, Andrews RH, Mayrhofer G, Ey PL. Molecular systematics of the parasitic protozoan Giardia intestinalis. Mol Biol Evol 1999;16:1135–44.
6. Adam RD. Biology of Giardia lamblia. Clin Microbiol Rev 2001;14:447–75.
7. Caccio SM, De Giacomo M, Pozio E. Sequence analysis of the [beta]-giardin gene and development of a polymerase chain reaction-restriction fragment length polymorphism assay to genotype Giardia duodenalis cysts from human faecal samples. Int J Parasitol 2002;32:1023–30.
8. Haque R, Roy S, Kabir M, et al. Giardia assemblage A infection and diarrhea in Bangladesh. J Infectious Diseases 2005;192:2171–3.
9. Oyerinde PO, Ogunbi O, Alonge AA. Age and sex distribution of infections with *Entamoeba histolytica* and *Giardia intestinalis* in the Lagos population. Int J Epidemiol 1977;6:231–4.
10. Ali SA, Hill DR. Giardia intestinalis. Curr Opin Infec Dis 2003;16:453–60.
11. Jelinek T, Loescher T. Epidemiology of giardiasis in German travelers. J Travel Med 2000;7:70–3.
12. Gardner TB, Hill DR. Treatment of giardiasis. Clin Microbiol Rev 2001;14:114–28.

13. Hiatt RA, Markell EK, Ng E. How many stool examinations are necessary to detect pathogenic intestinal protozoa? Am J Trop Med Hyg 1995;53:36–9.

14. Aldeen WE, Carroll K, Robison A, et al. Comparison of nine commercially available enzyme-linked immunosorbent assays for detection of Giardia lamblia in fecal specimens. J Clin Microbiol 1998;36:1338–40.

15. Nash TE, Ohl CA, Thomas E, et al. Treatment of patients with refractory giardiasis. Clin Infect Dis 2001; 33:22–8.

16. Ortiz JJ, Ayoub A, Gargala G, et al. Randomized clinical study of nitazoxanide compared to metronidazole in the treatment of symptomatic giardiasis in children from Northern Peru. Aliment Pharmacol Ther 2001;15:1409–15.

17. Rossignol JF, Ayoub A, Ayers MS. Treatment of diarrhea caused by Giardia intestinalis and Entamoeba histolytica or E. dispar: a randomized, double-blind, placebo-controlled study of nitazoxanide. J Infect Dis 2001;184: 381–4.

18. Adagu IS, Nolder D, Warhurst DC, Rossignol JF. In vitro activity of nitazoxanide and related compounds against isolates of Giardia intestinalis, Entamoeba histolytica and Trichomonas vaginalis. J Antimicrob Chemother 2002;49: 103–11.

19. Drugs for Parasitic Infections. Medical Letter Drugs Therapeutics 2004;46:e1–12.

20. Petri WA Jr. Therapy of intestinal protozoa. Trends Parasitol 2003;19:523–6.

21. Ramesh MA, Malik SB, Logsdon JM Jr. A phylogenomic inventory of meiotic genes; evidence for sex in Giardia and an early eukaryotic origin of meiosis. Current Biology 2005;15:185–91.

22. Haque R, Huston CD, Hughes M, et al. Current Concepts: amebiasis. New Engl J Med 2003;348:1565–73.

23. Diamond LS, Clark CG. A redescription of Entamoeba histolytica Shaudin, 1903 (Emended Walker, 1911) separating it from Entamoeba dispar Brumpt, 1925. J Eukaryot Microbiol 1993;40:340–44.

24. Ali IKM, Hossain MB, Roy S, et al. Entamoeba moshkovskii infections in children, Bangladesh. Emerg Infect. Dis. 2003;9:580–4.

25. Haque R, Mollah NU, Ali IKM, et al. Diagnosis of amebic liver abscess and intestinal infection with the Techlab Entamoeba histolytica II antigen detection and antibody tests. J Clin Microbiol 2000;38:3235–9.

26. Roy S, Kabir M, Mondal D, et al. Real-time PCR assay for the diagnosis of Entamoeba histolytica infection. J Clin Microbiol 2005;43:2168–72.

27. Barwick R, Uzicanin A, Lareau S, et al. Outbreak of amebiasis in Tbilisi, Republic of Georgia, 1998. Am J Trop Med Hyg 2002;67:623–31.

28. Gilchrist CA, Houpt E, Trapaidze N, et al. Impact of intestinal colonization and invasion on the E. histolytica transcriptome. Molec Biochem Parasitol 2006;147:163–76.

29. Ali IK, Mondal U, Roy S, et al. Evidence for a link between parasite genotype and outcome of infection with Entamoeba histolytica. J. Clin Microbiol 2007;45:285–9.

30. Duggal P, Haque R, Roy S, et al. Influence of human leukocyte antigen class II alleles on susceptibility to Entamoeba histolytica infection in Bangladeshi children. J Infect Dis 2004;189:520–6.

31. Mondal D, Petri WA Jr, Sack RB, Haque R. Entamoeba histolytica—associated diarrheal illness is negatively associated with the growth of preschool children: evidence from a prospective study. Trans R Soc Trop Med Hyg 2006;100:1032–38.

32. Haque R, Mondal D, Duggal P, et al. Entamoeba histolytica. Infection in children and protection from subsequent amebiasis. Infect Immun 2006;74:904–9.

33. Petri WA Jr, Mann BJ, Haque R. The bittersweet interface of parasite and host: lectin-carbohydrate interactions during human invasion by the parasite Entamoeba histolytica. Ann Rev Microbiol 2002;56:39–64.

34. Huston CD, Miller-Sims V, Petri WA Jr. Apoptotic killing and phagocytosis of host cells by the parasite Entamoeba histolytica. Infect Immun 2003;71:964–72.

35. Boettner DR, Huston CD, Sullivan J, Petri WA Jr. Entamoeba histolytica and Entamoeba dispar utilize externalized phosphatidylserine for recognition and phagocytosis of erythrocytes. Infect Immun 2005;73:3422–30.

36. Beck DL, Boettner DR, Dragulev B, et al. Identification and gene expression analysis of a large family of transmembrane kinases related to the Gal/GalNAc lectin in Entamoeba histolytica Eukaryotic Cell 2005;4:722–32.

37. Loftus B, Anderson I, Davies R, et al. The genome of the protist parasite Entamoeba histolytica, Nature 2005;433: 865–8.

38. Hamano S, Asgharpour A, Stroup SE, et al. Resistance of C57BL/6 mice to amoebiasis is mediated by nonhemopoietic cells but requires hemopoietic IL-10 production. J Immunol 2006;177:1208–13.

39. Asgharpour A, Gilchrist C, Baba D, et al. Resistance to intestinal Entamoeba histolytica infection is conferred by innate immunity and Gr-1+ cells. Infect Immun 2005;73: 4522–9.

40. Houpt ER, Glembocki DJ, Obrig TG, et al. The mouse model of amebic colitis reveals mouse strain susceptibility to infection and exacerbation of disease by CD4+ T cells. J Immunol 2002;169:4496–503.

41. Haque R, Duggal P, Ali IM, et al. Innate and acquired resistance to amebiasis in Bangladeshi children. J Infect Dis 2002;186:547–52.

42. Haque R, Mondal D, Roy S, et al. IFN-γamma production by peripheral blood mononuclear cells is associated with childhood resistance to amebiasis. Am J Trop Med Hyg 2007;76:340–4.

43. Houpt E, Barroso L, Lockhart L, et al. Prevention of intestinal amebiasis by vaccination with the Entamoeba histolytica Gal/GalNac lectin. Vaccine 2004;22:611–7.

44. Blessmann J, Ali IK, Nu PA, et al. Longitudinal study of intestinal Entamoeba histolytica infections in asymptomatic adult carriers. J Clin Microbiol 2003;41:4745–50.

45. Hira PR, Iqbal J, Al-Ali F, et al. Invasive amebiasis: challenges in diagnosis in a non-endemic country (Kuwait). Am J Trop Med Hyg 2001;65:341–5.

46. Hughes MA, Petri WA Jr. Amebic liver abscess. Infect Dis Clin North Am 2000;14:565–82.

47. Adams EB, MacLeod IN. Invasive amebiasis II: amebic liver abscess and its complications. Medicine 1977;56:325–34.

48. Katzenstein D, Rickerson V, Braude A. New concepts of amebic liver abscess derived from hepatic imaging, serodiagnosis, and hepatic enzymes in 67 consecutive cases in San Diego. Medicine 1982;61:237–46.

49. Solaymani-Mohammadi S, Lam MM, Zunt JR, Petri WA Jr. Entamoeba histolytica encephalitis diagnosed by PCR of cerebrospinal fluid. Tr Roy Soc Trop Med Hyg 2007;101:311–3.

50. Pillai DR, Keystone JS, Sheppard DC, et al. Entamoeba histolytica and Entamoeba dispar: epidemiology and comparison of diagnostic methods in a setting of nonendemicity. Clin Infect Dis 1999;29:1315–8.

51. McCarthy JS, Peacock D, Trown KP, et al. Endemic invasive amoebiasis in northern Australia. Med J Australia 2002;177:570.

52. Blessmann J, Tannich E. Treatment of asymptomatic intestinal Entamoeba histolytica infection. N Engl J Med 2002;347:1384.

53. Current WL, Reese NC, Ernst JV, et al. Human cryptosporidiosis in immunocompetent and immunodeficient persons: studies of an outbreak and experimental transmission. N Engl J Med 1983;308:1252–7.

54. Homan W, van Gorkom T, Kan YY, Hepener J. Characterization of Cryptosporidium parvum in human and animal feces by single-tube nested polymerase chain reaction and restriction analysis. Parasitol Res 1999;85:707–12.

55. Chauret C, Nolan K, Chen P, et al. Aging of Cryptosporidium parvum oocysts in river water and their susceptibility to disinfection by chlorine and monochloramine. Can J Microbiol 1998;44:1154–60.

56. Widmer G, Tchack L, Chappell CL, Tzipori S. Sequence polymorphism in the beta-tubulin gene reveals heterogeneous and variable population structures in Cryptosporidium parvum. Appl Environ Microbiol 1998;64:4477–81.

57. Widmer G, Tzipori S, Fichtenbaum CJ, Griffiths JK. Genotypic and phenotypic characterization of Cryptosporidium parvum isolates from people with AIDS. J Infect Dis 1998;178:834–40.

58. Okhuysen PC, Chappell CL, Crabb JH, et al. Virulence of three distinct Cryptosporidium parvum isolates for healthy adults. J Infect Dis 1999;180:1275–81.

59. Abrahamsen MS, Templeton TJ, Enomoto S, et al. Complete genome sequence of the apicomplexan, Cryptosporidium parvum. Science 2004;304:441–5.

60. Xu P, Widmer G, Wang Y, et al. The genome of Cryptosporidium hominis. Nature 2004;431:1107–12.

61. Koch KL, Phillips DJ, Aber RC, Current WL. Cryptosporidiosis in hospital personnel: evidence for personto-person transmission. Ann Intern Med 1984; 102:593–6.

62. Meinhardt PL, Casemore DP, Miller KB. Epidemiologic aspects of human cryptosporidiosis and the role of waterborne transmission. Epidemiol Rev 1996;18:118–36.

63. Foodborne outbreak of cryptosporidiosis—Spokane, Washington, 1997. MMWR Morb Mortal Wkly Rep 1998;47:565–7.

64. Outbreak of cryptosporidiosis associated with a water sprinkler fountain—Minnesota, 1997. MMWR Morb Mortal Wkly Rep 1998;47:856–60.

65. DuPont HL, Chappell CL, Sterling CR, et al. The infectivity of Cryptosporidium parvum in healthy volunteers. N Engl J Med 1995;332:855–9.

66. Chappell CL, Okhuysen PC, Sterling CR, et al. Infectivity of Cryptosporidium parvum in healthy adults with preexisting anti-C. parvum serum immunoglobulin G. Am J Trop Med Hyg 1999;60:157–64.

67. Moss DM, Chappell CL, Okhuysen PC, et al. The antibody response to 27-, 17-, and 15-kDa Cryptosporidium antigens following experimental infection in humans. J Infect Dis 1998;178:827–33.

68. Okhuysen PC, Chappell CL, Sterling CR, et al. Susceptibility and serologic response of healthy adults to reinfection with Cryptosporidium parvum. Infect Immun 1998;66:441–3.

69. Checkley W, Gilman RH, Epstein LD, et al. Asymptomatic and symptomatic cryptosporidiosis: their acute effect on weight gain in Peruvian children. Am J Epidemiol 1997; 145:156–63.

70. Dillingham RA, Lima AA, Guerrant RL. Cryptosporidiosis: epidemiology and impact. Microbes Infect 2002;4:1059.

71. Newman RD, Sears CL, Moore SR, et al. Longitudinal study of Cryptosporidium infection in children in northeastern Brazil. J Infect Dis 1999;180:167–75.

72. Ungar BL, Mulligan M, Nutman TB. Serologic evidence of Cryptosporidium infection in US volunteers before and during Peace Corps service in Africa. Arch Intern Med 1989;149:894–7.

73. Goodgame RW, Kimball K, Ou C-N, et al. Intestinal function and injury in AIDS-related cryptosporidiosis. Gastroenterology 1995;108:1075–82.

74. Laurent F, McCole D, Eckmann L, Kagnoff MF. Pathogenesis of Cryptosporidium parvum infection. Microbes Infect 1999;1:141–8.

75. Zhang Y, Lee B, Thompson M, et al. Lactulose-mannitol intestinal permeability test in children with diarrhea caused by rotavirus and cryptosporidium. Diarrhea Working Group, Peru. J Pediatr Gastroenterol Nutr 2000;31:16–21.

76. Kosek M, Alcantara C, Lima AA, Guerrant RL. Cryptosporidiosis: an update. Lancet Infect Dis 2001;1:262–9.

77. Jacyna M, Parkin J, Goldin R, Baron J. Protracted enteric cryptosporidial infection in selective immunoglobulin A and Saccharomyces opsonin deficiencies. Gut 1990;31: 714–6.

78. Hashmey R, Smith NH, Cron S, et al. Cryptosporidiosis in Houston, Texas. A report of 95 cases. Medicine (Baltimore) 1997;76:118–39.

79. Garcia LS, Shimizu RY. Evaluation of nine immunoassay kits (enzyme immunoassay and direct fluorescence) for detection of Giardia lamblia and Cryptosporidium parvum in human fecal specimens. J Clin Microbiol 1997;35:1526–9.

80. Stroup SE, Roy S, Mchele J, et al. Species-specific real-time PCR for Cryptosporidium in stool using Scorpion probes. J Medical Microbiol 2006;55:1217–22.

81. Haque R, Roy S, Siddique A, et al. Multiplex real-time PCR assay for detection of Entamoeba histolytica, Giardia lamblia and Cryptosporidium spp. Am J Trop Med Hyg 2007;76(4).

82. Rossignol JF, Ayoub A, Ayers MS. Treatment of diarrhea caused by Cryptosporidium parvum: a prospective randomized, double-blind, placebo-controlled study of Nitazoxanide. J Infect Dis 2001;184:103–6.

83. Rossignol JF, Hidalgo H, Feregrino M, et al. A double-'blind' placebo-controlled study of nitazoxanide in the treatment of cryptosporidial diarrhoea in AIDS patients in Mexico. Trans R Soc Trop Med Hyg 1998;92:663–6.

84. Okhuysen PC, Chappell CL, Crabb J, et al. Prophylactic effect of bovine anti-Cryptosporidium hyperimmune colostrum immunoglobulin in healthy volunteers challenged with Cryptosporidium parvum. Clin Infect Dis 1998;26:1324–9.

85. Hewitt RG, Yiannoutsos CT, Higgs ES, et al. Paromomycin: no more effective than placebo for treatment of cryptosporidiosis in patients with advanced human immunodeficiency virus infection. AIDS Clinical Trial Group. Clin Infect Dis. 2000;31:1084–92.

86. Kaplan JE, Masur H, Holmes KK. Guidelines for preventing opportunistic infections among HIV-infected persons–2002. Recommendations of the US Public Health Service and the Infectious Diseases Society of America. MMWR Recomm Rep 2002;51:1–52.

87. Eberhard ML, Nace EK, Freeman AR. Survey for Cyclospora cayetanensis in domestic animals in an endemic area in Haiti. J Parasitol 1999;85:562–3.

88. Sturbaum GD, Ortega YR, Gilman RH, et al. Detection of Cyclospora cayetanensis in wastewater. Appl Env-iron Microbiol 1998;64:2284–6.

89. Herwaldt BL, Beach MJ. The return of Cyclospora in 1997: another outbreak of cyclosporiasis in North America associated with imported raspberries. Cyclospora Working Group. Ann Intern Med 1999;130:210–20.

90. Drenaggi D, Cirioni O, Giacometti A, et al. Cyclosporiasis in a traveler returning from South America. J Travel Med 1998;5:153–5.

91. Varea M, Clavel A, Doiz O, et al. Fuchsin fluorescence and autofluorescence in Cryptosporidium, Isospora and Cyclospora oocysts. Int J Parasitol 1998;28:1881–3.

92. Didier ES, Weiss LM. Microsporidiosis: current status. Curr Opin Infect Dis 2006;19:485–92.

93. Xu Y, Takvorian PM, Cali A, et al. Glycosylation of the major polar tube protein of Encephalitozoon hellem, a microsporidian parasite that infects humans. Infect Immun 2004;72:6341–50.

94. Tan KS. Blastocystis in humans and animals: new insights using modern methodologies. Vet Parasitol 2004;126:121–44.

95. MacLean JD, Viallet J, Law C, Staudt M. Trichinosis in the Canadian arctic: report of five outbreaks and a new clinical syndrome. J Infect Dis 1989;160:513–20.

96. Tsai HC, Lee SS, Liu YC, et al. Clinical manifestations of strongyloidiasis in southern Taiwan. J Microbiol Immunol Infect 2002;35:29–36.

97. Genta RM, Gatti S, Linke MJ, et al. Endemic strongyloidiasis in Northern Italy: clinical and immunologic aspects. Q J Med 1988;257:679–90.

98. Siddiqui AA, Berk SL. Diagnosis of Strongyloides stercoralis infection. Clin Infect Dis 2001;33:1040–7.

99. Cross JH. Intestinal capillariasis. Clin Microbiol Rev 1992; 5:120–9.

100. Roca C, Balanzo X, Gascon J, et al. Comparative, clinico-epidemiologic study of Schistosoma mansoni infections in travellers and immigrants in Spain. Eur J Clin Microbiol Infect Dis 2002;21:219–23.

101. Guyatt H, Gryseels B, Smith T, Tanner M. Assessing the public health importance of Schistosoma mansoni in different endemic areas: attributable fraction estimates as an approach. Am J Trop Med Hyg 1995;53:660–7.

CHAPTER 5

BACTERIAL RESISTANCE TO ANTIMICROBIALS

JORDI VILA, MD, PhD

DAVID G. WHITE, PhD

PATRICK F. MCDERMOTT, PhD

STUART B. LEVY, MD, FAAM

Diarrhea incapacitates travelers to all parts of the world, but particularly in areas where clean water and optimal hygiene are lacking. Thus, the incidence of travelers' diarrhea ranges from 2% in low-risk geographical areas (the United States, Europe, Australia, and Japan) to 40% in high-risk geographical areas (Latin America, Southern Asia, and Africa).[1,2] All travelers from industrialized countries to developing countries develop a relatively rapid change in their intestinal flora. While most bacteria are harmless and represent local flora, some organisms can include potential enteric pathogens. Diarrhea follows ingestion of an inoculum of virulent organisms sufficiently large to overcome individual defense mechanisms. In patients traveling to high-risk areas, more than 60% of diarrheal illnesses are caused by a bacterial pathogen.[3] Knowing the antibiotic susceptibility profile of these enteric pathogens can help control the disease; however, information on the antimicrobial resistance of bacteria causing travelers' diarrhea is scarce. Considering that the highest risk areas are developing countries, resistance data on certain relevant enteropathogenic bacteria in these countries can be helpful in selecting an appropriate therapy when needed.

Factors Favoring the Emergence of Antimicrobial Resistance

Antimicrobial resistance has increased drastically in recent years in both developed and developing countries and can be spread through international travel (Figure 1). It has rapidly become a leading public health concern. Enteric infectious disease organisms are among those which are most affected by antimicrobial resistance. The prevalence of antimicrobial resistance varies greatly between and within countries and between different

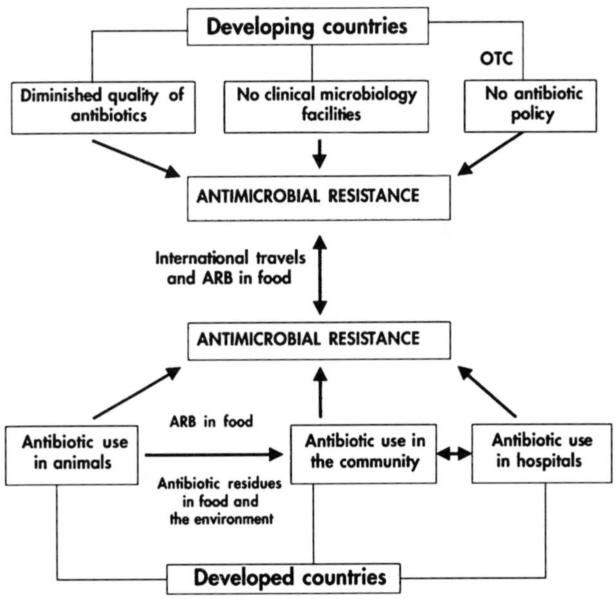

OTC = Over-the-counter
ARB = Antibiotic resistant bacteria

Figure 1 Main factors favoring the development of antibiotic resistance in bacteria.

pathogens. Three main factors favor the development of bacterial resistance to antibiotics in developing countries:

1. *Less potent activity*: Some of the antibiotics provided in developing countries have decreased potency because of degradation or adulteration of the drug, or because of the presence of a lower concentration of active substances.[4–6] For instance, substandard concentrations of ampicillin and tetracycline have been found in Nigeria.[7,8] Moreover, expired drugs, with altered or removed expiry dates, have also been detected in developing countries.[9–11] Some drugs produced in industrialized countries have been found to have expired on distribution in developing countries.[12] Finally, the antibiotics provided to these countries may be poorly transported and stored, leading to drug inactivation.[13–15]
2. *Lack of diagnostic laboratories:* Most of the hospitals in developing countries do not have clinical microbiology laboratories to perform routine analyses for microbiological diagnosis. Therefore, they have no information about either the etiology of the infectious diseases or antimicrobial susceptibility, both essential for clinical practice. Bacterial infections are often treated empirically with broad-spectrum antibiotics. Although they are not frequently performed, specific and periodic studies regarding the etiology and antimicrobial susceptibility of some important infectious disease agents would help clinicians decide on which antibiotics to choose to treat such infections.[16,17]
3. *Over-the-counter availability*: In most developing countries, antibiotics can be purchased without prescription in pharmacies, general stores, markets, and from street vendors. Because many drugs are expensive, some patients purchase incomplete regimens whenever possible and discontinue treatment when the symptoms disappear.[18] As in industrialized countries, unnecessary prescriptions of antibiotics, mainly in cases of acute infantile diarrhea and respiratory infections, have been reported in developing countries.[19–22] Health care personnel, who frequently have minimal training, are scarce and cannot serve the entire population, especially in rural areas. The infection control practices in many hospitals in developing countries are suboptimal or nonexistent and often compromised by the lack of resources and personnel trained in controlling infections in hospitals.[23]

Finally, although it may not seem to be an important problem in developing countries, where the practice is less applied, the excessive use of antimicrobials, especially as growth promoters in animals destined for human consumption, presents a growing risk to human health due to the emergence of bacteria resistant to the antibiotics fed to animals, which can then be transferred to humans through the food chain.[24–26] Spread of antibiotics and resistant bacteria into the environment is also a contributor to the problem (see Figure 1). Spread is also associated with the use of contaminated water from sewage runoff.[27]

The Use of Antimicrobial Agents in Animals

Because the vast majority of bacteria involved in travelers' diarrhea come through ingestion of contaminated food, it is of interest to discuss how resistance could emerge in this bacterial reservoir. Antimicrobials have been used extensively in livestock and poultry since their discovery, with significant beneficial effects on food animal health and production efficiency. This use is focused primarily on the treatment and/or prevention of animal diseases. Diseases requiring the most extensive use of antimicrobial drugs for treatment or prophylaxis in veterinary medicine are respiratory and enteric diseases in pigs and cattle, colibacillosis in poultry, and mastitis in dairy cattle. In fact, one of the earliest reports of antimicrobial use in veterinary medicine was for the treatment of mastitis in dairy cows in the mid 1940s.[28]

Most classes of antimicrobials used in animals have human analogues and are therefore capable of selecting for resistance to antibiotics. These include penicillins, cephalosporins, macrolides, lincosamides, streptogramins, aminoglycosides, fluoroquinolones, tetracyclines, folate pathway inhibitors (sulfonamides and potentiated sulfonamides, eg, trimethoprim/sulfamethoxazole), phenicols, and polypeptides. Other antimicrobial agents, which are mostly administered in feeds for growth promotion and prophylaxis, belong to classes used only in veterinary medicine, such as the ionophores (eg, monensin, salinomycin, lasalocid), arsenical compounds, pleuromutilins, quinoxalines (eg, olaquindox), and phosphoglycolipids (eg, flavomycin).

Antimicrobials are used in animal production primarily for: 1) therapy in animals that show overt signs of disease; 2) prophylaxis in healthy animals at risk for contracting an infection; 3) infection control (metaphylaxis) in a herd or flock that displays elevated morbidity or mortality; and 4) improved feed efficiency and weight gain (growth promotion) in healthy animals. In contrast to human medicine where treatment is customarily directed at the patient, entire groups of animals may be treated by the use of medicated feed and/or water.[29] For some food production animals (eg, fish and poultry), mass medication is the only practical means of antimicrobial treatment. Certain mass medication measures are aimed at treating sick animals while medicating others in the herd or flock to prevent disease.[29] Such practice is often initiated when illness is first detected in a small fraction of the animals. Other prophylactic antimicrobial treatments are typically used during high-risk or high-stress periods where illness is likely to occur (eg, during transport or after weaning).

It was the unexpected discovery in the 1950s that less than therapeutic amounts of antimicrobials increased growth rates and improved the efficiency of feed utilization in animals that led to their use as growth promoters. The latter use is the most controversial veterinary practice; it is complicated by the fact that nearly all licensed compounds may be administered for both growth promoting and prophylactic purposes, depending on the dosage. Growth promoting dosages are given to healthy cattle, pigs, and poultry, usually at low concentrations (2.5 to 50 ppm) for extended time periods. Past studies have shown that this practice is also a potentially significant driving force in accelerating the emergence of resistant bacteria in these animals that can be transferred through contact or food to infect humans.[30–32] To date, only the European Union has banned the use of "growth promoter" in-feed antibiotics because of their ability to select for resistance to antimicrobials of human importance.[33]

As a result of continued exposure to antibiotics, the prevalence of resistant bacteria in the fecal flora of food animals may be relatively high. Determining the impact of these resistant bacteria on the management of human infections is an ongoing challenge. Three scenarios have been previously proposed by which the use of antimicrobials in food animals could affect treatment of diarrheal diseases in humans: 1) antimicrobial-resistant zoonotic bacterial pathogens are selected and food is contaminated during slaughter and/or preparation. After consumption of the food, these pathogens cause an infection that requires antibiotic treatment and therapy is compromised; 2) antimicrobial-resistant bacteria non-pathogenic to humans are selected in the animal. When the contaminated food is ingested, the bacteria transfer resistance determinants to other bacteria in the human gut, commensal, and potential pathogens; and 3) antibiotics remain as residues in food products, which allows the selection of antibiotic-resistant bacteria after the food is consumed.[34]

Antimicrobial-resistant enteric pathogens can reach humans through direct animal contact or, more commonly, through ingestion of contaminated water or foods. Several studies have demonstrated an association between antimicrobial use in animals and the subsequent isolation of resistant bacteria from the same animal.[35–38] Epidemiological and microbiological data show that resistant isolates from food animals can reach humans via the food supply.[39–44] Other studies have demonstrated the spread of resistant fecal bacteria to humans living in close proximity to farm animals. One of the earliest studies showed the movement of antimicrobial resistant *Escherichia coli* from poultry to farm personnel following treatment with tetracycline.[45] The same study showed an increase in resistant fecal *E. coli* in farm workers on a farm that provided low levels of tetracycline to chickens.[46] Another study profiled the emergence of both gentamicin- and apramycin-resistant *E. coli* and *Salmonella* spp. following the use of these antibiotics in food animals, prompting the dissemination of a common plasmid carrying the resistance gene (animoglycoside-3-N-acetyltransferase) among bacteria from both the animals and the workers caring for them.[47] More recently, Fey and colleagues demonstrated that a ceftriaxone-resistant isolate of *S. enterica* serotype Typhimurium recovered from a child with diarrhea was indistinguishable from a cattle isolate[48] and was likely contracted by direct contact.

While contaminated animal-derived food products and exposure to farm animals are well established vehicles of transmission, less attention has been paid to the impact of fertilizing agricultural fields for crop production using untreated wastewater or manure, and the subsequent contamination of produce by resistant fecal pathogens. Wastewater is a known source of contamination in areas where it is used.[49] Because animal wastes are contaminated with significant levels of zoonotic pathogens,[50] the practice may provide a pathway for resistant enteric pathogens, selected in the farm environment, to disseminate to uncooked food products. The importance of this has yet to be quantified but is expected to vary in importance in different countries.

Information on the magnitude of the public health burden linked to antimicrobial-resistant zoonotic foodborne pathogens, and the hazard it poses to travelers, shows that the situation is complex and varies by country and region. It can be influenced by a number of variables such as antimicrobial use practices in farming and human medicine, process control at slaughter, hazard control in storage and distribution systems, the availability of clean water, and proper cooking and home/restaurant hygiene.[51] In regions where these variables are loosely controlled, indigenous exposure levels to multidrug-resistant salmonellae may be high. In Mexico, for example, the carriage rate of multidrug-resistant non-Typhi salmonellae in asymptomatic kindergarten children was estimated at 11.4%.[44] When resistant pathogens cause overt illness, evidence suggests that antimicrobial-resistant strains can lead to more intractable and severe disease compared to susceptible strains.[52–55]

It is very difficult to also ascertain the amount of antimicrobials used in animal production in both developed and developing economies, including many countries that are travel destinations. With the exception of several European countries, there is little public information available regarding the total amounts of antimicrobials used in various food animal species in different geographic regions. In the US, where modern meat and poultry production is intensive, nearly all animals will receive an antimicrobial at some stage in their growth. In addition, data on the prevalence of resistance among foodborne zoonotic pathogens in animals, foods, and human clinical cases is rarely available, particularly in developing economies. Additional quantitative information is therefore needed on the magnitude and nature of the contribution of agricultural antibiotic use and its impact on the severity of foodborne bacterial diseases.[56–58]

Ongoing surveillance of the antimicrobial susceptibility profiles of foodborne pathogens is needed to identify emerging antimicrobial-resistant phenotypes within the food production continuum. Available surveillance data on resistance from animal isolates of *Salmonella*, *E. coli* and *Campylobacter* can give some indication of the selective pressures being applied in food animal production (see <http://www.fda.gov/cvm/narms_pg.html>). Considering the magnitude of international travel and trade in agricultural products, global surveillance of antimicrobial susceptibility of foodborne pathogens is increasingly important to assist physicians in determining the appropriate treatment regimens.

Dissemination of Resistant Bacteria

Bacteria resistant to antibiotics can spread locally and internationally. The latter can occur bidirectionally between developed and developing countries (see Figure 1). Given that resistance determinants are often located on mobile genetic elements, resistance can be transferred to other bacteria. The dissemination of nonpathogenic antibiotic resistant bacteria is also important because they can serve as reservoirs of resistance genes that may be transferred to pathogens. For instance, investigators described the spread of a plasmid carrying a gentamicin-resistance gene among enteric bacteria isolated in Venezuela and the United States.[59] Apparently healthy people in developing countries carry potentially pathogenic antibiotic-resistant organisms asymptomatically,[17,60] which can be acquired from the local food supply[44] or spread person to person.

Crowding and unhygienic conditions are important factors favoring the dissemination of resistant bacteria. In Nigeria, resistant *E. coli* isolates from individuals in an urban metropolis were significantly more likely to be resistant to 4 to 6 of 7 antibiotics tested, than were strains from rural areas, which were resistant to only 3 antibiotics.[61] Similar findings were reported from Nepal.[62] The low level of sanitation of many of the developing countries may also contribute to the spread of antimicrobial-resistant bacteria.[12] Finally, warm and humid tropical climates are conducive to the propagation of bacteria in food and water.[63]

Visitors to developing countries acquire antibiotic resistant bacteria mainly in the intestinal tract.[64] Travelers from the United States to Mexico have acquired antimicrobial resistant bacteria without taking antibiotics and have returned to the United States with these resistant organisms.[64] Foodborne bacteria, such as *Shigella sonnei* and *Vibrio cholerae*, have been transmitted by contaminated meals served during international flights or aboard cruise ships.[65–67]

Diarrheagenic E. coli

ENTEROTOXIGENIC *E. COLI*

Enterotoxigenic *E. coli* (ETEC) are the most common causative agents of travelers' diarrhea in all countries where surveys have been conducted. However, they are an important cause of diarrhea among children in the developing world as well, usually at the time of weaning.[68,69]

Susceptibility data for ETEC in comparison with other enteric pathogens causing travelers' diarrhea are scarce because most clinical laboratories do not perform toxin detection tests. Overall, the percentages of resistance of ETEC bearing the stable toxins (ST) or labile toxins (LT) or both are very similar, with figures above 40% for ampicillin, tetracycline, and trimethoprim-sulfamethoxazole. Chloramphenicol shows activity against ETEC with percentages of resistance ranging from 13 to 25% (Table 1). There are no significant statistical differences among the different geographical areas analyzed and among those causing travelers' diarrhea in travelers abroad. Similar levels of resistance were observed among these recent reports and previously published studies in the 1980s.[70–74] Nalidixic acid or ciprofloxacin show the best activity against these microorganisms. However, a trend to a rise in quinolone resistance has recently been described, possibly following the increase in the use of

Table 1 Frequency of Antimicrobial Resistance of Diarrheagenic *Escherichia coli* from Different Developing Countries and in Those Causing Travelers' Diarrhea

	Resistance (%)						
Country	AMP	CHL	TET	SXT	NAL	CIP	Ref.
ETEC							
Mexico	---	---	81	31	---	---	70
Tanzania	84.1	25	68.2	79.5	2.3	0	71
Thailand	54	13	43	51	3	2	72
Vietnam	67	17	65	63	<1	<1	72
Vietnam	71	57	---	71	14.3	7.1	75
TD*	40.7	22.3	55.6	47	7.3	0.6	73
EAEC							
Nigeria	80.9	46.5	95.4	74.0	0	0	78
Tanzania	83.1	57	87.7	90.8	1.5	0	71
Vietnam	90	87	---	92	18.6	0	75
TD*	52	28	64	48	6	2	76
EPEC							
Tanzania	90.4	33.3	81	90.4	0	0	71
Uruguay	100	27	23	42	----	0	81
Vietnam	82	64	---	84	24	10	75

TD* = ETEC and EAEC causing travelers' diarrhea.
TD** = Data not published.
AMP = ampicillin; CHL = chloramphenicol; CIP = ciprofloxacin; EAEC = enteroaggregative E. coli; EPEC = enteropathogenic E. coli; ETEC = enterotoxigenic E. coli; NAL = nalidixic acid; SXT = trimethoprim-sulfamethoxazole; TET = tetracycline.

quinolones for other diseases resistant to quinolones. ETEC have been isolated from people who traveled to India.[73] Nalidixic acid was introduced a few years ago as the first line therapy for shigellosis in some areas of India and therefore ETEC strains resistant to nalidixic acid are now emerging. In a recent study performed in Hanoi (Vietnam), 14% of ETEC isolates were resistant to nalidixic acid whereas none of the *S. flexneri* isolates were.[75]

ENTEROAGGREGATIVE *E. COLI*

Enteroaggregative *E. coli* (EAEC) rank second among the diarrheagenic *E. coli* causing travelers' diarrhea.[68,69] In one study, resistance of EAEC to ampicillin was found to be 52%, to tetracycline 64%, to trimethoprim-sulfamethoxazole 48%, and to chloramphenicol 28%, whereas only 6% and 2% of the tested EAEC were resistant to nalidixic acid and ciprofloxacin, respectively.[76] The quinolone resistant EAEC strains were isolated from patients with travelers' diarrhea who have journeyed to India or to Mexico.[76] Multidrug-resistant EAEC have also been reported in Kenya, Nigeria, Tanzania, Mexico, Chile, Peru, Vietnam and Thailand (see Table 1).[71,77–79]

ENTEROPATHOGENIC *E . COLI*

Enteropathogenic *E. coli* (EPEC) cause diarrhea in infants in developing countries as well as in travelers.[69,71,80,81] The percentages of antimicrobial resistance are similar to those described for the other diarrheagenic E. coli, with high level of resistance (above 23%) to ampicillin, tetracycline, and trimethoprim-sulfamethoxazole, moderate resistance to chloramphenicol, and almost no strains resistant to quinolones (see Table 1).

VEROTOXIN-PRODUCING/ ENTEROHEMORRHAGIC *E. COLI*

Verotoxin-Producing/Enterohemorrhagic *E . coli* (VTEC/ EHEC), in particular, *E. coli* serotype O157:H7, are an important cause of diarrhea, which can sometimes be complicated by hemorrhagic colitis and hemolytic uremic syndrome (HUS).[68] No systematic search for VTEC has been conducted in developing countries. Moreover, they are not highly prevalent as a cause of travelers' diarrhea.[69] Therefore, little susceptibility data are available. However, two strains of verotoxin-producing *E. coli* O-rough:K1:H7 causing travelers' diarrhea were susceptible to ampicillin, chloramphenicol, and quinolones, whereas one was resistant to trimethoprim-sulfamethoxazole and both were resistant to tetracycline.[82]

Shigella SPP

Shigella are a well-known cause of bacillary dysentery affecting 5 to 15% of travelers. There are four species of *Shigella: Shigella dysenteriae, Shigella flexneri, Shigella boydii*, and *Shigella sonnei*. The percentages of resistance to several antimicrobial agents in the three main species of Shigella isolated from different geographical areas (mainly developing countries) as well as a cause of travelers' diarrhea are shown in Tables 2 through 4. Overall, *S. flexneri* and *S. dysenteriae* are more resistant than *S. sonnei*, at least when ampicillin and chloramphenicol are tested. It is also worth mentioning that in a recent study, 54% of the *S. flexneri* clinical isolates causing traveler's diarrhea were resistant to chloramphenicol, whereas none of the *S. sonnei* isolates were.[83] The prevalence of resistance to ampicillin for *S. sonnei* ranges from a low of 0% in Calcutta (India) to a high of 62% in Vietnam.[72,89] Similarly, the rate of chloramphenicol resistance is very wide, being from 0% in Western Kenya or Tanzania to 44.3% in Korea. [86,89,91]

In most of the geographic areas analyzed, resistance to trimethoprim-sulfamethoxazole in three species of *Shigella* ranged from 55 to 100% and was higher than that previously reported, showing a trend towards increased resistance to these antimicrobial agents in *Shigella* spp clinical isolates.[74] However, most of the scientific literature on antimicrobial resistance in *Shigella* spp do not analyze the epidemiological relationship among the isolates, and a predominant multiresistant clone is probably responsible for this high frequency of resistance.[89] A large percentage of *Shigella* is multiresistant, with two predominant resistance phenotypes: those resistant to ampicillin, tetracycline, and trimethoprim-sulfamethoxazole; and those resistant to ampicillin,

Table 2 Frequency of Antimicrobial Resistance of *Shigella flexneri* from Different Developing Countries and in Strains Causing Travelers' Diarrhea

	Resistance (%)						
Country	AMP	CHL	TET	SXT	NAL	CIP	Ref.
Brazil	100	---	---	55	0	---	84
India	87	58	100	100	21	0	85
Indonesia	90	83	94	80	---	0	103
Kenya	94	90	99	88	2	0	86
Kenya	84	92	98	93	3	0	87
Rwanda	83	80	—	75	0.5	0	88
Tanzania	92	92	99	92	0	0	89
Thailand	82	61	96	86	0	0	72
Vietnam	84	74	87	83	< 1	0	72
Vietnam	85	85	---	85	0	0	75
TD*	40.7	22.3	55.6	47	7.3	0.6	90
TD*	73	54	84	65	---	---	83

*TD = S. flexneri causing travelers' diarrhea.
AMP = ampicillin; CHL = chloramphenicol; CIP = ciprofloxacin; NAL = nalidixic acid; SXT = trimethoprim-sulfamethoxazole; TET = tetracycline.

Table 3 Frequency of Antimicrobial Resistance of *Shigella sonnei* from Different Developing Countries and in Strains Causing Travelers' Diarrhea

	Resistance (%)						
Country	AMP	CHL	TET	SXT	NAL	CIP	Ref.
India	0	25	100	100	25	0	85
Indonesia	27	17	83	76	---	0	103
Kenya	0	0	100	100	0	0	86
Kenya	5	0	98	100	0	0	87
Korea	11.4	44.3	96.6	95	45.5	100	91
Rwanda	13	7	---	38	0	---	88
Tanzania	25	0	100	100	0	0	89
Thailand	4	3	92	97	0	0	72
Vietnam	62	36	60	67	< 1	0	72
Vietnam	70	40	---	90	5	0	75
TD*	32	18	73	54	0	0	90
TD*	58	0	72	81	---	---	83

*TD = S. sonnei causing travelers' diarrhea.
AMP = ampicillin; CHL = chloramphenicol; CIP = ciprofloxacin; NAL = nalidixic acid; SXT = trimethoprim-sulfamethoxazole; TET = tetracycline.

Table 4 Frequency of Antimicrobial Resistance of *Shigella dysenteriae* from Different Developing Countries

	Resistance (%)						
Country	AMP	CHL	TET	SXT	NAL	CIP	Ref.
India	100	80	100	100	60	0	85
Indonesia	100	100	100	100	---	0	103
Kenya	100	100	92	100	4	0	86
Kenya	98	100	100	95	0	0	87
Rwanda	100	100	—	68	20	0	88
Tanzania	100	100	100	100	0	0	89
Thailand	0	0	33	0	0	0	72
Vietnam	50	17	50	50	0	0	72

AMP = ampicillin; CHL = chloramphenicol; CIP = ciprofloxacin; NAL = nalidixic acid; SXT = trimethoprim-sulfamethoxazole; TET = tetracycline.

tetracycline, chloramphenicol, and trimethoprim-sulfamethoxazole. Although no resistance to fluoroquinolones, such as ciprofloxacin, has been detected, the percentage of resistance to nalidixic acid ranges from 0% in several geographical areas to 100% in strains of *S. sonnei* isolated in Korea.[91] However, the latter figures may be attributed to the spread of a resistant clone. Moreover, a trend to quinolone resistance has been observed in *S. dysenteriae* strains isolated in Burundi.[92]

Campylobacter SPP

Campylobacter species associated with gastrointestinal infectious diseases include *Campylobacter jejuni, Campylobacter coli, Campylobacter lari,* and *Campylobacter upsaliensis.* The most common species implicated are *C. jejuni* and *C. coli. C. jejuni* is a common cause of diarrhea throughout the world.

The resistance frequency to tetracycline in *C. jejuni* causing travelers' diarrhea is approximately 66%. Macrolides, either erythromycin or azithromycin, are the most active antibiotics against *C. jejuni* (Table 5). Among 15 of 16 Peruvian children presenting with *C. jejuni* related dysentery, stools became normal within 5 days when treated with erythromycin, in contrast to only 6 of 12 children who received placebo.[94] Studies in adults with enteritis caused by *Campylobacter* have indicated that treatment with either ciprofloxacin or azithromycin shortened the duration of symptoms.[95] Resistance to ciprofloxacin in *C. jejuni* causing travelers' diarrhea is steadily increasing, ranging from 36% in the period of 1993 to 1998 to 57.8% in the period 1999 to 2003.[96] This significant increase has also been described for isolates in travelers returning to Finland and was also significant in Asia alone, suggesting a continual presence of selection pressure for the emergence of fluoroquinolone resistance on that continent.[97] This high figure is similar to that found in some industrialized countries, such as the US (18%). At the end of the 1980s, several studies showed minimal resistance to fluoroquinolones among *Campylobacter* species.[98] Recently there has been a trend toward an increased frequency of quinolone resistance concomitant with the increased use of fluoroquinolones in humans and animals.[99]

Erythromycin resistance rates remain low (< 2%) in most regions. Contrary to what was found with ETEC,

Table 5 Frequency of Antimicrobial Resistance of *Campylobacter jejuni* from Different Developing Countries and in Strains Causing Travelers' Diarrhea

	Resistance (%)							
Country	AMP	A/C	TET	ERI	AZIT	NAL	CIP	Ref.
Indonesia	65	---	65	0	---	---	35	103
Kenya	---	---	2	48**	---	26	7	87
Thailand	---	---	---	---	6	73	77	72
Vietnam	---	---	---	---	0	7	7	72
TD*	33	0	37.5	0	---	12.5	12.5	93
TD	66	20	42	2	---	52.2	46.7	96

*TD = C. jejuni causing travelers' diarrhea.
** These strains showed intermediate resistance to erythromycin.
A/C = amoxicillin plus clavulanic acid; AMP = ampicillin; AZIT = azithromycin; CIP = ciprofloxacin; ERI = erythromycin; NAL = nalidixic acid; TET = tetracycline.

EAEC, and *Shigella* spp, rifaximin did not show as good activity against *C. jejuni* because the MIC_{50} and MIC_{90} were 256 and 512 mg/L, respectively.[80]

Salmonella SPP

Salmonella gastroenteritis is a well-known disease that occurs throughout the world. In industrialized nations, this large group of organisms is the most common cause of outbreaks of food associated diarrhea. The proportion of travelers' diarrhea caused by *Salmonella* in those patients traveling to developing countries varies but is not high.[100]

Between 1980 and 1984, the susceptibility data for *Salmonella* strains from different tropical countries were compiled to predict significant patterns or trends.[74] The percentages of resistance to ampicillin, tetracycline, chloramphenicol, and trimethoprim-sulfamethoxazole were quite variable, with the lowest rates found in Sri Lanka, the percentages ranging from 3% (resistance to chloramphenicol) to 10% (resistance to trimethoprim).[74] In recent studies (Table 6), the resistance to the above-mentioned antibiotics among *Salmonella* spp has also varied among the different developing countries, with Vietnam showing the lowest rate.[72] Overall, the frequencies of resistance to ampicillin, trimethoprim-sulfamethoxazole, chloramphenicol and tetracycline in *Salmonella* spp causing travelers' diarrhea in a recent study were 19, 9, 8, and 21%, respectively. No resistance to fluoroquinolones or third-generation cephalosporins was observed (see Table 6). The antimicrobial resistances of travel-related and nontravel-related isolates of *Salmonella* are very similar.[100]

Other Microorganisms Associated with Travelers' Diarrhea

Other potential bacterial pathogens, including *Aeromonas* spp, *Plesiomonas shigelloides, Yersinia enterocolitica,* and *V. cholerae* are known to cause travelers' diarrhea at a low prevalence. Among the *Aeromonas* genospecies, those considered of clinical relevance are *Aeromonas hydrophila, Aeromonas caviae,* and *Aeromonas veronii* biotype sobria. *A. veronii* biotype sobria and *Aeromonas caviae* are most frequently related to travelers' diarrhea.[101] Although only 18 *Aeromonas* spp were analyzed, a high level of resistance to ampicillin (100%) and a moderate level of resistance to chloramphenicol (31%), tetracycline (37.5%), and trimethoprim-sulfamethoxazole (12.5%) were observed, with no resistance to quinolones.[101] Little is known about the antimicrobial resistance of *P. shigelloides* causing travelers' diarrhea. The microorganism is variably susceptible in vitro to chloramphenicol, tetracycline, trimethoprim-sulfamethoxazole, aminoglycosides, fluoroquinolones, imipenem, and third-generation cephalosporins, and is naturally resistant to several antimicrobial agents such as penicillins and some cephalosporins, such as cefoperazone, ceftazidime, and cefepime.[102]

There are not many reports on the antimicrobial susceptibility of *Y. enterocolitica* as a cause of travelers' diarrhea. All the isolates were resistant to ampicillin but susceptible to tetracycline, nalidixic acid, and ciprofloxacin. Resistance to chloramphenicol and trimethoprim-sulfamethoxazole was less frequent (8%) (Vila, November 2006).

In a recent study performed in Indonesia, the percentage of resistance to several antimicrobial agents in *V. cholerae* was very low.[103] However, some *V. cholerae* isolates causing outbreaks as well as sporadic strains have been shown to be tetracycline or trimethoprim-sulfamethoxazole resistant, mainly when the outbreaks are caused by O139 strains.

Resistance Gene Transfer[104]

Bacteria can acquire resistance by mutations in existing genetic material or the acquisition of new genetic

Table 6 Frequency of Antimicrobial Resistance of *Salmonella spp* from Different Developing Countries and in Strains Causing Travelers' Diarrhea

	Resistance (%)							
Country	AMP	CHL	TET	SXT	NAL	CIP	CFX	Ref.
Kenya	45	4	76	41	7	0	0	86
Kenya	53	36	59	53	13	1	0	87
Thailand	28	26	59	37	21	< 1	---	72
Vietnam	3	7	13	10	0	0	---	72
TD*	21	11	32	21	---	0	70	100
TD	19	8	21	9	16	0	---	111

*TD = Salmonella spp causing travelers' diarrhea.
AMP = ampicillin; CFX = ceftriaxone; CHL = chloramphenicol; CIP = ciprofloxacin; NAL = nalidixic acid; SXT = trimethoprimsulfamethoxazole; TET = tetracycline.

material by horizontal transference. Gene transfer by incorporation of naked deoxyribonucleic acid (DNA) involves a process called "transformation." Among the species in which transformation is a common mechanism for gene transfer are *Acinetobacter baumannii*, *Haemophilus influenzae*, and *Streptococcus pneumoniae*. Probably the most common mechanism for acquiring genes is transferring extrachromosomal pieces of DNA called "plasmids," through cell-to-cell contact, a process called conjugation. Plasmids may contain many non-chromosomal genes, including genes for antibiotic resistance. The resistance genes themselves may lie on even smaller pieces of DNA called "transposons" which can independently move or transpose from one DNA vehicle (such as a plasmid) to another (such as a chromosome). Bacteriophages offer another means of spreading resistance genes. These bacterial viruses can pick up pieces of DNA from one organism (generally from the same species or genus) and transfer it to another. This process, called "transduction," will often involve transposons, which then find a site to integrate into the new host genome. This mechanism of transfer is limited by the narrow host range of the bacteriophage.

Recently, a specialized kind of transposon called an "integron" has been discovered as the basis for multidrug resistance. In simple terms, this vehicle consists of an integrase and a single promoter upstream from a number of different genes that are members of cassettes integrated behind the single promoter. The acquisition of these different genes leads to a multidrug-resistance genetic element. Thus, bacteria causing travelers' diarrhea have at their disposal any one or more of these many genetic mechanisms for acquiring drug resistance.

Mechanisms of Resistance

1. *β-lactams*

   Although no studies on the mechanisms of resistance to β-lactam antibiotics in ETEC strains have been published, we can assume that they are the same mechanisms of resistance as found in nonenteropathogenic *E. coli.* Most of the *E. coli* and *Shigella* spp strains synthesize low concentrations of the chromosomal AmpC cephalosporinase, which is not inhibited by clavulanic acid.[105] However, in less than 3% of the *E. coli* strains, this cephalosporinase is constitutively derepressed, generating a resistance pattern characterized by resistance to ampicillin, amoxicillin plus clavulanic acid, and first- and second-generation cephalosporins. In about 75% of the *E. coli* clinical isolates, the main mechanism of resistance to ampicillin is the production of a plasmid-mediated β-lactamase type TEM-1.[106] Other β-lactamases such as OXA-1 have been found to have a prevalence of between 1 and 5% in *E. coli* strains resistant to ampicillin. The gene encoding the OXA-1 β--lactamase has been located in an integron.[107] In *Shigella* spp, the main mechanism of resistance to β--lactam antibiotics is the synthesis of TEM-1-type and OXA-1-type β--lactamases,[83] with OXA-1 also being located in an integron, whereas TEM-1 would be plasmid-mediated. In a recent study it was reported that genes for OXA-1 were abundant, particularly among *S. flexneri* strains, whereas *S. sonnei* mainly harbored genes encoding OXA-2 and OXA-5.[83] Overall, OXA-type β-lactamases are more prevalent in *Shigella* spp strains than those of TEM-1-type, and an OXA-30 β-lactamase has been described in an *S. flexneri* strain.[108] In *Salmonella* spp, and mainly in *Salmonella typhimurium*, OXA-1 and PSE-1 are the two β-lactamases that are more often detected (Table 7).[109, 110] However, TEM-1 has been found to be more prevalent than OXA or PSE-like β-lactamases in *Salmonella* spp. isolates causing traveler's diarrhea.[111]

   Although the emergence of extended-spectrum variants of TEM and SHV enzymes, so called extended spectrum β-lactamases (ESBLs), is of great clinical concern, to date this phenomenon either does not seem to be a problem in developing countries or it has not been studied in depth. Still, several extended-spectrum β-lactamases have been described in different countries. *E. coli* TLA-1 β-lactamase and VEB-1 β-lactamase, which have activity against ceftazidime, have been detected in Mexico and Vietnam/Thailand, respectively.[112, 113] Moreover, TEM-26 and SHV5 have also been described in *E. coli* strains isolated in South Africa.[114] A SHV-11 β-lactamase found in an *S. dysenteriae* strain isolated in India has recently been described. This β-lactamase hydrolyzed oxacillin, cloxacillin, and oxyiminocephalosporins such as cefotaxime.[115] A new family of ESBLs, displaying greater affinity for cefotaxime than ceftazidime (CTX-M) has been detected in *E. coli, S. sonnei*, and *S. typhimurium* in South America.[116] Although β-lactamases constitute the major form of β-lactam resistance in *E. coli* and *Shigella* spp, other mechanisms of resistance such as decrease in outer membrane permeability, increase of active efflux systems, or

Table 7 Main Mechanisms of Resistance to Several Antimicrobial Agents and Patterns of Resistance in *Escherichia coli, Shigella* spp, and *Salmonella* spp

Antimicrobial Agent		Resistant Patterns			
CTX	Mechanisms of Resistance	AMP	TIC	FOX	CXM
β-Lactam Antibiotics	A) TEM-1, OXA-1, PSE-1 R	R	S	S	S
	B) ESBLs (TLA-1, VEB-1, CTX-M)	R	S	R	R R
Trimethoprim	DHFR 1, 5, 7, 12, 14, 15 and 17				
Chloramphenicol	CAT, CmlA, FloR				
Tetracycline	tet (A), tet (B), tet (C), tet (D), tet (G)				
		NAL	CIP		
Quinolones	A) Mutations in the gyrA gene	R	S		
	B) Mutations in the gyrA and parC genes*	R	R		

AMP = ampicillin; TIC = ticarcillin; FOX = cefoxitin; CXM = cefuroxime; CTX = cefotaxime; NAL = nalidixic acid; CIP = ciprofloxacin.
*In some clinical isolates an overexpression of an efflux pump as a concomitant mechanism of resistance to quinolones has also been shown.

decrease in the affinity for target penicillin binding proteins may also contribute to the increase of β-lactam resistance.

2. *Co-trimoxazole*
Trimethoprim-sulfamethoxazole is one of the antibiotic therapies against which enteropathogens have developed increased frequency of resistance. Trimethoprim resistance may be linked to the presence of one or more of the following four different mechanisms: auxotrophy in thymine/thymidine; impaired permeability; efflux pumps; alterations in chromosomal dihydrofolate reductase (DHFR); and/or presence of a plasmid-encoded trimethoprim-resistant gene, *dfr*. The latter mechanism is the most common mechanism of trimethoprim resistance.[117] To date, at least twenty dfr genes have been reported.[117] The corresponding enzymes differ, and thus can be distinguished by biochemical and biophysical properties. DHFR 1 is considered the most frequently found DHFR in Enterobacteriaceae. However, DHFR 5, DHFR 7, DHFR 12, DHFR 14, and DHFR 15 have also been recently described in *S. flexneri* and *S. sonnei* [83] and some of these genes are also integron-borne (see Table 7).[94] Meanwhile, in *Salmonella* spp. causing traveler's diarrhea, DHFR 1, DHFR 12, DHFR 14, and DHFR 17 have recently been reported.[111]

3. *Chloramphenicol*
The major mechanism of resistance to chloramphenicol is its inactivation by acetylation in a reaction catalyzed by chloramphenicol acetyltransferase.[118] Three genetically distinct groups of chloramphenicol acetyltransferase have been found so far, some inducible and others constitutive. This mechanism has been described in both *Shigella* spp and *Salmonella* spp.[83,89,111] Alternately, *cml*A and *flo*R genes, encoding chloramphenicol efflux pumps have recently been found in *S. typhimurium* and *S. kiambu* causing traveler's diarrhea, respectively.[111]

4. *Tetracyclines*
The two most important mechanisms of tetracycline resistance involve an inducible active efflux system that prevents the intracellular accumulation of this antibiotic, and a protein that protects the ribosome from tetracycline inhibition. The latter is exemplified by tet(O), which was originally described in *Campylobacter* spp.[119] Many genes encoding these efflux systems in gram-negative bacteria have been identified. Among them, *tet(A)*, *tet(B)*, *tet(C)*, and *tet(D)* are frequently found in *E. coli, Shigella* spp, *Salmonella* spp, *Aeromonas* spp, *P. shigelloides*, and *Vibrio* spp.[119] The majority of the Tet determinants are often associated with transferable genetic elements such as transposons.[120]

5. *Quinolones*
Quinolone resistance has been steadily rising over the last decade.[121] The main mechanisms of resistance to this family of antimicrobial agents are mutations in the *gyr*A and *par*C genes encoding the A subunits of the DNA gyrase and topoisomerase IV, which are the protein targets for quinolones; and reduced quinolone accumulation in the cells caused by increased efflux of the drug out of the cell.[121] In ETEC and EAEC strains, a low level of resistance to ciprofloxacin and a high level of resistance to nalidixic acid have been associated with a mutation of the amino acid codon Ser-83 of the *gyr*A gene, which produces a change from Ser to Leu or Ala. Meanwhile, the high level of

resistance to both ciprofloxacin and nalidixic acid is associated with a double mutation in the amino acid codons Ser-83 and Asp-87 of the *gyr*A gene plus a double mutation in the amino acid codons Ser-80 and Glu-84 of the *par*C gene.[73] A similar mechanism can explain the quinolone resistance in *Shigella* spp and in *Salmonella* spp (see Table 7).[110,122]

However, in *C. jejuni*, the situation is slightly different because a mutation in the *gyr*A gene (Thr86 to Ile or Lys) is enough to produce a high level of resistance to both ciprofloxacin and nalidixic acid.[123] A multidrug efflux mechanism has been reported in *C. jejuni*,[124] which can explain the intrinsic resistance to several antimicrobial agents including quinolones. Therefore, in *C. jejuni*, which shows this basal intrinsic quinolone resistance, a mutation in the *gyr*A gene is enough to generate a high level of resistance to these antimicrobial agents, explaining the difference from *Enterobacteriaceae*. Multidrug efflux systems similar to that described above for *C. jejuni* have been shown in *E. coli*, *Shigella* spp, and *Salmonella* spp. Among the *Enterobacteriaceae*, the most in-depth studies have been performed on AcrAB, which consists of an inner membrane pump (AcrB) and an outer membrane protein (TolC) linked together by a membrane fusion protein (AcrA). This system affects a wide range of substrates such as quinolones, tetracycline, chloramphenicol, ampicillin, and rifampicin.[125,126] Several transcriptional factors (eg, MarA, SoxS, and Rob) can induce expression of the AcrAB efflux pump.[127] Two plasmid-mediated quinolone resistance mechanisms have recently been described. The first is associated with the presence of the *qnr* gene, encoding the Qnr protein, which can protect the DNA gyrase from quinolones. This mechanism has been detected in several *Enterobacteriaceae* including *E. coli*, *Shigella spp.* and *Salmonella spp.* The other mechanism is related to a variant aminoglycoside acetyltransferase (AAC(6')-Ib-cr) capable of modifying ciprofloxacin. This second mechanism seems to be more prevalent than the Qnr proteins.[128] However, the prevalence of both mechanisms has not been investigated in *Enterobacteriaceae* causing travelers' diarrhea.

Conclusion

Drug resistance among bacteria associated with travelers' diarrhea continues to increase, particularly to inexpensive, first-line, broad-spectrum antibiotics. High frequency of resistance to trimethoprim-sulfamethoxazole in many parts of the developing world now limits the effective use of this drug for persons traveling to such areas. Furthermore, the introduction of newer drugs, such as fluoroquinolones, has been followed relatively quickly by the emergence and dissemination of resistant strains. In the meantime, azithromycin and new fluoroquinolones show promise as possible replacements for the older antimicrobial agents. However, it should be taken into consideration that a significant percentage of quinolone resistance has been reported in isolates, mainly *C. jejuni*, in travelers returning from India. Therefore, empiric treatment with fluoroquinolones should be avoided when treating diarrhea in these travelers. Nonabsorbable antibiotics, such as rifaximin, may supplant "classical" antibiotic treatment, although more studies are needed to assure its reliability.

References

1. DuPont HL, Ericsson CD. Prevention and treatment of travelers' diarrhea. N Engl J Med 1993;328:1821–7.
2. Ericsson CD. Travelers' diarrhea: epidemiology, prevention and self-treatment. Infect Dis Clin North Am 1998; 12:285–303.
3. Gascón J, Vila J, Valls ME. Etiology of travelers' diarrhea in Spanish travellers to developing countries. Eur J Epidemiol 1993;9:217–23.
4. Land T. Combating counterfeit drugs. Nature 1992;355: 192.
5. McGregor A. Counterfeit drugs flood developing world. Lancet 1997;350:1690.
6. Pecoul B, Chirac P, Trouiller P, Pinel J. Access to essential drugs in poor countries: a lost battle? J Am Med Assoc 1999;281:361–7.
7. Okeke I, Lamikanra A. Quality and bioavailability of tetracycline capsules in a Nigerian semi-urban community. Int J Antimicrob Agents 1995;5:245–50.
8. Agom JK, Akannii AO, Dawodu TO. Quality of ampicillin/cloxacillin preparations on the Nigerian market. Nigerian J Pharmacol 1990;21:36–8.
9. Gustafsson LL, Wide K. Marketing of obsolete antibiotics in Central America. Lancet 1981;1:31–3.
10. Ali HM, Homeida MM, Abdeen MA. Drug dumping in donations to Sudan. Lancet 1988;333:538–9.
11. Kigotho AW. Kenya's government tackles influx of substandard drugs. Lancet 1997;350:1690.
12. Okeke IN, Lamikanra A, Edelman R. Socioeconomic and behavioral factors leading to acquired bacterial resistance to antibiotics in developing countries. Emerg Infect Dis 1999;5:18–27.
13. Hogerzel HV, Battersby A, Srdanovic V, Stjernstrom NE. Stability of essential drugs during shipment to the tropics. Br Med J 1992;304:210–2.

14. Shakoor O, Taylor RB, Behrens RH. Assessment of the incidence of substandard drugs in developing countries. Trop Med Int Health 1997;2:839–45.

15. Ballereau F, Prazuck T, Schrive I, et al. Stability of essential drugs in the field: results of a study conducted over a two-year period in Burkina-Faso. Am J Trop Med Hyg 1997;57:31–6.

16. Ringerts S, Nuhe L, Krantz I, et al. Prevalence of potential respiratory disease bacteria in children in Ethiopia: antimicrobial susceptibility of the pathogens and use of antibiotics among the children. Acta Pediatr 1993;82:843–9.

17. Gascón J, Vargas M, Schellenberg D, et al. Diarrhea in children under 5 years of age from Ifakara, Tanzania: a case-control study. J Clin Microbiol 2000;38:4459–62.

18. Lansang MA, Lucas-Aquino R, Tupasi TE, et al. Purchase of antibiotics without prescription in Manila, Philippines. Inappropriate choices and doses. J Clin Epidemiol 1990; 43:61–7.

19. Guyon AB, Barman A, Ahmed JU, et al. A baseline survey on use of drugs at the primary health care level in Bangladesh. Bull World Health Organ 1994;72:265–71.

20. Bojalil R, Calva JJ. Antibiotic misuse in diarrhea. A household survey in a Mexican community. J Clin Epidemiol 1994;47:147–56.

21. Hui L, Li XS, Zeng XJ, et al. Patterns and determinants of use of antibiotics for acute respiratory tract infection in children in China. Pediatr Infect Dis J 1997;16:560–4.

22. Reyes H, Guiscafre H, Muñoz O, et al. Antibiotic noncompliance and waste in upper respiratory infections and acute diarrhea. J Clin Epidemiol 1997;50:1297–304.

23. Meers PD. Infection control in developing countries. J Hosp Infect 1988;11Suppl A:406–10.

24. Rasniraul L, Suthienkul O, Echevarria PD, et al. Foods as a source of enteropathogens causing childhood diarrhea in Thailand. Am J Trop Med Hyg 1988;39:97–102.

25. Rahim Z, Aziz KM. Enterotoxigenic, hemolytic activity and antibiotic resistance of Aeromonas spp isolated from freshwater prawn marketed in Dhaka, Bangladesh. Microbiol Immunol 1994;38:773–8.

26. Barza M, Gorbach SL. The need to improve antimicrobial use in agriculture: ecological and human health consequences. Clin Infect Dis 2002;34Suppl 3:S71–144.

27. Sokari TG, Ibiebele DD, Ottih RM. Antibiotic resistance among coliforms and Pseudomonas spp. from bodies of water around Port Harcourt, Nigeria. J Appl Bacteriol 1988;64:355–9.

28. Johnston AM. Animals and antibiotics. Int J Antimicrob Agents 2001;18:291–4.

29. McEwen SA, Fedorka-Cray PJ. Antimicrobial use and resistance in animals. Clin Infect Dis 2002;34Suppl 3:S93–106.

30. Wegener HC. Antibiotics in animal feed and their role in resistance development. Curr Opin Microbiol 2003;6:439–45.

31. Kelly L, Smith DL, Snary EL, et al. Animal growth promoters: to ban or not to ban? A risk assessment approach. Int J Antimicrob Agents 2004;24:205–12.

32. Dibner JJ, Richards JD. Antibiotic growth promoters in agriculture: history and mode of action. Poult Sci 2005;4: 634–43.

33. Turnidge J. Antibiotic use in animals--prejudices, perceptions and realities. J Antimicrob Chemother. 2004;53:26–7.

34. Piddock LJ. Does the use of antimicrobial agents in veterinary medicine and animal husbandry select antibiotic-resistant bacteria that infect man and compromise antimicrobial chemotherapy? J Antimicrob Chemother 1996;38:1–3.

35. McDermott PF, Bodeis SM, English LL, et al. Ciprofloxacin resistance in Campylobacter jejuni evolves rapidly in chickens treated with fluoroquinolones. J Infect Dis 2002;185:837–40.

36. Delsol AA, Sunderland J, Woodward MJ, et al. Emergence of fluoroquinolone resistance in the native Campylobacter coli population of pigs exposed to enrofloxacin. J Antimicrob Chemother 2004;53:872–4.

37. Delsol AA, Woodward MJ, Roe JM. Effect of a 5 day enrofloxacin treatment on Salmonella enterica serotype Typhimurium DT104 in the pig. J Antimicrob Chemother 2004;53:396–8.

38. McDermott PF, Cullen P, Hubert SK, et al. Changes in antimicrobial susceptibility of native Enterococcus faecium in chickens fed virginiamycin. Appl Environ Microbiol 2005;71:4986–91.

39. Smith KE, Besser JM, Hedberg CW, et al. Quinolone-resistant Campylobacter jejuni infections in Minnesota, 1992–1998. Investigation Team. N Engl J Med 1999;340: 1525–32.

40. White DG, Zhao S, Sudler R, et al. The isolation of antibiotic-resistant salmonella from retail ground meats. N Engl J Med 2001;345:1147–54.

41. Zhao S, Qaiyumi S, Friedman S, et al. Characterization of Salmonella enterica serotype newport isolated from humans and food animals. J Clin Microbiol 2003;41: 5366–71.

42. Gupta A, Fontana J, Crowe C, et al. Emergence of multidrug-resistant Salmonella enterica serotype Newport infections resistant to expanded-spectrum cephalosporins in the United States. J Infect Dis 2003;188:1707–16.

43. Berge AC, Adaska JM, Sischo WM. Use of antibiotic susceptibility patterns and pulsed-field gel electrophoresis to compare historic and contemporary isolates of multi-drug-resistant Salmonella enterica subsp. enterica serovar Newport. Appl Environ Microbiol 2004;70:318–23.

44. Zaidi MB, McDermott PF, Fedorka-Cray P, et al. Nontyphoidal Salmonella from human clinical cases, asymptomatic children, and raw retail meats in Yucatan, Mexico. Clin Infect Dis 2006;42:21–8.

45. Levy SB, FitzGerald GB, Macone AB. Changes in intestinal flora of farm personnel after introduction of a tetracycline-supplemented feed on a farm. N Engl J Med 1976; 295:583–8.

46. Levy SB, FitzGerald GB, Macone AB. Spread of antibiotic resistance plasmids from chicken to chicken and from chicken to man. Nature 1976;260:40–2.

47. Chaslus-Dancla EP, Pohl P, Meurisse M, et al. High genetic homology between plasmids of human and animal origins conferring resistance to the aminoglycosides gentamicin and apramycin. Antimicrob Agents Chemother 1991;35:590–3.

48. Fey PD, Safranek TJ, Rupp ME, et al. Ceftriaxone-resistant Salmonella infection acquired by a child from cattle. N Engl J Med 2000;342:1242–9.

49. Ait Melloul A, Hassani L, Rafouk L. Salmonella contamination of vegetables irrigated with untreated wastewater. World J Microbiol Biotechnol 2001;17:207–9.

50. Hutchison ML, Walters LD, Avery SM, et al. Levels of zoonotic agents in British livestock manures. Lett Appl Microbiol 2004;39:207–14.

51. World Health Organization. Joint FAO/OIE/WHO expert workshop on non-human antimicrobial usage and antimicrobial resistance: scientific assessment. Geneva, Switzerland. 2004.

52. Helms M, Vastrup P, Gerner-Smidt P, Molbak K. Excess mortality associated with antimicrobial drug-resistant Salmonella typhimurium. Emerg Infect Dis 2002;8:490–5.

53. Martin LJ, Fyfe M, Dore K, et al. Increased burden of illness associated with antimicrobial-resistant Salmonella enterica serotype typhimurium infections. J Infect Dis 2004;189:377–84.

54. Nelson JM, Smith KE, Vugia DJ, et al. Prolonged diarrhea due to ciprofloxacin-resistant Campylobacter infection. J Infect Dis 2004;190:1150–7.

55. Varma JK, Molbak K, Barrett TJ, et al. Antimicrobial-resistant nontyphoidal Salmonella is associated with excess bloodstream infections and hospitalizations. J Infect Dis 2005;191:554–61.

56. Lipsitch M, Singer RS, Levin BR. Antibiotics in agriculture: when is it time to close the barn door? Proc Natl Acad Sci U S A 2002;99:5752–4.

57. Smith DL, Harris AD, Johnson JA, et al. Animal antibiotic use has an early but important impact on the emergence of antibiotic resistance in human commensal bacteria. Proc Natl Acad Sci U S A 2002;99:6434–9.

58. Phillips I, Casewell M, Cox T, et al. Antibiotic use in animals. J Antimicrob Chemother 2004;53:885.

59. O'Brien T, Pla MP, Mayer KH, et al. Intercontinental spread of a new antibiotic resistance gene on an epidemic plasmid. Science 1985;230:87–8.

60. Lamikanra A, Fayinka ST, Olusanya O. A study of low trimethoprim resistance in faecal isolates obtained from apparently healthy Nigerian students. FEMS Microbiol Lett 1989;50:275–8.

61. Lamikanra A, Okeke IN. A study of the effect of the urban/rural divide on the incidence of antibiotic resistance in Escherichia coli. Biomed Lett 1997;55:91–7.

62. Walson JL, Marshall B, Pokrel BM, et al. Fecal carriage of antibiotic resistance in Nepal reflects proximity to Katmandu. J Infect Dis 2001;184:1163–9.

63. Rosas I, Salinas E, Yela A, et al. Escherichia coli in settled-dust and air samples collected in residential environments in Mexico City. Appl Environ Microbiol 1997;63: 4093–5.

64. Murray BE, Mathewson JJ, DuPont HL, et al. Emergence of resistant fecal Escherichia coli in travelers not taking prophylactic antimicrobial agents. Antimicrob Agents Chemother 1990;34:515–8.

65. Wenzel P. Airline travel and infection. N Engl J Med 1996; 334:981–2.

66. Hedberg CW, Levine WC, White KE, et al. An international foodborne outbreak of shigellosis associated with a commercial airline. J Am Med Assoc 1992;268:3208–12.

67. Minoose A, Rickman L. Infectious diseases on cruise ships. Clin Infect Dis 1999;29:737–44.

68. Nataro JP, Kaper JB. Diarrheagenic Escherichia coli. Clin Microbiol Rev 1998;11:142–201.

69. Vargas M, Gascón J, Gallardo F, et al. Prevalence of diarrheagenic Escherichia coli strains detected by PCR in patients with travelers' diarrhea. Clin Microbiol Infect 1998;4:682–8.

70. Jiang ZD, Mathewson JJ, Ericsson CD, et al. Characterization of enterotoxigenic Escherichia coli strains in patients with travelers' diarrhea acquired in Guadalajara, Mexico, 1992–1997. J Infect Dis 2000;181: 779–82.

71. Vila J, Vargas M, Casals C, et al. Antimicrobial resistance of diarrheagenic Escherichia coli isolated from children under the age of 5 years from Ifakara, Tanzania. Antimicrob Agents Chemother 1999;43:3022–4.

72. Isenbarger DW, Hoge CW, Srijan A, et al. Comparative antibiotic resistance of diarrheal pathogens from Vietnam and Thailand, 1996–1999. Emerg Infect Dis 2002;8:175–80.

73. Vila J, Vargas M, Ruiz J, et al. Quinolone resistance in enterotoxigenic Escherichia coli causing diarrhea in travelers to India in comparison with other geographical areas. Antimicrob Agents Chemother 2000;44: 1731–3.

74. Murray BE. Resistance of Shigella, Salmonella, and other selected enteric pathogens to antimicrobial agents. Rev Infect Dis 1986;8Suppl 2:S172–81.

75. Nguyen TV, Le PV, Le CH, Weintraub A. Antibiotic resistance in diarrheagenic Escherichia coli and Shigella strains isolated from children in Hanoi, Vietnam. Antimicrob Agents Chemother 2005;49:816–9.

76. Vila J, Vargas M, Ruiz J, et al. Susceptibility patterns of enteroaggregative Escherichia coli associated with traveller's diarrhoea: emergence of quinolone resistance. J Med Microbiol 2001;50:996–1000.

77. Sang WK, Oundo JO, Mwituria JK, et al. Multidrug-resistant enteroaggregative Escherichia coli associated with persistent diarrhea in Kenyan children. Emerg Infect Dis 1997;3:373–4.

78. Okeke IN, Lamikanra A, Czeczulin J, et al. Heterogeneous virulence of enteroaggregative Escherichia coli strains isolated from children in Southwest Nigeria. J Infect Dis 2000;181:252–60.

79. Yamamoto T, Echeverria P, Yokota T. Drug resistance and adherence to human intestines of enteroaggregative Escherichia coli. J Infect Dis 1992;165:744–9.

80. Sierra JM, Ruiz J, Navia MM, et al. In vitro activity of rifaximin against enteropathogens producing travelers' diarrhea. Antimicrob Agents Chemother 2001;45:643–4.

81. Torres ME, Pirez MC, Schelotto F, et al. Etiology of children's diarrhea in Montevideo, Uruguay: associated pathogens and unusual isolates. J Clin Microbiol 2001;39: 2134–9.

82. Vila J, Vargas M, Ruiz J, et al. Isolation of verotoxin-producing Escherichia coli O-rough:K1:H7 from two patients with travelers' diarrhea. J Clin Microbiol 1997; 35:2279–82.

83. Navia MM, Gascón J, Vila J. Analysis of the mechanisms of resistance to several antimicrobial agents in Shigella spp. causing travellers' diarrhoea. Clin Microbiol Infect 2005;11:1044–6.

84. Lima AAM, Lima NL, Pinho MCN, et al. High frequency of strains multiply resistant to ampicillin, trimethoprim-sulfamethoxazole, streptomycin, chloramphenicol, and tetracycline isolated from patients with shigellosis in Northeastern Brazil during the period 1988 to 1993. Antimicrob Agents Chemother 1995;39:256–9.

85. Dutta S, Sinha T, Dutta P. Serotypes and antimicrobial susceptibility patterns of Shigella species isolated from children in Calcutta, India. Eur J Clin Microb Infect Dis 1998;17:298–9.

86. Shapiro RL, Kumar L, Phillips-Howard P, et al. Antimicrobial-resistant bacterial diarrhea in rural western Kenya. J Infect Dis 2001;183:1701–4.

87. Brooks JT, Chieng JB, Kumar L, et al. Surveillance for bacterial diarrhea and antimicrobial resistance in rural Western Kenya, 1997–2003. Clin Infect Dis 2006;43:393–401.

88. Bogaerts J, Verhaegen J, Munyabikali JP, et al. Antimicrobial resistance and serotypes of Shigella isolates in Kigali, Rwanda (1983 to 1993): increasing frequency of multiple resistance. Diagn Microbiol Infect Dis 1997;28: 165–71.

89. Navia MM, Capitano L, Ruiz J, et al. Typing and characterization of mechanisms of resistance of Shigella spp isolated from feces of children under 5 years of age from Ifakara, Tanzania. J Clin Microbiol 1999;37:3113–7.

90. Vila J, Gascón J, Abdalla S, et al. Antimicrobial resistance of Shigella isolates causing travelers' diarrhea. Antimicrob Agents Chemother 1994;38:2668–70.

91. Lee JC, Oh JY, Kim KS, et al. Antimicrobial resistance of Shigella sonnei in Korea during the last two decades. APMIS 2001;109:228–34.

92. Ries AA, Wells JG, Olivola MD, et al. Epidemic Shigella dysenteriae type 1 in Burundi: panresistance and implications for prevention. J Infect Dis 1994;169:1035–41.

93. Gallardo F, Gascón J, Ruiz J, et al. Campylobacter jejuni as a cause of traveller's diarrhea: clinical features and antimicrobial susceptibility. J Travel Med 1998;5:23–6.

94. Salazar-Lindo E, Sack RB, Chea-Woo E, et al. Early treatment with erythromycin of Campylobacter jejuni-associated dysentery in children. J Pediatr 1986;109:355–60.

95. Kuschner Trofa AF, Thomas RJ. Use of azithromycin for the treatment of Campylobacter enteritis in travelers to Thailand, an area where ciprofloxacin resistance is prevalent. Clin Infect Dis 1995;21:536–41.

96. Ruiz J, Marco F, Oliveira I, et al. Trends in antimicrobial resistance in Campylobacter spp. causing traveler's diarrhea., APMIS; 2007.

97. Hakanen A, Jousimies-Somer H, Siitonen A, et al. Fluoroquinolone resistance in Campylobacter jejuni isolates in travelers returning to Finland: association of ciprofloxacin resistance to travel destination. Emerg Infect Dis 2003;9:267–70.

98. Goosens H, DeMol P Coignan H, et al. Comparative in vitro activities of aztreonam, ciprofloxacin, norfloxacin, ofloxacin, HR 810 (a new cephalosporin), RU 28965 (a new macrolide) and other agents against enteropathogens. Antimicrob Agents Chemother 1985;27:388–92.

99. Endtz HP, Ruijs GJ, Van Klingeren B, et al. Quinolone resistance in Campylobacter isolates from man and poultry following the introduction of fluoroquinolones in veterinary medicine. J Antimicrob Chemother 1991;27: 199–208.

100. Vila J, Gascón J, Abdalla S, et al. Antimicrobial resistance of nontyphoidal Salmonella isolates in traveller's diarrhea. J Travel Med 1995;2:45–7.

101. Vila J, Ruiz J, Gallardo F, et al. Aeromonas spp. and traveler's diarrhea: clinical features and antimicrobial resistance. Emerg Infect Dis 2003;9:552–5.

102. Stock I, Wiedemann B. Natural antimicrobial susceptibilities of Plesiomonas shigelloides strains. J Antimicrob Chemother 2001;48:803–11.

103. Tjaniadi P, Lesmana M, Subekti D, Machpud N, et al. Antimicrobial resistance of bacterial pathogens associated with diarrheal patients in Indonesia. Am J Trop Med Hyg 2003;68:666–70.

104. Levy SB, BMarshall. Antibacterial resistance worldwide: causes, challenges and responses. Nature Med 2004;10: S122–9.

105. Normak S, Gundstrom T, Bergstrom S. Susceptibility to penicillins and cephalosporins in lactamase producing strains of Escherichia coli and relative amount of β-lactamase produced by these strains. Scand J Infect Dis 1980;25:23–9.

106. Liu PYF, Gur D, Hall LMC, Livermore DM. Survey of the prevalence of β-lactamases amongst 1,000 gram-negative bacilli isolated consecutively at the Royal London Hospital. J Antimicrob Chemother 1992;30:429–47.

107. Hall RM, Collins CM. Antibiotic resistance in gram-negative bacteria: the role of gene cassettes and integrons. Drug Resist Updates 1998;1:109–19.

108. Siu LK, Lo JYC, Yuen KY, et al. β-lactamases in Shigella flexneri isolates from Hong Kong and Shanghai and a novel OXA-1-like β-lactamase, OXA-30. Antimicrob Agents Chemother 2000;44:2034–8.

109. Gallardo F, Ruiz J, Marco F, et al. Increase in the incidence of resistance to ampicillin, chloramphenicol and trimethoprim in clinical isolates of Salmonella serotype typhimurium with investigation of molecular epidemiology and mechanisms of resistance. J Med Microbiol 1999; 48:367–74.

110. Ruiz J, Capitano L, Nuñez L, et al. Mechanisms of resistance to ampicillin, chloramphenicol and quinolones in multiresistant Salmonella typhimurium strains isolated from fish. J Antimicrob Chemother 1999;43:699–701.

111. Cabrera R, Ruiz J, Marco F, et al. Mechanism of resistance to several antimicrobial agents in Salmonella clinical isolates causing traveler's diarrhea. Antimicrob Agents Chemother 2004;48:3934–9.

112. Silva J, Aguilar C, Ayala G, et al. TLA-1: a new plasmid-mediated extended spectrum β-lactamase from Escherichia coli. Antimicrob Agents Chemother 2000;44: 997–1003.

113. Poirel L, Naas T, Guibert M, et al. Molecular and biochemical characterization of VEB-1, a novel class A extended spectrum β-lactamase encoded by an Escherichia coli integron gene. Antimicrob Agents Chemother 1999;43:573–81.

114. Pitout JDD, Thomson KS, Hanson ND, et al. β-Lactamases responsible for resistance to expanded spectrum cephalosporins in Klebsiella pneumoniae, Escherichia coli, and Proteus mirabilis isolates recovered in South Africa. Antimicrob Agents Chemother 1998;42: 1350–4.

115. Ahamed J, Kundu M. Molecular characterization of the SHV-11 β-lactamase of Shigella dysenteriae. Antimicrob Agents Chemother 1999;43:2081–3.

116. Radice M, Power P, Di Conza J, Gutkind G. Early dissemination of CTX-M-derived enzymes in South America. Antimicrob Agents Chemother 2002;46:602–3.

117. Amyes SGB, Towner KJ. Trimethoprim resistance: epidemiology and molecular aspects. J Med Microbiol 1990;31:1–19.

118. Lovett PS. Translational attenuation as the regulator of inducible cat genes. J Bacteriol 1990;172:1–6.

119. Levy SB, McMurry LM, Barbosa TM, et al. Nomenclature for new tetracycline resistance determinants. Antimicrob Agents Chemother 1999;43:1523–4.

120. Chopra I, Roberts M. Tetracycline antibiotics: mode of action, applications, molecular biology, and epidemiology of bacterial resistance. Microbiol Mol Biol Rev 2001;65: 232–60.

121. Vila J. Fluoroquinolone resistance. In: White DG, Alekshun MN, McDermott PF, editors. Frontiers in Antimicrobial Resistance. Washington: ASM Press; 2005. p. 41–52.

122. Rahman M, Mauf G, Levy J, et al. Detection of 4-quinolone resistance mutations in the gyrA gene of Shigella dysenteriae type 1 by PCR. Antimicrob Agents Chemother 1994;38:2488–91.

123. Ruiz J, Goñi P Marco F, et al. Increased resistance to quinolones in Campylobacter jejuni: a genetic analysis of gyrA gene mutations in quinolone-resistant clinical isolates. Microbiol Immunol 1998;42:223–6.

124. Lin J, Michel LO, Zhang Q. CmeABC functions as a multidrug efflux system in Campylobacter jejuni. Antimicrob Agents Chemother 2002;46:2124–31.

125. Ma D, Cook DN, Hearst JE, Nikaido H. Efflux pumps and drug resistance in gram-negative bacteria. Trends Microbiol 1994;2:489–93.

126. Nikaido H, Basina M, Nguyen VY, Rosenberg EY. Multidrug efflux pump AcrAB of Salmonella typhimurium excretes only those β-lactam antibiotics containing lipophilic side chains. J Bacteriol 1998;180:4686–92.

127. Alekskun MN, Levy SB. The mar regulon: multiple resistance to antibiotics and other toxic chemicals. Trends Microbiol 1999;7:410–3.

128. Robicsek A, Jacoby GA, Hooper DC. The worldwide emergence of plasmid-mediated quinolone resistance. Lancet Infect Dis 2006;6:629–40.

CHAPTER 6

PATHOGENESIS

DAVID B. HUANG, MD, PhD

JAMES P. NATARO, MD, PhD

The pathogenesis of infectious disease involves a complex and still mysterious interplay among the pathogen's virulence factors and determinants of the host's susceptibility. The pathogen's attack is mediated by colonization factors, host-damaging toxins, and sinister mechanisms of immune evasion. On the host side, an intact integument is the most reliable anti-infective defense, though the mucosal surfaces are buttressed by secreted antibodies and the cellular components of the immune system. To comprehend the picture of human disease, we must also grasp variations in virulence among pathogenic strains, the ecology of microorganisms, factors influencing the transmissibility and infectious dose, as well as the myriad vagaries of host susceptibility including but not limited to age, gastrointestinal (GI) physiology, and innate and acquired mucosal immunity. Thus, despite over a century of research in bacterial pathogenesis, we have only begun to understand the nature of pathogenicity. Here, we consider pathogenesis from the side of the pathogen; a more thorough discussion of host susceptibility and genetic risk factors in enteric disease will be discussed in Chapter 16, "Genetic Susceptibility to Enteric Infections."

A long list of microbial agents can produce infection of the human GI tract. In travelers' diarrhea, the most commonly implicated organisms are enterotoxigenic *E. coli* (ETEC), enteroaggregative *E. coli* (EAEC), *Campylobacter jejuni*, and Shigella spp., though a large number of other organisms are implicated in various settings.[1,2] In this chapter, we will focus on the most common organisms that cause travelers' diarrhea, as well as several that elicit particularly severe infections. However, common causes of acute infectious diarrhea that are not important causes of travelers' diarrhea are not discussed here. Both the species and strain of the organism are important in predicting the virulence of the pathogen. The majority of *E. coli* strains are normal aerobic colonic flora. They become pathogenic when they acquire genes or plasmids that encode various toxins or confer invasiveness. The six major pathotypes of diarrheagenic *E. coli* are ETEC, enteropathogenic *E. coli* (EPEC), EAEC, enterohemmorhagic *E. coli* (EHEC), enteroinvasive *E. coli* (EIEC), and diffusely adherent *E. coli* (DAEC).[3] ETEC and EAEC are commonly reported causes of traveler's diarrhea; EPEC may cause severe and persistent traveler's diarrhea in infants.

The number of microorganisms consumed, their inherent virulence, and the susceptibility of the host are the key determinants for development of disease. All enteric pathogens infect by the fecal-oral route. Those with particularly low infectious doses (e.g., Shigella spp. and EHEC) are capable of person-to-person spread, whereas those with lower infectivity are more commonly spread via a food or water vehicle. Volunteer challenge studies have demonstrated that fewer than 200 viable cells of Shigella readily produce disease in healthy adults.[4] This low infective dose of Shigella may allow the transmission of Shigella spp. through the touch of an infected person or indirect contamination of food, which may occur via contaminated flies or utensils.[5,6] Some intestinal parasites also feature a low infectious dose. Only 10 to 100 cysts of *Entamoeba histolytica* and *Giardia lamblia* are required to cause diarrhea. Fortunately, other enteric pathogens typically cause disease only after exposure to higher infectious doses. For example, over 10^7 of pathogenic *Vibrio cholerae* and ETEC are required for efficient infection.[7]

Pathogenesis of Infectious Diarrhea

Enteric pathogens cause diarrhea by a small number of general strategies, typically described as mucosal adherence with elaboration of enterotoxins and cytotoxins, invasion of the epithelium, and signal transduction. The pathogenic schema of enteric pathogens is summarized in Table 1.

Table 1 Pathogenic Mechanism of Various Microorganisms

Pathogen	Attachment, HEp-2 Cell Adherence	Invasiveness	Toxin Production	Primary Mechanism of Diarrhea
ETEC		No	Yes (LT, ST)	Stimulation of cellular kinases
EPEC	Intimate attachment, localized adherence	No	No	Signal transduction
EHEC	Intimate attachment	No	Yes (Shiga toxin)	Selective killing of absorptive villus, inflammatory response
EAEC	Aggregative	Perhaps	Cytotoxin	Enhancement of mucous secretion, exfoliation of epithelial cells
Shigella spp.		Yes	Yes (Shiga toxin)	Selective killing of absorptive villus, inflammatory response
Salmonella spp.		Yes	Yes	Unclear, possible inflammatory response
Campylobacter spp.		Yes	Cytotoxin	Enterocyte damage, inflammatory response
V. parahemolyticus		Yes	Cytotoxin	Unclear
Aeromonas spp.		Yes	Yes	Unclear
Plesiomonas spp.		Yes	Yes	Unclear
B. fragilis		Yes	Yes (BFT)	Stimulation of Cl– secretion
Rotavirus		No	Yes (NSP4)	Inhibition of Na+-D-glucose symporter
Norovirus		Yes	No	Unclear
Cryptosporidium parvum		No	Yes	Reduction of nutrient transporters
Cyclospora		No	Unknown	Unclear
G. lamblia		Rarely	No	Mechanical irritation, inflammatory response
E. histolytica		Yes	Yes	Degradation of matrix proteins, inflammatory response and mucosal ulceration

BFT = bacteroides fragilis toxin; EAEC = enteroaggregative E. coli; EHEC = enterohemorrhagic E. coli; EPEC = enteropathogenic E. coli; ETEC, enterotoxigenic E. coli; LT = heat-labile toxin; NSP4 = nonstructural protein 4; ST = heat-stable toxin.

ADHERENCE

Regardless of their ultimate strategy, all enteric pathogens must begin by colonizing the epithelial surface. Several adherence mechanisms have been described. Most notable are the adherence fimbriae, the prototypes of which are the Colonization Factor Antigens (CFAs) of ETEC. These organelles bind to specific ligands on enterocytes in a lectin-like fashion.[8] Whereas the CFAs are thought to simply tether the bacterium to the epithelium, the Bundle-forming Pilus of EPEC may execute a complex phenotype including retraction and dispersion. In addition to the fimbrial antigens, outer membrane proteins may also contribute to adherence and colonization. The EPEC outer membrane protein intimin binds to one or more cellular receptors (and the translocated intimin receptor Tir), whereupon it contributes to an intimate and subversive bacteria-cell interaction.[3,9]

INVASION OF THE MUCOSA

Enteric pathogens such as Shigella spp. and some enteroinvasive strains of *E. coli* cause diarrhea by adhering to and invading the intestinal mucosa. Shigella is able to induce phagocytosis by the intestinal epithelial cells, enter the cytoplasm, and co-opt the epithelial cell cytoskeleton by virtue of a panoply of enterotoxins secreted through a molecular syringe, termed the type III secretion system (T3SS).[10,11] After entry, Shigella organisms lyse the phagosomes, multiply in the cytoplasm, and spread to contiguous epithelial cells. This movement is medicated by polymerization of filamentous actin (F-actin); the bacteria thereby project themselves into adjacent host cells, ultimately causing destruction and inflammation of the mucosa.[12] Shigella spp. and some strains of *E. coli* are also able to produce cytotoxins, notably Shiga toxin. The absorption of Shiga toxin into the systemic circulation is responsible for the hemolytic uremic syndrome (HUS), seen after infection with *S. dysenteriae* 1 and EHEC.

TOXIN PRODUCTION

Infectious diarrhea can be divided into two clinical syndromes. Noninflammatory diarrhea is generally caused by viruses or enterotoxin-producing bacteria. It affects primarily the small intestine rather than the large intestine. The pathogen typically adheres to the intestinal mucosa, secretes enterotoxins and/or cytotoxins, but does not invade or damage the enterocytes or epithelial cells. The toxins in turn elicit a complex series of biochemical reactions inside the epithelial cells, which ultimately lead to excessive water and ion secretion. In this type of diarrhea, fecal leukocytes may not be present due to an absence of significant mucosal destruction.

Inflammatory diarrhea generally affects the large intestine and is commonly caused by invasive or cytotoxin-producing bacteria and protozoa. The pathogen invades and disrupts the colonic mucosal lining, which leads to extravasation of blood and serous fluid into the intestinal lumen. Microscopic examination of the stool reveals the presence of fecal leukocytes. Inflammatory diarrhea is more commonly associated with systemic manifestations of enteric disease compared to noninflammatory diarrhea. Patients with inflammatory diarrhea may have febrile illness and may appear toxic.

Diarrhea Due to ETEC

ETEC is the most common cause of travelers' diarrhea.[3] A dose of 10^8 of ETEC organisms is sufficient to cause diarrheal illness in healthy adults. After entry into the host intestinal tract, these bacteria adhere and colonize the surface of the intestinal mucosa through an array of colonization factor antigens (CFAs).[13] One or more of the least 18 defined CFAs are found on the surfaces of at 50 to 80% of ETEC strains found worldwide. Once on the intestinal mucosa, ETEC elaborate enterotoxins, and diarrhea results. Two ETEC enterotoxins are known: heat-labile toxin (LT) and heat-stable toxin (ST). ETEC strains may express LT only, ST only, or both LT and ST.[3] In epidemiologic studies, ST producers are more virulent.

LT has a structure and mechanism of action similar to cholera toxin.[14] The toxins share many characteristic structures including similarity in protein sequence, primary receptor, and enzymatic activity.[15] Also similar to cholera toxin, LT is secreted by a type II secretion pathway.[16] LT enterotoxins can be divided into two immunologically distinct serogroups, LT-I and LT-II. LT-1 is expressed by ETEC strains pathogenic in humans and animals. LT-II is secreted primarily by animals infected with ETEC.[3] LT-I is a 86 kDa protein, composed of one 28 kDa subunit and 5 identical 11.5 kDa B subunits. LT consists of an A and a B subunit. The B subunit binds to their receptor, ganglioside GM1 (monosialoganglioside GM1), on the host cell surface.[17] GD1b ganglioside and some other glycoproteins may also act as LT receptors.[17] After binding to the host cell membrane, the A subunit is endocytosed and translocated to the cytoplasm through a trans-Golgi vesicular transport.[18] Similar to cholera toxin, the A subunit catalyzes the adenosine diphusphate (ADP)-ribosylation of a regulatory subunit of mucosal adenylate cyclase (the enzyme that converts adenosine triphosphate (ATP) to cyclic adenosine monophosphate (cAMP)) inside the cytoplasm of the epithelial cells. Increased levels of the intracellular cyclic AMP activates Protein A kinase, which results in the abnormal phosphorylation of chloride channels on the apical enterocyte membranes.[17] This process leads to excessive Cl- secretion from the crypt epithelial cells and inhibition of NaCl absorption. The increase in luminal Cl- content draws water passively into the intestinal lumen.[19]

Despite its importance in ETEC pathogenicity, less is known of the mechanism of action of ST. ST is a small monomeric toxin. It activates guanylate cyclase and leads to increased intracellular cyclic guanosine monophosphate (GMP) levels.[19] The abnormal activation of guanylate cyclase allows stimulation of chloride secretion and inhibition of intestinal fluid uptake, resulting in net intestinal fluid secretion and diarrhea.

Diarrhea Due to EPEC

EPEC were classically associated with outbreaks of diarrhea among infants in hospital nurseries, but are now common causes of infant diarrhea in developing regions of the world. EPEC may cause diarrhea among infant travelers. EPEC pathogenesis research centers on the characteristic attaching and effacing (A/E) lesion. This process involves intimate adherence of EPEC to the intestinal epithelial cell, followed by an effacing process that is characterized by formation of a cuplike pedestal on the enterocyte membrane upon which the bacteria sit.[20] The A/E process is initiated by EPEC's outer member protein intimin, which binds to a protein called Tir in the host cell membrane. Remarkably, the Tir receptor is of bacterial origin, as it is one of the first proteins secreted into the cell by EPEC's T3SS. Intimin-Tir binding is essential for the tight epithelial attachment, loss of mivrovilli, and establishment of the secretory state. Binding of intimin to Tir recruits several cytoskeletal proteins, including the adaptor protein Nck and the Wiskott-Aldrich syndrome protein (WASP), which in turn activate the Arp2/3 complex, resulting in nucleation and polymerization of actin.[21] By using immunofluorescence actin staining, cytoskeletal changes, including accumulation of polymerized F-actin, can be seen directly beneath the adherent bacteria.[22]

EPEC bind to the membrane of HEp-2 or HeLa cells in culture in a characteristic pattern called "localized adherence." In this pattern, bacteria bind to localized areas of the cell surface, forming compact microcolonies or bacterial clusters.[23] The localized adherence (LA) pattern is associated with the presence of a large EPEC adherence factor (EAF) plasmid, encoding bundle-forming pili (BFP). The major structural subunit of BFP is bundlin. BFP interconnect EPEC within microcolonies and function to maintain its stabilization. BFP are required for bacterial aggregation and localized adherence to epithelial cells. As infection proceeds, the bacteria detach from the pilus fibers, disaggregate, and become connected to the host cell through a surface appendage erected by components of the T3SS.[24]

EPEC activate a variety of signal transduction pathways. The bacterial genes responsible for this signal transduction activity are encoded on a 35 kb pathogenicity island called the locus of enterocyte effacement (LEE), which harbors the T3SS.[3] LEE secreted proteins include Tir, as well as the *E. coli* secreted protein (Esp) B, EspG and EspF. The T3SS translocates these proteins directly into the host cell cytoplasm. Both EspB and Tir are required for attaching and effacing activity. In vitro studies have shown that EPEC strains increase intracellular calcium levels in cultured epithelial cells to which they are attached.[25] Increases in intracellular calcium inhibit Na+ and Cl- absorption and stimulate chloride secretion by enterocytes.[26] The changes in calcium (Ca2+) metabolism mediate the intestinal secretory response due to EPEC infection. In addition, EPEC elicit a drop in transepithelial resistance, which may lead to leakage of fluid via the paracellular spaces.[27]

Diarrhea Due to EAEC

EAEC are increasingly recognized as causes of diarrhea both in developing and developed countries. EAEC is characterized by its distinctive aggregative or "stacked brick pattern" (Figure 1) of adherence to cultured human epithelial cells.[28] After their ingestion, EAEC strains adhere to the intestinal mucosa through aggregative adherence fimbriae (AAF), of which several antigenically distinct alleles have been described. EAEC strains are able to enhance mucus secretion from the intestinal mucosa[29]; the secreted mucus may thereupon bind to the bacteria, resulting in the formation of a tenacious mucus-bacteria biofilm. This biofilm has been postulated to lead to prolonged colonization by EAEC and persistent enteric symptoms.

Once EAEC colonizes mucosa, it elaborates one or more enterotoxins and cytotoxins, which leads to exfoliation of enterocytes and induction of a net secretory state.[30] These toxins include the Pet cytotoxin, the enteroaggregative *E. col.* heat-stable enterotoxin 1 (EAST1) and the Shigella enterotoxin 1 (ShET1).[31,32] Pet is a member of the autotransporter family of secreted proteins. The toxin enters epithelial cells, where it acts to cleave the cytoskeletal protein spectrin.[31] Cleavage of spectrin

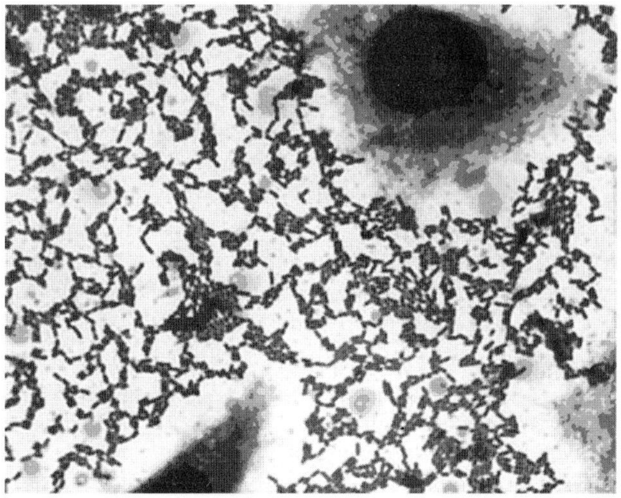

Figure 1 Aggregative pattern of adherence of enteroaggregative *E. coli* in the HEp-2 assay.

induces cell rounding and may directly or indirectly lead to intestinal secretion. The roles of EAST and ShET1 in EAEC diarrhea are as yet unknown.

A large set of EAEC plasmid and chromosomally encoded virulence factors are under the control of a transcriptional activator called AggR,[33] including the AAF adhesions. Also under AggR control is expression of a surface protein called dispersin; mutation of the dispersin-encoding gene leads to collapse of the AAF pili onto the bacterial cell surface and loss of their ability to mediate intestinal colonization. AggR also directs expression of a two secretion systems: a plasmid-born translocator of dispersin and chromosomal genes called *aai*, which secretes at least one cryptic protein.[34]

There is clinical evidence that EAEC infection may induce a mild inflammatory enteritis manifested by presence of fecal lactoferrin and cytokines (IL-8, IL-1b) during infection.[35] The EAEC flagellin has been suggested as a mediator of this effect,[36] though more recently an additional factor under AggR control has been suggested.[37]

Shigella

Shigella infection is associated with a spectrum of watery to bloody diarrhea. Early in the disease, the small bowel may be involved, as patients experience watery diarrhea. Later in the disease, a colitis develops and patients develop fever, urgency, tenesmus, and dysentery. There are four species of Shigella:

- Group A: *Shigella dysenteriae* (or Shiga bacillus, 13 serotypes)
- Group B: *Shigella flexneri* (6 serotypes, 15 subtypes)

- Group C: *Shigella boydii* (18 serotypes)
- Group D: *Shigella sonnei* (1 serotype)

In developing countries, *Shigella flexneri* and *Shigella dysenteriae* type 1 are the predominant species causing diarrhea, whereas in developed countries, *Shigella sonnei* is the predominant isolate.[38] *Shigella boydii* is most commonly encountered in the Indian subcontinent.[39] *Shigella dysenteriae* and *Shigella flexneri* most commonly cause dysentery, while *Shigella sonnei* and *Shigella boydii* are more associated with watery diarrhea.[40] Shigella is pathogenic only to humans and primates. As few as 10 to 100 organisms of *Shigella dysenteriae* type 1 are sufficient to cause clinical dysentery in healthy adults. Shigella is transmitted through contaminated food and water, person-to-person spread, and potentially, a fly vector.[41] *Shigella dysenteriae* species produce a potent cytotoxin known as Shiga toxin.

The physiopathologic effects of Shigella can be divided into three processes: 1) invasion of epithelial cells, 2) invasion of the underlying tissue, and 3) toxin production. Shigella pathogenesis has been the subject of several excellent reviews.[42,43]

INVASION OF EPITHELIAL CELLS

The entry of Shigella may occur at the basolateral surface of the epithelial cells, and/or via specialized structures known as M cells, which are devoid of brush border and associated with the mucosal lymphatic follicle.[44,45] Intracellular replication and intracellular spread leads to an amplified inflammatory cascade at the initial site of entry. As this inflammation persists and expands, infiltration of polymorphonuclear (PMN) facilitates the entry of additional bacteria into the epithelium. A number of plasmid- and chromosomally encoded proteins facilitate the entry of pathogenic Shigella into host epithelial cells. These proteins are generally effectors of its T3SS, including the invasion plasmid antigens (ipa), surface presentation of invasion plasmid antigens (spa), membrane excretion of Ipa (mxi), and virulence (vir) proteins. Other proteins include outer surface proteins (Osp) F and OspC1, which are T3SS effectors that are required for postinvasion aspects of virulence.[46] Through a process of transcytosis, Shigella are deposited into the subepithelial space. Bacterial entry involves a complex of IpaB and IpaC proteins. This protein complex induces actin polymerization and is followed by the entry of several other T3SS effectors. After entry, Shigella escapes the phagocytic vacuole and moves through the cytoplasm via nucleation of actin filaments. These specialized actin filaments, induced by an outer membrane protein called IcsA (VirG), promote intracellular motility, thus facilitating cell-to-cell spreading.[47]

INVASION OF THE UNDERLYING TISSUE

Once Shigella penetrates the epithelial layer, it is phagocytosed by macrophages. The infected macrophages undergo apoptosis (programmed cell death) in a process dependent upon the IpaB protein, resulting in the release of the bacteria, which in turn are free to infect adjacent enterocytes at their basolateral surface. The effect of IpaB is via activation of the cysteine protease caspase-1.[48] Infected host cells produce an inflammatory response, which is mediated most importantly through interleukin-8 (IL-8) and interleukin-10 (IL-10) production. IL-8 and IL-10 are responsible for the chemotaxis of polymorphonuclear leukocytes, which cause disruption of the epithelial barrier's integrity.[49] This inflammatory response causes degeneration of the epithelium and inflammation of the lamina propria. These changes induce disruption of epithelial absorption, resulting in diarrhea and abdominal cramps. Shigella may cause mucosal destruction in the form of focal hemorrhage and ulcerations of the colonic mucosa, which explains the presence of blood in the stools. Eradication of Shigella infection occurs when a T helper 1 (Th1) response is elicited, typically late in infection. Both T cells and NK cells contribute to the early control of *S. flexneri* infection through production of IFN-γ.[50]

TOXIN PRODUCTION

Shigella dysenteriae type 1 produces a toxin referred to as Shiga toxin, which is active in Vero cells. This toxin has enterotoxic activity in rabbit ileal loops and causes capillary destruction and focal hemorrhage that exacerbates dysentery in rhesus monkeys inoculated with these bacteria.[45] Shiga toxin belongs to the family of A-B toxins, so named because they consist of two parts—an A subunit (active) and a B subunit (binding); Shiga toxin consists of one A subunit and five B subunits. The B component of the exotoxin binds to a receptor on the surface of the host cell. The A subunit then enters the host cell by endocytosis, where it modifies a host cell target protein through depurination. Subunit A of Shiga toxin inactivates the 60S subunit of the host cell ribosomes and prevents the attachment of charged tRNA, resulting in inhibition of host cell protein synthesis and cell death. Shiga toxin increases release of tumor necrosis factor alpha (TNF-α) and IL-1, which is responsible for HUS.[51]

Salmonella

Nontyphoid Salmonella infections are an important cause of morbidity and mortality around the world. The distal ileum and colon are sites of infection. Salmonella ingested in food may survive the gastric acid barrier, travel through the mucus layer overlying the epithelium of the small intestine, and evade intestinal defenses such as specific IgA to result in infection. A dose of 10^9 of *Salmonella typhimurium* bacteria are needed to cause symptoms of a toxic infection in healthy adults. Salmonella interact with both the enterocytes and M cells that overlie the ileal Peyer's patches. Salmonella are then internalized and transported into the submucosal lymphoid tissue. The lymphoid tissue has the ability to induce enterocytes to take *Salmonella* into their cytoplasm in a process known as bacteria-mediated endocytosis.[52] This process is an important pathway for invasive *Salmonella* to reach deeper tissues. Once *Salmonella* invade the intestinal epithelial barrier, the organisms interact with macrophages and lymphocytes in Peyer's patches, where bacterial multiplication occur, which results in marked enlargement and necrosis of the lymphoid tissue.[53] Invasion of epithelial cells also stimulates the release of proinflammatory cytokines which induce an inflammatory reaction. The acute inflammatory response causes diarrhea and leads to ulceration and destruction of the mucosa. From the submucosal lymphoid tissue or Peyer's patches, the organism can enter the systemic circulation or release lipopolysaccharide (LPS) (endotoxin) into the blood stream causing fever and other systemic symptoms and diseases.

Salmonella are intracellular pathogens and are able to invade and replicate in epithelial cells of the gut and in cultured cell lines. *Salmonella* survive and replicate in macrophages, but do not survive in neutrophils. The ability of *Salmonella* to survive within macrophages plays an important role in typhoid fever pathogenesis and in the spread of the organisms beyond the bowel to the systemic circulation. In the bloodstream, the organisms are contained in the mononuclear cell fraction, especially tissue macrophages in the bone marrow, liver, and spleen.[54] Symptoms of typhoid fever occur due to the secretion of cytokines by macrophages in response to bacterial infection and endotoxin exposure.[54] The enlargement of the liver and the spleen found in patients with typhoid fever is related to *S. typhi* survival or replication within reticuloendothelial cells, recruitment of mononuclear cells, and the development of a cell-mediated immune response. Endotoxins evoke fever, activate the serum complement—kinin and clotting systems, depress myocardial function and alter lymphocyte function, and are responsible for many of the manifestations of septic shock.

Several Salmonella genes required for virulence have been identified. Chromosomal invasion (inv) genes are encoded on a pathogenicity island, which includes a T3SS.[55] Genes encoding macrophage survival have been identified on a second such island. These genes are controlled in part by phoP/phoQ, a two-component regulator that senses low Mg2+ inside the macrophage and turns on genes to allow survival in the macrophage.[56] The same genes also encode resistance to cationic antimicrobial proteins and acid pH.[56]

The Salmonella T3SS injects protein toxins that together induce uptake by epithelial cells. Some of the effectors required for this phenotype are homologous to the Ipa proteins of Shigella. Salmonella has a second T3SS, which is induced upon uptake into macrophages. The bacteria induce membrane ruffling in macrophages similar to that observed in enterocytes. They enter macrophages by induction of generalized macropinocytosis rather than by receptor-mediated endocytosis.[57] Salmonella are initially internalized in membrane-bound vacuoles called macropinosomes, formed by fusion of the ends of membrane ruffles. After endocytosis, fusion with other macropinosomes can result in the formation of large vacuoles called spacious phagosomes.[57] Salmonella then induce macrophage cell death, and this ability allows them to survive after phagocytosis and may contribute to the inflammation seen in lymphoid tissue. Salmonella's ability to induce phagocytosis by macrophages and enterocytes protect them from phagocytosis by neutrophils. The organisms are rapidly killed by neutrophils, with less than 10% of an initial inoculum surviving after phagocytosis.[56] Liver biopsy specimens from patients with typhoid show Kupffer's cell hyperplasia and erythrophagocytosis.[58] Therefore, *Salmonella* stimulation of hemophagocytosis may be an important mechanism in producing anemia, neutropenia, and thrombocytopenia in typhoid fever.

The surface molecules of Salmonella are important in pathogenesis. The Vi antigen of *S. typhi* prevents antibody-mediated opsonization, increases resistance to peroxide, and confers resistance to complement activation by the alternative pathway and to complement-mediated lysis.[59] The Vi antigen inhibits phagocytosis of Salmonella by neutrophils while not interfering with the induction of phagocytosis by more permissive macrophages and epithelial cells. Salmonella lacking the complete outer O-sugar repeat units have a rough appearance of colonies and are usually avirulent or less virulent than smooth strain, which possess a full complement of O-sugar repeat units.[60] The lipid A component of lipopolysaccharide is a potent toxin for mammalian cells, and lipopolysaccharide is an essential virulence determinant in a *S. typhimurium* infection.[61,62]

Cell-mediated immunity is important in controlling intracellular pathogens such as *Salmonella*. The risk of invasive salmonellosis is increased in patients with acquired immunodeficiency syndrome (AIDS), organ transplantation, and lymphoproliferative disease.[63–65] Individuals deficient in the IL-12 receptor are also extremely susceptible to *Salmonella* infections.[66] Interleukin-12 induces Th1-type cell responses and interferon-γ production, which is important in resistance to salmonellosis. Patients who have splenic dysfunction, such as those with sickle cell disease, also have an increased incidence of salmonellosis.[67]

Campylobacter

Campylobacter is the most common bacterial cause of foodborne illness in the United States; it is responsible for 46% of reportable causes of bacterial diarrhea. A dose of 10^3 to 10^6 of Campylobacter organisms is sufficient to cause diarrheal illness in humans.[68] The rates of illness increase when inocula are ingested in a suspension buffered to reduce gastric acidity.[68] Similar to *S. typhimurium*, *C. jejuni* is susceptible to hydrochloric acid.[69] Milk and fatty foods that favor passage through the gastric acid barrier may permit some infections to occur at low doses.

The pathogenesis of *C. jejuni* infection is not well understood. Cell invasion and perhaps cytotoxin production with subsequent tissue destruction are key elements in pathogenesis.[70,71] Enterocyte damage results in a loss of net fluid absorption and eventual perturbation of epithelial integrity, which leads to leakage of serous fluid and diarrhea. A heat-labile enterotoxin may contribute to the diarrheal response. An outer membrane protein (PEB1) may be a major adhesin,[72] and it is conserved among *C. jejuni* strains. Many *C. jejuni* strains are invasive and proliferate within the intestinal epithelium of the jejunum, ileum, and colon, resulting in cell damage and an inflammatory response. The affected intestine reveals diffuse, edematous, and exudative enteritis.[73] Microscopic examination of the affected mucosa generally reveals a colitis with an inflammatory infiltrate of neutrophils, mononuclear cells, and eosinophils in the lamina propria. Degeneration, atrophy, loss of mucus, crypt abscesses in the epithelial glands, and ulceration of the mucosal epithelium can also be observed.[70,73]

Guillain-Barre syndrome (GBS), irritable bowel syndrome, and reactive arthritis are postinfectious complications of *C. jejuni* infection. Many *C. jejuni* O antigens possess sialic acid-containing structures.[74] The antigen mimicry of *C. jejuni*'s sialic acid with human ganglioside GM1 and their presence in strains (eg, serotype O:19) isolated from patients who developed the GBS suggest their role in inducing an autoimmune response that leads to motor neuron injury.[74,75] It is estimated that one case of GBS occurs for every 1,000 cases of campylobacteriosis.[75] Reiter's syndrome has been associated with *C. jejuni* and *C. fetus* infections through stimulation of autoimmune response due to cross reactivity of exogenous *Campylobacter* antigens with endogenous antigens.[76]

Vibrio Parahemolyticus

V. parahemolyticus is a halophilic (salt requiring) gram-negative bacillus that lives in seawater. This organism is a cause of diarrhea after ingestion of seafood in the Northwest Pacific.[77] *V. parahemolyticus* has also caused outbreaks of diarrhea along the Atlantic and Gulf Coast of the United States and on Caribbean cruise ships.[78,79] This pathogen is an invasive organism and can cause bacteremia, particularly in patients with an immunocompromised state, such as those with leukemia and cirrhosis. Within 24 hours of ingestion, *V. parahemolyticus* causes symptoms of watery diarrhea, abdominal cramping, nausea, vomiting, fever, and chills. *V. parahemolyticus* can also cause an infection of the skin when an open wound is exposed to warm seawater. There is very little published about this organism; hence, its mechanism to cause diarrhea and invasive disease is unclear. However, putative virulence factors of *V. parahaemolyticus* have been described. Thermostable direct hemolysin (TDH) is associated with *V. parahaemolyticus* strain's ability to cause gastroenteritis and to cause beta-hemolysis on Watgatsuma blood agar, referred to as the Kanagawa phenomenon (KP).[80] TDH acts on cellular membranes as a pore-forming toxin that alters ion influx in intestinal cells resulting in a secretory response and diarrhea. Another putative virulence factor is TDH-related hemolysin (TRH), which was first identified in a KP-negative strain.[81] TRH induces Ca 2+-activated Cl- channels, which also results in altered ion flux in intestinal cells and subsequent diarrhea. Other proposed virulence markers for some pathogenic *V. parahaemolyticus* include urea hydrolysis, vibrioferrin (a sideophore), a pathogenicity island, and a type III secretion system.[82] Evidence linking the presence of these virulence factors with *V. parahaemolyticus* and its pathogenesis of diarrhea is limited and remain unclear.

Aeromonas

Aeromonas are ubiquitous inhabitants of freshwater, especially in tropical areas. Aeromonas spp. are classified into two major groups: those bacteria that cause septicemia and those that cause gastroenteritis. Aeromonas has been increasingly associated with travelers' diarrhea.[83–85] Occasionally, they cause soft tissue infections and sepsis in immunocompromised hosts. A number of virulence factors are liked to Aeromonas associated pathogenesis, including matrix-binding proteins, elastases, proteases, cytotonic and cytotoxic enterotoxins, hemolysins, aldolase, chitinase, lipases/phospholipases, type III secretion system, a ToxR-regulated lipoprotein called TagA (which potentates the activity of C1- esterase inhibitor), type IV pili, and a bundle-forming pili.[86,87] However, the role of these putative virulence factors in the pathogenesis of Aeromonas-induced diarrhea is unclear.

Plesiomonas

P. shigelloides has been implicated as a cause of travelers' diarrhea.[88–90] *P. shigelloides* is a water- and soil-associated organism that replicates at temperatures above 8°C. It is found primarily in freshwater or estuary environments within temperate and tropical climates but can exist in seawater during summer. The usual vehicles of transmission of Plesiomonas to humans are water, food such as oysters, shrimp, or chicken, and a variety of animals that may be colonized with the organism.[88] When germ-free piglets were fed with 10^{10} *P. shigelloides* strain P012, mild to moderate diarrhea resulted in 3 of 3 piglets.[91] The organisms were found in the jejunum and distal small intestine of the piglets. However, when 33 human volunteers were challenged with 10^9 *P. shigelloides* strain P012, 36% of the volunteers shed the organisms but none of them developed diarrhea.[91] Negative results were also found in monkey and adult rabbits fed with *P. shigelloides* strain P012.[91] Potential virulence factors involved in the pathogenesis of *P. shigelloides* associated infections include elastase, hemolysin, proteinase, histidine decarboxylase, and triacylglycerol lipase.[92] The role each of these virulence factors and the mechanism of *Plesiomonas* in causing diarrhea remains unclear.

Rotavirus

Rotaviruses are the single most important cause of pediatric (6 months to 3 years of age) diarrhea in many regions of the world. Rotaviruses primarily infect and kill cells via lysis of the mature villous epithelial cells that line the small intestine.[93,94] Rotavirus serotypes are defined by two outer proteins, P (VP4) and G (VP7). The virus outer capsid protein (VP4) attaches to the glycolipid receptor on the host cell surface and enters the cytoplasm by direct plasma membrane penetration.[95–97]

Several mechanisms of rotavirus-induced diarrhea have been proposed, including malabsorption that occurs secondary to the destruction of enterocytes, villus ischemia, and activation of the enteric nervous system that may be evoked by release of vasoactive agent from infected epithelial cells in the absence of significant pathologic lesions or enterocyte damage,[98] and intestinal secretion stimulated by the intracellular or extracellular action of the rotavirus nonstructural protein, NSP4, which serves as an enterotoxin and a secretory agonist. NSP4 is produced in the early replication cycle and is able to induce diarrhea in mice.[99,100] The NSP4 enterotoxin activates a Ca2+-dependent signal transduction pathway resulting in cell permeability or inhibits the Na+-D-glucose symporter and consequently impairs Cl- and Na+ transport into and out of epithelial cells, which results in diarrhea.[99,101] Lysis of mature enterocytes at villous tips of the small intestine cause atrophy of the villous cell, detachment of absorptive cells from the basement membranes, and hyperplasia of the crypt cells, which subsequently leads to diarrhea.[102] Rotavirus infection can also cause a loss of intestinal permeability to macromolecules such as lactose, which is associated with decreased levels of intestinal disaccharidases via a cyclic AMP protein kinase A-dependent mechanism.[103,104] This rotavirus-induced lactase deficiency may last for 10 to 14 days.[103]

Norovirus (Norwalk and Norwalk-Like Virus)

Norovirus belong to the Calciviridae family. Norovirus was recently approved as the official genus name for the group of viruses previously referred to as Norwalk and Norwalk-like viruses. Noroviruses produce institutional or community-wide outbreaks and are important causes of diarrheal and vomiting outbreaks in cruise ships and nursing homes for the elderly.[105] Less than 100 norovirus particles are sufficient to cause diarrheal illness.[106] Transmission and outbreaks of Norovirus-related gastroenteritis occur by drinking contaminated water or ingestion of any type of food that has contact with contaminated water.[107,108] A surrogate for norovirus (feline calicivirus) is inactivated by $> 4 \log_{10}$ within 5 minutes with a dose of 30 mg of applied chlorine.[109] Vomitus has been implicated as a vehicle of transmission, and virus has been detected in vomitus by electron microscopy and polymerase chain reaction (PCR).[110–112]

Two Norovirus genogroups exist. Norovirus G1 preferentially bind to histo-blood group antigens A and O, and Norovirus G2 preferentially bind to blood group antigens A and B. Studies show that volunteers who are ABO nonsecretors are resistant to infection when challenged with large amounts of norovirus.[113] The P domain of norovirus capsid protein is responsible for binding to viral receptors, and a highly conserved arginine (R) cluster at the C terminus of the P domain is critical for norovirus receptor binding.[114] Increased levels of fecal IL-2 and IFN-γ have been identified in travelers with norovirus infection suggesting a predominant Th1 immune response to this virus.[115] Acute infection with noroviruses generally results in histopathologic lesions in the duodenum and jejunum.[116] In gnotobiotic pigs, structural and nonstructural norovirus proteins were identified in enterocytes by immunofluorescence indicating viral replication in epithelial cells.[116] The infection apparently spares the stomach and rectum.[117] Under microscopy, the infected villi are blunted, but the mucosa is otherwise intact. Round cell and polymorphonuclear leukocytic infiltration can be seen in the lamina propria. Under electron microscopy, the epithelial cells are intact, microvilli are shortened, and widened intercellular spaces can be observed. These histopathologic changes are temporary and generally resolved within two weeks after the onset of illness. During an acute episode of illness, a variable amount of intestinal fluid is produced. Diarrhea induced by the norovirus can be associated with transient malabsorption of D-xylose and fat and with decreased activity of brush-border enzymes, including alkaline phosphatase and trehalase.[118,119] Absorption and brush-border enzyme levels generally return to normal values within 2 weeks after the infection.

Infection with the norovirus has not been associated with detectable enterotoxin production. Adenylate cyclase levels in jejunal biopsy specimens appear to be normal during infection.[120] The precise pathogenesis of norovirus-induced diarrhea and vomiting remains unclear.

Cryptosporidium Parvum

Cryptosporidium is a noninvasive intracellular protozoan parasite belonging to the phylum Apicomplexa, subclass Coccidia. Cryptosporidium can infect the respiratory or the GI tracts of fish, birds, reptiles, and mammals. Cryptosporidium causes diarrheal diseases in immunocompetent and immunocompromised patients. Genotype 1 causes human infection and genotype 2 is associated with zoonotic transmission.[121]

The parasite is transmitted via the fecal-oral route. The infection may be acquired through contaminated water or foods, farm animals, person-to-person contact, or unpasteurized milk.[122] Since 1980, Cryptosporidium had been recognized as a cause of travelers' diarrhea in individuals returning from Russia.[123] There are also reports of disease acquired by travelers visiting the Caribbean, Mexico, Mauritius, Egypt, Central Africa, New Guinea, and Pakistan.[124–127]

The parasite undergoes asexual reproduction in the small intestine, and oocysts—each containing four sporozoites—are produced (Figure 2). The infected host excretes the sporulated oocysts by feces and respiratory secretions. A suitable host is infected following ingestion or inhalation of these sporulated oocysts. The excystation process occurs in the small intestine and is enhanced by proteolytic enzymes and bile salts. The four sporozoites are then released from each oocyst and parasitize the epithelial cells of the GI tract or the respiratory tract. The released sporozoites invade the microvillous border of enterocytes and replicate either asexually to become merozoites, or sexually with the subsequent development of gametocytes in the brush-border epithelial cell surface. After fertilization of macrogamonts (female) by the microgametes (male), the oocysts are produced and the sporulation process occurs inside the infected host, whereafter the sporulated oocysts are excreted or begin a new cycle inside the host and autoinfection can occur.[122]

Data from 29 healthy volunteers indicate that the median infective dose of Cryptosporidium is 132 oocysts and a dose of 10 to 1,000 oocysts is able to produce infection in 50% of volunteers exposed.[128,129] The incubation period is 1 to 2 weeks. Cryptosporidium infection is characterized by watery diarrhea with abdominal pain, nausea, weight loss, and occasionally low-grade fever. The mechanism by which Cryptosporidium causes diarrhea is poorly understood. Illness in humans is localized to the jejunum, but in immunocompromised patients, organisms may be found in the epithelium of the GI tract from the pharynx to the rectum, and in the respiratory tracts from the sinuses to the lungs.

Three important changes of the enterocyte cytoskeleton in Cryptosporidium infection have been described: 1) the microvilli are absent in the area of parasite invasion, 2) columnar epithelial cells shortened after the parasite invasion, and 3) there is development of a unique structure at the host-parasite interface during invasion. *Cryptosporidium parvum* induces a rearrangement of the host enterocyte cytoskeleton, reducing the membrane expression of nutrient transporters and causing impaired absorption and osmotic diarrhea.[130] The voluminous watery diarrhea in Cryptosporidium infection is caused by hypersecretion of fluids and electrolytes due to a cholera-like cryptosporidial enterotoxin. Studies using piglet ileal mucosa and human jejunum show that the loss of vacuolated villous tip epithelium is accompanied by an approximately 50% reduction in glucose-coupled sodium cotransport in the ileum.[131] Experimental studies have shown that these effects are due to the decrease in permeability to solute and macromolecules with impaired transcellular nutrient transport.[131]

In Cryptosporidium-infected piglet epithelium, glutamine drives Na+ and Cl- absorption. The absorption is inhibited by prostaglandins. There is an increase in macrophage-produced tumor necrosis factor (TNF) in

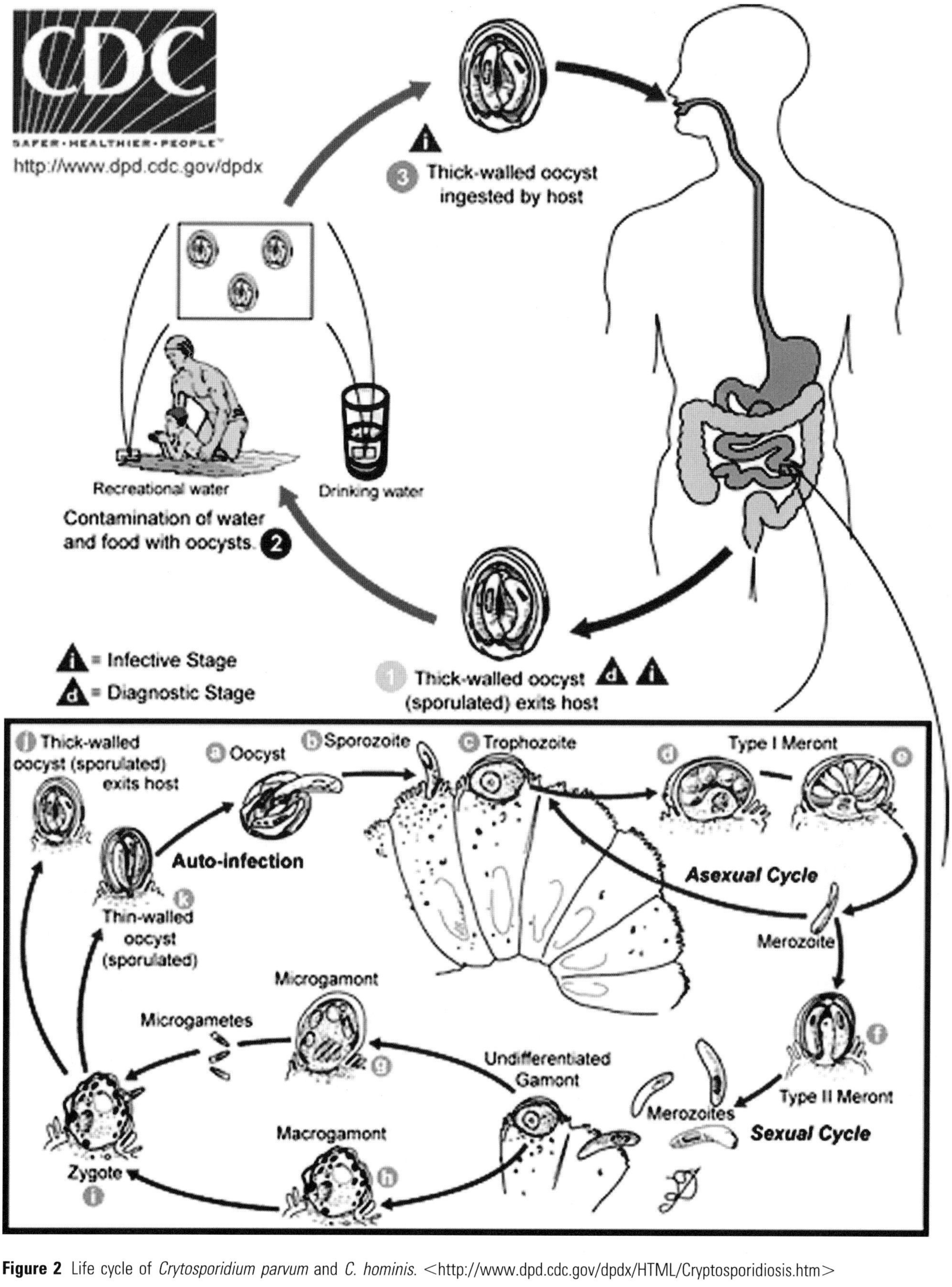

Figure 2 Life cycle of *Crytosporidium parvum* and *C. hominis*. <http://www.dpd.cdc.gov/dpdx/HTML/Cryptosporidiosis.htm>

the lamina propria of infected piglets.[132] TNF does not directly affect epithelial transport, but when fibroblasts are present, a secretory effect is noted. This effect is inhibited by indomethacin. Researchers propose a prostaglandin-mediated secretory effect by crypt cells in a chloride secretory pathway and through the inhibition of neutral sodium chloride absorption by the Na+:H+ exchanger.

Nitric oxide synthase stimulates prostaglandin secretion at the junctional or transitional epithelium during active cryptosporidial infection.[133] All the inflammatory changes produce reduced xylose and B-12 absorption. In children and in human immunodeficiency virus (HIV)-infected patients, increased permeability to lactulose and mannitol has been described.

CD4+ intraepithelial lymphocytes at the mucosal level are important in the control of cryptosporidial infection. These lymphocytes produce IFN-γ, which has a direct inhibitory effect on parasite development in enterocytes.[134] IFN-γ inhibits the parasite's development by inhibiting parasite invasion and modification of the intracellular Fe2+ concentration. In addition, infection results in increased intestinal expression of proinflammatory cytokines such as IL-12, IFN-γ, and TNF-α.[134, 135] Secretory IgA is an important defense mechanism against Cryptosporidium infection. Basolateral secretion of IL-8 and GRO-α contributes to the mucosal inflammatory cell infiltrate in the underlying intestinal mucosa in vivo.[136]

Cyclospora

Cyclospora is highly endemic in many developing regions of which Nepal, Haiti, and Peru have been the best studied. *C. cayetenensis* causes diarrhea among travelers and is an opportunistic infection in those with HIV infection.[137–139]

Cyclospora is not infectious when first passed in stool of an infected person. The oocyst, measuring about 8 to 10 microns in diameter, requires 5 to 11 days for sporulation before becoming infectious. The oocyst contains two sporocysts that each hold two sporozoites, and are variably acid-fast. Oocysts in the environment are quite resilient, surviving freezing and chlorination.[140–142] Transmission occurs by contaminated food and water. Cyclospora oocysts in freshly excreted stool are noninfectious. Under favorable conditions, the oocysts require several days to weeks outside the host to sporulate and become infective.[143] The sporozoites invade the enterocytes, resulting in the release of cytokines from epithelial cells. Cytokine activate and recruit phagocytes and then in turn release histamine, prostaglandins, and platelet-aggregating factors that increase intestinal secretion of chloride and water and inhibit absorption.

Cyclospora can be detected in jejunal aspirates or in biopsy specimens of patients with diarrheal illness.[144] They are generally located in the supranuclear location of the cytoplasm, distinguishing them from Cryptosporidium, which are found on the surface of the enterocytes.[144] Electron microscopy reveals the presence of the Cyclospora organisms and its various stages in the cytoplasm of jejunal epithelial cells.[144] T cells, mast cells, and proteases elicit an inflammatory response to Cyclospora infection. Under endoscopy, the small bowel may appear normal, but the histologic architecture of the small bowel is altered, with villous atrophy, crypt hyperplasia, infiltration of the lamina propria by inflammatory cells, vascular dilatation, and the presence of electron-dense phospholipid membrane/myelin-like material.[145,146] Destruction of enterocytes cause nutrient malabsorption and increased secretion of fluid and electrolytes from the gut, which results in a secretory and osmotic diarrhea.

Blastocytis Hominis

Blastocystis hominis is an intestinal protozoan that can cause traveler's diarrhea. The prevalence of *B. hominis* infection is 30 to 50% in developing countries and 1.5 to 10% in developed countries.[147,148] Traveler's diarrhea caused by *B. hominis* infection should be a diagnosis of exclusion. A careful examination of the stool for other causes of the diarrheal illness should be conducted because *B. hominis* is often found along with other bacterial, viral, and parasitic organisms that actually may be the cause of symptoms associated with diarrheal illness. However, clinical studies and case reports have shown an association between identification of the organism and symptoms and a decrease in symptoms with antiparasitic therapy and parasite clearance.[149,150] In patients infected with *B. hominis*, endoscopy and biopsy results reveal that this parasite does not invade the colonic mucosa in infected individuals.[147] Edema and inflammation of the intestinal mucosa may be observed.[151] The pathogenesis of *B. hominis* remains unclear due to the presence of uncertainty in studies that other microbial causes of symptoms have been eliminated and the inability of studies to determine a strong association of this low-grade pathogen with disease.

Giardia

Giardia lamblia (also known as *Giardia intestinalis* or *G. duodenalis*) is a protozoan flagellate that infects the small intestine of humans. Giardia is one of the most common causes of waterborne (drinking and recreational) and foodborne diseases among travelers to developing regions.[122,152] *G. lamblia* has a fecal-oral mode of transmission via cysts; oral ingestion of as few as 10 to 25 cysts is sufficient to cause infection. *G. lamblia* trophozoites usually remain in the intestinal lumen.

Giardia lamblia cysts germinate in the GI tract and may produce symptoms of acute or chronic diarrhea associated with weight loss and growth retardation in children.[153] In developing regions, carriage is often asymptomatic. A direct correlation exists between the genotype of *G. lamblia* and the type of clinical picture it manifests. Genotype A isolates are detected in patients with intermittent diarrhea, while Genotype B isolates are associated with persistent diarrhea.[154]

The Giardia life cycle involves two stages: the trophozoite, or the free living stage, and the cyst. The ingested cyst, each of which produces two trophozoites, passes through the stomach and excystation takes place in the duodenum. The excystation releases the trophozoites. In vitro excystation can be induced after a brief exposure of the cysts to acidic pH or other sources of hydrogen ions. The breakdown of the cyst wall is mediated by stimulation of parasite-derived proteases. Flagellar activity begins within 5 to 10 minutes following the acid treatment and the trophozoite emerges through a break in the cyst wall. The trophozoite undergoes cytokinesis (cell division without nuclear replication) within 30 minutes after emerging from the cyst, resulting in two binucleated trophozoites. In the lumen of the proximal small intestine, the trophozoites can be free or attached to the mucosa by a ventral sucking disk. Some of the trophozoites then undergo encystation when the parasites transit toward the colon. During encystation, three cyst wall proteins (CWPs) are specifically expressed and concentrated within encystation-specific secretory vesicles (ESVs).[155] This encystation process is enhanced by multiple factors such as an alkaline pH and excess bile salts. Encystation is the completion of the life cycle, and new infectious cysts pass into the environment.[122]

Giardia lamblia attach to the brush border of enterocytes by either suction or a clasping mechanism with its adhesive disk.[156] The adhesive disk is a rigid structure made up of microtubules and microribbons. A major component of microribbons is proteins called giardins.[157,158] Attachment of trophozoites to the brush border causes diffuse border microvillous alterations and disaccharidase deficiencies, which are responsible for intestinal malabsorption, particularly of fat and carbohydrates.[159] Attachment of the large numbers of trophozoites to the brush border can produce mechanical irritation or obstruction. Villus blunting (atrophy), crypt cell hypertrophy, and increased inflammatory cell infiltration in the lamina propria have been observed with Giardia infection. The deficiencies of lactase and other enzymes in the microvilli suggest damage at the enzymatic level. There is a correlation between the infectious load and the extent of enzyme inhibition. As a result, reduced digestion and absorption of solutes lead to an osmotic diarrhea.

Experimental giardiasis in immunocompetent mice showed that the enterocyte brush-border injury was mediated by T lymphocytes. The mechanisms of T cells' effects on microvillus structure are unknown.[160] The epithelial injury is caused by a reduced transepithelial electrical resistance and is due, at least in part, to trophozoite products.[161] The reduced absorption of solutes may lead to osmotic diarrhea. Giardia-induced lactose intolerance can occur and may persist for a variable time following elimination of the parasite.

The immune response plays an important role in the host's defenses against Giardia.[122] It starts when Giardia are taken up and processed by macrophages residing in Peyer's patches. Giardia reside strictly in the lumen of the intestine and do not invade the mucosa. IgA antibodies are important for controlling and clearing Giardia infection. The protective mechanism of IgA against *Giardia lamblia* prevents the trophozoites' adherence to the intestinal mucosa. Cellular immunity including T lymphocytes and macrophages are components of the host's immune response to Giardia infection. The cellular immune response helps to clear parasites by coordinating the production of anti-Giardia secretory IgA. Experimental Giardia infections in mice with ablation of CD4+ T cells and B cells lead to chronic giardiasis.[162] Polarized intestinal epithelial cells produce nitric oxide (NO). NO inhibits both encystation and excystation of Giardia and thus could interfere with parasite transmission.[162]

Normal flora have protective effects against *Giardia lamblia* infection. Experimental studies suggest that the resident flora block infection with this pathogen.[163] Experimental studies have also shown that the intestinal microbiota are important for the pathogenicity, but not for the multiplication of *G. lamblia* in the intestinal lumen.[164]

Entamoeba Histolytica

Entamoeba histolytica is a protozoan parasite of humans that causes 40,000 to 100,000 deaths annually.[165] The robust *E. histolytica* cyst is the primary reason for the extensive prevalence of its infection throughout the world. The cysts move from one person to another through fecal contamination of water and vegetables or ano-genital or direct fecal-oral contact. The excreted cysts can survive for weeks in a hospitable environment. Ingestion of the cyst results in excystation in the small intestine and ends with trophozoite infection of the colon, most often in the cecum or sigmoid colon. A number of virulence factors of *E. histolytica* have been identified, including a Gal-specific adhesion, cysteine proteinases, and a family of small ampiphatic pore-forming peptide called amoebapores.[166] The cysteine proteases secreted from the amoeba disrupt the mucin polymeric network, thereby overcoming the protective mucus barrier.[167]

E. histolytica has an adherence molecule identified as a lectin.[168] Lectin can bind to either of two common carbohydrate components of the cell membrane—galactose and N-acetyl glactosemaine. After attachment, amebas invade the colonic epithelium directly.[165,169] On light and electron microscopic studies, lysis of mucosal cells are found before amebic invasion or after contact with amebas.[170] Amebic trophozoite membranes are coated with a glycocalyx layer. A lipid-anchored glycolipid called lipophosphoglycan (LPG) and lipopeptid ophosphoglycan (LPPG) play an important role for the invasiveness of the ameba.[171] A direct correlation is observed between the relative abundance of LPG and LPPG in different amebic strains and their virulence. The glycolipids extracted from avirulent *E. histolytica* contained extremely low levels of LPG molecules and an LPPG of smaller molecular weight.[171] *E. histolytica* release a pore-forming protein (amoebapore), soluble toxic molecules, and a cysteine proteinase that degrades matrix proteins. These virulence factors cause intestinal inflammation, damage mucosal cells, and enable the invasion of *E. histolytica*. Epithelial cells express pro-inflammatory IL-2, IL-6, IL-8, MIP-1alpha, MCP-1, RANTES, GRO-α and GMCSF in response to *E. histolytica* infection.[172]

E. histolytica have the capacity to destroy leukocytes.[173] Lysis of host neutrophils by *E. histolytica* results in the release of toxic nonoxidative neutrophil products that contribute to the destruction of host tissues.[174,175] Macroscopically, ulcerative lesions in the intestinal mucosa may become the characteristic flask-shaped, chronic amebic ulcer, which involves a moderate inflammatory response. Advanced lesions have necrotic centers, with ameba concentrated at the outer zone of normal tissue.

E. histolytica infection can manifest as a dysenteric syndrome with production of small volumes of bloody, mucoid stools without fecal leukocytes. A more severe form of amebiasis colitis may occur which is characterized by ulcerations of the colonic mucosa with typical flask-shaped abscesses. Occasionally, the formation of a fibrotic mass (ameboma) may occur in the intestinal wall.

After invading the intestinal mucosa, *E. histolytica* can migrate hematogenously to the liver, causing abscess formation. In a hamster model, mRNA levels of a protein tyrosine phosphatase (PTP) gene are up-regulated in trophozoites recovered after 96 hours of liver abscess development.[176] PTP is an essential signal transduction mechanism that regulates cell growth, differentiation, mobility, metabolism, and survival. Patients infected with *E. histolytica* may present clinically with abdominal pain, jaundice, and fever. Adjacent internal organs, such as the pulmonary parenchyma, peritoneum, and pericardium, can be affected. Occasionally, *E. histolytica* may disseminate to the brain and cause brain abscess. Immunocompromised patients are especially at risk for this invasive form of amebiasis.

Conclusion

There are myriad bacterial, viral, and parasitic causes of infectious diarrhea. The factors most important in causing infectious diarrhea are the virulence or toxicity of the organism, the transmissibility and number of organisms (infectious dose), and the host status (age, decreased gastric physiology, innate, and acquired mucosal immunity). An understanding of these factors is essential in elucidating the pathogenesis of traveler's diarrhea. The pathogenesis of the common enteric organisms has been better elucidated over the past few decades; however, additional research is still needed, especially to understand the pathogenesis of less common and emerging enteric organisms.

References

1. Riddle MS, Sanders JW, Putnam SD, Tribble DR. Incidence, etiology, and impact of diarrhea among long-term travelers (US military and similar populations): a systematic review. Am J Trop Med Hyg 2006;74:891–900.
2. Monteville MR, Riddle MS, Baht U, et al. Incidence, etiology, and impact of diarrhea among deployed US military personnel in support of Operation Iraqi Freedom and Operation Enduring Freedom. Am J Trop Med Hyg 2006;75:762–7.
3. Nataro JP, Kaper JB. Diarrheagenic Escherichia coli. Clin Microbiol Rev 1998;11:142–85.
4. DuPont HL, Levine MM, Hornick RB, et al. Inoculum size in shigellosis and implications for expected mode of transmission. J Infect Dis 1989;159:1126.
5. Richard CS, Jackson WB, Decapito WB, Maier PP. Studies on rates of recovery of Shigella from domestic files and

from humans in southwestern United States. Am J Trop Med Hyg 1961;10:44–8.

6. Barro N, Aly S, Tidiane OC, Sababenedjo TA. Carriage of bacteria by proboscises, legs, and feces of two species of flies in street food vending sites in Ouagadougou, Burkina Faso. J Food Prot 2006;69:2007–10.
7. Pitisuttithum P, Cohen MB, Phonrat B, et al. A human volunteer challenge model using frozen bacteria of the new epidemic serotype, V. cholerae O139 in Thai volunteers. Vaccine 2001;20:920–5.
8. Ofek I, Beachey EH. Mannose binding and epithelial cell adherence of Escherichia coli. Infect Immun 1978;22:247.
9. Michgehl S, Heusipp G, Greune L, et al. Esp-independent functional integration of the translocated intimin receptor (Tir) of enteropathogenic Escherichia coli (EPEC) into host cell membranes. Cell Microbiol 2006;8:625–33.
10. Clerk P, Sansonetti PJ. Entry of Shigella flexneri into HeLa cells: evidence for directed phagocytosis involving actin polymerization and myosin accumulation. Infect Immun 1987;55:2681–8.
11. Ogawa M, Yoshimori T, Suzuki T, et al. Escape of intracellular Shigella from autophagy. Science 2005;307: 727–31.
12. Bernardini ML, Mounier J, d'Hauteville H, et al. Identification of icsA, a plasmid locus of Shigella flexneri that governs bacterial intra- and intercellular spread through interaction with F-actin. Proc Natl Acad Sci USA 1989;86:38–67.
13. Jansson L, Tobias J, Lebens M, et al. The major subunit, CfaB, of colonization factor antigen i from enterotoxigenic Escherichia coli is a glycosphingolipid binding protein. Infect Immun 2006;74:3488–97.
14. Sixma TK, Kalk KH, van Zanten BA, et al. Refined structure of Escherichia coli heat-labile enterotoxin, a close relative of cholera toxin. J Mol Biol 1993;230:890–918.
15. Dickinson BL, Clements JD. Dissociation of Escherichia coli heat-labile enterotoxin adjuvanticity from ADP-ribosyltransferase activity. Infect Immun 1995;63:1617–23.
16. Tauschek M, Gorrell RJ, Strugnell RA, Robins-Browne RM. Identification of a protein secretory pathway for the secretion of heat-labile enterotoxin by an enterotoxigenic strain of Escherichia coli. Proc Natl Acad Sci U S A 2002;99:7066–71.
17. Teneberg S, Hirst TR, Angstrom J, Karlsson KA. Comparison of the glycolipid-binding specificities of cholera toxin and porcine Escherichia coli heat-labile enterotoxin: identification of a receptor-active non-ganglioside glycolipid for the heat-labile toxin in infant rabbit small intestine. Glycoconjugate J 1994;11:533–40.
18. Lencer WI, Constable C, Moe S, et al. Targeting of cholera toxin and Escherichia coli heat labile toxin in polarized epithelia: role of COOH-terminal KDEL. J Cell Biol 1995; 131:951–62.
19. Parkinson SJ, Alekseev AE, Gomez LA, et al. Interruption of Escherichia coli heat-stable enterotoxin-induced guanylyl cyclase signaling and associated chloride current in human intestinal cells by 2-chloroadenosine. J Biol Chem 1997;272:754–8.
20. Patel A, Cummings N, Batchelor M, et al. Host protein interactions with enteropathogenic Escherichia coli (EPEC): 14-3-3tau binds Tir and has a role in EPEC-induced actin polymerization. Cell Microbiol 2006;8:55–71.
21. Lommel S, Benesch S, Rohde M, et al. Enterohaemorrhagic and enteropathogenic Escherichia coli use different mechanisms for actin pedestal formation that converge on N-WASP. Cell Microbiol 2004;6: 243–54.
22. Knutton S, Baldwin T, Williams PH, McNeish AS. Actin accumulation at sites of bacterial adhesion to tissue culture cells: basis of a new diagnostic test for enteropathogenic and enterohemorrhagic Escherichia coli. Infect Immun 1989;57:1290–8.
23. Scaletsky ICA, Silva MLM, Trabulsi LR. Distinctive patterns of adherence of enteropathogenic Escherichia coli to HeLa cells. Infect Immun 1984;45:534–6.
24. Abe A, Nagano H. Functional analysis of the type III secretion system in enteropathogenic Escherichia coli O157:H45. Microbiol Immunol 2000;44:857–61.
25. Dytoc M, Fedorko L, Sherman PM. Signal transduction in human epithelial cells infected with attaching and effacing Escherichia coli in vitro. Gastroenterology 1994;106:1150–61.
26. Field M, Rao MC, Chang EB. Intestinal electrolyte transport and diarrheal disease, part 1. N Engl J Med 1989;321:800–6.
27. Shifflett DE, Clayburgh DR, Koutsouris A, et al. Enteropathogenic E. coli disrupts tight junction barrier function and structure in vivo. Lab Invest 2005;85:1308–24.
28. Nataro JP, Kaper JB, Robins-Browne R, et al. Patterns of adherence of diarrheagenic Escherichia coli to HEp-2 cells. Pediatr Infect Dis J 1987;6:829–31.
29. Sheikh J, Hicks S, Dall'Agnol M, et al. Roles for Fis and YafK in biofilm formation by enteroaggregative Escherichia coli. Mol Microbiol 2001;41:983–97.
30. Nataro JP, Hicks S, Phillips AD, et al. T84 cells in culture as a model for enteroaggregative Escherichia coli pathogenesis. Infect Immun 1996;64:4761–8.
31. Villaseca JM, Navarro-Garcia F, Mendoza-Hernandez G, et al. Pet toxin from enteroaggregative Escherichia coli produces cellular damage associated with fodrin disruption. Infect Immun 2000;68:5920–7.

32. Vila J, Vargas M, Henderson IR, et al. Enteroaggregative Escherichia coli virulence factors in travelers' diarrhea strains. J Infect Dis 2000;182:1780–3.

33. Dudley EG, Thomson NR, Parkhill J, et al. Proteomic and microarray characterization of the AggR regulon identifies a pheU pathogenicity island in enteroaggregative Escherichia coli. Mol Microbiol 2006;61:1267–82.

34. Sheikh J, Czeczulin JR, Harrington S, et al. A novel dispersin protein in enteroaggregative Escherichia coli. J Clin Invest 2002;110:1329–37.

35. Greenberg DE, Jiang ZD, Steffen R, et al. Markers of inflammation in bacterial diarrhea among travelers, with a focus on enteroaggregative Escherichia coli pathogenicity. J Infect Dis 2002;185:944–9.

36. Steiner TS, Nataro JP, Poteet-Smith CE, et al. Enteroaggregative Escherichia coli expresses a novel flagellin that causes IL-8 release from intestinal epithelial cells. J Clin Invest 2000;105:1769–77.

37. Harrington SM, Strauman MC, Abe CM, Nataro JP. Aggregative adherence fimbriae contribute to the inflammatory response of epithelial cells infected with enteroaggregative Escherichia coli. Cell Microbiol 2005;7:1565–78.

38. Ekdahl K, Andersson Y. The epidemiology of travel-associated shigellosis—regional risks, seasonality and serogroups. J Infect 2005;51:222–9.

39. Lopez EL, Prado-Jimenez V, O'Ryan-Gallardo M, Contrini MM. Shigella and shiga toxin-producing Escherichia coli causing bloody diarrhea in Latin America. Infect Dis Clin North Am 2000;14:41–65.

40. Procop GW. Gastrointestinal infections. Infect Dis Clin North Am 2001;15:1073–108.

41. Cohen D, Green M, Block C, et al. Reduction of transmission of shigellosis by control of houseflies (Musca domestica). Lancet 1991;337:993–7.

42. Sansonetti PJ. The bacterial weaponry: lessons from Shigella. Ann N Y Acad Sci 2006;1072:307–12.

43. Sansonetti PJ. Shigellosis: an old disease in new clothes? PLoS Med 2006;3:e354.

44. Sansonetti PJ, Tran Van Nhieu G, Pgile C. Rupture of the intestinal epithelial barrier and mucosal invasion by Shigella flexneri. Clin Infect Dis 1999;28:466–75.

45. Chopra P, Verma D, Khullar M, et al. Shiga toxin exposure modulates intestinal brush border membrane functional proteins in rabbit ileum. Mol Cell Biochem 2006;283:85–92.

46. Zurawski DV, Mitsuhata C, Mumy KL, et al. OspF and OspC1 are Shigella flexneri type III secretion system effectors that are required for postinvasion aspects of virulence. Infect Immun 2006;74:5964–76.

47. Goldberg MB, Theriot JA. Shigella flexneri surface protein IcsA is sufficient to direct actin-based motility. Proc Natl Acad Sci U S A 1995;92:6572–6.

48. Hilbi H, Moss JE, Hersh D, et al. Shigella-induced apoptosis is dependent on caspase-1 which binds to IpaB. J Biol Chem 1998;273:32895–900.

49. Sansonetti PJ. Microbes and microbial toxins: paradigms for microbial-mucosal interactions III. Shigellosis: from symptoms to molecular pathogenesis. Am J Physiol Gastrointest Liver Physiol 2001;280:G319–23.

50. Le-Barillec K, Magalhaes JG, Corcuff E, et al. Roles for T and NK cells in the innate immune response to Shigella flexneri. J Immunol 2005;175:1735–40.

51. Harrison LM, van Haaften WC, Tesh VL. Regulation of proinflammatory cytokine expression by Shiga toxin 1 and/or lipopolysaccharides in the human monocytic cell line THP-1. Infect Immun 2004;72:2618–27.

52. Drecktrah D, Knodler LA, Ireland R, Steele-Mortimer O. The mechanism of Salmonella entry determines the vacuolar environment and intracellular gene expression. Traffic 2006;7:39–51.

53. Hackett J, Kotlarski I, Mathan V, et al. The colonization of Peyer's patches by a strain of Salmonella typhimurium cured of the cryptic plasmid. J Infect Dis 1986;153:1119–25.

54. Huang DB, DuPont HL. Problem pathogens: extra-intestinal complications of Salmonella enterica serotype Typhi infection. Lancet Infect Dis 2005;5:341–8.

55. Li J, Ochman H, Groisman EA, et al. Relationship between evolutionary rate and cellular location among the Inv/Spa invasion proteins of Salmonella enterica. Proc Natl Acad Sci U S A 1995;92:7252–6.

56. Weiss J, Victor M, Stendhal O, Elsbach P. Killing of gram-negative bacteria by polymorphonuclear leukocytes: role of an O2-independent bactericidal system. J Clin Invest 1982;69:959–70.

57. Alpuche-Aranda CM, Racoosin EL, Swanson JA, Miller SI. Salmonella stimulate macrophage macropinocytosis and persist within spacious phagosomes. J Exp Med 1994;179:601–8.

58. Calva JJ, Ruiz-Palacios GM. Salmonella hepatitis: detection of Salmonella antigens in the liver of patients with typhoid fever. J Infect Dis 1986;154:373–4.

59. Looney RJ, Steigbigel RT. Role of the Vi antigen of Salmonella typhi in resistance to host defense in vitro. J Lab Clin Med 1986;108:506–16.

60. Yethon JA, Gunn JS, Ernst RK, et al. Salmonella enterica serovar typhimurium waaP mutants show increased susceptibility to polymyxin and loss of virulence In vivo. Infect Immun 2000;68:4485–91.

61. Lindberg AA. Bacterial virulence factors with particular reference to Salmonella bacteria. Scand J Infect Dis Suppl 1980;24:86–92.

62. Kawasaki K, Ernst RK, Miller SI. Purification and characterization of deacylated and/or palmitoylated lipid A species unique to Salmonella enterica serovar Typhimurium. J Endotoxin Res 2005;11:57–61.

63. Wolfe MS, Louria DB, Armstrong D, Blevins A. Salmonellosis in patients with neoplastic disease. A review of 100 episodes at Memorial Cancer Center over a 13-year period. Arch Intern Med 1971;128:546–54.

64. Mussche MM, Lameire NH, Ringoir SM. Salmonella typhimurium infections in renal transplant patients. Report of five cases. Nephron 1975;15:143–150.

65. Levine WC, Buehler JW, Bean NH, Tauxe RV. Epidemiology of nontyphoidal Salmonella bacteremia during the human immunodeficiency virus epidemic. J Infect Dis 1991;164:81–7.

66. de Jong R, Altare F, Haagen IA, et al. Severe mycobacterial and Salmonella infections in interleukin-12 receptor-deficient patients. Science 1998;280:1435–8.

67. Workman MR, Philpott-Howard J, Bellingham AJ. Managing patients with an absent or dysfunctional spleen: guidelines should highlight risk of Salmonella infection in sickle cell disease. Br Med J 1996;312:1359–60.

68. Black RE, Levine MM, Clements ML, et al. Experimental Campylobacter jejuni infection in humans. J Infect Dis 1988;157:472.

69. Blaser MJ, Hardesty HL, Powers B, et al. Survival of Campylobacter fetus subsp. jejuni in biological milieus. J Clin Microbiol 1980;11:309.

70. Russell RG, O'Donnoghue M, Blake DC Jr, et al. Early colonic damage and invasion of Campylobacter jejuni in experimentally challenged infant Macaca mulatta. J Infect Dis 1993;168:210–5.

71. Babakhani FK, Joens LA. Primary swine intestinal cells as a model for studying Campylobacter jejuni invasiveness. Infect Immun 1993;61:2723–6.

72. Leon-Kempis Mdel R, Guccione E, Mulholland F, et al. The Campylobacter jejuni PEB1a adhesin is an aspartate/glutamate-binding protein of an ABC transporter essential for microaerobic growth on dicarboxylic amino acids. Mol Microbiol 2006;60:1262–75.

73. Van Spreeuwel JP, Duursma GC, Meijer CJLM, et al. Campylobacter colitis: histologic, immunohistochemical and ultrastructural findings. Gut 1985;26:945–51.

74. Aspinall GO, Fujimoto S, McDonald AG, et al. Lipopolysaccharides from Campylobacter jejuni associated with Guillain-Barrio syndrome patients mimic human gangliosides in structure. Infect Immun 1994;62: 2122–5.

75. Allos BM. Association between Campylobacter infection and Guillain-Barré syndrome. J Infect Dis 1997;176:S125–8.

76. Peterson MC. Rheumatic manifestation of Campylobacter jejuni and C. fetus infections in adults. Scand J Rheumatol 1994;23:167–70.

77. Zen-Yoji H, Sakai S, Terayama T, et al. Epidemiology, enteropathogenicity, and classification of Vibrio parahemolyticus. J Infect Dis 1965;115:436.

78. Barker WH, Mackowick PA, Fishbein M, et al. Vibrio parahemolyticus gastroenteritis outbreak in Covington, Louisiana, in August 1972. Am J Epidemiol 1974;100:316.

79. Centers for Disease Control and Prevention. Gastroenteritis caused by Vibrio parahemolyticus aboard a cruise ship. MMWR Morb Mortal Wkly Rep 1978;27: 67.

80. Okuda J, Nishibuchi M. Manifestation of the Kanagawa phenomenon, the virulence-associated phenotype, of Vibrio parahaemolyticus depends on a particular single base change in the promoter of the thermostable direct haemolysin gene. Mol Microbiol 1998;30:499–511.

81. Yoh M, Miwatani T, Honda T. Comparison of Vibrio parahaemolyticus hemolysin (Vp-TRH) produced by environmental and clinical isolates. FEMS Microbiol Lett 1992;71:157–61.

82. Maluping RP, Lavilla-Pitogo CR, DePaola A, et al. Occurrence, characterisation and detection of potential virulence determinants of emerging aquatic bacterial pathogens from the Philippines and Thailand. New Microbiol 2004;27:381–9.

83. Hanninen ML, Salmi S, Mattila L, et al. Association of Aeromonas spp with travelers' diarrhoea in Finland. J Med Microbiol 1995;42:26–31.

84. Jones BL, Wilcox MH. Aeromonas infections and their treatment. J Antimicrob Chemother 1995;35:453–61.

85. Vila J, Ruiz J, Gallardo F, et al. Aeromonas spp. and traveler's diarrhea: clinical features and antimicrobial resistance. Emerg Infect Dis 2003;9:552–5.

86. Ebanks RO, Knickle LC, Goguen M, et al. Expression of and secretion through the Aeromonas salmonicida type III secretion system. Microbiology 2006;152:1275–86.

87. Yu HB, Zhang YL, Lau YL, et al. Identification and characterization of putative virulence genes and gene clusters in Aeromonas hydrophila PPD134/91. Appl Environ Microbiol 2005;71:4469–77.

88. Brenden RA, Miller MA, Janda JM. Clinical disease spectrum and pathogenic factors associated with Plesiomonas shigelloides infections in humans. Rev Infect Dis 1988;10:303–16.

89. Rautelin H, Sivonen A, Kuikka A, et al. Enteric Plesiomonas shigelloides infections in Finnish patients. Scand J Infect Dis 1995;27:495–8.

90. Kain KC, Kelly MT. Clinical features, epidemiology, and treatment of Plesiomonas shigelloides diarrhea. J Clin Microbiol 1989;27:998–1001.

91. Herrington DA, Tzipori S, Robins-Browne RM, et al. In vitro and in vivo pathogenicity of Plesiomonas shigelloides. Infect Immun 1987;55:979–85.

92. Ciznar I, Hostacka A, Gonzalez-Rey C, Krovacek K. Potential virulence-associated properties of Plesiomonas shigelloides strains. Folia Microbiol 2004;49:543–8.

93. Bishop R, Davidson G, Holmes I, et al. Virus particles in epithelial cells of duodenal mucosa from children with acute non-bacterial gastroenteritis. Lancet 1973;2:1281–3.

94. Davidson G, Goller J, Bishop R, et al. Immunofluorescence in duodenal mucosa of children with acute enteritis due to a new virus. J Clin Pathol 1975;28:263–6.

95. Willoughby R, Yolken R, Schnaar R. Rotaviruses specifically bind to the neutral glycosphingolipid asialo-GM1. J Virol 1990;64:4830–5.

96. Fukuhara N, Yoshie O, Kitaoka S, et al. Evidence for endocytosis-independent infection by human rotavirus. Arch Virol 1987;97:93–9.

97. Kaljot K, Shaw R, Rubin D, et al. Infectious rotavirus enters cells by direct cell membrane penetration, not by endocytosis. J Virol 1988;62:1136–44.

98. Lundgren O, Peregrin AT, Persson K, et al. Role of the enteric nervous system in the fluid and electrolyte secretion of rotavirus diarrhea. Science 2000;287:491–5.

99. Ball JM, Tian P, Zeng CQ, et al. Age-dependent diarrhea induced by a rotaviral nonstructural glycoprotein. Science 1996;272:101–4.

100. Berkova Z, Crawford SE, Trugnan G, et al. Rotavirus NSP4 induces a novel vesicular compartment regulated by calcium and associated with viroplasms. J Virol 2006;80: 6061–71.

101. Halaihel N, Lievin V, Ball JM, et al. Direct inhibitory effect of rotavirus NSP4(114–135) peptide on the Na-D-glucose symporter of rabbit intestinal brush border membrane. J Virol 2000;74:9464–70.

102. Osborne MP, Haddon SJ, Worton KJ, et al. Rotavirus-induced changes in the microcirculation of intestinal villi of neonatal mice in relation to the induction and persistence of diarrhea. J Pediatr Gastroenterol Nutr 1991;12:111–20.

103. Hyams J, Krause P, Gleason P. Lactose malabsorption following rotavirus infection in young children. J Pediatr 1981;99:916–8.

104. Martin-Latil S, Cotte-Laffitte J, Beau I, et al. A cyclic AMP protein kinase A-dependent mechanism by which rotavirus impairs the expression and enzyme activity of brush border-associated sucrase-isomaltase in differentiated intestinal Caco-2 cells. Cell Microbiol 2004;6:719–31.

105. Enserink M. Infectious diseases. Gastrointestinal virus strikes European cruise ships. Science 2006;313:747.

106. Johnson PC, Mathewson JJ, DuPont HL, Greenberg HB. Multiple-challenge study of host susceptibility to Norwalk gastroenteritis in US adults. J Infect Dis 1990;161:18–21.

107. Baron RC, Murphy FD, Greenberg HB. Norwalk gastrointestinal illness: an outbreak associated with swimming in a recreational lake and secondary person-to-person transmission. Am J Epidemiol 1982;115:163–72.

108. Koopman JS, Eckert EA, Greenberg HB. Norwalk virus enteric illness acquired by swimming exposure. Am J Epidemiol 1982;115:173–7.

109. Tree JA, Adams MR, Lees DN. Disinfection of feline calicivirus (a surrogate for Norovirus) in wastewaters. J Appl Microbiol 2005;98:155–62.

110. Patterson W, Haswell P, Fryers PT, et al. Outbreak of small round structured virus gastroenteritis arose after kitchen assistant vomited. Commun Dis Rep CDR Rev 1997;7:R101–3.

111. Chadwick PR, McCann R. Transmission of a small round structured virus by vomiting during hospital out-break of gastroenteritis. J Hosp Infect 1994;26:251–9.

112. Greenberg HB, Wyatt RG, Kapikian AZ. Norwalk virus in vomitus. Lancet 1979;1:55.

113. Rockx BH, Vennema H, Hoebe CJ, et al. Association of histo-blood group antigens and susceptibility to norovirus infections. J Infect Dis 2005;191:749–54.

114. Tan M, Meller J, Jiang X. C-terminal arginine cluster is essential for receptor binding of norovirus capsid protein. J Virol 2006;80:7322–31.

115. Ko G, Jiang ZD, Okhuysen PC, DuPont HL. Fecal cytokines and markers of intestinal inflammation in international travelers with diarrhea due to Noroviruses. J Med Virol 2006;78:825–8.

116. Cheetham S, Souza M, Meulia T, et al. Pathogenesis of a genogroup II human norovirus in gnotobiotic pigs. J Virol 2006;80:10372–81.

117. Widerlite L, Trier J, Blacklow N, et al. Structure of the gastric mucosa in acute infectious nonbacterial gastroenteritis. Gastroenterology 1975;70:321–5.

118. Agus SG, Dolin R, Wyatt RG, et al. Acute infectious nonbacterial gastroenteritis: intestinal histopathology. Ann Intern Med 1973;79:18–25.

119. Blacklow NR, Dolin R, Feson DS, et al. Acute infectious nonbacterial gastroenteritis: etiology and pathogenesis. Ann Intern Med 1972;76:993–1000.

120. Levy AG, Widerlite L, Schwartz CJ, et al. Jejunal adenylate cyclase activity in human subjects during viral gastroenteritis. Gastroenterology 1976;70:321–5.

121. Okhuysen P. Traveler's diarrhea due to intestinal protozoa. Clin Infect Dis 2001;33:110–4.

122. Huang DB, White AC. An updated review on Cryptosporidium and Giardia. Gastroenterol Clin North Am 2006;35:291–314.

123. Jokipii L, Pohjola S, Jokipii AM. Cryptosporidium: a frequent finding in patients with gastrointestinal symptoms. Lancet 1983;2:358–61.

124. Ma P, Kaufman DL, Helmick CG, et al. Cryptosporidiosis in tourists returning from the Caribbean. N Engl J Med 1985;312:647–8.

125. Gatti S, Cevini C, Bruno A, et al. Cryptosporidiosis in tourists returning from Egypt and the Island of Mauritius. Clin Infect Dis 1993;16:344.

126. Flegg PJ. Crypstosporidium in travelers from Pakistan. Trans R Soc Trop Med Hyg 1987;81:171.

127. Guerrant RL. Cryptosporidiosis: an emerging, highly infectious threat. Emerg Infect Dis 1997;48:329–40.

128. Du Pont HL, Chappell CL, Sterling CR, et al. The infectivity of Cryptosporidium parvum in healthy volunteers. N Engl J Med 1995;332:855–60.

129. Okhuysen PC, Chappell CL, Crabb JH, et al. Virulence of three distinct Cryptosporidium parvum isolates for healthy adults. J Infect Dis 1999;180:1275–81.

130. Elliot DA, Clark DP. Cryptosporidium parvum induces host cell actin accumulation at the host-parasite interface. Infect Immun 2000;68:2315–22.

131. Capet C, Kapel N, Huneau JF, et al. Cryptosporidium parvum infection in suckling rats: impairment of mucosal permeability and Na(+)-glucose cotransport. Exp Parasitol 1999;91:119–25.

132. Kandil HM, Berschneider HM, Argenzio RA. Tumour necrosis factor alpha changes porcine intestinal ion transport through a paracrine mechanism involving prostaglandins. Gut 1994;35:934–40.

133. Gookin JL, Duckett LL, Armstrong MU, et al. Nitric oxide synthase stimulates prostaglandin synthesis and barrier function in C. parvum-infected porcine ileum. Am J Physiol Gastrointest Liver Physiol 2004;287:G571–81.

134. Pollok RC, Farthing MJ, Bajaj-Elliot M, et al. Interferon gamma induces enterocyte resistance against infection by the intracellular pathogen. Gastroenterology 2001;120:99–107.

135. McDonald V. Host cell-mediated responses to infection with Cryptosporidium. Parasite Immnunol 2000;22:597–604.

136. Rehg JE. Effect of interferon-gamma in experimental Cryptosporidium parvum infection. J Infect Dis 1996;174:229–32.

137. Jelinek T, Lotze M, Eichenlaub S, et al. Prevalence of infection with Cryptosporidium parvum and Cyclospora cayetanensis among international travellers. Gut 1997;41:801–4.

138. Hart AS, Ridinger MR, Soundarajan R, et al. Novel organism associated with chronic diarrhoea in AIDS. Lancet 1990;335:169–70.

139. Pape JW, Verdien RI, Boncy M, et al. Cyclospora infections in adults with HIV: clinical manifestations, treatment and prophylaxis. Ann Intern Med 1994;121:654–7.

140. Rabold JG, Hoge CW, Shlim DR, et al. Cyclospora outbreak associated with chlorinated drinking water [letter]. Lancet 1994;344:1360–1.

141. Huang P, Weber JT, Sosin DM, et al. The first reported outbreak of diarrheal illness associated with Cyclospora in the United States. Ann Intern Med 1995;123:409–14.

142. el-Karamany EM, Zaher TI, el-Bahnasawy MM. Role of water in the transmission of cyclosporiarsis in Sharkia Governorate, Egypt. J Egypt Soc Parasitol 2005;35:953–62.

143. Shlim DR. Cyclospora cayetanesis. Clin Lab Med 2002;22:927–36.

144. Sun T, Ilardi CF, Asnis D, et al. Light and electron microscopic identification of Cyclospora species in the small intestine. Evidence of the presence of asexual life cycle in human host. Am J Clin Pathol 1996;105:216–20.

145. Connor BA, Reidy J, Soave R. Cyclosporiasis: clinical and histopathologic correlates. Clin Infect Dis 1999;28:1216–22.

146. Ortega YR, Nagle R, Gilman RH, et al. Pathologic and clinical findings in patients with cyclosporiasis and a description of intracellular parasite life-cycle stages. J Infect Dis 1997;176:1584–9.

147. Doyle PW, Helgason MM, Mathias RG, Proctor EM. Epidemiology and pathogenicity of Blastocystis hominis. J Clin Microbiol 1990;28:116–21.

148. Graczyk TK, Shiff CK, Tamang L, et al. The association of Blastocystis hominis and Endolimax nana with diarrheal stools in Zambian school-age children. Parasitol Res 2005;98:38–43.

149. Jelinek T, Peyerl G, Loscher T, et al. The role of Blastocystis hominis as a possible intestinal pathogen in travellers. J Infect 1997;35:63–6.

150. Nigro L, Larocca L, Massarelli L, et al. A placebo-controlled treatment trial of Blastocystis hominis infection with metronidazole. J Travel Med 2003;10:128–30.

151. Russo AR, Stone SL, Taplin ME, et al. Presumptive evidence for Blastocystis hominis as a cause of colitis. Arch Intern Med 1988;148:1064.

152. Adkins H, Merrell B, O'Rourke T, Echeverria P. Travelers' diarrhea among U.S. Navy and Marine Corps personnel during a Western Pacific deployment. Mil Med 1990;155:111–6.

153. Hjelt K, Paerregaard A, Krasilnikoff PA. Giardiasis causing chronic diarrhea in suburban Copenhagen: incidence,

physical growth, clinical symptoms and small intestine abnormality. Acta Paediatr 1992;81:881–6.

154. Homan WL, Mank TG. Human giardiasis: genotype linked differences in clinical symptomatology. Int J Parasitol 2001;31:822–6.

155. Gottig N, Elias EV, Quiroga R, et al. Active and passive mechanisms drive secretory granule biogenesis during differentiation of the intestinal parasite Giardia lamblia. J Biol Chem 2006;281:18156–66.

156. Erlandsen SL, Russo AP, Turner JN. Evidence for adhesive activity of the ventrolateral flange in Giardia lamblia. J Eukaryot Microbiol 2004;51:73–80.

157. Weiland ME, McArthur AG, Morrison HG, et al. Annexin-like alpha giardins: a new cytoskeletal gene family in Giardia lamblia. Int J Parasitol 2005;35:617–26.

158. Peattie DA, Alonso RA, Hein A, Caulfield JP. Ultrastructural localization of giardins to the edges of disk microribbons of Giarida lamblia and the nucleotide and deduced protein sequence of alpha giardin. J Cell Biol 1989;109:2323–35.

159. Mohammed SR, Faubert GM. Disaccharidase deficiencies in Mongolian gerbils (Meriones unguiculatus) protected against Giardia lamblia. Parasitol Res 1995;81: 582–90.

160. Scott KG. Jejunal brush border microvillous alterations in Giardia muris-infected mice: role of T lymphocytes and interleukin-6. Infect Immun 2000;68:3412–8.

161. Teoh DA, Kamieniecki D, Pang G, Buret AG. Giardia lamblia rearranges F-actin and alpha-actinin in human colonic and duodenal monolayers and reduces transepithelial electrical resistance. J Parasitol 2000;86:800–6.

162. Eckman L, Gillin FD. Microbes and microbial toxins: paradigms for microbial-mucosal interactions I. Pathophysiological aspects of enteric infections with the lumen-dwelling protozoan pathogen Giardia lamblia. Am J Physiol Gastrointest Liver Physiol 2001;280:G1–6.

163. Singer SM, Nash TE. The role of normal flora in Giardia infection in mice. J Infect Dis 2000;181:1510–2.

164. Torres MF, Uetanabaro AP, Costa AF, et al. Influence of bacteria from the duodenal microbiota of patients with symptomatic giardiasis on the pathogenicity of Giardia duodenalis in gonotoxemic mice. J Med Microbiol 2000; 49:209–15.

165. Ackers JP, Mirelman D. Progress in research on Entamoeba histolytica pathogenesis. Curr Opin Microbiol 2006;9:367–73.

166. Winkelmann J, Leippe M, Bruhn H. A novel saposin-like protein of Entamoeba histolytica with membrane-fusogenic activity. Mol Biochem Parasitol 2006;147:85–94.

167. Lidell ME, Moncada DM, Chadee K, Hansson GC. Entamoeba histolytica cysteine proteases cleave the MUC2 mucin in its C-terminal domain and dissolve the protective colonic mucus gel. Proc Natl Acad Sci U S A 2006;103:9298–303.

168. Frederick JR, Petri WA Jr. Roles for the galactose-/N-acetylgalactosamine-binding lectin of Entamoeba in parasite virulence and differentiation. Glycobiology 2005;15: 53R–9R.

169. Pittman FE, El Hashimi WK, Pittman JC. Studies of human amebiasis. Light and electromicroscopic observations of colonic mucosa and exudate in acute amebic colitis. Gastroenterology 1973;65:588–603.

170. Takeuchi A, Phillips BP. Electron microscopic studies of experimental Entamoeba histolytica infection in the guinea pig. I. Penetration of the intestinal epithelium by trophozoites. Am J Trop Med Hyg 1975;24:34–48.

171. Moody S, Becker S, Nuchamowitz Y, Mirelman D. Identification of significant variation in the composition of lipophosphoglycan-like molecules of E. histolytica and E. dispar. J Eukaryot Microbiol 1998;45:9S–12S.

172. Sharma M, Vohra H, Bhasin D. Enhanced pro-inflammatory chemokine/cytokine response triggered by pathogenic Entamoeba histolytica: basis of invasive disease. Parasitology 2005;131:783–96.

173. Guerrant RL, Brush J, Ravdin JI, et al. Interaction between Entamoeba histolytica and human polymorphonuclear neutrophils. J Infect Dis 1981;143:83–93.

174. Tsutsumi V, Mena-Lopez R, Anaya-Velazquez F, et al. Cellular basis of experimental amebic liver abscess formation. Am J Pathol 1984;117:81–91.

175. Salata RA, Ravdin JI. The interaction of human neutrophils and Entamoeba histolytica increases cytopathogenicity for liver cell monolayers. J Infect Dis 1986;154:19–26.

176. Herrera-Rodriguez SE, Baylon-Pacheco L, Talamas-Rohana P, Rosales-Encina JL. Cloning and partial characterization of Entamoeba histolytica PTPases. Biochem Biophys Res Commun 2006;342:1014–21.

CHAPTER 7

RELATIVE IMPORTANCE OF PATHOGENS AND NONINFECTIOUS CAUSES

ANNELIES WILDER-SMITH, MD, PhD

JAIME BELKIND-GERSON, MS, MD

The yield of causal enteropathogens has improved over the years, and approximately 60 to 80% of cases of travelers' diarrhea are now associated with an identified pathogen.[1–7] This chapter attempts to put these pathogens into perspective as they relate to causing travelers' diarrhea: eg, the relative importance of bacterial, viral, and parasitic pathogens as well as noninfectious causes, their relation to geographical distribution, season, activities during travel, and risk groups. The intent is to help the travel medicine practitioner make an evidence-based risk assessment and guide the decision for empiric treatment or prevention.

Relative Importance of Pathogens

Bacterial pathogens are the most common cause of travelers' diarrhea (50 to 80%), followed by viruses (0 to 36%) and parasites (0 to 36%) (Table 1). In approximately 20% of cases, no pathogen is identified. The geographic distribution of pathogens in travelers' diarrhea is summarized in Table 1.

Relative Importance of Pathogens Depending on Destination, Season, and Travel Activities

Destination of travel and season have a major impact on the risk of travelers' diarrhea and the etiology. A recent report based on surveillance data of GeoSentinel—a global provider network of travel medicine practitioners on six continents (data for 17,353 ill returned travelers)—showed that acute diarrhea was disproportionately higher among those returning from south central Asia.[8] However, specific pathogens were not identified in this study. Even at a single destination, there are highly significant differences in traveler's diarrhea incidence rates for different risk groups.[1] Factors such as the selection of a hotel, younger age, increased duration of travel, origin from industrialized countries, more adventurous travel style, eating at street vendors, lack of avoidance of potentially contaminated food and beverages, decreased gastric acidity, immunodeficiency, genetic factors, and excessive alcohol consumption are all are associated with a higher risk.[1,9,10] In the following, the relative importance of pathogens related to destination, season, and travel activities will be examined.

BACTERIA

Bacteria are the enteropathogens most frequently incriminated (50 to 80%) as a cause of travelers' diarrhea.[11] Enterotoxigenic Escherichia coli (ETEC) was shown to be the most important cause of travelers' diarrhea worldwide, accounting for 5 to 60% of cases in all developing tropical and subtropical regions,[4,12–14] two–thirds of which involve heat-labile toxin (LT)-ETEC.[2] ETEC is more prevalent in most regions of Latin America and the Caribbean than in Asia and Africa. Figure 1 depicts the relative risk of ETEC in the world. ETEC in some studies was shown to have a seasonal pattern with a higher prevalence in summer and fall than in winter.[15,16] Rainy seasons also appear to be associated with a higher risk of ETEC diarrhea.[17] ETEC strains show geographic and seasonal variation in the expression of different toxin types (heat-labile versus heat-stable toxin production), colonization-factor antigens, plasmid, serotypes and antibiotic susceptibility.[18,19] The annual attack rate in

Table 1 Relative Importance of Pathogens Depending on Geographic Distribution

Pathogen	Latin America	Carribean	Asia	Africa	Total
ETEC	15–60	15–40	5–40	5–40	5–60
EAEC	0–40	0–30	0–20	0–15	0–40
Campylobacter	0–5	0–5	0–40	0–30	0–40
Salmonella	0–15	0–15	0–30	5–25	0–30
Shigella	0–30	0–15	0–15	0–10	0–30
Others	0–5	0–5	0–40	0–10	0–40
Viruses	0–20	0–20	0–10	0–30	0–20
Rotavirus	0–20	0–20	0–10	0–30	0–20
Protozoa	0–5	0–5	0–10	0–10	0–10
Mixed	0–20	0–10	0–30	0–20	0–20
No pathogen	20–60	20–70	10–55	10–55	10–60

EAEC = enteroaggregative E. coli; ETEC = enterotoxigenic E. coli; NR = not reported.

adult ex-patriots staying in Nepal for < 2 years was 43%.[20]

Enteroaggregative Escherichia coli (EAEC) have recently been identified as the second most common cause of travelers' diarrhea in a multi-site study, accounting for an average of 26% compared with 30% for ETEC.[21] EAEC appears to account for a substantial proportion of cases where previously no pathogen was identified. Diarrhea due to enteroaggregative Escherichia coli occurs significantly more often in individuals with the AA genotype than in individuals with the T genotype or the TT genotype in the interleukin-8 promotor region.[9] Enteropathogenic and Shiga toxin-producing E. coli strains are not common causes of travelers' diarrhea.

Campylobacter jejuni is overall the third most common cause of infection, but there is a great variation (0 to 40%) depending on destination and season. In

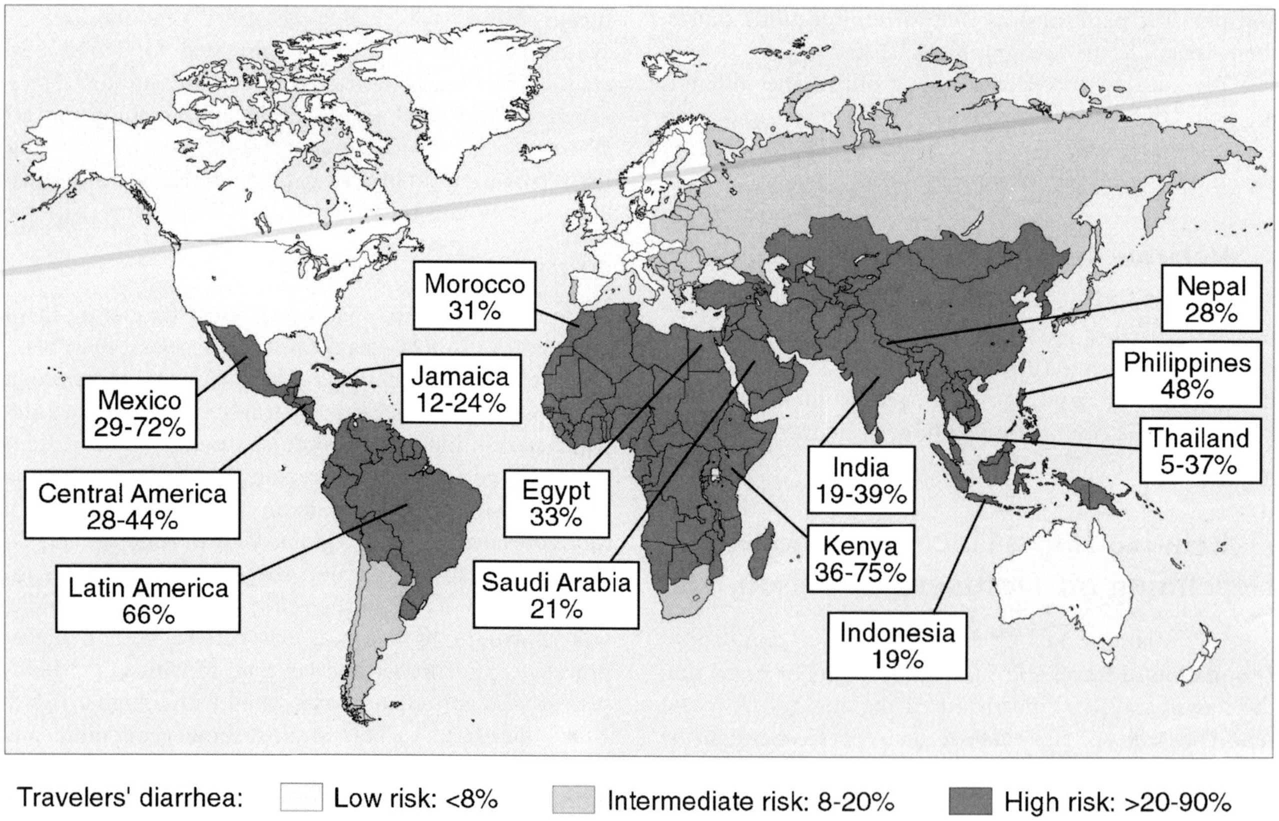

Figure 1 Percentage incidence of travelers' diarrhea caused by enterotoxigenic Escherichia coli. Reprinted with permission from Robert Steffen.[2]

some parts of Asia, Campylobacter is now more common than ETEC.[22,23] Campylobacter was reported to be the most common cause in military populations in Thailand.[22] C. *jejuni* was shown to be an important antecedent illnesses in patients with Guillain-Barre syndrome in India.[24] The epidemiology of travel-associated campylobacteriosis was studied using data from 28,704 notifications of travel-associated campylobacteriosis in Sweden from 1997 to 2003.[25] This large study showed that the highest risk for Campylobacter infection was seen in returning travelers from the Indian subcontinent (1,253/100,000 travelers), and the lowest in travelers from the other Nordic countries (3/100,000 travelers). In Africa, large differences in risk between regions were noted, with 502/100,000 in travelers from East Africa compared to 76/100,00 from West Africa and 50/100,000 from Central Africa.[25] A distinct seasonal pattern was seen in all temperate regions with peaks in the summer, while no or less distinct seasonality was seen in tropical regions. In travelers to the tropics, the highest risk was seen in children below the age of six.[25] C. jejuni is resistant to trimethoprim-sulfamethoxazole, and its resistance to fluoroquinolones is rapidly increasing in Southeast Asia.[23] The ofloxacin-resistance rate among Campylobacter isolates in a Dutch study increased from 11% to 29%; resistance against tetracycline fluctuated between 7 and 15%, and resistance against erythromycin remained low.[26] Increasingly, fluoroquinolone resistant Campylobacter are also reported from India, Japan, and United Arab Emirates.[27–29] Azithromycin therapy may be an effective alternative to ciprofloxacin therapy in areas where ciprofloxacin-resistant Campylobacter species are prevalent.[22]

The prevalence of shigellosis in travelers' diarrhea (0 to 30%) is similar to Campylobacter.[12] Shigellosis is more common in Mexico and India than in Jamaica.[30]

The relative prevalence of other bacteria such as *Aeromoas spp.*, *Salmonella spp.*, or *Vibrio species* varies greatly according to different studies, mainly due to the different techniques used for microbial identification and the seasonal variations and geographical distribution studied.[11] Nontyphoid salmonella is not common, but depending on studies may account for up to 3 to 30% of cases and is more common in Asia and Africa. Aeromonas and plesiomonas account for up to 10% of travelers' diarrhea cases, and non-vibrio cholera occurs occasionally, particularly in coastal Asian regions.[12]

VIRAL ENTERIC PATHOGENS

Viruses have been less studied except for the easily diagnosed rotavirus with a wide spectrum of prevalence (0 to 36%) in different series. Norwalk Virus and Norwalk-like viruses (NLVs) are reportedly responsible for 2.5 to 4.0% of nonbacterial acute gastroenteritis (NBAG) worldwide.[31–34] One study showed a substantial proportion of NLVs in troops on exercises in South East Asia.[32] Noroviruses (NoVs) were the second most commonly identified enteric pathogen in diarrheal stool samples (21/124, 17%) in 124 travelers to Mexico, exceeded only by enterotoxigenic Escherichia coli (50/106, 47%). This study indicates that NoV is an under-appreciated cause of traveler's diarrhea.[35] NLVs are primarily associated with cruise ship travel.[36,37] Dramatic improvements in sanitary engineering and especially operational procedures aboard cruise ships began in the mid-1970s after several large outbreaks of acute gastroenteritis. The significant increase in median ship sanitation scores over the past decade has been concomitant with a reduction in outbreak frequency to 3.7 per 1,000 cruises.[38] Although norovirus outbreaks may begin as food borne or waterborne disease, easy person-to-person transmission occurs through fecal- or vomitus-splattered surfaces, other items, clothing, and especially hands. Control of person-to-person spread of illness among crew and passengers becomes the major objective. Rigorous hand washing, environmental disinfection, and other food service job-related restrictions are required to prevent multiple outbreaks on the same ship. Vigilance by public health and industry officials has prevented many thousands of illnesses and some associated deaths. Clinicians providing pre-travel health advice and post-travel diagnoses and care can benefit from and contribute to epidemiologic investigations and thereby enhance the health of cruise passengers individually and collectively.[38]

Astroviruses and enteric adenoviruses cause a great disease burden in young children in cohort studies in different settings, but are not a frequent cause of diarrhea in travelers, most likely because these viruses primarily affect children.

Rotavirus is the principal cause of dehydrating diarrhea of young children in the world. Almost all children are infected at least once by the age of 3 years.[39] The first licensed rotavirus vaccine, RRV-TV, was removed from the market shortly after licensure because of an unexpected serious adverse event, intussusception. A pentavalent rotavirus vaccine, pentavalent rotavirus vaccine (PRV), is the second rotavirus vaccine licensed by the Food and Drug Administration and does not signal the risk observed with RRV-TV.[40] There is also a live attenuated human rotavirus vaccine in use in Latin America and the countries of the European Union that also appears to be safe and protective for severe rotavirus diarrhea.[41] With the recent advent of safe and effective rotavirus vaccines, the incidence of rotavirus-associated disease in travelers, in particular in pediatric travelers, needs to be investigated further to determine whether this vaccine would be indicated in the traveling population.

INTESTINAL PROTOZOA

Protozoal enteric pathogens are identified in 0 to 5% of travelers with diarrhea.[12] Intestinal protozoa account for a minority of cases of acute traveler's diarrhea, but they are common pathogens in travelers who experience protracted diarrhea during or after travel. Evaluation of the travelers with chronic diarrhea should include a careful examination for typical infecting organisms, such as Giardia and Entamoeba species, as well as for emerging parasites, such as Cryptosporidium species, Cyclospora species, and microsporidia.[42] Entamoeba histolytica accounts for less than 1% of travelers' diarrhea[43] and cryptosporidium for 1 to 2%. Cyclospora has been reported in travelers to Nepal.[44] In a study on adult expatriates staying in Nepal for < 2 years, the annual attack rate of specific pathogens was 32% for Cyclospora species and 16% for Giardia lamblia, and 6% for Entamoeba histolytica, showing the increasing importance of protozoal pathogens, in particular Cyclospora.[20] Cyclospora cayetanensis was reported to be more frequent during the rainy season in Nepal.[20] Cryptosporidiosis in travelers has been poorly studied. One survey of Peace Corps volunteers in West Africa demonstrated a 13.6% increase in seroprevalence over a 2-year period.[45] Cryptosporidiosis was reported in travelers to Leningrad and seemed to be acquired from similar sources as giardiasis.[46]

Noninfectious Causes

In approximately 20% of cases, causative pathogens are not identified. A substantial proportion of these cases represent undetected bacterial or viral agents. Stress, changes in dietary habits, excessive alcohol consumption, and eating oily foods can cause changes in stool consistency or frequency. However, these bowel changes are usually minor, with passage of often only one or two loose movements per day. Food allergies may present as acute diarrhea. A drug history needs to be taken because certain drugs can cause diarrhea, such as antibiotics, nonsteroidal anti-inflammatory drugs, antiarrhythmics (eg, quinidine), certain antihypertensives (eg, beta-adrenergic receptor blocking drugs), antacids (eg, those containing magnesium), acid-reducing agents (proton pump inhibitors, H2-receptor antagonists), colchicine, misoprostol, theophylline, etc. Laxative abuse (in particular stimulant laxatives) may be a cause of acute diarrhea in those travelers who self treated their constipation because constipation is a frequent problem during travel. Clostridium difficile- associated colitis should be considered (or excluded) in those who recently took a course of antibiotics.

Among noninfectious causes, ciguatoxin is prominent as an intoxication in travelers to the Caribbean and the Pacific areas.[47] Destination, season, and especially food habits have a great influence on its presence. Ciguatera poisoning causes early diarrhea followed by neurological and, less frequently, cardiovascular symptoms.

Prolonged stays in the tropics are associated with celiac sprue that requires specific diagnostic procedures and treatment.

Diarrhea due to noninfectious systemic illnesses may incidentally commence during travel but not be related to travel. This should particularly be considered if diarrheal symptoms persist. Examples include diarrhea-predominant irritable bowel syndrome (IBS), diarrhea due to endocrine dysfunction (such as hypothyroidism, Addison's disease, diabetic autonomic neuropathy), tumors (such as colon carcinoma, lymphoma, villous adenoma), inflammatory bowel disease etc.[48] It is also possible that undiagnosed conditions such as IBS and disaccharidase deficiencies, which are very common, may lead to diarrheal symptoms that become more evident with stress and dietary changes related to travel. A thorough work-up by the gastroenterologist is warranted. Infectious diseases that do not primarily affect the gastrointestinal tract can also cause severe diarrhea. Of the travel-associated systemic infections presenting with fever, diarrhea occurs in patients with malaria, dengue fever, and SARS.[49,50]

The proportion of diarrhea not associated with an enteropathogen or responsive to antimicrobial therapy deserves additional study. Perhaps new nonbacterial pathogens will be discovered, and search for new viruses, protozoa, and bacteria, including strict anaerobes, should continue.

Implications For the Travel Medicine Practitioner

Travel medicine practitioners need to be aware that certain travel activities are associated with certain pathogens. For example, the risk of norovirus infections is high on cruise ships. Trekking in Canada, New Zealand, or Nepal is associated with Giardia. The risk of fluoroquinolone-resistant campylobacter is associated with travel to Thailand. Cyclospora is a higher risk for travelers to Nepal or Peru. Giardia and cryptosporidium have been associated with tap water in St Petersburg, Russia (Table 2).[46] Certain preferences for food may be associated with a higher risk, such as Mexican sauces, excessive beer, ceviche, etc.[1]

Table 2 Rough Associations between Certain Activities, Destinations and Pathogens

Pathogen	Destination	Travel activities
Bacterial enteropathogens, particularly ETEC and EAEC	All tropical and subtropical areas	Any travel
Parasitic pathogens such as giardia, cyclospora, cryptosporidium	Nepal, Peru, Haiti	Trekking. Long term stay
Cryptosporidium and Giardia	Russia, particularly St Petersburg	Drinking tap water
Fluoroquinolone-resistant Campylobacter jejuni	Thailand, possibly many other parts in Asia	Any travel
Norovirus	Cruise ships anywhere	Cruise ship travel

Early empirical therapy with antibacterial drugs, including rifaximin, a fluoroquinolone, or azithromycin, will decrease the duration of illness and return travelers more quickly to their planned activities.[51] It is important to identify regions of highest risks in order to target appropriate empiric antimicrobial therapy. Because E. coli continues to be the leading cause of travelers' diarrhea, empiric treatment with fluoroquinolones for most parts of the world remains justified. However, in some parts of Asia, Campylobacter is now more common than ETEC, and resistance to fluoroquinolones is high in Asia.[22,23] This is particularly well described for Thailand. With increasing reports of resistance in other parts of Asia, it is prudent to select azithromycin as the empiric antimicrobial agent of choice for treatment of travelers' diarrhea.

Salmonella is often thought to be best managed without antibiotics to prevent prolonged excretion of the pathogen.[52] Expert consensus is that antimicrobial therapy is appropriate for treatment of travelers' diarrhea even when the etiology is uncertain, recognizing that a proportion of illness may be caused by nontyphoid salmonella. As the prolongation of excretion stimulated by antimicrobial therapy is often short lasting, this is of little consequence to the usual traveler. *S. dysenteriae* requires 3 or more days of antimicrobial therapy and would therefore not be adequately covered by the commonly given single dose therapy for most cases of travelers' diarrhea. *S. dysenteriae* remains such a rare cause of travelers' diarrhea that it has not driven the choice of a preferred treatment regimen.

Dietary restrictions for patients with traveler's diarrhea are often recommended; however, the benefit of this therapy is not proven.[53] Similarly, the use of lactobacillus as preventive therapy has so far not be shown to be beneficial.[54]

The presence of parasitic agents should be strongly considered in travelers who present with diarrhea after traveling to Nepal or Russia or in those with persistent ($>$ 14 days) or recurrent symptoms.

In conclusion, the travel medicine practitioner needs to inform the traveler about risk factors associated with traveler's diarrhea per se, as well as risk factors for certain pathogens in terms of travel destination and activities and their implications on empiric self treatment.

References

1. Steffen R. Epidemiology of traveler's diarrhea. Clin Infect Dis 2005;41 Suppl 8:S536–40.
2. Steffen R, Castelli F, Dieter Nothdurft H, et al. Vaccination against enterotoxigenic Escherichia coli, a cause of travelers' diarrhea. J Travel Med 2005;12:102–7.
3. Steffen R, deBernardis C, Banos A. Travel epidemiology—a global perspective. Int J Antimicrob Agents 2003;21:89–95.
4. Steffen R, Tornieporth N, Clemens SA, et al. Epidemiology of travelers' diarrhea: details of a global survey. J Travel Med 2004;11:231–7.
5. Gorbach SL, Kean BH, Evans DG, et al. Travelers' diarrhea and toxigenic Escherichia coli. N Engl J Med 1975;292:933–6.
6. DuPont AW, DuPont HL. Travelers' diarrhea: modern concepts and new developments. Curr Treat Options Gastroenterol 2006;9:13–21.
7. DuPont HL. Diarrhoeal disease: current concepts and future challenges. Antimicrobial therapy and prophylaxis. Trans R Soc Trop Med Hyg 1993;87 Suppl 3:31–4.
8. Freedman DO, Weld LH, Kozarsky PE, et al. Spectrum of disease and relation to place of exposure among ill returned travelers. N Engl J Med 2006;354:119–30.
9. Jiang ZD, Okhuysen PC, Guo DC, et al. Genetic susceptibility to enteroaggregative Escherichia coli diarrhea: polymorphism in the interleukin-8 promotor region. J Infect Dis 2003;188:506–11.
10. Huang DB, Sanchez AP, Triana E, et al. United States male students who heavily consume alcohol in Mexico are at greater risk of travelers' diarrhea than their female counterparts. J Travel Med 2004;11:143–5.
11. Gascon J. Epidemiology, etiology, and pathophysiology of traveler's diarrhea. Digestion 2006;73 Suppl 1:102–8.
12. Jiang ZD, Lowe B, Verenkar MP, et al. Prevalence of enteric pathogens among international travelers with diarrhea acquired in Kenya (Mombasa), India (Goa), or Jamaica (Montego Bay). J Infect Dis 2002;185:497–502.
13. Echeverria P, Blacklow NR, Sanford LB, Cukor GG. Travelers' diarrhea among American Peace Corps volunteers in rural Thailand. J Infect Dis 1981;143:767–71.
14. Steffen R, Mathewson JJ, Ericsson CD, et al. Travelers' diarrhea in West Africa and Mexico: fecal transport systems

and liquid bismuth subsalicylate for self-therapy. J Infect Dis 1988;157:1008–13.

15. Steffen R, Collard F, Tornieporth N, et al. Epidemiology, etiology, and impact of traveler's diarrhea in Jamaica. Jama 1999;281:811–7.

16. Mattila L, Siitonen A, Kyronseppa H, et al. Seasonal variation in etiology of travelers' diarrhea. Finnish-Moroccan Study Group. J Infect Dis 1992;165:385–8.

17. Ericsson CD, DuPont HL. Travelers' diarrhea: approaches to prevention and treatment. Clin Infect Dis 1993;16:616–24.

18. Jiang ZD, Mathewson JJ, Ericsson CD, et al. Characterization of enterotoxigenic Escherichia coli strains in patients with travelers' diarrhea acquired in Guadalajara, Mexico, 1992–1997. J Infect Dis 2000;181:779–82.

19. Stenderup J, Orskov I, Orskov F. Changes in serotype and resistance pattern of the intestinal Escherichia coli flora during travel. Results from a trial of mecillinam as a prophylactic against travellers' diarrhoea. Scand J Infect Dis 1983;15:367–73.

20. Shlim DR, Hoge CW, Rajah R, et al. Persistent high risk of diarrhea among foreigners in Nepal during the first 2 years of residence. Clin Infect Dis 1999;29:613–6.

21. Adachi JA, Jiang ZD, Mathewson JJ, et al. Enteroaggregative Escherichia coli as a major etiologic agent in traveler's diarrhea in 3 regions of the world. Clin Infect Dis 2001;32:1706–9.

22. Kuschner RA, Trofa AF, Thomas RJ, et al. Use of azithromycin for the treatment of Campylobacter enteritis in travelers to Thailand, an area where ciprofloxacin resistance is prevalent. Clin Infect Dis 1995;21: 536–41.

23. Hoge CW, Gambel JM, Srijan A, et al. Trends in antibiotic resistance among diarrheal pathogens isolated in Thailand over 15 years. Clin Infect Dis 1998;26:341–5.

24. Gorthi SP, Kapoor L, Chaudhry R, et al. Guillain-Barre syndrome: association with Campylobacter jejuni and Mycoplasma pneumoniae infections in India. Natl Med J India 2006;19:137–9.

25. Ekdahl K, Andersson Y. Regional risks and seasonality in travel-associated campylobacteriosis. BMC Infect Dis 2004; 4:54.

26. Talsma E, Goettsch WG, Nieste HL, et al. Resistance in Campylobacter species: increased resistance to fluoroquinolones and seasonal variation. Clin Infect Dis 1999;29: 845–8.

27. Jumaa PA, Neringer R. A survey of antimicrobial resistance in a tertiary referral hospital in the United Arab Emirates. J Chemother 2005;17:376–9.

28. Takahashi T, Ishihara K, Kojima A, et al. Emergence of fluoroquinolone resistance in Campylobacter jejuni in chickens exposed to enrofloxacin treatment at the inherent dosage licensed in Japan. J Vet Med B Infect Dis Vet Public Health 2005;52:460–4.

29. Jain D, Sinha S, Prasad KN, Pandey CM. Campylobacter species and drug resistance in a north Indian rural community. Trans R Soc Trop Med Hyg 2005;99:207–14.

30. von Sonnenburg F, Tornieporth N, Waiyaki P, et al. Risk and aetiology of diarrhoea at various tourist destinations. Lancet 2000;356:133–4.

31. Corwin AL, Soderquist R, Edwards M, et al. Shipboard impact of a probable Norwalk virus outbreak from coastal Japan. Am J Trop Med Hyg 1999;61:898–903.

32. Oyofo BA, Soderquist R, Lesmana M, et al. Norwalk-like virus and bacterial pathogens associated with cases of gastroenteritis onboard a US Navy ship. Am J Trop Med Hyg 1999;61:904–8.

33. Subekti D, Lesmana M, Tjaniadi P, et al. Incidence of Norwalk-like viruses, rotavirus and adenovirus infection in patients with acute gastroenteritis in Jakarta, Indonesia. FEMS Immunol Med Microbiol 2002;33:27–33.

34. Subekti DS, Tjaniadi P, Lesmana M, et al. Characterization of Norwalk-like virus associated with gastroenteritis in Indonesia. J Med Virol 2002;67:253–8.

35. Ko G, Garcia C, Jiang ZD, et al. Noroviruses as a cause of traveler's diarrhea among students from the United States visiting Mexico. J Clin Microbiol 2005;43:6126–9.

36. Lang L. Acute gastroenteritis outbreaks on cruise ships linked to Norwalk-like viruses. Gastroenterology 2003;124: 284–5.

37. Gastroenteritis outbreaks on two Caribbean cruise ships. MMWR Morb Mortal Wkly Rep 1986;35:383–4.

38. Lawrence DN. Outbreaks of gastrointestinal diseases on cruise ships: lessons from three decades of progress. Curr Infect Dis Rep 2004;6:115–123.

39. Matson DO, Estes MK. Impact of rotavirus infection at a large pediatric hospital. J Infect Dis 1990;162:598–604.

40. Matson DO. The pentavalent rotavirus vaccine, RotaTeq(trade mark). Semin Pediatr Infect Dis 2006;17: 195–9.

41. DI B. Live attenuated human rotavirus vaccine, Rotarix. Semin Pediatr Infect Dis 2006;17:188–94.

42. Okhuysen PC. Traveler's diarrhea due to intestinal protozoa. Clin Infect Dis 2001;33:110–4.

43. Frachtman RL, Ericsson CD, DuPont HL. Seroconversion to Entamoeba histolytica among short-term travelers to Mexico. Arch Intern Med 1982;142:1299.

44. Hoge CW, Shlim DR, Rajah R, et al. Epidemiology of diarrhoeal illness associated with coccidian-like organism among travelers and foreign residents in Nepal. Lancet 1993;341:1175–9.

45. Ungar BL, Mulligan M, Nutman TB. Serologic evidence of Cryptosporidium infection in US volunteers before and during Peace Corps service in Africa. Arch Intern Med 1989;149:894–7.

46. Jokipii L, Pohjola S, Jokipii AM. Cryptosporidiosis associated with traveling and giardiasis. Gastroenterology 1985;89:838–42.

47. Gascon J, Macia M, Oliveira I, Corachan M. [Ciguatera poisoning in Spanish travellers]. Med Clin (Barc) 2003;120: 777–9.

48. Feldman LF, Sleisinger MH. In: Feldman M, Friedman LS, Sleisinger MH, editors. Gastrointestinal and liver disease. 7th ed. Elsevier; 2004.

49. Helbok R, Dent W, Gattringer K, et al. Imported Dengue fever presenting with febrile diarrhoea: report of two cases. Wien Klin Wochenschr 2004;116 Suppl 4:58–60.

50. Reisinger EC, Fritzsche C, Krause R, Krejs GJ. Diarrhea caused by primarily non-gastrointestinal infections. Nat Clin Pract Gastroenterol Hepatol 2005;2:216–22.

51. DuPont HL. Travellers' diarrhoea: contemporary approaches to therapy and prevention. Drugs 2006;66:303–14.

52. Neill MA, Opal SM, Heelan J, et al. Failure of ciprofloxacin to eradicate convalescent fecal excretion after acute salmonellosis: experience during an outbreak in health care workers. Ann Intern Med 1991;114:195–9.

53. Huang DB, Awasthi M, Le BM, et al. The role of diet in the treatment of travelers' diarrhea: a pilot study. Clin Infect Dis 2004;39:468–71.

54. Briand V, Buffet P, Genty S, et al. Absence of efficacy of nonviable Lactobacillus acidophilus for the prevention of traveler's diarrhea: a randomized, double-blind, controlled study. Clin Infect Dis 2006;43:1170–5.

CHAPTER 8

DIARRHEA ASSOCIATED WITH NONENTERIC INFECTIONS

ISRAEL POTASMAN, MD

DAVID O. FREEDMAN, MD

Studies conducted over the past two decades have indicated that the causative pathogens of diarrhea in either travelers or expatriates residing in developing countries are still not identified in approximately 20 to 40% of cases.[1–3] Thus, nonenteric pathogens should always be considered in the differential diagnoses of "travelers' diarrhea." Despite these well-known figures, only a handful of papers have dealt with these pathogens.[1,4,5] This chapter will focus on diarrhea caused by infectious agents that are not primarily enteropathogens.

The pathogenesis of diarrhea in systemic infections is not clearly understood. Several cytokines, such as interferon-gamma (INF-γ), IL-6 and IL-10 were found to be elevated in children with rotavirus.[6] Tumor necrosis factor-α (TNF- α), as well as IL-6 were found to correlate with the presence of fever.[6,7] Other mediators of diarrhea include direct invasion of gut epithelial cells by bacteria, inflammation of the lamina propria, sequestration of red blood cells, which causes ischemia and apoptosis with resultant increased permeability of endothelial cells.

The range of etiologies of nonenteropathogen-induced diarrhea goes through viral-bacterial-parasitic agents, toxins, stress, alcohol and drugs, endocrine disorders, and diseases with as yet unknown etiology. This chapter will try to outline the gamut of etiologies involved in these disorders and provide hints towards the diagnosis.

Viral Diseases

Nonenteric viruses may certainly cause diarrhea; however, diarrhea is rarely the hallmark in these entities, but rather a part of the clinical spectrum (Table 1). Some of these viruses may be acquired during travel to tropical areas (eg, Monkeypox and Dengue), while the majority have a worldwide distribution (Cytomegalovirus, Adenovirus).

Dengue fever is a classic example of a nonenteric viral disease that may present with fever. Dengue is endemic in most tropical and subtropical countries, many of which are popular tourist destinations.[8] The risk of dengue among travelers, long-term expatriates, aid workers, and military troops ranges between 2 to 16%.[9–11] Travelers may both acquire dengue virus infection and spread it in their home countries. Dengue virus is transmitted by mosquitoes of the genus Aedes, such as *Aedes aegypti* and *A. albopictus.*[12] After an incubation period of 2 to 7 days, patients typically develop symptoms of high fever, headache, retro-orbital pain, fatigue, myalgia, and arthralgia (break-bone fever).[13] There is often a macular or maculopapular rash that appears towards defervescence. Additional symptoms and signs include anorexia, nausea, vomiting, diarrhea, flushed facies, and scleral injection.

Diarrhea is not a prominent symptom of dengue fever, but has been reported in up to 41% in carefully studied outbreaks.[14,15] Interestingly, a large study from Thailand (n = 4,595) found that diarrhea, as part of dengue hemorrhagic fever, was much more common among infants (13.1%) than children (2.0%).[16] Few case reports have described patients returning from the tropics with "febrile diarrhea," which eventually turned out to be dengue.[17] Laboratory findings commonly associated with dengue fever include thrombocytopenia, leukopenia with lymphopenia, mild-to-moderate elevations of hepatic aminotransferases[18] and lactate dehydrogenase, and hyponatremia.[19] Quite often, these tests help clinicians reach the correct diagnosis well before serology is available. Ultimate diagnosis is usually based on virus isolation or, more commonly, on serology.

Another example of nonenteric viral disease that may present with diarrhea is the severe acute respiratory syndrome (SARS). SARS is a new infectious disease, first

Table 1 Diarrhea in Nonenteric Viral Diseases

Agent	Diagnostic Hints	Rate of Diarrhea	Reference
Monkeypox	Diffuse vesicular rash in young children Recent US outbreak	5–18%	56,57
Chickenpox	Typical rash	Few case reports	58
Cytomegalovirus	Mononucleosis-like syndrome	Was common in AIDS, pre-HAART era. Rare in immuno-competent	59,60
HHV-6	Ubiquitous, almost all infected by age 2 exanthem subitum	21/81=26%	61
HHV-7	Similar to HHV-6	Rare	62
HHV-8	Kaposi sarcoma agent Common in HIV+	unknown	63,64
Adenovirus, serotype 2,3,5,40,41	Watery diarrhea+ fever Causes outbreaks	18/417 (4.3%) of children's ER specimens tested positive	65,66
Parvovirus	Slapped cheek	Probably rare	67
Dengue	"Breakbone fever"	16/39=41% in Singapore outbreak	14
West-Nile virus	Fever, headache, arthralgia, encephalitis	Up to 14%	68
SARS-CoV	Severe pneumonia, profuse diarrhea	73%	23
Human Metapneumovirus	Fever, cough, rhinorrhea	5%	69
Measles	Fever, rash, conjunctivitis, Koplik's spots	42% in Iran; 215/401 (53.6%) in India	34,35
Marburg virus	Rare small outbreaks in Africa	Rare	70
Ebola virus	Confined to Africa Abrupt onset of fever, headache, arthralgia, vomiting	85%, many with bloody diarrhea	31
Influenza (H5N1)	Pneumonia +diarrhea as presenting symptom	Common	71
Bunyaviridae	High fever, chills, and severe headache	Up to 22% in Saudi Arabia	72,73
Arenavirus (Lassa fever)	Severe infection occurs in only 5–10% Chest pain, backache, cough	26%	74

CoV = coronavirus; ER = emergency room; HAART = highly active antiretroviral therapy; HHV = human herpesvirus; HIV = human immunodeficiency virus; SARS = severe acute respiratory disease.

recognized in the Guangdong province of China in November 2002. From there, via Hong-Kong, SARS rapidly spread around the world to five continents and 30 countries. Final data for this mini-pandemic indicate that more than 8,000 people were infected and ~10% died.[20] SARS is caused by a newly discovered Coronavirus: SARS-CoV. Sequencing of the entire viral RNA was completed in several laboratories and demonstrated that the virus was only distantly related to all previously characterized human or animal coronaviruses. Although the risk is small, a few cases of SARS were probably associated with air-travel.[21,22] The incubation period of SARS is, on average, 2 days, and the peak of respiratory symptoms and viral shedding occur 2 days later.

SARS is usually manifested by fever, headache, malaise, or myalgia. One week later, respiratory symptoms such as nonproductive cough and dyspnea ensue. Chest radiograph at this stage is frequently abnormal. Up to three-quarters of infected people may develop diarrhea during their illness. In the study by Peiris and colleagues[23] in China, 55 of 75 patients (73%) had watery diarrhea after 7.5 days. Another study from Taiwan has found that diarrhea was an initial symptom in 31.6% of their patients.[24] In contrast, Chong and colleagues[25] found that diarrhea was reported by only 2.7 to 7.7% of their patients with possible or probable SARS, respectively. Patients with SARS who present with diarrhea pose a special diagnostic and epidemiologic challenge.[26]

Avian influenza is an infectious disease of birds caused by type A strains of the influenza virus. The disease occurs worldwide. Apart from being highly contagious among poultry, avian influenza viruses are readily transmitted from farm to farm by the movement of live birds, people, and contaminated vehicles, equipment, etc. The highly pathogenic H5N1 virus can survive in bird feces for at least 35 days at low temperature (4°C). At a much higher temperature (37°C), H5N1 viruses have been shown to survive in fecal samples for 6 days. Scientists are increasingly convinced that at least some migratory waterfowl are now carrying the H5N1 virus in its highly pathogenic form, sometimes over long distances. Almost all cases of avian influenza have been linked to sick or dead poultry. [27] The current epidemic of avian influenza that began in south-east Asia in mid-2003 and have now spread to a few parts of Europe and Africa. Nine Asian countries have reported outbreaks: Vietnam,

Thailand, Korea, Japan, Cambodia, Laos, Indonesia, China, and Malaysia.

The clinical features of H5N1 influenza in humans follow an unusually aggressive clinical course, with rapid deterioration and high fatality. The incubation period of avian influenza may be longer than that for normal seasonal influenza (2 to 3 days). Current data for H5N1 infection indicate an incubation period ranging from 2 to 8 days. Initial symptoms include a high fever, usually higher than 38°C, and influenza-like symptoms. Diarrhea, vomiting, abdominal pain, chest pain, and bleeding from the nose and gums are also common. Watery diarrhea without blood appears to be more common (up to 70%[28]) in H5N1 avian influenza than in normal seasonal influenza. Diarrhea as a presenting symptom was also found in 5 of 12 Thai patients.[29] Because avian influenza is generally conceived as a respiratory illness, presentation with gastrointestinal (GI) symptoms alone may be worrisome, and the diagnosis in such cases may be easily delayed.[30] Because avian influenza shows a worldwide distribution, clinicians caring for returning travelers should be aware of these subtleties.

Perhaps the most devastating nonenteric viral disease that may present with diarrhea is Ebola. First recognized in 1976, in two unrelated epidemics in northern Zaire and southern Sudan, the disease quickly became one of the most dreaded ailments of Africa, and suspected cases are subject to quarantine. The death rate in these two epidemics reached 88% and 53%, respectively. The disease has an incubation period of 5 to 10 days and starts abruptly with fever, myalgia, and headache. In the 1995 outbreak in Kikwit, the democratic republic of Congo, 103 cases were analyzed by Bwaka and colleagues[31] Additional symptoms and signs included diarrhea (85%), nausea/vomiting (71%), sore throat (54%), and conjunctival injection (41%). Eight patients presented with melena and 7 with bloody stools.

Measles is one of those "older" viral diseases that are still linked to overseas or in-flight acquisition.[32,33] Measles is also one of the nonenteric viral diseases that may present with diarrhea. A study of 824 clinically confirmed cases during the years 1997 to 2003 in Iran found that complications such as vomiting and diarrhea occurred in 45.5% and 42.4%, respectively.[34] Diarrhea was also common among children in India.[35] In this latter study the overall rate of diarrhea was 53.6%. The authors point out that the children with measles-associated-diarrhea had significantly more "dysenteric" type of stools than controls.

The rate of diarrhea and diagnostic hints for other viral diseases are given in Table 1.

Bacterial Diseases

Nonenteric bacterial diseases in travelers may present with diarrhea in a non-negligible rate of cases. Because the incubation period may be prolonged, and the GI symptoms may dominate the clinical picture, the accurate diagnosis may be delayed, as is the appropriate treatment.

A classical example of diarrhea as a major symptom in nonenteric disease is leptospirosis. In the 1998 outbreak of leptospirosis among triathlon competitors in Wisconsin and Illinois,[36] the rate of diarrhea was 58%, while the rate among the eco-challenge participants in Borneo 2000 was 36%.[37] Leptospirosis is a zoonosis with a worldwide distribution. Rodents, especially rats, are the most important reservoir. Leptospirosis is characterized by broad spectrum clinical manifestations varying from unapparent infection to fulminant, fatal disease. Following an incubation period that usually lasts 1 to 2 weeks, an influenza-like illness develops: fever, chills, headache, nausea, vomiting, and myalgia. Some travelers may return from the tropics with a clinical picture dominated by GI complaints, which instinctively raise the suspicion of travelers' diarrhea.[38]

Q fever is an acute febrile illness with a worldwide distribution. Consequently, travelers to all parts of the globe may "import" the disease.[39–41] Humans are infected by inhalation of contaminated aerosols. The disease manifests mainly as a febrile disease with symptoms of pneumonia and hepatitis, but may be complicated by endocarditis, osteomyelitis, or encephalitis). GI symptoms are not rare in Q fever. In a recent outbreak in Turkey the authors have found that 100% of the patients vomited, 57% had diarrhea, and 43% had abdominal pain.[42] Other uncommon manifestations of Q fever include acalculous cholecystitis[43] and acute abdomen.[44]

Diarrhea also occurs in patients with community-acquired pneumonia, such as legionellosis. In an outbreak of Legionnaires' disease among cruise ship passengers, Jernigan and colleagues found diarrhea to occur in up to 25% of cases.[45] The infectious aerosol in these cases came from whirlpool spas. The association of diarrhea with legionellosis goes back to the earlier reports of the disease.[46]

Human ehrlichiosis was first described in 1987. The disease, which is transmitted to humans mainly from dogs via tick vectors, was known to veterinarians for decades. The disease usually manifests as a febrile disease with chills and rigors and a prominent headache. However, GI symptoms are not rare: nausea and vomiting occur in more than one-third of patients and diarrhea in 25%.[47] Similar figures were reached at a series of 12 children from Arkansas.[48] The GI manifestations of tickborne diseases in the US have been thoroughly reviewed by Zaidi and Singer.[49] It appears that in fact each one of these diseases is capable of eliciting diarrhea.

The rates of diarrhea caused by the above-mentioned and other bacterial pathogen that are not primarily enteropathogens are detailed in Table 2.

Parasitic Diseases

The "classical" intestinal parasites, such as Giardia, Ameba, or tapeworms, often cause GI symptoms. The fact that nonenteric parasites may also present with diarrhea is less well recognized. Furthermore, people in the tropics may be co-infected with both an intraluminal and extra-intestinal parasites, which may hinder the diagnosis.

Malaria is probably the most recognized disease in the tropics. The reported incidence of diarrhea during malaria varies from 5 to 38%. This combination is thought to be more common among children and nonimmune adults.[50] The mechanisms that underlie diarrhea in malaria are complex. They include sequestration of red blood cells and capillary occlusion, cytokine activation by parasitized red blood cells, inflammatory response, apoptosis, and capillary leakage.[4] This is followed by edema, increased permeability, and malabsorption of dietary elements. That being said, it is hard to estimate the prevalence of diarrhea in malaria. In a small study of neonatal malaria in Nigeria, 4 of 16 neonates suffered from diarrhea.[51] Another study among children in Indonesia found *P. falciparum* in all cases of diarrhea + malaria. The majority of these cases were younger than 1 year, and hospitalization was longer for concurrent malaria and diarrhea.[52]

Schistosomiasis is estimated to infect 200 million people in 74 countries. Approximately 120 million have symptoms and 20 millions have severe disease.[53] People acquire schistosomiasis after bathing in waters infected with cercaria. The acute disease associated with Schistosomiasis, which occurs 2 to 8 weeks after exposure, is sometimes called Katayama fever. It consists of fever, chills, headache, myalgia, abdominal pain, diarrhea, and occasionally bloody stools. Diarrhea is a common feature of this entity. A recent publication by a French group[54] found that diarrhea had been reported by 40% of their patients. Similarly, investigators from Spain found diarrhea in 4 of 14 travelers returning with schistosomiasis.[55]

Additional nonintestinal parasites that have been associated with diarrhea are detailed in Table 3.

Table 2 Diarrhea in Nonenteric Bacterial Diseases

Agent	Diagnostic Hints	Rate of Diarrhea	Reference
Rocky mountain spotted fever	Fever, myalgia, headache, rash	20%	75
Q fever	Fever, cough, hepatitis	57% (outbreak in Turkey)	42
Louse borne typhus	Fever, headache, cough, nausea	13%	76
Ehrlichia/ Anaplasma	Fever, chills, headache, myalgia	22–25%	47
S. aureus	Food poisoning Heat stable toxin		77,78
Pneumonia	Diarrhea, especially in children		79
Listeria	High attack rate in elderly and pregnancy and immune-deficient	79% in Illinois outbreak	80
Anthrax	Oropharyngeal painful adenopathy Intestinal low grade fever, syncope, abdominal pain, N/V	< 5% of all cases	81–83
Brucella	Uncooked goat milk/cheese, osteoarticular manifestations	6%; GI manifestations present in 67%	84–86
Tularemia	Abrupt onset fever, chills, cough, myalgia Direct or vector contact with animals.		87
Legionnaires'	Fever, chills, headache, myalgia, nausea/vomiting	20–25%	45
Leptospira	Fever, chills, headache, myalgia, nausea	11–53%	37
Botulism	Acute bilateral cranial neuropathy	Type A =35%, Type B =8%, Type E =39%	88
Tuberculosis	Ascites, change in bowel habits, acute abdomen	17%	89

GI = gastrointestinal; NV = nausea, vomiting.

Table 3 Diarrhea in Nonenteric Parasitic Diseases

Agents	Diagnostic Hints	Rate of Diarrhea	Reference
Malaria	Stayed in malarious area, no prophylaxis, fever + chills, splenomegaly	5–38%	4
Toxoplasmosis (congenital)	Abdominal pain, dry cough	Rare	90,91
Trichinosis	Eating raw pork meat, fever, myalgia, periorbital edema	0–48% (mean = 16%)	92–94
Schistosomiasis	Katayama fever: chills, headache, myalgia, abdominal pain		54

References

1. Felton JM, Harries AD, Beeching NJ, et al. Acute gastroenteritis: the need to remember alternative diagnoses. Postgrad Med J 1990;66:1037–9.
2. Hoge CW, Shlim DR, Echeverria P, et al. Epidemiology of diarrhea among expatriate residents living in a highly endemic environment. JAMA 1996;275:533–8.
3. Ko G, Garcia C, Jiang ZD, et al. Noroviruses as a cause of traveler's diarrhea among students from the United States visiting Mexico. J Clin Microbiol 2005;43:6126–9.
4. Reisinger EC, Fritzsche C, Krause R, Kreis GJ. Diarrhea caused by primarily non-gastrointestinal infections. Nat Clin Pract Gastroenterol Hepatol 2005;2:216–22.
5. Sibal A, Patwari AK, Anand VK, et al. Associated infections in persistent diarrhoea—another perspective. J Trop Pediatr 1996;42:64–7.
6. Jiang B, Snipes-Magaldi L, Dennehy P, et al. Cytokines as mediators for or effectors against rotavirus disease in children. Clin Diagn Lab Immunol 2003;10:995–1001.
7. Oprins JC, Meijer HP, Groot JA. TNF-alpha potentiates the ion secretion induced by muscarinic receptor activation in HT29cl.19A cells. Am J Physiol Cell Physiol 2000;278:C463–72.
8. Jelinek T. Dengue fever in international travelers. Clin Infect Dis 2000;31:144–7.
9. Potasman I, Srugo I, Schwartz E. Dengue seroconversion among Israeli travelers to tropical countries. Emerg Infect Dis 1999;5:824–7.
10. Doherty JF, Grant AD, Bryceson AD. Fever as the presenting complaint of travellers returning from the tropics. QJM 1995;88:277–81.
11. O'Brien D, Tobin S, Brown GV, Torresi J. Fever in returned travelers: review of hospital admissions for a 3-year period. Clin Infect Dis 2001;33:603–9.
12. Gubler DJ. The global emergence/resurgence of arboviral diseases as public health problems. Arch Med Res 2002;33:330–42.
13. Wilder-Smith A, Schwartz E. Dengue in travelers. N Engl J Med 2005;353:924–32.
14. Seet RC, Ooi EE, Wong HB, Paton NI. An outbreak of primary dengue infection among migrant Chinese workers in Singapore characterized by prominent gastrointestinal symptoms and a high proportion of symptomatic cases. J Clin Virol 2005;33:336–40, Epub 2005 Apr 25.
15. Pancharoen C, Mekmullica J, Thisyakorn U. Primary dengue infection: what are the clinical distinctions from secondary infection? Southeast Asian J Trop Med Public Health 2001;32:476–80.
16. Kalayanarooj S, Nimmannitya S. Clinical presentations of dengue hemorrhagic fever in infants compared to children. J Med Assoc Thai 2003;86,Suppl 3:S673–80.
17. Helbok R, Dent W, Gattringer K, et al. Imported Dengue fever presenting with febrile diarrhoea: report of two cases. Wien Klin Wochenschr 2004;116,Suppl 4:58–60.
18. Kularatne SA, Gawarammana IB, Kumarasiri PR. Epidemiology, clinical features, laboratory investigations and early diagnosis of dengue fever in adults: a descriptive study in Sri Lanka. Southeast Asian J Trop Med Public Health 2005;36:686–92.
19. Gibbons RV, Vaughn DW. Dengue: an escalating problem. BMJ 2002;324:1563–6.
20. Summary of Probable SARS cases with onset of illness from 1 November 2002 to 31 July 2003. http://www.who.int/csr/sars/country/table2004_04_21/en/index.html (accessed March 13, 2007).
21. Olsen S, Chang HL, Cheung TY, et al. Transmission of the severe acute respiratory syndrome on aircraft. N Engl J Med 2003;349:2416–22.
22. Wilder-Smith A, Paton NI, Goh KT. Low risk of transmission of severe acute respiratory syndrome on airplanes: the Singapore experience. Trop Med Int Health 2003;8:1035–7.
23. Peiris JH, Chu CM, Cheng VC, et al. Clinical progression and viral load in a community outbreak of coronavirus-associated SARS pneumonia: a prospective study. Lancet 2003;361:1767–72.
24. Wang JT, Sheng WH, Fang CT, et al. Clinical manifestations, laboratory findings, and treatment outcomes of SARS patients. Emerg Infect Dis 2004;10:818–24.
25. Chong WC, Tham KY, Goh HK, Seow E. Presentation of severe acute respiratory syndrome (SARS) patients in a screening centre. Singapore Med J 2005;46:161–4.

26. Kwan YW, Leung CW, Chiu MC. Diarrhoea as the presenting sign in an adolescent suffering from severe acute respiratory syndrome. Eur J Pediatr 2005;164:227–30.

27. Dinh PN, Long HT, Tien NTK, et al. Risk factors for human infection with avian influenza A H5N1, Vietnam, 2004. Emerg Infect Dis 2006;12:1841–7.

28. Tran TH, Nguyen TL, Nguyen TD, et al. Avian influenza A (H5N1) in 10 patients in Vietnam. N Engl J Med 2004;350: 1179–88.

29. Wiwanitkit V. Diarrhoea as a presentation of bird flu infection: a summary on its correlation to outcome in Thai cases. Gut 2005;54:1506.

30. Apisarnthanarak A, Kitphati R, Thongphubeth K, et al. Atypical avian influenza (H5N1). Atypical avian influenza (H5N1). Emerg Infect Dis 2004;10:1321–4.

31. Bwaka MA, Bonnet MJ, Calain P, et al. Ebola hemorrhagic fever in Kikwit, Democratic Republic of the Congo: clinical observations in 103 patients. J Infect Dis 1999;179,Suppl 1: S1–7.

32. de Barros FR, Danovaro-Holliday MC, Toscano C, et al. Measles transmission during commercial air travel in Brazil. J Clin Virol 2006;36:235–6.

33. Anon. Import-associated measles outbreak—Indiana, May–June 2005. MMWR 2005;54:1073–5.

34. Asefzadeh M, Peyrovian B. Epidemiological study of measles in Ghazvin, Islamic Republic of Iran, April 1997–April 2003. East Mediterr Health J 2006;12:14–22.

35. Deivanayagam N, Mala N, Ahmed SS, et al. Measles associated diarrhea and pneumonia in south India. Indian Pediatr 1994;31:35–40.

36. Morgan J, Bornstein SL, Karpati AM, et al. Outbreak of leptospirosis among Triathlon Participants and Community Residents in Springfield, Illinois, 1998. Clin Infect Dis 2002;34:1593–9.

37. Sejvar J, Bancroft E, Winthrop K, et al. Leptospirosis in "Eco-Challenge" athletes, Malaysian Borneo, 2000. Emerg Infect Dis 2003;9:702–7.

38. Paz A, Krimerman S, Potasman I. Leptospirosis masquerading as infectious enteritis. Travel Med Infect Dis 2004;2: 89–91.

39. Potasman I, Rzotkiewicz S, Pick N, KeysaryA. Outbreak of Q fever following a safari trip. Clin Infect Dis 2000;30:214–5.

40. Kawamoto T, Ogawa M, Kishimoto T, et al. Three imported cases of acute Q fever after an inspection tour to Australia and New Zealand. Kansenshogaku Zasshi 2002; 76:1030–4.

41. Brouqui P, Rolain JM, Foucault C, Raoult D. Q fever and Plasmodium falciparum malaria co-infection in a patient returning from the Comoros archipelago. Am J Trop Med Hyg 2005;73:1028–30.

42. Gozalan A, Esen B, Rolain JM. Is Q fever an emerging infection in Turkey? East Mediterr Health J 2005;11:384–91.

43. Rolain JM, Lepidi H, Harle JR, et al. Acute acalculous cholecystitis associated with Q fever: report of seven cases and review of the literature. Eur J Clin Microbiol Infect Dis 2003;22:222–7.

44. Modol JM, Llamazares JF, Mate JL, et al. Acute abdominal pain and Q fever. Eur J Clin Microbiol Infect Dis 1999;18: 158–60.

45. Jernigan DB, Hofmann J, Cetron M, et al. Outbreak of Legionnaires' disease among cruise ship passengers exposed to a contaminated whirlpool spa. Lancet 1996;347: 494–9.

46. Kirby BD, Snyder KM, Meyer RD, Finegold SM. Legionnaires' disease: clinical features of 24 cases. Ann Intern Med 1978;89:297–309.

47. Nutt AK, Raufman J. Gastrointestinal and hepatic manifestations of human ehrlichiosis: 8 cases and a review of the literature. Dig Dis 1999;17:37–43.

48. Schutze GE, Jacobs RF. Human monocytic ehrlichiosis in children. Pediatrics 1997;100:E10.

49. Zaidi SA, Singer C. Gastrointestinal and hepatic manifestations of tickborne diseases in the United States. Clin Infect Dis 2002;34:1206–12.

50. Prasad RN, Virk KJ. Malaria as a cause of diarrhoea—a review. P N G Med J 1993;36:337–41.

51. Ibhanesebhor SE. Clinical characteristics of neonatal malaria. J Trop Pediatr 1995;41:330–3.

52. Laurentz R, Manoempil PS. Malaria diarrhoea in children. Asia Pac J Public Health 1995;8:186–9.

53. Maguire JH. Trematodes (schistosomes and other flukes). In: Mandell GL, Bennett JE, Dolin R, editors. Principles and Practice of Infectious Diseases. 6th ed. Philadelphia: Elsevier; 2005. p. 3276–85.

54. Agbessi CA, Bourvis N, Fromentin M, et al. Acute schistosomiasis in French travelers. Rev Med Interne 2006;27:595–9.

55. Roca C, Balanzo X, Gascon J, et al. Comparative, clinico-epidemiologic study of Schistosoma mansoni infections in travellers and immigrants in Spain. Eur J Clin Microbiol Infect Dis 2002;21:219–23.

56. Damon I. Orthopoxviruses: Vaccinia, Variola, Monkeypox and Cowpox. In: Mandell GL, Bennett JE, Dolin R, editors. Principles and Practice of Infectious Diseases. 6th ed. Philadelphia: Elsevier; 2005. p. 1742–51.

57. Reed KD, Melski JW, Graham MB, et al. The detection of monkeypox in humans in the Western Hemisphere. N Engl J Med 2004;350:342–50.

58. Whitley RJ. Varicella-Zoster virus. In: Mandell GL, Bennett JE, Dolin R, editors. Principles and Practice of

Infectious Diseases. 6th ed. Philadelphia: Elsevier; 2005. p. 1780–6.

59. Klauber E, Briski LE, Khatib R. Cytomegalovirus colitis in the immunocompetent host: an overview. Scand J Infect Dis 1998;30:559–64.

60. Meunier YA. Infectious mononucleosis-like syndrome and gastrointestinal disorders in acute acquired cytomegalovirus infection. Singapore Med J 2005;46:421–3.

61. Zerr DM, Meier AS, Selke SS, et al. A population-based study of primary human herpesvirus 6 infection. N Engl J Med 2005;352:768–76.

62. Asano Y, Suga S, Yoshikawa T, et al. Clinical features and viral excretion in an infant with primary human herpesvirus 7 infection. Pediatrics 1995;95:187–90.

63. Kaye KM. Kaposi's Sarcoma associated herpesvirus (HHV type 8). In: Mandell GL, Bennett JE, Dolin R, editors. Principles and Practice of Infectious Diseases. 6th ed. Philadelphia: Elsevier; 2005. p. 1827–32.

64. Wang QJ, Jenkins FJ, Jacobson LP, et al. Primary human herpesvirus 8 infection generates a broadly specific CD8(+) T-cell response to viral lytic cycle proteins. Blood 2001;97: 2366–73.

65. Klein EJ, Boster DR, Stapp JR, et al. Diarrhea etiology in a Children's Hospital Emergency Department: a prospective cohort study. Clin Infect Dis 2006;43:807–13.

66. Jalal H, Bibby DF, Tang JW, et al. First reported outbreak of diarrhea due to adenovirus infection in a hematology unit for adults. J Clin Microbiol 2005;43: 2575–80.

67. Brown KE. Parvovirus B19. In: Mandell GL, Bennett JE, Dolin R, editors. Principles and Practice of Infectious Diseases. 6th ed. Philadelphia: Elsevier; 2005. p. 1891–98.

68. Klein C, Kimiagar I, Pollak L, et al. Neurological features of West Nile virus infection during the 2000 outbreak in a regional hospital in Israel. J Neurol Sci 2002;200:63–6.

69. Falsey AR. Human Metapneumovirus. In: Mandell GL, Bennett JE, Dolin R, editors. Principles and Practice of Infectious Diseases. 6th ed. Philadelphia: Elsevier; 2005. p. 2026–31.

70. Peters CJ. Marburg and Ebola virus hemorrhagic fevers. In: Mandell GL, Bennett JE, Dolin R, editors. Principles and Practice of Infectious Diseases. 6th ed. Philadelphia: Elsevier; 2005. p. 2057–60.

71. De Jong MD, Bach VC, Phan TQ, et al. Fatal avian influenza A (H5N1) in a child presenting with diarrhea followed by coma. N Engl J Med 2005;352:686–91.

72. Flick R, Whitehouse CA. Crimean-Congo hemorrhagic fever virus. Curr Mol Med 2005;5:753–60.

73. Madani TA, Al-Mazrou YY, Al-Jeffri MH, et al. Rift Valley fever epidemic in Saudi Arabia: epidemiological, clinical, and laboratory characteristics. Clin Infect Dis 2003;37: 1084–92.

74. McCormick JB, King IJ, Webb PA, et al. A case-control study of the clinical diagnosis and course of Lassa fever. J Infect Dis 1987;155:445–55.

75. Walker DH, Raoult D. *Rickettsia rickettsi* and other spotted fever group Rickettsiae (RMSF and other spotted fevers). In: Mandell GL, Bennett JE, Dolin R, editors. Principles and Practice of Infectious Diseases. 6th ed. Philadelphia: Elsevier; 2005. p. 2287–95.

76. Raoult D, Ndihokubwayo JB, Tissot-Dupont H, et al. Outbreak of epidemic typhus associated with trench fever in Burundi. Lancet 1998;352:353–8.

77. Miwa N, Kawamura A, Masuda T, Akiyama M. An outbreak of food poisoning due to egg yolk reaction-negative Staphylococcus aureus. Int J Food Microbiol 2001; 20:361–6.

78. de Jong JT, ten Brinke JM, van Ouwerkerk IM, et al. Large-scale, acute, bacterial gastroenteritis caused by the enterotoxin of *Staphylococcus aureus* after a barbecue. Ned Tijdschr Geneeskd 2004;148:2136–40.

79. Medarov BI, Siddiqui AK, Mughal T, et al. Legionella micdadei infection presenting as severe secretory diarrhea and a solitary pulmonary mass. Clin Infect Dis 2004;38: e63–5.

80. Dalton CB, Austin CC, Sobel J, et al. An outbreak of gastroenteritis and fever due to Listeria monocytogenes in milk. N Engl J Med 1997;336:100–5.

81. Sirisanthana T, Brown AE. Anthrax of the gastrointestinal tract. Emerg Infect Dis 2002;8:649–51.

82. Kanafani ZA, Ghossain A, Sharara AI, et al. Endemic gastrointestinal anthrax in 1960s Lebanon: clinical manifestations and surgical findings. Emerg Infect Dis 2003;9: 520–5.

83. Friedlander AM. Clinical aspects, diagnosis and treatment of anthrax. J Appl Microbiol 1999;87:303.

84. Potasman I, Even L, Banai M, et al. Brucellosis: an unusual diagnosis for a seronegative patient with abscesses, osteomyelitis, and ulcerative colitis. Rev Infect Dis 1991; 13:1039–42.

85. al-Aska AK. Gastrointestinal manifestations of brucellosis in Saudi Arabian patients. Trop Gastroenterol 1989;10: 217–9.

86. Ablin J, Mevorach D, Eliakim R. Brucellosis and the gastrointestinal tract. The odd couple. J Clin Gastroenterol 1997;24:25–9.

87. Sanders CV, Hahn R. Analysis of 106 cases of tularemia. J La State Med Soc 1968;120:391–3.

88. Bleck TP. *Clostridium botulinum* (Botulism). In: Mandell GL, Bennett JE, Dolin R, editors. Principles and Practice of Infectious Diseases. 6th ed. Philadelphia: Elsevier; 2005. p. 2822–8.

89. Bolukbas C, Bolukbas FF, Kendir T, et al. Clinical presentation of abdominal tuberculosis in HIV seronegative adults. BMC Gastroenterol 2005;5:21.

90. Ganji M, Tan A, Maitar MI, et al. Gastric toxoplasmosis in a patient with acquired immunodeficiency syndrome. A case report and review of the literature. Arch Pathol Lab Med 2003;127:732–4.

91. Yang M, Perez E. Disseminated toxoplasmosis as a cause of diarrhea. South Med J 1995;88:860–1.

92. Turk M, Kaptan F, Turker N, et al. Clinical and laboratory aspects of a trichinellosis outbreak in Izmir, Turkey. Parasite 2006;13:65–70.

93. Garcia E, Mora L, Torres P, et al. First record of human trichinosis in Chile associated with consumption of wild boar (Sus scrofa). Mem Inst Oswaldo Cruz 2005;100:17–8.

94. Greenbloom SL, Martin-Smith P, Isaacs S, et al. Outbreak of trichinosis in Ontario secondary to the ingestion of wild boar meat. Can J Public Health 1997;88:52–6.

PART TWO

EPIDEMIOLOGY AND SPECIAL POPULATIONS

CHAPTER 9

EPIDEMIOLOGY OF TRAVELERS' DIARRHEA

FRANCESCO CASTELLI, MD

ROBERT E. BLACK, MD

Nearly 80 million international travelers from industrialized countries annually cross the borders of tropical countries, and many of them suffer from travelers' diarrhea (TD).[1] The clear definition of the epidemiological and etiological characteristics of the syndrome is certainly of the utmost importance for the followings reasons:

- it allows monitoring of the phenomenon over time;
- it permits planning interventions for the protection of the traveler; and
- it motivates countries to reduce the problem that may affect economically important tourism revenues.

Many valuable contributions have been published in the past on the epidemiology of TD.[2–6] Unfortunately, the precise description of the epidemiology of TD is hindered by numerous factors:

- it deals with a syndrome and not a unique pathologic entity;
- the available studies have often used different definitions of the same syndrome;
- TD is caused by a considerable number of enteropathogens, whose clinical picture may differ;
- the epidemiology of enteropathogens may vary from continent to continent, making the description of the global picture difficult; and
- consequently, the majority of the studies only describe a small fragment of truth, especially relevant for the geographical area where the study has been conducted, but not necessarily applicable to the entire world.

Despite such difficulties, some studies have attempted to offer a global picture of the epidemiological characteristics of TD, offering a remarkable contribution to its understanding.[1,7]

Aside from the important repercussion in the field of travel medicine, the understanding of the determinants of TD can also offer precious information for the control of the far more important health problem of childhood diarrhea in the developing world.[8] Diarrhea causes almost 2 million deaths in children below 5 years of age, nearly all in developing countries.[9] In fact, the microbiological causes of TD and diarrhea in childhood in specific locations in developing countries are remarkably similar, particularly in regard to enterotoxigenic *Escherichia* coli infection.[10,11]

Despite the substantial current knowledge on the etiologic, pathophysiologic, and clinical aspects of the phenomenon of TD, more remains to be done so that diarrhea can be better controlled in travelers and in children in developing countries.[12]

Case Definition

TD is the most common medical disturbance of international travelers, occurring in a considerable proportion of people crossing borders from industrialized to developing countries. Several definitions of TD have been proposed in the past. The definition most commonly used encompasses the distinction of classical, moderate, and mild diarrhea,[13] defined as follows:

- Classical diarrhea: three or more loose stools per day, together with at least 1 gastrointestinal symptom among nausea, vomiting, abdominal pains or cramps, fever, blood in the stools;

- Moderate diarrhea: one or two loose stools per day, accompanied by at least 1 gastrointestinal symptom or three liquid stools per day in the absence of gastrointestinal symptoms;
- Mild diarrhea: one or two loose stools per day in the absence of gastrointestinal symptoms.

The proportion of classical diarrhea cases out of the total cases of TD differs in the different studies, especially in relationship to the destination, resulting in values of 50% or more in high-risk destinations.[1]

The clinical evolution of acute TD is generally benign and usually self limits in 2 to 3 days. However, when the traveler suffers from a preexisting clinical condition, such as diabetes, cardiopathy, or immunosuppression, diarrheal disease may follow a more severe course. In case the classical symptoms continue for more than 14 or 30 days (about 1% of travelers), the terms persistent or chronic diarrhea should be used, respectively.[14,15]

Although its course is usually mild, the available evidence suggests that more than 11 million cases of TD occur every year. Among them, 1% requires hospitalization, 20% are confined to bed, and 40% have no other way than changing their itinerary; this also has a significant impact on the tourism industry.[16]

Studies show that the incidence of TD peaks 3 days after arrival. This period of time, together with the evidence of good response to antibacterial therapy, suggests that the syndrome is mainly caused by infection, even though there are usually no symptoms that are specific to particular infectious agents.[17]

Etiology of TD

TD recognizes an infectious origin in the great majority of the cases, up to 85%,[18] although the proportion of cases where no specific enteropathogen is isolated is substantial, especially in earlier studies.[4] This fact reflects, at least in part, how microbiologically difficult it is to isolate microorganisms in the field. The use of new diagnostic techniques has in recent years reduced the proportion of cases of TD without an enteropathogen found,[19] allowing the identification of microorganisms in the majority of all cases of TD with significant regional variations in pathogens' detection according to location.[20] However, a proportion of cases might still be ascribed to noninfectious causes such as travel-related stress, changes in eating habits, or jet lag.

The traveler is exposed, in fact, to a new microbiologic environment and to a new enteric flora that may colonize the bowel and cause the symptoms of TD. Bacteria are the most frequently involved microorganisms in the pathogenesis of acute TD, up to 80% of cases.[21] Enterotoxigenic *Escherichia* strains (ETEC, producing either heat-labile or heat-stable enterotoxin or both) are the most frequently isolated pathogen in all geographic area.[22] Other *E. coli* strains, including enteroinvasive *E. coli* (EIEC), enteropathogenic *E. coli* (EPEC) and enteroaggregative *E. coli* (EAEC)[23] are increasingly being recognized as responsible agents for TD.[24,25] Enterohemorragic *E. coli* (EHEC) have not yet become a substantial cause of, but continued surveillance is needed in light of the severe disease that can result from this agent.

Finally, despite the fact that the spectrum of enteropathogens that causes TD has long been considered to be fairly constant throughout the world, specific pathogens are preferentially isolated in specific geographic locations, such as *Campylobacter spp.* and *Salmonella spp.* in Asia.

The clinical picture of TD is often undifferentiated, making etiologic diagnosis virtually impossible on the basis of the clinical assessment of the symptoms alone.[17]

In the case of prolonged diarrhea, the possible role on nonbacterial microorganisms should be investigated, with particular reference to helminthic and protozoan agents.[12,26] The importance of the parasitic nature of TD has been recently underlined by an extensive assessment of the spectrum of imported diseases in international travelers carried out by the international Geosentinel Network. According to the data of the Geosentinel study, parasites are the prevailing agents of those cases of diarrheal diseases in returning international travelers sick enough to look for medical advice after return from all continents except for South East Asia, where bacteria were more frequent as enteropathogens.[27]

Sources of Infection

As a rule, the enteropathogens causing TD are ingested through the consumption of foods and contaminated water and beverages containing a number of microorganisms high enough to trigger the infection and pathogenetic mechanisms of diarrhea. Inoculum size is important in causing diarrhea symptoms.[28] It has been estimated that the ingestion of as few as 10 to 100 cysts of *Giardia* or *Cryptosporiudium* are enough to cause diarrhea, while the ingestion of at least 1.000 *Shigellas*, 10,000 to 100.000 *Salmonellas* or 1.000.000 cholera vibrios are needed to overcome the defenses of the host and cause the appearance of symptoms.

Many food items and beverages may be contaminated by enteropathogens and may be classified according to their specific risk (Table 1).

Enteropathogens may also contaminate the environment and surface water,[29] and contamination may also occur via bathing and swimming.[11,30]

Table 1 Risk for Travelers' Diarrhea on Selected Foods and Beverages

Often Safe	Probably safe	Frequently Unsafe
Food: • Piping hot • Peeled fruit • Processed/packaged • Cooked vegetables (served steaming hot)	Food: • Dry • Jelly/syrup • Washed vegetables	Food: • Cold salads/desserts • Hamburgers • Hot sausages (served at room temperature) • Unpeeled fruits • Fresh cheese • Raspberries/strawberries
Beverages: • Irradiated milk • Boiled water • Iodized water • Carbonated	Beverages: • Fresh citrus juices • Packaged ice • Bottled water	Beverages • Tap water • Uncarbonated, bottled fruit juices • Chipped ice • Alcohol and chipped ice • Unpastorized milk/butter

Adapted from Ericsson CD et al.[98]

FOOD

It is generally estimated that any food may be potentially contaminated by enteropathogens, and the role of food as the vehicle of microorganism-causing TD is crucial. Contamination of any food may occur at source or during handling and/or preparation. The risk of food contamination is obviously higher when hygienic standards and sanitary systems are poor and fecal pollution in the environment is common. This is particularly true in those locations where untreated human sewage is used for irrigation purposes, thus contaminating vegetables and salads.

Cooking to sufficient temperature for an adequate amount of time is the best way to eliminate the risk of bacterial and viral contamination. It is also to be stressed that food that has been allowed to cool at room temperatures for hours after cooking may become a suitable bacterial-growing medium and must be heated again before being ingested. This is a typical situation of food sold by street vendors and contributes to adding a remarkable risk of ingesting a significant load of enteropathogens that may lead to the intestinal symptoms. However, it is to be recognized that is not always feasible to have complete control of the adequacy of food preparation and storage, eg, in restaurant and hotel kitchens.

Certainly to avoid are raw shellfish and dairy products (fresh cheese, cream, milk, etc.). Any vegetables need to be disinfected or boiled. Fruits that may be peeled personally are preferred.

Apart from carefully choosing the food, it should be stressed that personal hygienic measures by the traveler, with particular regard to proper hand washing, are to be implemented with particular care.

It should also be noted that catered food served onboard airplanes is generally considered safe; however, its consumption has led to diarrheal diseases and outbreaks. The best way to protect children below 6 months of age is breastfeeding. For older children, commercial formula should be prepared with boiled water.

WATER

Water may also be a vehicle of transmission of the microorganisms responsible for TD. Few milliliters of contaminated water can contain a sufficient number of enteropathogens to cause diarrhea. It is to be remembered that water contamination is usually not detectable on the basis of its physical characteristics (odor, taste, color).[31]

Tap water, even if too hot to touch, is best to be considered potentially contaminated because the evaluation is hazardously subjective,[32] and consequently, it is to be considered unsafe unless disinfection is assured. Adequate water chlorination drastically diminishes the risk of bacterial and viral contamination. However, it may not be sufficient to eliminate all viruses and certainly is less effective against parasites that have cystic stages, such as giardiasis, amoebiasis, and cryptosporidiosis.[31,33,34]

In those areas where chlorinated water is not certainly available, travelers should remember that only the following beverages may be considered safe[30]:

- beverages prepared by boiled water, such as tea and coffee, if drunk when still piping hot;
- bottled or packed beverages (water, soft drinks, etc.), especially carbonated beverages (carbonation lowers the pH, which kills or inhibits bacteria), although the contamination of locally bottled water is possible[21];
- bottled alcoholic beverages (such as wine and beer), especially if their pH is decreased by carbonation.

Where tap water is suspected to be contaminated, ice cubes are also unsafe and should not be added to beverages. If drinking vessels have been in contact with ice cubes, they need to be washed carefully with hot water and soap and dried. As a general rule, it is better to drink directly from bottles and cans than from doubtfully clean glasses. In doubtful situations, bottled water should be preferred to tap water for teeth washing.

Apart from microbiologic and other biological contaminants, surface water may be polluted due to the presence of organic or inorganic material and industrial pollutants.[35] From the microbiological point of view, the goal of water disinfection is to make water safe and drinkable by the removal of dangerous pathogens or the drastic reduction (3 to 5 logs) of their number.[36]

The following physical and chemical treatments may make water safe for drinking and other purposes:

Boiling

Boiled water is considered microbiologically safe when boiling lasts for at least 1 minute. Water may then be cooled at room temperatures and ice should not be added unless also made with boiled water. Boiling time should be increased to 3 minutes at high altitudes (2,000 meters or more over sea level), where boiling temperatures is 90°C.[37] Alternatively, additional chemical treatments should be used after 1 minute of boiling.

Chemical Disinfection

Chemical disinfection of water may yield good short-term results. The most commonly used agents are halogens (iodine and chlorine), which are active against nonspore-forming bacteria by causing oxidation of bacterial cell structures and metabolic processes,[38] while cysts and spores are usually resistant. Viruses have intermediate susceptibility. The particular water taste conferred by the use of halogens may be minimized by subsequent filtration[39] or by the addition of ascorbic acid.[40] The most commonly used halogens are iodine and chlorine, which have similar disinfection activity.[41]

Iodine

Iodine (tablets or solution) disinfection is a good alternative to obtain safe water when boiling is not feasible. However, *Cryptosporidium* spp. and some parasitic cysts may resist iodine. To obtain better results, iodine-treated water has to decant for a long time, approximately 15 hours, making it a very cumbersome procedure. Iodine tincture or tetraglicine idroperiodide may also be used, but their effectiveness is limited in the case of cold water below 5°C. In these cases, water has to be preliminarily heated or contact time increased. To avoid the risk of toxicity, the World Health Organization (WHO) advises against the use of iodine as a disinfection method for periods longer than 3 weeks.[42] However, a recent review of the available evidence has suggested that the use of the recommended dose of iodine for water disinfection should not exceed 1 month, while lower doses may be used for prolonged period of time, provided that thyroid function is monitored carefully.[43]

Chlorine

Chlorine (chlorination-flocculation or chlorine bleach tablets) may also be used to treat water, even if its antimicrobial effectiveness varies greatly according to pH, temperature, and organic content of the water to be treated. It is, however, to be remembered that *Cryptosporiudium* and *Giardia* are highly and moderately resistant to chlorine, respectively. Whenever possible, methods combining chlorine disinfection and coagulation-flocculation are recommended because their activity against protozoa is significan.[21] Chlorine use for water disinfection is considered safe for humans.[31]

Filtration

The protection conferred by the many commercially available filters varies greatly according to their quality and their pores' dimensions. Preliminary filtration is also indicated before chemical treatment if water turbidity is high. Most portable filtration devices use membranes, or ceramic or carbon blocks to remove impurities. However, only reverse osmotic filters or ultrafiltration offer good protection against viruses, while filter membranes with pores 0.1 to 0.3 μm are effective against protozoa and bacteria, but not viruses. To avoid any viral danger, chemical disinfection is indicated after filtration. Iodine-impregnated resins may increase filters' activity against bacteria and viruses, but contact time is usually too short to act against *Cryptosporidium* spp. and *Giardia*, especially in cold water. It is important to remind the traveler that filters claiming their capability to remove *Giardia* or *Cryptosporidium* (such as NFS standard 53 or 58 filters) must be adequately certified. Filter membranes may easily be filled and stopped by dirty material and microorganisms. Maintenance and membranes removal should follow manufacturers' recommendations and should be carried out with precaution, wearing protective gloves. Additional practical information on the selection and use of the different filters available are provided by the CDC Division of Parasitic Diseases <*http://www.cdc.gov/ncidod/dpd/parasites/cryptosporidiosis/factsht_crypto_prevent_water.htm*> Table 2 reports WHO recommendations on the use of the various disinfection methods.

Incidence of Travelers' Diarrhea

Travelers' diarrhea certainly represents the most frequent sanitary trouble for the international traveler. The

Table 2 Recommendations for Use of Disinfection Methods

Method	Recommendation (1 L or 1 Qt of water)	What it DOES	What it Does NOT Do
Boiling	• Bring water to a rolling boil and allow to cool	• Kills all pathogens	• Does not remove turbidity/ cloudiness
Chlorine compounds • Household bleach (sodium hypochlorite) • Sodium dichloroisocyanurate tablet • Calcium hypochlorite	• For typical room temperature and water temperature of 25°C (77°F), minimum contact time should be 30 minutes; increase contact time for colder water; eg, 1 hour at less than 10° C • Prepare according to package instructions • Should be added to clear water or after settling or clarification to be most effective • Type and typical dosage: • Household bleach (5%)—4 drops • Sodium dichloroisocyanurate—1 tablet (per package directions)-15 mg per liter of clear water • Calcium hypochlorite (1% stock solution)—4 drops	• Very effective for killing most bacteria and viruses • Longer contact time required to kill *Giardia* cysts, especially when water is cold	• Not effective against *Cryptosporidium* or some other parasites; not as effective as iodine when using turbid water
Chlorinating-flocculating tablets or sachets	• Chlorinating-flocculating tablet or sachet (per package directions)	• Very effective for killing or removing all waterborne pathogens	• Flocculated water must be decanted into a clean container, preferably through a simple fabric filter
Iodine • Tincture of iodine (2% solution) • Iodine (10% solution) • Iodine tablet • Iodinated resin Caution: for pregnant women who may be more sensitive, a carbon filter should be used to remove excess iodine after iodine treatment	• 25°C (77°F)—minimum contact for 30 minutes; increase contact time for colder • Not recommended for pregnant women, people with thyroid problems, or for more than a few months continuous use • Prepare according to package instructions • Type and typical dosage: • Tincture of iodine 2% solution—5 drops • Iodine 10% Solution—8 drops • Iodine Tablets—1 or 2 tablets • Triiodide or pentaiodide resin—room temperature according to directions and stay within rated capacity	Kills most pathogens; • Longer contact time is required to kill *Giardia* cysts, especially when water is cold • Carbon filtration after an iodine resin will remove excess iodine from the water, replace the carbon filter regularly	• Not effective against *Cryptosporidium*
Portable filtering devices • Ceramic filters • Carbon filters Some carbon block filters will remove cryptosporidia—only if tested and certified for cyst removal • Reverse osmosis and ultrafilter type devices • Membrane filter devices	• Filter media pore size must be rated at 1 micron (absolute) or less for filtration of clear unsafe water	• 1-micron or less filter pore size will remove *Giardia lamblia, Cryptosporidium* and other protozoa • Reverse osmosis and ultrafilter devices can remove almost all pathogens	• Most bacteria and viruses will not be removed • Many carbon-block filters do not remove pathogens, other than possibly protozoa, even if carbon is impregnated with silver They must have a specified pore size and be certified for microbe removal

To make a 1% stock solution of calcium hypochlorite, add to 1 L of water, 28 g if chlorine content is 35%, 15.4 g if 65%, or 14.3 g if 70%.
Adapted from World Health Organization.[21]

incidence of TD may be as high as 60% in certain high-risk destinations and greatly varies in relationship to numerous risk factors that will be reviewed in this chapter. The exact assessment of the incidence of TD in the different geographical areas is made nevertheless complex both by the different definitions used in the past to define the syndrome and by the different methodologies used to calculate incidence. Furthermore, the results of many of the studies that have investigated the role of the different risk factors for TD have exclusively been analyzed by univariate analysis, an inadequate way to clearly discriminate the independent role of specific factors that are tightly interconnected, such as age, the way the travel was performed, and the standard of the hotel, etc.

Conventionally, the term of incidence should exclusively be reported to a precise time of exposure. The majority of the available studies have used the period of 14 days, corresponding to 2 weeks of stay,[1] although the study recently published by the international Geosentinel network shows that the median time spent abroad by international travelers range from 14 days in the Caribbean to 35 days in travelers to Latin America.[27]

At the beginning of the third millennium, significant reductions of the incidence rates of TD are registered in southern European countries,[44] although the international epidemiological panorama of the TD in the other areas of the world does not seem to have undergone substantial modifications since the initial assessment in wide-scale studies showing incidence rates varying from 20 to 60% in relationship to the different geographical areas of destination.[2,45] The incidence of TD certainly depends upon a number of risk factors, some of which are related to the travel characteristics (destination, country of origin, motivations of the trip, duration and season of the stay, way of travel and standard of accommodation, place of consumption of the meals), while others are related to the unique and specific characteristics of the single traveler (age, sex, previous travels, predisposing personal baseline conditions, alimentary errors, etc.).[46] Such risk factors of risk are discussed below.

A) Travel-Related Risk Factors

DESTINATION

Travel destination is certainly the single most important factor influencing the risk of diarrhea among travelers from industrialized to developing countries in the tropics. Classically, three geographical areas have been identified with different risk of TD[6,45,47–49] (Figure 1):

- low-risk areas (incidence rate of TD estimated as < 8% for 2 weeks of stay): central and northern Europe, USA, Canada, Japan, Australia;
- intermediate-risk areas: (incidence rate of 8 to 20%): southern and eastern Europe, Russia, China, Israel, Caribbean, and South Africa;
- high-risk areas (incidence rate of 20 to 90%) risk: Middle-East, southern Asia, central and south America, Africa.

Some studies have tried to define a global picture of the risk of TD (Goa, India; Fortaleza, Brazil; Mombasa, Kenya; Montego Bay, Jamaica) by using the same methodology.[6,7] Such studies, which have involved a high number of travelers, have pointed out that the incidence rates of TD (classical, moderate, and mild) may be even higher than those normally considered. The incidence rate for TD for 2 weeks of stay was in fact higher than 60% in Goa and Mombasa, 37 to 39% in Montego Bay, and 19 to 20% in Fortaleza.

The correlation between destination and incidence of TD is certainly connected to warm climate that favours bacterial multiplication, but also, and more importantly, to the hygienic standard at destination. For such reason,

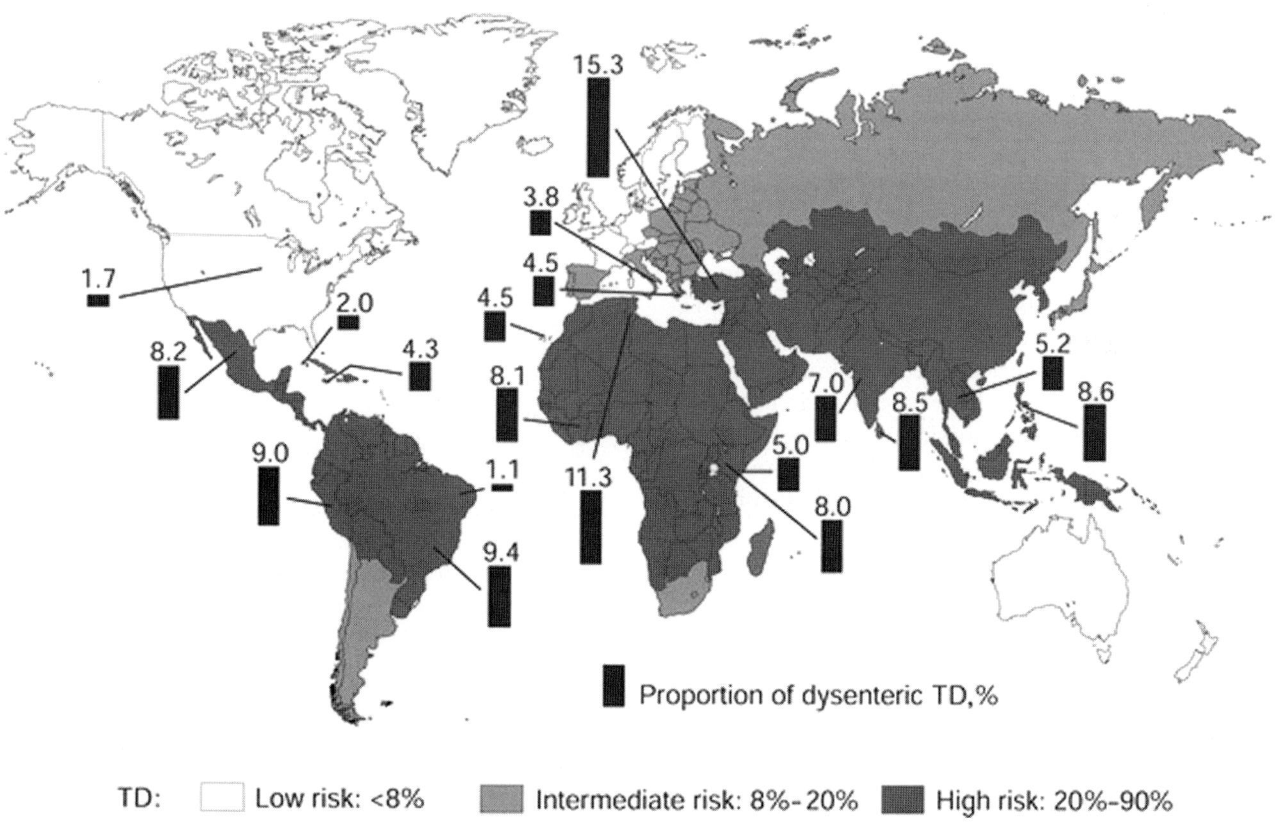

Figure 1 Risk areas for travelers' diarrhea (2-week incidence rates) and proportion of dysentery.[6]

the places of higher incidence of TD correspond to the places where more important it is the problem of high morbidity and mortality rates of childhood diarrhea in the local population in developing countries.[50]

However, apart from international travels, even traveling within one's country may be considered a risk factor for the occurrence of diarrhea. The role of travel itself on the occurrence of diarrhea was also recently confirmed by a large nationwide case-control study carried out among general practitioners in France, which demonstrated that French subjects living away from their usual residence had a significantly higher risk (OR = 3.0) of developing symptoms of acute diarrhea than residents.[51]

COUNTRY OF ORIGIN

Kean and Merson first demonstrated the influence of the traveler's country of origin on diarrhea attack rates. They noticed at two congress venues in Teheran and Mexico City, respectively, that delegates from industrialized countries suffered from higher diarrhea attack rates than their colleagues from developing countries.[52,53] This observation has later been confirmed by many other studies.

Several recent studies also concluded that the origin country of the the traveled is an important factor to determine the risk of TD. In the classical study of Steffen and colleagues in Jamaica, the travelers coming from northern countries (USA, UK, Canada) showed a significantly higher attack rate of classical diarrhea (11.1 to 24.3%) in comparison to travelers coming from southern European countries (Italy, 3.8%) or from Latin America (1.4%). It is nevertheless interesting to note that the attack rates of mild diarrhea were substantially similar regardless of the origin of the traveler.[54] The influence of provenance on diarrhea attack rates is probably due to a stronger protective immunity in those travelers coming from areas where the circulation of enteropathogens is somehow widespread.[55]

Being British, for example, involves a significantly higher risk of TD,[1,7,51,56] even if no biologically plausible explanation has been postulated.

DURATION OF STAY

The attack rates of TD shows a complex relationship with the duration of the period of time spent abroad in the tropics.[57] Certainly more elevated in the first days after the arrival in tropical area, TD appears to decrease subsequently.[54]

Data from retrospective case-control studies indicate that the risk of TD tends to decrease after about 12 months of permanence at destination, probably as a consequence of growing immunity to enteropathogens.[58,59] In the same line, a prospective study of US medical students in Mexico shows a 34% attack rate of diarrhea upon arrival in August that dropped to 5% later in January, which resulted to be equivalent to the diarrhea attack rate observed in control Mexican-residing students and significantly lower if compared to the attack rates reported in a group of US students newly arrived in January.[60] Nevertheless, if this observation has been substantiated in those locations where ETEC is the leading cause of TD, a prospective study in Nepal pointed out that diarrhea due to parasitic causes remained persistently high for as long as 2 years in long-term expatriates, with a yearly number of cases (3.2/year) equivalent to the yearly number of cases observed in children from the same area.[61]

Furthermore, a recent systematic review of the available studies on long-term travelers (military and non-military populations) has revealed the significant impact of diarrhea even in these populations, with higher incidence rates reported in those studies that used self-reported estimates than those based on passive surveillance or clinic assessment (29 versus 7 versus 6 episodes for 100 person-months, respectively).[20] However, generalization of the results of the review is somehow limited by high the number of studies carried out in the particular population of soldiers whose food supply is not comparable to typical long-term travelers for other reasons. A recent review of the available evidence deals particularly with risk factors for TD in military population, an increasingly important issue.[62]

SEASON OF TRAVEL

The influence of the season and, in particular, temperature- and rainfall-related humidity on the incidence of TD has been repeatedly suggested.[58] This is probably due to the different replication rate and circulation of enteropathogens according to microclimatic conditions and applies to both travelers and local population.[11] As many as 28% of cases of TD in Finnish tourists in Morocco were due to *Campylobacter* during the winter (7% during autumn), while enterotoxigenic *E. coli* strain and *Salmonella* spp. prevailed during the autumn (32% and 25% versus 8% and 10%, respectively).[63] We can observe the same differences in seasonality for Mexico.[60] Significant relationships between the incidence of specific pathogens and rainfall periods were underlined in other studies, as in the case of *Cyclospora cayetanensis* in Nepal.[64]

Nevertheless, in other studies, the correlation between the incidence of TD and seasonality was less evident. As an example, the wide-scale epidemiological study carried out in three different continents has shown significant seasonal differences in the incidence of TD in those travelers to Goa, India and Montego Bay, Jamaica, but not in travelers to Fortaleza, Brazil and to Mombasa, Kenya.[1] In this study, nevertheless, the seasonal differences in the incidence of TD could not be explained on the basis of different prevalence rates of isolated enteropathogens.[65]

MODE OF TRAVEL AND STANDARD OF ACCOMMODATION

Given the infectious origin of the overwhelming majority of cases of TD, it is not surprising that a particular style of travel or low standards of accommodation are in a close relationship with higher TD attack rates if compared with vacation in beach resorts.[6] In fact, Dutch people traveling on package tours reported a significantly lower incidence of attack rates than Dutch people traveling on self-arranged holidays (OR = 0.67).[66] The same was true for Austrian tourists camping or trekking in southern destinations.[48] The importance of structural factors, such as standard of accommodation, food quality, and hygiene was suggested by the different attack rates reported in different Jamaican hotels settings.[54] However, other works failed to confirm the association between hotel quality and diarrhea attack rates. More recent observations show that luxury hotels that offers gourmet foods (eg, complicated hand-prepared food, buffets, and cold dishes) are not at a lesser risk than ordinary hotels[6] and outbreaks of TD have been reported in resort hotels.[67] It is interesting to note that structural and training interventions aimed at reducing the incidence rate of the TD in the guests of hotels can have a significant impact.[50,68,69]

Travelers on cruise ships may experience high attack rates of TD should a common source food- or water-borne outbreak occur.[70]

PLACE OF EATING

Eating outside one's house is by itself a risk factor for the acquisition of TD, independently from the trip to the foreign countries.[71] This has also been shown inside the same nation.[51] In particular, it appears risky to consume food purchased by street vendors because food can be contaminated with feces and may contain a sufficient enteropathogens load to cause diarrhea.[72] In a recent microbiologic survey carried out in Mexico City, 14 of 18 raw oysters samples from street vendors, 4 of 12 ceviches fish and 3 of 18 shrimps cocktails yielded positive culture results for various enteropathogens, including not-01 vibrios, *V. parahaemolyticus* and *A. hydrophyla.*[73] If the majority of the available studies underline this risk, it is nevertheless notable that other studies have failed to detect significant differences in attack rates of TD in relationship to the place of purchase of the food.[1,54]

B) Traveler-Related Risk Factors

AGE AND GENDER

The available studies could not detect differences in the incidence of TD in relationship to gender.[1,54,74] On the contrary, robust scientific evidence suggests a great rate of attack of TD in young subjects, perhaps because of a greater appetite with consequent ingestion of a greater bacterial load.[1,54] The most affected is the 20- to 29-year-old age group.[45,75] It has also been postulated that young age can be associated with an adventurous travel style, implying a higher risk of encountering contaminated food or water. However, a higher incidence of TD in younger traveling people has also been observed when meals had been consumed together with the travelers of older ages.[1] In resident population in developing countries, the incidence and severity of diarrhea due to *enterotoxinogenic E. coli* decreases after childhood and increases later in adult life, probably as a consequence of environmental and immunologic factors.[11]

PREVIOUS TRAVELS

The role of previous travels in tropical areas in reducing the susceptibility of travelers to diarrheal symptoms has been much debated. In reality, the available data point out that the history of trips to tropical or subtropical area in the 6 preceding months significantly decreases the risk of the occurrence of TD in comparison to those people who had not traveled (16,7% versus 24.1%).[54] Solid evidence suggests that previous experiences in the tropics in the last 12 months may protect travelers from suffering from the clinical manifestations of diarrhea.[66]

PERSONAL PREDISPOSING CONDITIONS OF THE TRAVELER

The incidence and the severity of TD can also depend to a large extent on the genetic and physiopathological individual characteristics of the traveler. Among the factors of genetic predisposition, it is to be reminded that carriers of the blood group O may more susceptible to norovirus infection and *Shigella* spp. infections.[49,76] The increased susceptibility of blood group O carriers to the most severe forms of *Vibrio cholerae* infection, previously suggested,[77] has recently been counter-balanced by the evidence that these persons may actually be somehow less likely to be affected by choleric infection.[78] Likewise, the presence of a particular polymorphism in the promoter gene of interleukin 8 could increase the susceptibility to the infection from *enteroaggregative E. coli* .[79]

Some studies have pointed out a greater susceptibility to TD in travelers of British origin,[7] although no risky behavioral pattern was detected to explain such a difference.

It has long been recognized that any disruption or alteration of the gastric acid barrier may influence susceptibility to TD,[80] in particular when antacid, proton pump inhibitors, or H2 blockers are used by travelers.[66,81] Travelers with preexisting gastrointestinal illnesses who use antacid drugs should pay particular attention to their eating and drinking habits and might profit from chemoprophylaxis. The same might be true for persons with secretory immunoglobulin A deficiency, even if a conclusive demonstration of their higher susceptibility to diarrhea is lacking.[82] It has also been suggested that pregnant women are at increased risk for TD, probably due to transient immune impairment and slower intestinal transit time.[83]

Last but not least, the increasing number of human immunodeficiency virus (HIV)-infected travelers or otherwise immunocompromised travelers are at a greater risk of acquiring severe diarrhea,[84,85] especially when their CD4+ lymphocyte count is low. Such patients are more often affected by parasitic TD.[86]

REASON FOR TRAVELING

The motivations of the trip inevitably imply different styles of travel and behavior and consequently result in different risk of acquiring TD.

If the typical business trip is usually easier to control, holiday trips are often an opportunity to escape routine life with exotic experiences, including dining, translating to a higher risk of encountering enteropathogens causing TD. The high diarrhea attack rates observed among honeymooners might perhaps be related to the consumption of particularly elaborate food during ceremonies.[1,54]

DIETARY ERRORS

The often quoted aphorism: "*boil it, cook it, peel it or forget it,*"[87] suggests that dietary mistakes are in close relation with the attack rate of TD. This statement has a strong rational in the confirmed infectious nature of the syndrome. It is true that carefully self-prepared food carries little risk of ingesting enteropathogens, while eating in outside restaurants implies a significant risk. On the other hand, most studies agree that advising dietary self-control is of little use in preventing TD because very few short-term travelers comply with safe eating behavior.[15,88]

In his review of the available evidence on the effectiveness of personal hygiene precautions, Shlim notes that a significant proportion of compliant travelers do nevertheless develop diarrhea and concludes that "*... the risk of acquiring TD cannot be diminished significantly by teaching travelers simple rules to follow with regard to food choices*" and that new approaches to control the problem are needed.[89] This statement finds further support from the results of a recent questionnaire study that failed to identify any correlation between adherence to hygienic precautions as suggested by WHO[90] and the incidence of TD in India. Despite the low proportion of questionnaires returned (30%), which may limit its statistical value, the nonfeasibility of respecting such hygienic rules was also demonstrated by the fact that none of the travelers were able to adhere strictly to them.[91] Entheropathogens causing TD may simply be too ubiquitous in a poorly hygienic settings to be avoided.[92]

The fact that travelers' practice in tropical areas does not respect the norms of food hygiene is disheartening. Of all the participants to the study carried out in the returning travelers from the Jamaica, 95% added ice to their drinks, 90% ate salad, 80% consumed fresh dairy products and drank water from a faucet, while only 3% of the participants in the study declared a complete and rigorous adhesion to safe alimentary rules.[54] Such data are also confirmed by the results of a recent and ample airport investigation that demonstrated that only the 5.5% of the travelers departing for tropical destinations showed a positive attitude and willingness to abstain from all the dangerous foods.[93,94] It is also important to stress that the relationship between the history of consumption of dangerous foods and the occurrence of TD has not always been shown whereas sought after.[1]

Some studies have suggested an antidiarrheal protective effect of preventive predeparture counseling.[74] However, offer investigation have shown opposite results, revealing a greater incidence of TD in those people who had received predeparture counseling in comparison to those people who had not received it.[1,95] In the classical global study carried out by Steffen and colleagues, such paradoxical incidence difference was constantly observed in all studied sites (Goa, India 59% versus 36%; Mombasa, Kenya 57% versus 44%; Montego Bay, Jamaica 34% versus 22%; and Fortaleza, Brazil 17% versus 14%).[1] Such results, apparently paradoxical, could result from the greatest sensitivity of the travelers who had received predeparture information, thus leading to a recall bias and to a higher reporting rate of diarrheal episodes. Furthermore, curiously, the same study underlines that having consumed a significant number of meals out of the hotel constitutes a risk factor in Goa, but contrarily a protective factor in Mombasa.

Lastly, one cannot forget the importance of alcohol abuse as a cause of TD. In some studies, in fact, the availability of "free" alcoholic drinks within "all inclusive" tours has shown a correlation with the incidence rate of TD,[1] in particular with men.[96] Contrarily, the moderate consumption of red wine could have a protective effect.[97]

Impact

Although usually benign and self limiting, TD has a significant public health importance for several reasons:

- It represents a mirror (even though partial) of the more important phenomenon of diarrheal diseases in childhood in developing countries.
- It constitutes an important limiting factor in terms of comfort in the mobile population. The duration of diarrhea, with its subsequent incapacitation of greater or smaller entity in relationship to the type of diarrhea (classical, moderate, light), can constitute an important proportion of the stay to the foreign countries, causing a substantial loss in the quality of life. In the classical study by Steffen,[1] the duration of diarrhea covered 32.5% of the period of stay in Kenya, 39.3% in Jamaica, 27.7% in Brazil, and 27.1% in India.
- It represents a huge social cost for the countries of destination, whose revenues are often closely related to travelers, sometimes leading to political and structural interventions to decrease its incidence.[50,54]

Acknowledgments

The secretarial help of Mr. Giovanni Zoppi is gratefully acknowledged.

References

1. Steffen R, Tornieporth N, Costa Clemens S-A, et al. Epidemiology of travelers' diarrhea: details of a global survey. J Trav Med 2004;11:231–8.
2. Steffen R, van der Linde F, Gyr K, Schar M. Epidemiology of diarrhea in travelers. JAMA 1983;249:1176–80.
3. McDonald KL, Cohen ML. Epidemiology of travelers' diarrhea: current perspectives. Rev Infect Dis 1986;8(suppl 2):S117–21.
4. Black RE. Epidemiology of travelers' diarrhea and relative importance of various pathogens. Rev Infect Dis 1990; 12(suppl 1):S73–9.
5. Castelli F, Pezzoli C, Tomasoni L. Epidemiology of travelers' diarrhea. J Trav Med 2001;8(suppl 2):S26–S30.
6. Steffen R. Epidemiology of traveler's diarrhea. Clin Infect Dis 2005;41:S536–40.
7. von Sonnenburg F, Tornieporth N, Waiyaki P, et al. Risk and etiology of diarrhea at various tourist destinations. Lancet 2000;3562:133–4.
8. Guerrant RL, Oria R, Bushen OY, et al. Global impact of diarrheal diseases that are sampled by travelers: the rest of the hippopotamus. Clin Infect Dis 2005;41(suppl 8):S524–30.
9. Kosek M, Bern C, Guerrant RL. The global burden of diarrheal diseases, as estimated from studies published between 1992 and 2000. Bull. World Health Organization 2003;81:197–204.
10. Rao MR, Abu-Elyazeed R, Savarino SJ, et al. High disease burden of diarrhea due to enterotoxinogenic *Escherichia coli* among rural Egyptian infants and young children. J Clin Microbiol 2003;41:4862–4.
11. Qadri F, Svennerholm AM, Faruque ASG, Sack RB. Enterotoxinogenic *Escherichia coli* in developing countries: epidemiology, microbiology, clinical features, treatment and prevention. Clin Microbiol Rev 2005;18:465–83.
12. Okhuysen PC. Traveler's diarrhea due to intestinal protozoa. Clin Infect Dis 2001;33:110–4.
13. Steffen R, Sack RB. Epidemiology in: Ericsson CD, DuPont HL, Steffen R, editors. Travelers' diarrhea. 1st ed, Hamilton: BC Decker, 2003. p. 112–23.
14. DuPont HL, Capsuto EG. Persistent diarrhea in travelers. Clin Infect Dis 1996;22:124–8.
15. Taylor DN, Connor BA, Shlim DR. Chronic diarrhea in the returned traveler. In Med Clin North Am 1999;4:1033–52.
16. Ericsson CD. Travelers' Diarrhea. Infect Dis Clin North Am 1998;12:285–303.
17. Svenungsson B, Lagergren A, Ekwall E, et al. Enteropathogens in adult patients with diarrhea and healthy control subjects. A 1-year prospective study in to Swedish clinic for infectious diseases. Clin Infect Dis 2000; 30:770–8.
18. DuPont HL. What's new in enteric infectious diseases at home and abroad. Curr Opin Infect Dis 2005;18:407–12.
19. Caeiro JP, Estrada-Garcia MT, Jiang ZD, et al. Improved detection of enterotoxigenic *Escherichia coli* among patients with travelers' diarrhea by use of the Polymerase Chain Reaction technique. J Infect Dis 1999;180:2053–5.
20. Riddle MS, Sanders JW, Putnam SD, Tribble DR. Incidence, etiology, and impact of diarrhea among long-term travelers (US military and similar populations): to systematic review. Am J Trop Med Hyg 2006;74:891–900.

21. World Health Organization. Preventing travelers' diarrhea: how to make drinking water safe. Doc. WHO/SDE/WHS/05.07, Geneva, 2005.

22. World Health Organization. New frontiers in the development of vaccines against enterotoxigenic (ETEC) and enterohaemorragic (EHEC) *Escherichia coli* infections. Wkly Epidemiol Rec 1999;13:98–100.

23. Adachi JA, Jiang Z-D, Mathewson JJ, et al. Enteroaggregative *Escherichia coli* as to major etiologic agent in traveler's diarrhea in 3 regions of the world. Clin Infect Dis 2001;32:1706–9.

24. Glandt M, Adachi JA, Mathewson JJ, et al. Enteroaggregative *Escherichia coli* as a cause of travelers' diarrhea: clinical response to ciprofloxacin. Clin Infect Dis 1999;29:335–8.

25. Vila J, Vargas M, Henderson IR, et al. Enteroaggregative *Escherichia coli* virulence factors in travelers' diarrhea strains. J Infect Dis 2000;182:1780–3.

26. Ericsson CD, Steffen R. Traveler's diarrhea two to intestinal protozoa. Clin Infect Dis 2001;33:110–4.

27. Freedman DO, Weld LH, Kozarsky PE, et al. Spectrum of disease and relation to place of exposure among ill returned travelers. N Engl J Med 2006;354:119–30.

28. Hurst C. Estimating the risk of acquiring infectious diseases from ingestion of water. In: Hurst C, editor. Modeling disease transmission and its prevention by disinfection. Melbourne: Cambridge University Press, 1996. p. 99–139.

29. Begum YA, Talukder KA, Nair GB, et al. Enterotoxigenic *Escherichia coli* isolated from surface water in urban and rural areas of Bangladesh. J Clin Microbiol 2005;43:3582–3.

30. Centers for Disease Control and Prevention (CDC). Risks from food and water. In: Arguin PM, Kozarsky PE, Navin AW, editors. Health Information for International Travel 2005–2006. Atlanta: US Department of Health and Human Services, Public Health Service, 2005.

31. Backer H. Water disinfection for international and wilderness travelers. Clin Infect Dis 2002;34:355–64.

32. Groh C, McPherson D, Groves D. Effect of heath on the sterilization of artificially contaminated water. J Trav Med 1996;3:11–3.

33. Juranek D, Luby S, Maguire J, Mintz E. Risks from food and drink. In: Arguin PM, Navin AW, Kozarsky PE, Cetron MS, editors. Health Information for International Travel 2003–2004. Department of Health and Human Sciences, Centers for Disease Control and Prevention (CDC Yellow Book); 2003. p. 180–4.

34. Rossanese A, Nguyen TMD, Castelli F, et al. Guidelines for prevention and treatment of travelers' diarrhea. Italian Journal of Tropical Medicine (in Italian); 2005. p. 1–23.

35. Geldreich E. Microbiological quality of sources waters for water supply. In: McFeters G, editor. Drinking water microbiology. New York: Springer-Verlag; 1990. p. 3–32.

36. Regli S. Regulations on filtration and disinfection. In: Sorg TJ, Manwaring JF, editors. Proceedings of the Conference on Current Research in Drinking Water Treatment (Cincinnati). Springfield, VA: National Technical Information Service, US Department of Commerce; 1987. p. 151–70.

37. Centers for Disease Control and Prevention (CDC). Treatment of water to make it safe for drinking. www.cdc.gov/travel/water_treatment.htm (accessed November 6, 2006).

38. White G. Handbook of chlorination. 3rd ed. New York: Van Nostrand Reinhold; 1992.

39. Krym VF, McDonald RD. Safe water for travelers. CMAJ 2003;169:317–8.

40. Rogers MR, Vitaliano JJ. Military and small group water disinfecting systems: an assessement. Mil Med 1979;7:267–77.

41. Powers E. Efficacy of flocculating and other emergency water purification tablets. Report Natick/TR-93/033. Natick, MA: United States Army Natick Research, Development and Engineering Center, 1993.

42. Zoeteman B. The suitability of iodine and iodine compounds as disinfectant for small water supplies. The Hague: WHO International Reference Center for Community water supplies. 1972.

43. Backer H, Hollowell J. Use of iodine for water disinfection: iodine toxicity and maximum recommended dose. Environ Health Perspect 2000;108:679–84.

44. Cartwright RY. Food and waterborne infections associated with package holidays. J Applied Microbiol 2003;94:12S–24S.

45. Steffen R. Epidemiological studies of travelers' diarrhea, severe gastrointestinal infections and cholera. Rev Infect Dis 1986;8(suppl. 2):S122–30.

46. Castelli F, Carosi G. Epidemiology of travelers' diarrhea. Chemother 1995;41(suppl 1):20–32.

47. Steffen R. Travel medicine. Prevention based on epidemiological data. Trans R Soc Trop Med Hyg 1991;85:156–62.

48. Kollaritsch H. Travelers' diarrhea among Austrian tourists in warm climate countries: I. Epidemiology. Eur J Epidemiol 1989;5:74–81.

49. Al-Abri SS, Beeching NJ, Nye FJ. Traveler's diarrhea. Lancet Infect Diseases 2005;5:349–60.

50. Ashley DV, Walters C, Dockery-Brown C, et al. Interventions to prevent and control food-borne diseases associated with a reduction in traveler's diarrhea in tourists to Jamaica. J Trav Med 2004;11:364–9.

51. Yazdanpanah Y, Beaugerie L, Boelle PY, et al. Risk factors of acute diarrhea in summer—a nation-wide French case-control study. Epidemiol Infect 2000;124:409–16.

52. Kean BH. Tourist in Teheran. Travelers' Diarrhea at the 8th International Congress of Tropical Medicine and Malaria. Lancet 1969;2:583–4.

53. Merson MH, Morris GK, Sack DA, et al. Travelers' Diarrhea in Mexico. A prospective study of physicians and family members attending a Congress. N Engl J Med 1976;294:1299–305.

54. Steffen R, Collard F, Tornieporth N, et al. Epidemiology, etiology and impact of travelers' diarrhea in Jamaica. JAMA 1999;281:811–7.

55. Farthing MJG, DuPont HL, Guandalini S, et al. Treatment and prevention of travelers' diarrhea. Gastroenterol Int 1993;5:162–65.

56. Cartwright RY. Epidemiology of travelers' diarrhea in British package holiday tourists. Public Health Lab Serv Microbiol Digest 1992;9:121–4.

57. Cavalcanti A, Costa Clemens SA, von Sonnenburg F, et al. Traveler's diarrhea; epidemiology and impact on visitors to Fortaleza, Brazil. Rev Panam Salud Publica 2002;11:245–52.

58. Hoge CW, Shlim DR, Echeverria P, et al. Epidemiology of diarrhea among expatriate residents living in a highly endemic environment. JAMA 1996;275:533–8.

59. Herwaldt B, de Arroyave K, Roberts J, Juranek D. A multiyear prospective study of the risk factors for and incidence of diarrheal illness in to cohort of Peace Corps Volunteers in Guatemala. Ann Intern Med 2000;132:982–8.

60. Ericsson CD, DuPont HL, Mathewson JJ. Epidemiologic observations on diarrhea developing in US and Mexican students living in Guadalajara, Mexico. J Trav Med 1994;2: 6–10.

61. Shlim DR, Hoge CW, Rajah R, et al. High persistent risk of diarrhea among foreigners in Nepal during the first 2 years of residence. Clin Infect Dis 1999;29:613–6.

62. Putnam SD, Sanders JW, Frenck RW, et al. Self-reported description of diarrhea among military populations in operation Iraqi Freedom and Enduring Freedom. J Trav Med 2006;13:92–9.

63. Mattila L, Siitonen A, Kyronseppa H, et al. Seasonal variations in etiology of traveler' diarrhea. J Infect Dis 1992;165:385–8.

64. Hoge CW, Shlim DR, Rajah R, et al. Epidemiology of diarrheal illness associated with coccidian-like organisms among travelers and foreign residents in Nepal. Lancet 1993;341:1175–9.

65. Jiang ZD, Lowe B, Verenkar MP, et al. Prevalence of enteric pathogens among international travelers with diarrhea acquired in Kenya (Mombasa), India (Goa) or Jamaica (Montego Bay). J Infect Dis 2002;185:497–502.

66. Cobelens FGJ, Leentvaar-Kuijpers A, Kleijnen J, Coutinho RA. Incidence and risk factors of diarrhea in Dutch travelers: consequences for priorities in pre-travel health advice. Trop Med Int Health 1998;3:896–903.

67. Hardie RM, Wall PG, Gott P, et al. Infectious diarrhea in tourists staying in a resort hotel. Emerg Infect Dis 1999;5: 168–71.

68. Cartwright RY, Chahed M. Foodborne diseases in travelers. World Health Stat Q 1997;50:102–10.

69. Cartwright RY. The role of hygiene and public health programs in reducing the incidence of travelers' diarrhea. Comment on consensus paper by Steffen et al. J Trav Med 2004;11:189–90.

70. Widdowson MA, Cramer EH, Hadley L, et al. Outbreaks acute of gastroenteritis on cruise ships and on land: identification of a predominant circulating strain of norovirus. United States 2002. J Infect Dis 2002 2004;190: 27–36.

71. Jones TF, Angulo FJ. Eating in restaurants: a risk factor for foodborne disease. Clin Infect Dis 2006;43:1324–8.

72. Estrada-Garcia T, Cerna JF, Thompson MR, Lopez-Saucedo C. Faecal contamination and enterotoxinogenic *Escherichia coli* in street-vended chili sauces in Mexico and its public health relevance. Epidemiol Infect 2002;129:223–6.

73. Estrada-Garcia T, Lopez-Saucedo C, Arevalo C, et al. Street-vended seafood: a risk for foodborne diseases in Mexico. Lancet Infect Dis 2005;5:69–70.

74. Evans MR, Shickle D, Morgan MZ. Travel illness in British package holiday tourists: prospective cohort study. J Infect 2001;43:140–7.

75. Reinthaler FF, Feierl G, Stunzner D, Marth E. Diarrhea in returning Austrian tourists: epidemiology, etiology, and cost-analyses. J Trav Med 1998;5:65–72.

76. Hutson AM, Atmar RL, Graham DY, Estes MK. Norwalk virus infection and disease is associated with ABO histo-group type. J Infect Dis 2002;185:1335–7.

77. Glass RI, Holmgren J, Haley CE, et al. Predisposition for cholera of individuals with O blood group. Possible evolutionary significance. Am J Epidemiol 1985;121:791–6.

78. Harris JB, Khan AI, LaRocque RC, et al. Blood group, immunity, and risk of infection with *Vibrio cholerae* in an area of endemicity. Infect Immun 2005;73:7422–7.

79. Jiang ZD, Okhuysen PC, Guo DC, et al. Genetic susceptibility to enteroaggregative *Escherichia coli* diarrhea: polymorphism in the interleukin-8 promoter region. J Infect Dis 2003;188:506–11.

80. Giannella RA, Broitman SA, Zamchek N. Influence of gastric acidity on bacterial and parasitic enteric diseases. Ann Intern Med 1973;78:271–6.

81. Neal KR, Scott HM, Slack RC, Logan RFA. Omeprazole as risk factor for campylobacter gastroenteritis: house-control study. Br Med J 1996;312:414–5.

82. Diemert DJ. Prevention and self-treatment of travelers' diarrhea. Clin Microbiol Rev 2006;19:583–94.

83. DuPont AW, DuPont HL. Travelers' diarrhea: modern concepts and new developments. Curr Treat Options Gastroenterol 2006;9:13–21.

84. Castelli F, Patroni A. The HIV-infected traveler. Clin Infect Dis 2000;31:1403–8.

85. Castelli F, Pizzocolo C. The traveler with HIV. In: Keystone J, Kozarsky PE, Freedman DO, Nothdurft HD, Connor BD, editors. Travel Medicine. St. Louis: Mosby; 2004. p. 257–67.

86. Brink AK, Mahe C, Watera C, et al. Diarrhea, CD4 counts and enteric infections in a community-based cohort of HIV-infected adults in Uganda. J Infect 2002;45:99–106.

87. Kozicki M, Steffen R, Schar M. "Boil it, cook it, peel it or forget it." Does this rule prevent travelers' diarrhea? Int J Epidemiol 1985;14:169–72.

88. Peltola H, Gorbach SL. Travelers' diarrhea. Epidemiology and clinical aspects. In: DuPont HL, Steffen R, editors. Textbook of travel medicine and health. 2nd ed. Hamilton: B.C. Decker Inc.; 2001. p. 151–9.

89. Shlim DR. Looking for evidence that personal hygiene precautions prevent traveler's diarrhea. Clin Infect Dis 2005;41(suppl 8):S531–5.

90. Nuttal I. In International Travel and Health Geneva: World Health Organization; 2004.

91. Hillel O, Potasman I. Correlation between adherence to precautions issued by the WHO and diarrhea among long-term travelers to India. J Trav Med 2005;12:243–7.

92. Mattila L, Siitonen A, Kyronseppa H, et al. Risk behavior for travelers' diarrhea among Finnish travelers. J Trav Med 1995;2:77–84.

93. Castelli F. Human mobility and disease: a global challenge. J Trav Med 2004;11:1–2.

94. Van Herck K, Castelli F, Zuckermann J, et al. Knowledge, attitudes and practices in travel-related infectious diseases: the European airport survey. J Trav Med 2004;11: 3–7.

95. Peetermans WE, Van Wijngaerden E. Implementation of pre-travel advice: good for malaria, bad for diarrhea. Acta Clin Belg 2001;56(5):284–8.

96. Huang DB, Sanchez AP, Triana E, et al. United States male students who heavily consume alcohol in Mexico are at greater risk of travelers' diarrhea than their female counterparts. J Trav Med 2004;11:143–7.

97. Weisse ME, Eberly B, Person DA. Wine as a digestive aid: comparative antimicrobial effect of bismuth salicylate and red and white wine. BMJ 1995;311:1657–60.

98. Ericsson CD, Mattila L. Prevention of travelers' diarrhea: risk avoidance and chemoprophylaxis. In: DuPont HL, Steffen R, editors. Textbook of travel medicine and health. Hamilton: B.C. Decker Inc.; 2001. p. 159–64.

Chapter 10

Special Hosts: Children, Pregnant Women, and the Elderly

Richard A. Oberhelman, MD

Deborah J. Nicolls, MD

Phyllis Kozarsky, MD

While most research studies of travelers' diarrhea (TD) have focused on healthy adults, who compose the vast majority of overseas travelers, there are increasing numbers of travelers in other groups who require special consideration. International air travel has increased significantly in the last decade, and with this increase many more children are traveling overseas, posing special considerations for evaluation and management of TD.[1] Pregnant women also deserve special consideration because of the risks of placental insufficiency with dehydration and limitations on drugs that can be used therapeutically. Immunocompromised hosts present other challenges, complicated by the fact that varying degrees and types of immune suppression make it impossible to define a single approach that is universally applicable. Special considerations for the evaluation, diagnosis, and management of TD in children, pregnant women, and elderly travelers are discussed in separate sections of this chapter. Information on the management of TD in immunocompromised hosts is discussed in Chapter 11.

Travelers' Diarrhea in Children

EPIDEMIOLOGY AND CLINICAL MANIFESTATIONS

While there are very few published studies of the epidemiology of TD in children, there is indirect evidence to suggest that children are at increased risk for TD compared to normal adults. Children from affluent societies in developed countries have very limited exposure to the bacterial and parasitic organisms prevalent in developing countries, so they rarely develop partial immunity from repeated early exposures to enteropathogens. Child travelers may also develop TD from organisms such as Rotavirus, which are common in developed countries as well, but cause relatively little TD in adults with prior immunity. While children from developing areas with poor sanitation may experience many more episodes of diarrhea and more adverse health consequences from diarrhea than children from developed areas traveling abroad, the child traveler is probably at increased risk of developing diarrhea with a given pathogen exposure than either children from developing countries or normal adult travelers.

The few published studies on the subject suggest that the epidemiology of TD in children and adolescents is similar to that seen in adults, but varies somewhat by age group. Pitzinger and colleagues described the incidence, clinical features, and management of TD in a group of 363 children and young adults aged 0 to 20 years, recruited from the Zurich University Vaccination Center in Switzerland and traveling to a variety of destinations in developing countries.[2] The duration of travel was less than or equal to 2 weeks in 41%, and in the remainder, the duration of travel varied from 3 to 28 weeks. Overall, 142 participants (39.1%) were reported to have suffered from at least one episode of TD, an attack rate that is slightly higher than in adults from the same population. When stratified by age groups, the TD attack rate was significantly higher in the 0 to 2-year-old group (60%) than in all other age groups. The second-highest rate was found in adolescents aged 15 to 20 years (44.8%), followed by the 7- to 14-yearold group (21.7%) and the 3- to 6-year-old group (17%). Multiple episodes of TD were reported in 28% of those who had at least one episode. When calculated as incidence of TD per 14-day travel period, the lowest rates by far were reported for the 3- to 6-year-olds (8.5%). Significantly higher rates were found in the 0- to 2-year-old subjects (40%) and in adults aged 20 and older (22 to 36%). TD rates were highest in young infants in spite of the fact that their parents often claimed that they consistently practiced dietary precautions. Most episodes (72%) were reported as watery diarrhea, and other common clinical features included abdominal cramping (43%) and vomiting (14%). Fever was reported by 14.1%, mucus in the stools by 4.9%, and blood in the stools by 2.1%. The mean duration of TD in this study was 11.5 days, although children aged 0 to 2 years often had a prolonged illness (mean duration 29.5 days). Twenty-seven patients (19.0%) were confined to a bed, 21 (14.8%) were evaluated by a physician, and 2 were hospitalized. Illness attack rates were highest for children traveling to North Africa (73%) and India (61%), whereas attack rates for children traveling to East or West Africa, Southeast Asia, or Latin America varied from 31 to 39%. Etiologic agents of TD cases were not reported in this study.

In contrast to the extensive literature on TD in adults, the etiology of TD in children has not been well studied. While it is tempting to extrapolate based on numerous studies of endemic pediatric diarrhea in children from developing countries, the causes of TD may be quite different because of differing nutritional status, level of sanitation, and preexisting immunity. However, it is likely that many common causes of endemic diarrhea will also cause TD in child travelers, especially those that are food-borne or waterborne such as enterotoxigenic Escherichia coli, Shigella spp, and Campylobacter jejuni. In contrast, agents that are spread by direct fecal–oral contact linked to crowding in environments like day care centers, such as Rotavirus, may be less frequent causes of TD in children unless the child's family are long-term travelers who have integrated more completely into the host country society.

DIAGNOSTIC TESTING AND THERAPY

Criteria for deciding which children should have a diagnostic evaluation for TD are similar to those for adults. Generally, stool culture and parasitologic evaluation are only recommended for children with frank dysentery, severe diarrhea, or persistent diarrhea lasting more than 14 days.

The mainstay of therapy for TD in children, as for pediatric diarrhea in general, is oral rehydration therapy (ORT).[3] This therapy is the most important intervention regardless of the etiology of diarrhea. In determining how best to use ORT for TD in children, one must consider the type of solution to use, volume to deliver, and method of delivery. Current medical standards advocated by both the World Health Organization (WHO) and the American Academy of Pediatrics state that ORT should be used for mild, moderate, and severe dehydration. In general, intravenous hydration is only necessary for very severe dehydration (eg, >15% dehydration, often with relative hypotension) and in certain medical conditions such as stomatitis or altered mental status that can predispose to aspiration. ORT was first developed in the 1970s, and the original formulation with 90 mMol/liter of sodium and an osmolarity of 330 mOsmols/l, similar to concentrations in stools from patients with cholera, was the preferred solution for all diarrhea cases for three decades. However, research conducted in the 1990s (reviewed in the chapter on oral rehydration) suggested that low-osmolarity ORT (245 mOsmols/l) containing 75 mEq/l of sodium, 75 mEq/l of glucose, was superior to standard ORT in children with noncholera diarrhea, and was similar in efficacy to standard ORT in children and adults with cholera. In 2001 WHO endorsed this low-osmolarity ORT solution as the preferred method of treatment, and starting in 2002, most countries adapted it into their packaged preparations. However, both the original WHO ORT solution and the newer low-osmolarity ORT solution are safe and effective for treating dehydration in children. ORT is usually administered by small, frequent sips using a cup and spoon, and target volumes to rehydrate children over 4 to 6 hours are based on clinical estimates of the degree of dehydration, ranging from 50 to 60 cc/kg (mild to moderate dehydration) to 80 to 100 cc/kg (moderate to severe dehydration). Single doses of antiemetics, such as ondansetron, have been shown to reduce vomiting during oral rehydration and may improve outcome in treating dehydration.[4,5] Further details on ORT may be found in Chapter 25, "Nonspecific Treatment: Diet and Oral Rehydration Therapy."

One medical dilemma that has evolved in recent years is whether to use empiric antibiotics for treatment of dysentery of unknown etiology because studies suggest that antibiotic treatment of inflammatory colitis due to E. coli O157 may predispose people to hemolytic uremic syndrome (HUS).[6] While there is no fail-safe approach to this dilemma, several facts and guidelines may be useful in making this decision. First, it is important to recognize that E. coli O157 is rarely described as an agent of TD, although by the same token, it is often not detected because special isolation techniques are required to identify it. Most E. coli O157 infections are associated with outbreaks and not sporadic cases of diarrhea. In contrast, common agents of dysentery such as Shigella and Campylobacter are often identified in cases of TD with dysentery.

If possible, child travelers with dysentery should be seen by a local physician who will be more knowledgeable about the risk of E. coli O157 in the particular area. Certain geographical locations, such as Argentina, are associated with higher rates of E. coli O157 infections in children, and greater restraint in using empiric antibiotics should be used in these areas. If it is not a high-risk area and the case of dysentery is sporadic (or limited to a family cluster), then the next step is the feasibility of stool culture for E. coli O157 and for other bacterial agents (which, if found, would make E. coli O157 less likely). While culture for E. coli O157 is possible within 24 hours, the availability of laboratory resources for rapid detection (or any detection at all) is doubtful in most locations where TD is prevalent. If culture is obtainable and reliable, it may be advisable to wait for the culture result to initiate directed therapy. If no reliable culture is available and the traveler is not in a known high-risk area, then in most cases it is reasonable to use empiric antibiotic therapy for shigellosis and/or campylobacteriosis, depending on the epidemiological associations. In general, Campylobacter is a more common etiology for dysentery in children under 12 months of age, while both Campylobacter and Shigella are common in older children and adolescents.

Once a decision is made to treat a case of TD with antibiotics, the distinction between dysentery and watery diarrhea becomes less important since the agents used for empiric therapy should cover common causes of both types of diarrhea. Trimethoprim–sulfamethoxazole (TMP–SMX) has been the mainstay of antimicrobial therapy for TD in children for years due to extensive experience in children and data from the 1980s suggesting efficacy against many pathogens causing TD. Widespread resistance to TMP–SMX, however, makes it a poor choice for TD in both children and adults today. While reports from Thailand frequently reflect extremes for antimicrobial resistance of enteropathogens (and malaria parasites), it is still significant that a recent report from Thailand demonstrated TMP–SMX resistance in 90% of Shigella, and 40% of enterotoxigenic E. coli and nontyphoidal Salmonella strains.[7] Although resistance to TMP–SMX in other locations is likely to be less, it is still a poor choice based on average levels of resistance among common TD pathogens. Because of this increasing resistance and the risk of rare but serious side effects (Stevens-Johnson Syndrome, blood dyscrasia), the Committee on Safety in Medicine (United Kingdom) recommends that use of this antibiotic combination be restricted to specific indications.[8] One should keep in mind, however, that certain protozoan agents of TD are still treated preferentially with TMP–SMX, such as Cyclospora cayetanensis and Isospora belli.

If not TMP–SMX, then what antibiotics should be used? Fluoroquinolones such as ciprofloxacin are standard empiric therapy in adults because they cover most of the common enteropathogens causing TD, but common pediatric practice precludes use of this category of antibiotic because of quinolone-associated cartilage toxicity in juvenile animals. However, the risk of this type of toxicity in children seems to be low, and some experts use short course fluoroquinolones (such as 3 to 5-day courses for TD) in children without concern.[9] While cefixime is an attractive choice because of substantial safety data in children and studies showing efficacy in vitro and in vivo against most enterobacteriaceae (including TMP–SMX-resistant Shigella strains isolated from children), caution is warranted because it was ineffective against shigellosis in adults from Bangladesh.[10–12] As in the case of other third-generation cephalosporins, cefixime is ineffective against most Campylobacter strains, limiting its use for empiric treatment of TD. Also, cefixime is no longer manufactured in the United States as of early 2003. Azithromycin appears to be a better choice because it was found to be effective against Shigella, Campylobacter, and other enterobacteriaciae-causing TD, but resistance is emerging in some locations.[13,14] Rifaximin (Xifaxin, Salix Pharmaceuticals) is a poorly absorbable rifamycin derivative that shows great promise as an agent for empiric treatment of TD in children. Rifaximin was approved by the US Food and Drug Administration (FDA) for treatment of TD due to noninvasive strains of E. coli in patients $\geq$ 12 years in 2004, but experience with this drug in children is limited.[15] Toxicity appears to be low, and rifaximin has been shown to be more effective than TMP–SMX and paromomycin and as effective as ciprofloxacin and azithromycin against a variety of common TD pathogens in both children and adults.[16–20] Clinical efficacy of rifaxamin for infectious diarrhea in children has also been shown in a few recent studies.[21–23] Rifaximin may become an important tool in the armamentarium of antibiotics for TD in children.

Nonspecific therapies for TD in children have not been well studied and are generally not recommended. Bismuth subsalicylate may be effective for treatment of

TD in children as it is in studies of adult travelers, and salicylate levels in Chilean children receiving therapeutic doses for diarrhea are well below therapeutic doses for aspirin.[24,25] Salicylate toxicity has not been demonstrated in adults or children taking bismuth subsalicylate for TD and is probably not an appropriate concern. However, concern over the occurrence of Reye Syndrome has prompted some clinicians to avoid any salicylates in children. Synthetic opiates as antiperistaltic agents (eg, loperamide) are not advisable in young children for several reasons. Classic concerns include delayed clearance of organisms and microbial toxins (though this has not been found to be of clinical significance in adults), occult dehydration that can occur in the lumen of the bowel in spite of reduced stool volume, unpredictable neurologic toxicity in young children, and their role as a potential risk factor for HUS.[26] In some cases, loperamide may be used in older children and adolescents, as it is in adults for symptomatic relief in difficult travel situations, such as long bus rides with limited restroom facilities.

PREVENTION

Most experts on TD in children advocate good hygienic practices as the best method of preventing TD. Prophylactic antibiotics are usually not recommended for adults except in special situations where TD would be especially problematic, such as short business trips or special personal situations such as honeymoons. This type of special situation is rarely applicable to children, and antibiotics that have been studied for prevention of TD either have very limited efficacy with current antibiotic resistance patterns (TMP–SMX) or are not usually recommended for prolonged therapy in children (eg, fluoroquinolones). Bismuth subsalicylate may be effective, but it has not been studied for prevention of TD in children. Probiotic agents such as Lactobacillus GG have been shown to significantly reduce diarrhea rates in undernourished Peruvian children, but studies of probiotics to prevent TD in adults have either shown no effect or only modest benefits.[27, 28] Current evidence does not support the widespread use of commonly available probiotics for prevention of TD.

Pregnant Women

The choice to travel while pregnant, especially to areas of poor sanitation, is one that should not be taken lightly. The well-being of both mother and child must be taken into consideration. The pregnant woman is in a state of relative immune deficiency and is therefore more susceptible to certain infectious pathogens. The developing fetus also has specific risks.

CLINICAL FEATURES

Gastrointestinal complaints, such as heartburn, abdominal bloating, and constipation, are common during pregnancy. Hormonal changes cause alterations in gastrointestinal motility and smooth muscle function. Increasing levels of progesterone and reduced levels of motilin, particularly during the second and third trimesters of pregnancy, are associated with a prolongation of gastrointestinal transit time that normalizes postpartum.[29–31] These hormones may also cause relaxation in the lower esophageal sphincter, thereby predisposing the pregnant woman to gastroesophageal reflux.

The effects of pregnancy on gastric acidity are inconsistent. Some reports demonstrate significant increases in gastric acid production during pregnancy, while others show significantly reduced secretion.[32,33] Furthermore, gastroesophageal reflux may lead the pregnant woman to use antacids frequently, thereby reducing gastric acidity and possibly increasing her risk of developing TD.

The immediate concern with TD, regardless of etiology, is the maintenance of adequate hydration. Pregnant women are more susceptible to the effects of dehydration because of physiological changes that occur during normal pregnancy. These physiological and changes include a significant increase in blood volume, which is brought about by salt and water retention, a lower thirst threshold, and the release of arginine vasopressin (formerly called antidiuretic hormone), and heart rate, resulting in greater cardiac output. However, systemic vascular resistance decreases in pregnancy, resulting in lower blood pressure.[34,35] Volume depletion due to diarrhea further stresses these physiologic processes. Preexisting nausea and vomiting may also increase the pregnant traveler's susceptibility to dehydration from even a mild diarrheal illness. Mild dehydration causes fatigue, muscle cramps, postural dizziness, and increased thirst. More severe dehydration can put the pregnant woman at risk for renal insufficiency, shock and, premature labor.

In general, although the pregnant woman is more susceptible to severe dehydration and the consequences thereof, the bacterial agents of TD are unlikely to follow a more fulminant course; however, a few exceptions have been observed. In endemic countries, cholera causes more severe disease in women during the third trimester of pregnancy, with greater evidence of dehydration and larger stool output compared to nonpregnant women or women in earlier stages of pregnancy. In one study, 50% of women who developed cholera during the third trimester of pregnancy had stillborn infants early in the course of disease, compared with 8% of women who developed cholera during the second trimester.[36] The majority of women in both groups presented within 24 hours of diarrhea onset. Fetal heart-sounds were absent on admission in 90% of women who later miscarried. No deaths occurred in the mothers, who received rehydration therapy with or without antibiotics. Fetal deaths were believed to have occurred within the first 24-hours of the onset of illness, when fulminant diarrhea results in significant dehydration and metabolic acidosis. *Entamoeba histolytica* also has been observed to cause severe disease, especially colitis, during pregnancy and the postpartum period.[37–40] The development of an amebic liver abscess is rare in pregnancy, but worrisome because of the risk for rupture.

There are other enterically acquired pathogens that are worth mentioning here because they pose a special risk to the pregnant woman or her child, although they are not typically causes of travelers' diarrhea. Chief among these is hepatitis E, which carries a fatality rate of 10 to 42% during pregnancy, especially when acquired during the third trimester, and may be transmitted through the consumption of contaminated drinking water that has been treated with chlorine.[41–43] No vaccine is available, and the only protection is meticulous care with food and water. Listeria monocytogenes leads to severe disease in the pregnant woman as well as the possibility of miscarriage. Approximately, 70% of women in the United States are susceptible to toxoplasmosis, which can be acquired through the consumption of undercooked meats.[44] Toxoplasmosis is endemic in the tropics and can cause severe congenital problems.

TREATMENT AND PREVENTION OF TD IN PREGNANT WOMEN

As with other persons at special risk, the pregnant traveler should be scrupulously attentive to dietary hygiene. One unique issue for the pregnant woman is the use of iodine compounds for water treatment. The use of iodine-containing drugs and even topical iodine-containing antiseptics has been associated with reports of congenital hypothyroidism.[45,46] Although brief exposure to iodine at the concentrations used for water purification is probably innocuous, repeated consumption of iodinated water may put the infant at risk for congenital hypothyroidism. Boiled water is most reliably safe.

Immunization against hepatitis A and typhoid can be achieved with inactivated vaccines and is generally considered safe. The Vi capsular polysaccharide vaccine against typhoid is preferred because of the lower rate of febrile reactions. An oral killed vaccine against cholera is available outside of the United States and offers some cross-protection against travelers' diarrhea, but it has not been tested for safety in pregnancy.

Because of the need to maintain adequate placental blood flow, aggressive oral rehydration is the most important intervention for management of TD in pregnant women. Dehydration may result in premature labor or shock, so it should be avoided as much as possible. It is prudent for pregnant women traveling to isolated areas to carry packets of oral rehydration salts (ORS) with them. Either standard WHO formula ORS or low-osmolarity ORS (as described above) may be used safely in pregnancy, although many experts suggest that women receiving the WHO formula should switch to a low-osmolarity formula; that is, a maintenance solution with lower salt concentrations (eg, Pedialyte [Abbott Laboratories, Abbott Park, Illinois] in bottles or CeraLyte 50 [Cera Products Inc., Columbia, Maryland] in packets to mix with water), after initial rehydration is complete to avoid fluid retention. Low-osmolarity ORS solutions are not widely available in developing countries, so these should be purchased before traveling.

Management of diarrheal disease in the pregnant woman is complicated by the concerns regarding teratogenicity of certain medications. For this reason, in any case of serious diarrheal illness, an attempt should be made to make a specific diagnosis if empiric therapy with a safe antimicrobial fails. Routine stool culture and parasitologic examinations are appropriate, and further investigation is warranted if the diarrhea does not improve. Comprehensive information on the safety of various drugs in pregnancy can be found in recent literature reviews[47] and textbooks.[48] Risk factor categories for use of drugs in pregnancy as defined by the US FDA are summarized in Table 1.

In general, it is recommended that the pregnant woman avoid the use of any unnecessary medications, and routine prophylactic antimicrobials are not recommended. Chemoprophylaxis with bismuth salicylate is also to be avoided because the salicylate is well absorbed and may have adverse effects on the fetus.[49] Loperamide is a category B drug and can be used if necessary. The fluoroquinolones and tetracyclines are contraindicated in pregnancy and should not be used for the self-treatment of diarrhea. TMP–SMX is a category C drug, but has been used in early pregnancy (there is a risk of kernicterus in the newborn in late pregnancy). Amoxicillin (category B) is also commonly used in early pregnancy, but high levels of resistance to both TMP–SMX and amoxicillin have limited their utility. While erythromycin is effective against some Campylobacter strains, azithromycin (a category B drug) is more commonly used due to increasing quinolone resistance and because it has reliable activity against

Table 1 Risk Factor Categories for Use of Drugs in Pregnancy*

Category A: Controlled studies failed to demonstrate risk to fetus, and the possibility of fetal harm appears remote.
Category B: Animal studies suggest a potential risk in the first trimester, only it is not confirmed in pregnant women; stud-ies in animals that did not demonstrate fetal risk have not been confirmed.
Category C: Animal studies to suggest adverse effects on the fetus and humans are not available; studies in women and ani-mals are also not available. Drugs should only be used if the potential benefit justifies the potential risk to the fetus.
Category D: Positive evidence of human fetal risk exists, but benefits for use in pregnancy may be acceptable despite the risk in certain situations (eg, life threatening situation, serious disease without safer alternatives).

*Federal Register 1980;44:37434–67.

other agents of TD. Other options include the oral second- and third-generation cephalosporins, such as cefixime. Rifaximin and oral aztreonam are poorly absorbed antimicrobials that offer promise but have not been evaluated in pregnant women.[15] However, rifaximin appears to be safe in animal studies, and intravenous aztreonam is a category B drug.[50] Metronidazole is a category B drug and may also be used empirically for amebiasis and giardiasis, although some experts advise against its use in the first trimester. Tinidazole was approved by the US FDA in 2004 for the treatment of giardiasis and amebiasis in adults and children over 1 year of age. As a category C drug, it is not approved for use in pregnancy.[47] Paromomycin is thought to be safe in pregnancy and can be used as an alternative agent for amebiasis, but not giardiasis. Nitazoxanide is also FDA approved for the treatment of giardiasis and cryptosporidiosis in persons 1 year of age or older; it is a category B drug.[51,52] Many other antiparasitics and antihelminthics, however, are contra-indicated in pregnancy or should be used only if the benefits outweighs the risk.

Exacerbations of underlying inflammatory bowel disease are also seen in pregnancy and should be considered in pregnant women who are not responding to antimicrobial therapy.[44] As well, C. difficile must be considered if the woman has received antibiotics.

Travelers' Diarrhea in the Elderly Traveler

Two notable trends in clinical practice are the increasing number of travelers with preexisting medical problems and the fact that many more "over 65s" are exploring the wider world. An estimated 13 to 15% of travelers are over 65 years of age, and in some studies, nearly half of travelers seeking pretravel care in the US are 50 years or older.[53] These trends mean that travel advice needs to focus on the unique hazards faced by these groups and the interventions available to reduce their particular risks.

EPIDEMIOLOGY AND CLINICAL MANIFESTATIONS

In general, age is not a contraindication to most travel or activities. However, with age comes an increasing likelihood of chronic medical conditions, including heart disease, hypertension, gastrointestinal disorders, and diabetes. To a great extent, it is these medical conditions that dictate whether an elderly person will be at increased risk from diarrheal disease. The impact of these specific conditions is discussed in Chapters 10 and 11.

If anything, it appears that the elderly may have a somewhat lower risk of developing TD than the younger set. In one cohort of 1,469 travelers, the highest rate of diarrhea was in the 15 to 34-year-old age group.[54] A study of visitors to Paris seen in an emergency room found rates of gastrointestinal problems of persons over 60 to be close to half of those in the 20- to 39-year-old group.[55] The same pattern was found in a multicenter study of TD carried out in Jamaica, Kenya, India, and Brazil, and in a study of travelers returning from southern Turkey.[56,57] A recent review of Dutch travelers found a reduced risk of developing TD in those with extensive travel history.[58] Decreased incidence in older age groups may be related to increased likelihood of past exposure to pathogens, with development of some degree of residual immunity; more cautious eating habits; or greater chance of traveling in luxury accommodations with controlled food sources.

Decreasing gastric acidity with age is often cited as a potential risk factor for developing TD. Several studies have shown than gastric acidity is an important line of defense against infection from a number of bacterial and possibly parasitic causes of TD. Hypochlorhydria and achlorhydria are associated with more severe and prolonged illness due to cholera, enterotoxigenic *E. coli* (ETEC), and salmonella.[59,60] Furthermore, lower gastric acidity may allow a lower inoculum of a potential pathogen to result in disease.[59] Recent studies looking at the effect of age on basal acid production and gastric acidity measured by 24-hour ambulatory pH monitoring did not show variations in gastric acidity with increasing age.[61,62] Katelaris and others looked at the association between gastric acid production and histological changes in gastric mucosa. Reduced gastric acid secretion was not seen in older subjects with normal gastric mucosa; however, lower gastric acid secretory volume was observed in those with atrophic gastritis and evidence of *Helicobacter pylori* infection.[63] Thus, aging per se probably does not result in a reduction in gastric acidity; it is more likely that comorbid conditions, such as atrophic gastritis and H. pylori infection, cause a reduction in gastric acid production with increased age.

The deleterious consequences of diarrheal disease are often more pronounced in the elderly because of their increased susceptibility to dehydration and electrolyte imbalance. A tendency toward reduced renal function and decreased sensitivity to thirst may contribute to this susceptibility. Dehydration can compound the effects of heatstroke, to which older travelers are also more prone.[64] The elderly traveler is also more likely to have underlying medical conditions, such as diabetes or heart disease, which may be adversely affected by dehydration, changes in caloric intake (due to nausea), or fever. Medications routinely taken by persons with underlying conditions such as hypertension may potentiate dehydration (diuretics), blunt the physiologic tachycardiac response to volume deficit (beta-blockers), or predispose to renal insufficiency in the face of volume deficit (angiotensin converting enzyme inhibitors and diuretics).

In general, the pathogens causing diarrheal disease in the elderly are not significantly different from those affecting younger adults. In terms of other enterically acquired pathogens, many elderly travelers may be immune to hepatitis A due to childhood infection; however, illness caused by hepatitis A is more severe in older travelers, with a fatality rate of approximately 2% in people over 40 years of age.[53] Older travelers are also at much higher risk of severe disease due to Listeria monocytogenes, which can be acquired through the consumption of unpasteurized dairy products.

TREATMENT AND PREVENTION

Avoiding severe dehydration and its consequences is probably the most important aspect of the management of acute diarrhea in the elderly. Oral rehydration therapy should be initiated aggressively. Intravenous hydration may be necessary if oral rehydration and maintenance fails. Laboratory evaluation for renal dysfunction and electrolyte disorders should be performed early if diarrhea is voluminous or lasts more than a day or two despite self treatment. Antimotility agents can be used, but caution must be used as the development of ileus may be more likely.

Recommendations for vaccines to protect against enterically acquired pathogens are the same for older travelers as for younger travelers, although studies on vaccine efficacy and immune response after vaccination in the elderly are limited. In a recent article, Leder and colleagues reviewed the published information regarding the use of pretravel vaccines in older individuals.[53] Following vaccination with an inactivated hepatitis A vaccine, older recipients (40 years and older) had slower rises in antibody response compared with travelers 29 to 39 years of age. Furthermore, older vaccine recipients reached lower peak antibody titers following immunization compared to younger recipients. The clinical significance of these findings is unclear. All vaccine recipients reached antibody titers above the level believed to be seroprotective; the differences in seroconversion rates that was observed at 2 weeks following vaccination disappeared by 1 month following vaccination. It is possible that greater attention should be given to the timing of hepatitis A vaccination prior to travel in older individuals during the pretravel visit.

Information on the efficacy of typhoid vaccine, both the purified polysaccharide vaccine and the live-attenuated vaccine, in older travelers is extremely limited. Most studies on the efficacy of these vaccines involve young individuals living in areas endemic for typhoid fever. In general, both vaccines have low protective efficacy. One study from Nepal showed seroconversion rates of 77% for children aged 5 to 14 years, 79% for adults aged 15 to 44 years, and 62% for adults aged 45 to 55 years.[53]

Diagnostic studies would be similar to those conducted in other adults (stool culture, parasitologic examination, and toxin assay for C. difficile). However, in an elderly population, more consideration must be given to the possibility of a noninfectious cause, such as neoplasm or inflammatory bowel disease. Antibiotics recommended for self therapy will be similar to those for other adults, with care to avoid potential drug interactions.

Because the consequences of disease may be more severe in the elderly, older travelers should be encouraged to be particularly careful with dietary hygiene. They should travel with a well-prepared medical kit and specific instruction on the use of oral rehydration solutions and self treatment. They should have appropriate medical insurance and should be encouraged to seek appropriate care early if self treatment fails.

References

1. Statistical Abstract of the United States. US Census Bureau; 2001. p. 667.
2. Pitzinger B, Steffen R, Tschopp A. Incidence and clinical features of TD in infants and children. Pediatr Infect Dis J 1991;10:719–23.

3. Hirshhorn N, Greenough WB. Progress in oral rehydration therapy. Sci Am 1991;264:50.

4. Thillainayagam AV, Hunt JB, Farthing MJ. Enhancing clinical efficacy of oral rehydration therapy: is low osmolarity the key? Gastroenterology 1998;114:197–210.

5. Freedman SB, Adler M, Seshadri R, Powell EC. Oral ondansetron for gastroenteritis in a pediatric emergency department. NEJM 2006;354:1698–705.

6. Acheson DWK, Sears CL. Dangers of empiric ciprofloxacin in the treatment of acute inflammatory diarrhea in children [letter]. Pediatr Infect Dis J 2001;20:817–8.

7. Hoge CW, Gambel JM, Srijan A, et al. Trends in antibiotic resistance among diarrheal pathogens isolated in Thailand over 15 years. Clin Infect Dis 1998;26:341–5.

8. British National Formulary (BNF); 2002. Section 5.1.8. http://www.bnf.org/webnf/lform1/ bnf/index.html (accessed September 1, 2002).

9. Schaad UB. Use of quinolones in pediatrics. Eur J Clin Microbiol Infect Dis 1991;10:355–60.

10. Ashkenazi S, Amir J, Wiasman Y, et al. A randomized double-blind study comparing cefixime and trimethoprim–sulfamethoxazole in the treatment of childhood shigellosis. J Pediatr 1993;123:817–21.

11. Fuchs PC, Jones RN, Barry AL, et al. In vitro evaluation of cefixime (FK027, FR17027, CL284635): spectrum against recent clinical isolates, comparative antimicrobial activity, beta-lactamase stability, and preliminary susceptibility testing criteria. Diagn Microbiol Infect Dis 1986;5: 151–62.

12. Salam MA, Seas C, Khan WA, Bennish ML. Treatment of shigellosis: IV. Cefixime is ineffective in shigellosis in adults. Ann Intern Med 1995;123:505–8.

13. Khan WA, Seas C, Dhar U, et al. Treatment of shigellosis: V. Comparison of azithromycin and ciprofloxacin: a double-blind, randomized, placebo-controlled trial. Ann Intern Med 1997;126:697–703.

14. Hoge CW, Gambel JM, Srijan A, et al. Trends in antibiotic resistance among diarrheal pathogens isolated in Thailand over 15 years. Clin Infect Dis 1998;26:341–5.

15. Gillis JC, Brogden RN. Rifaximin. A review of its antibacterial activity, pharmacokinetic properties and therapeutic potential in conditions mediated by gastrointestinal bacteria. Drugs 1995;49:467–84.

16. DuPont HL, Jiang ZD, Ericsson CD, et al. Rifaximin vs. ciprofloxacin for the treatment of travelers' diarrhea: a randomized, double-blind clinical trial. Clin Infect Dis 2001;33:1807–15.

17. Gomi H, Jiang ZD, Adachi JA, et al. In vitro antimicrobial susceptibility testing of bacterial enteropathogens causing TD in four geographic regions. Antimicrob Agents Chemother 2001;45:212–6.

18. Beseghi U, De'Angelis GL. Comparison of two non-absorbable antibiotics for treatment of bacterial enteritis in children. Eur Rev Med Pharmacol Sci 1998;2:131–6.

19. DuPont HL, Ericsson CD, Mathewson JJ, et al. Rifaximin: a nonabsorbed antimicrobial in the therapy of travelers' diarrhea. Digestion 1998;59:708–14.

20. Frisari L, Viggiano V, Pelagalli M. An open, controlled study of two non-absorbable antibiotics for the oral treatment of paediatric infectious diarrhoea. Curr Med Res Opin 1997;14:39–45.

21. Sanfilippo A, Racitti Longo G, Racitti Longo A. Clinical experience with rifaxamin in pediatric diarrhoeal syndrome. Med Praxis 1984;5:375–83.

22. DeCastro R, Domecheli di Lorenzo FP, Pestripino ML. Rifaxamin treatment for acute recurrent diarrhea in children with genitourinary disorders. Curr Ther Res 1998;59:746–52.

23. Macias M, Gonzalez N, Ramirez P, et al. Eficacia y seguridad de rifaximina en el tratamiento de episodio diarreico agudo en ninos de seis meses a cinco anos. Rev Enferm Infecc Pediatr 2002;16:23–8.

24. Figueroa-Quintanilla D, Salazar-Lindo E, Sack RB, et al. A controlled trial of bismuth subsalicylate in infants with acute watery diarrheal disease. N Engl J Med 1993;328: 1653–8.

25. Soriano-Brucher H, Avendano P, O'Ryan M, et al. Bismuth subsalicylate in the treatment of acute diarrhea in children: a clinical study. Pediatrics 1991;87:18–27.

26. Bell BP, Griffin PM, Lozano P, et al. Predictors of hemolytic uremic syndrome in children during a large outbreak of Escherichia coli O157:H7 infections. Pediatrics 1997;100:E12.

27. Oberhelman RA, Gilman RH, Taylor DN, et al. A placebo-controlled trial of Lactobacillus GG to prevent diarrhea in Peruvian children. J Pediatr 1999;134:15–20.

28. Alvarez M, Oberhelman RA. Probiotic agents and infectious diseases: a modern perspective on a traditional therapy. Clin Infect Dis 2001;32:1567–76.

29. Wald A, Van Thiel DH, Hoechstetter L, et al. Effect of pregnancy on gastrointestinal transit. Dig Dis Sci 1982;27: 1015–8.

30. Lawson M, Kern F, Everson GT. Gastrointestinal transit time in human pregnancy: prolongation in the second and third trimesters followed by postpartum normalization. Gastroenterol 1985;89:996–9.

31. Christofides ND, Ghatel MA, Bloom SR, et al. Decreased plasma motilin concentrations in pregnancy. Brit Med J 1982;285:1453–4.

32. Hong J, Park J, Oh J. Comparison of preoperative gastric contents and serum gastrin concentrations in pregnant and nonpregnant women. J Clin Anesth 2005;17:451–5.

33. Hytten F. The alimentary system in pregnancy. Midwifery 1990;6:201–4.

34. Theunissen IM, Parker JT. Fluid and electrolytes in pregnancy. Clin Obst Gyn 1994;37:3–15.

35. Davison JM, Gilmore EA, Dürr J, et al. Altered osmotic thresholds for vasopressin secretion and thirst in human pregnancy. Am J Physiol 1984;246:F105–9.

36. Hirschhorn N, Chowdhury A, Lindenbaum J. Cholera in pregnant women. Lancet 1969;1:1230–2.

37. Abioye A. Fatal amoebic colitis in pregnancy and peurperium. J Trop Med Hyg 1973;76:97–100.

38. Rivera R. Fatal postpartum amoebic colitis with trophozoites present in peritoneal fluid. Gastroenterol 1972;62:314–7.

39. Armon PJ. Amoebiasis in pregnancy and the puerperium. Brit J Obst Gyn 1978;85:264–9.

40. Read K, Kennedy-Andrews S, Gordon D. Amoebic liver abscess in pregnancy. Aus NZ J Obst Gyn 2001;41:236–7.

41. Mast EE, Krawczynski K. Hepatitis E: an overview. Annu Rev Med 1996;47:257.

42. Boccia D, Guthmann JP, Klovstad H, et al. High mortality associated with an outbreak of hepatitis E among displaced persons in Darfur, Sudan. Clin Inf Dis 2006;42:1679–84.

43. Guthmann JP, Klovstad H, Boccia D, et al. A large outbreak of hepatitis E among displaced population in Darfur, Sudan, 2004: the role of water treatment methods. Clin Inf Dis 2006;42:1685–91.

44. Barbieri R, Repke J. Medical disorders during pregnancy. In: Kasper DL, Fauci AS, Longo DL, Braunwald E, Hauser SL, Jameson JL, editors. Harrison's Principles of Internal Medicine. 16th ed. New York: McGraw-Hill; 2005. p. 36–7.

45. Crepin G, Delahousse G, Decocq J, et al. Danger of iodine drugs in the pregnant woman [in French]. Phlebologie 1978;31:279–85.

46. Stubbe P, Heidemann P, Schurnbrand P, Ulbrich R. Transient congenital hypothyroidism after amniofetography. Eur J Pediatr 1980;135:97–9.

47. Jones J, Schulkin J, Maguire JH. Therapy for common parasitic diseases in pregnancy in the United States: a review and a survey of obstetrician/gynecologists' level of knowledge about these diseases. Obst Gyn Sur 2005;60:386–93.

48. Briggs GG, Freeman RK, Yaffe SJ, editors. Drugs in pregnancy and lactation. 4th ed. Baltimore: Williams and Wilkins; 1994.

49. Samuel B, Barry M. The pregnant traveler. Infect Dis Clin North Am 1998;12:325–54.

50. Bertoli D, Borelli G. Fertility study of rifaximin (L/105) in rats. Chemioterapia 1986;5:204–7.

51. Fox LM, Saravolatz LD. Nitazoxanide: a new thiazolide antiparasitic agent. Clin Infect Dis 2005;40:1173–80.

52. Alinia prescribing information. Tampa, FL: Romark Laboratories, L.C. June 2005. Available at http://www.romark.com (accessed 10/29/2006).

53. Leder K, Weller PF, Wilson ME. Travel vaccines and elderly persons: review of vaccines available in the United States. Clin Inf Dis 2001;33:1553–66.

54. Evans MR, Shickle D, Morgan MZ. Travel illness in British package holiday tourists: prospective cohort study. J Infect 2001;43:140–7.

55. Fisch A, Prazuck T, Semaille C, et al. Emergency consultations of foreign tourists in Paris in the month of August. 5 years of prospective surveillance (1992–1996) [in French]. Bull Soc Pathol Exot 1998;91(5 Pt 1–2):461–3.

56. Steffen R. La turista: acquisitions et lecons tirees d'enquetes recentes [in French]. Bull Soc Pathol Exot 1998;91(5 Pt 1–2):450–1.

57. Oksanen PJ, Salminen S, Saxelin M, et al. Prevention of travelers' diarrhoea by Lactobacillus GG. Ann Med 1990;22:53–6.

58. Cobelens F, Leentvaar-Kuijpers A, Kleinjnen J, Coutinho R. Incidence and risk factors of diarrhea in Dutch travelers: consequences for priorities in pre-travel health advice. Trop Med Int Health 1998;3:896–903.

59. Giannella R, Broitman S, Zamcheck N. Influence of gastric acidity on bacterial and parasitic enteric infections. Ann Int Med 1973;78:271–6.

60. Evans C, Gilman R, Rabbani G, et al. Gastric acid secretion and enteric infection in Bangladesh. Trans Royal Soc Trop Med Hyg 1997;91:681–5.

61. Collen M, Abdulian J, Chen Y. Age does not affect basal gastric acid secretion in normal subjects or in patients with acid-peptic disease. Am J Gastroenterol 1994;89:712–6.

62. Shih G, Brensinger C, Katzka D, Metz D. Influence of age and gender on gastric acid secretion as estimated by integrated acidity in patients referred for 24-hour ambulatory pH monitoring. Am J Gastroenterol 2003;98:1713–8.

63. Katelaris P, Seow F, Lin B, et al. Effect of age, Helicobacter pylori infection, and gastritis with atrophy on serum gastrin and gastric acid secretion in healthy men. Gut 1993;34:1032–7.

64. Dessery BL, Robin MR, Pasani W. The aged, infirm, or handicapped traveler. In: DuPont HL, Steffen R, editors. The textbook of travel medicine and health. Hamilton: BC Decker Inc; 1997. p. 320–8.

CHAPTER 11

IMMUNOCOMPROMISED PATIENTS INCLUDING AIDS

SUSAN L.F. MCLELLAN, MD, MPH

FRANK VON SONNENBURG, MD, MPH

While most research studies of travelers' diarrhea have focused on healthy adults, who comprise the vast majority of overseas travelers, there are increasing numbers of travelers in other groups that require special consideration. The proportion of persons living with compromised immune systems due to human immunodeficiency virus (HIV), transplantation, chemotherapy, and treatment of auto-immune diseases has increased due to improved therapeutic modalities, which have improved the quality and duration of life, and many such persons are now part of the traveling population. However, they remain at increased risk of certain problems, and preparation and evaluation of the immunocompromised host is complicated by the fact that varying degrees and types of immune suppression make it impossible to define a single approach that is universally applicable. Special considerations for the evaluation, diagnosis, and management of travelers' diarrhea in immunocompromised hosts are discussed in this chapter.

Diarrheal disease, an important cause of morbidity in the healthy traveler, is even more of a concern in the immunocompromised traveler. Depending on pathogen and the specific type of immune deficit, the traveler may have increased susceptibility to a pathogen, reduced ability to tolerate the physiologic consequences of gastrointestinal disorders or dehydration, increased likelihood of severe manifestations of disease, or increased risk of chronic manifestations from certain travelers' diarrhea agents that act as opportunists. Specific data on travelers' diarrhea in immunocompromised travelers is sparse, and much of the information on diarrhea in immunocompromised travelers has been provided from studies in proxy populations such as adults living in endemic regions or from studies of diarrheal illness in immunocompromised patients living in developed countries.

Travelers' Diarrhea in Persons with HIV Infection

EPIDEMIOLOGY AND CLINICAL FEATURES

The traveler infected with HIV faces all of the above concerns with regards to diarrheal disease. However, an HIV-infected person whose virus is well suppressed and whose immune status is relatively stable may be considered to be at only mildly increased risk from foodborne infection. The primary indicator of risk faced by the HIV-infected traveler is the degree of immunodeficiency due to HIV infection. The patient whose CD4 cell count remains in the normal to near-normal range may have little increased risk of immediate disease due to diarrheal pathogens. However, once the CD4 count begins to drop, the risk of suffering symptomatic disease from an exposure increases. Adults whose CD4 cells are less than 200 fulfill the criteria for Acquired Immune Deficiency Syndrome (AIDS) and are at significantly increased risk for infection and disease due to both common and opportunistic pathogens.

Persons whose CD4 counts have rebounded from an AIDS-defining level to above 200, and whose viral load is controlled on highly active antiretroviral therapy (HAART), are much less likely to acquire symptomatic opportunistic infections. Nonetheless, it cannot be assumed that immunity is normal in such persons, even if the CD4 count has rebounded to near-normal levels. Several studies have shown persistent aberrations in various indicators of immune function even after years of successful HAART.[1,2] There is also the risk that the traveler could become colonized with a potential opportunist such as microsporidium, which could become manifest much later should viral suppression be lost, either by failure of the HAART regimen or intentional or inadvertent discontinuation of HIV therapy.

Although many HIV-infected persons travel, it is difficult to find any studies that address the actual incidence of travel-related illness in this population, particularly in the era of HAART. However, knowledge of the underlying defect in AIDS and the prevalence of specific pathogens in diverse geographic areas allows us to predict common problems. Patients with HIV and AIDS are at increased risk of infectious disease primarily as a result of decreased cell-mediated immunity, although decreased humoral immunity occurs. A reduction in gastric acidity may also play a role in increased rates of infection and disease in patients with AIDS because achlorhydria frequently is a consequence of chronic HIV infection and may permit the development of disease with a low inoculum of organisms.

The consequences of even the typical traveler's diarrhea may be more profound for the HIV-infected patient. Borderline nutritional status may be further compromised if appetite is suppressed. For patients taking antiretroviral therapy, the traveler may not be able to tolerate his or her usual drug regimen due to nausea. Many antiretrovirals must be taken with food for appropriate absorption. Some studies have shown diminished absorption of nucleoside analog antivirals in patients with diarrhea,[3,4] although the effect on non-nucleoside analogs and protease inhibitors is less apparent.[5,6] Persons taking indinavir, a protease inhibitor, are susceptible to the development of renal stones if they become dehydrated.

The specific agents of traveler's diarrhea in the HIV/AIDS patient will include all of the same pathogens known to cause diarrhea in healthy travelers, but the risk of both infection and of severe disease may be higher. Common bacterial pathogens seem to be an important cause of chronic as well as acute diarrhea for persons with AIDS in the developing world,[7,8] and the HIV-infected traveler would certainly be at risk from these. In a study of *Shigella* isolates in San Francisco, HIV infection was found to be a significant risk for shigellosis. HIV-infected persons were also more likely to be hospitalized.[9] *Campylobacter* has been found to occur in HIV-positive patients at rates of 39 times the general population in Los Angeles,[10] and salmonellosis has been seen to be 20 times more prevalent.[11] These studies included many gay men, and the role of sexual activity in the spread of these diseases was not well defined. However, in some heterosexual African populations, nontyphoidal *Salmonella* were the most common cause of severe bacterial infections in HIV-infected patients, suggesting that these organisms may pose an increased risk for HIV+ travelers to developing countries.[12] In the developed world as well, nontyphoidal *Salmonella* infections have been recognized as a cause of recurrent disease and invasive infection including bacteremia in AIDS patients.[13,14]

Certain coccidian parasites are also more likely to cause serious disease in patients who are immunocompromised. HIV-infected patients who have low (< 200) CD4 counts are well-known to be at risk for chronic, debilitating diarrhea from *Isospora belli* and *Cryptosporidium parvum*.[15] These parasites, as well as microsporidium, are common causes of chronic diarrhea in AIDS patients in the developing world.[16–18] Microsporidium, specifically *Enterocytozoon bieneusi*, has been described as a cause of travelers' diarrhea, which can follow a chronic course in the HIV-infected traveler[19] *Cyclospora cayetanensis* is also known to cause acute and chronic diarrhea in travelers and may affect HIV infected patients more profoundly.[20,21] Both *Isospora* and *Cyclospora* are susceptible to treatment with trimethoprim/sulfamethoxazole (TMP-SMX), so persons with AIDS who are taking that medication as prophylaxis against *Pneumocystis carinii* pneumonia may have some protection against those agents also. Chronic diarrhea due to *Cryptosporidium parvum*, however, is refractory to most forms of therapy unless the person's immune status improves with antiretroviral therapy.

Giardia lamblia is a common cause of diarrhea in the HIV-infected person even without a history of travel. Because it is one of the most common protozoan intestinal parasites, it should be looked for in any HIV-infected patient with persistent diarrhea. *Entamoeba histolytica/dispar* as well as *Giardia* have been reported in higher frequency in men who have sex with men, so behavioral factors may have a role in the prevalence of these pathogens.[22] Although invasive and unusual presentations of amebiasis are occasionally reported in AIDS patients, it appears that the spectrum of disease due to *E. histolytica* is similar to that in non-AIDS patients.[23]

The same appears to be true of *Strongyloides stercoralis*. This helminth has sometimes been reported in higher frequency in persons infected with HIV,[24] but other studies have not found an increased prevalence of *Strongyloides* carriage or disease in such patients,[25] and *Strongyloides* does not seem to be a common cause of severe illness in areas highly endemic for both diseases.[23] However, infection with *Strongyloides* may result in persistent autoinfection, which (although asymptomatic) can set the stage for subsequent disseminated disease when triggered by other conditions. The most important of these is exposure to corticosteroids, which are indicated in the treatment of several HIV-related conditions, including severe *Pneumocystis jiroveci* pneumonia and drug reactions. With regard to other helminth infections, although there is evidence for some interesting immunologic interactions, there is currently no good evidence suggesting higher prevalence or increased severity of disease in HIV-infected persons.[26]

PREVENTION AND EMPIRIC THERAPY

HIV-infected travelers should be scrupulous about following dietary guidelines to avoid enteric pathogens, in particular avoidance of inadequately treated water, undercooked meats, and raw unpeeled fruits and vegetables. Because iodination without filtration may not remove protozoan agents such as *Cryptosporidium*, HIV+ travelers with low CD4 counts should be careful to use bottled water that is adequately treated, or to boil their water. Inactivated parenteral vaccines are available against Hepatitis A and typhoid, and these should be safe for the HIV infected traveler to receive, although data are lacking and the response to vaccine may not be reliable if the patient is severely immunocompromised. Live vaccines, such as oral typhoid vaccine and the oral cholera vaccine available in Europe, should be avoided, although they are felt to be probably safe if the traveler has no AIDS defining conditions.[27]

For relatively immunocompromised HIV-infected travelers, it may be appropriate to prescribe an antimicrobial to be taken routinely for the prevention of traveler's diarrhea. This strategy is generally recommended only if the length of travel is less than 3 weeks, but in fact persons with HIV infection frequently are prescribed antimicrobials for opportunistic infections for considerably longer without ill effect. Rifaximin, a nonabsorbable antibiotic, has shown some utility as prophylaxis against travelers' diarrhea although it is not approved for that use and avoids the issue of long-term systemic exposure to an antimicrobial. In some cases, the HIV-infected traveler will already be taking some form of antimicrobial for the prevention of opportunistic infection, such as TMP/SMX to prevent *Pneumocystis carinii* or azithromycin for prophylaxis against *Mycobacterium avium-intracellulare.* In all cases, the traveler should be thoroughly counseled about the use of oral rehydration solutions, antiperistaltics such as loperamide, and standby therapy of diarrhea, as well as indications to seek medical care.

Appropriate antimicrobials for prophylaxis or self treatment will be similar to those recommended for non–HIV-infected travelers. The flouroquinolones have been the most commonly recommended agents for this use in recent years due to evidence of the development of resistance to earlier compounds in many of the agents of traveler's diarrhea.[28] However, in some areas of the world (such as South East Asia) flouroquinolone-resistant *Campylobacter* is becoming prevalent.[29] For travelers going to these areas, especially during winter or dry season, azithromycin may be a more appropriate choice.[28] In general, the antimicrobials used in the prevention and self treatment of traveler's diarrhea should not have significant interactions with most antiretrovirals, but the traveler taking such medication should be prepared to discuss the issue of potential drug interactions with health care providers he or she may seek out overseas.

The most important preparation that the HIV-infected traveler can make is to assure that his HIV care provider is aware of his plans, and, if appropriate given his stage of illness, that he is on a stable and effective HAART regimen.

DIAGNOSTIC APPROACH

The approach to travelers' diarrhea in HIV-infected travelers will initially be similar to that in other travelers. Empiric antimicrobial therapy with a quinolone or azithromycin is reasonable early in the course of relatively mild illness. If an HIV-infected traveler is taking antibiotic chemoprophylaxis, empiric treatment for travelers' diarrhea should not be done with a drug in the same class of antibiotics used for prophylaxis. However, in many cases it will be appropriate to aggressively seek the etiologic agent, especially if the diarrhea threatens to become chronic. Stool cultures may reveal nontyphoidal *Salmonella*, which would warrant antimicrobial therapy in the AIDS patient to avoid recurrent bacteremia and invasive complications. A finding of *Cryptosporidium* would prompt an aggressive approach to management of underlying HIV infection because specific therapy for this pathogen is disappointing. *Isospora* and *Cyclospora*, although self limited in the normal host, may cause chronic diarrhea in the AIDS patient and warrant treatment with TMP/SMX. A combination of albendazole and ornidazole has also been used to treat *Isospora.*[30] *Enterocytozoon bieneusi* can sometimes be treated with nitazoxanide, which has also been used as an empiric therapy for AIDS patients in Zambia[31] Diagnosis of coccidian parasites may require the use of special techniques such as acid-fast stain of the stool or immunoflourescence.

If an empiric course with flouroquinolones or azithromycin is unsuccessful and no diagnosis is immediately forthcoming, an empiric course of metronidazole is reasonable because *Clostridium (C.) difficile,*

Escherichia (E.) histolytica, and *Giardia* are all potential pathogens and may be difficult to detect. Newer stool antigen tests for the two protozoans may help in that regard. If diarrhea persists, colonoscopy and specialist consultation are appropriate, as the differential diagnosis of chronic diarrhea in the setting of HIV infection becomes very broad and may in the end be unrelated to prior travel.

Special Features of Travelers' Diarrhea in Other Immunocompromised Hosts

DISORDERS OF THE STOMACH

Gastric acid is one of the more important barriers to enteric infection and the low pH present in the stomach is capable of killing many enteric pathogens within minutes of exposure. Any interference with the production of gastric acid secretion either pharmacologically or surgically can increase the risk of bacterial and parasitic infections.[32,33] The most detailed study of susceptibility to enteric infection in the presence of reduced gastric acid was undertaken by Evans and colleagues, who demonstrated that patients suffering from enterotoxigenic *E. coli* (ETEC) or cholera diarrhea had significantly lower gastric acid levels than control subjects, and that low acid was associated with more severe disease.[34] Somewhat unexpectedly, low gastric acid in this study did not appear to influence susceptibility to shigellosis, amoebic dysentery, giardiasis, or hookworm infestation. In a case control study of 743 Dutch travelers, Cobelens and colleagues,[35] described how previous gastric surgery and recent treatment for gastrointestinal (GI) disorders were significant risk factors associated with developing diarrhea during travel. A similar effect was noted in travelers using antacids, but the confidence limits on the odds ratio were too large to be reliable. The interpretation of this data suggests that travelers with reduced gastric acid secretion are significantly more susceptible to infections with the toxin-producing bacteria ETEC and cholera but susceptibility to other pathogens has not been confirmed.

DIABETES

Diabetic patients have a relatively high rate of GI disorders even in the absence of travel. In the general population, type 2 diabetics are reported to be twice as likely to have watery loose stools than controls.[36] However, this association is likely to be consequent to poor glycemic control or medication, especially metformin,[37] rather than following an increase in infections of the intestinal tract. Information on specific GI infections of diabetic travelers is not readily available, but there is no clear reason to suspect a widely different spectrum of pathogens.

The diabetic patient is at risk of both hyper- and hypoglycemia as a consequence of the rigors of travel, and dehydration makes glucose concentrations more difficult to control. The diabetic who develops diarrhea must be prepared to monitor glucose levels more frequently and adjust insulin doses if necessary. A switch to short-acting insulin preparations for the duration of an acute illness might be appropriate, especially if nausea and vomiting result in decreased caloric intake. As hypoglycemia is more immediately life threatening than hyperglycemia, the diabetic traveler should carry rapid sources of glucose and consider a glucagon emergency kit.

Maintenance of hydration is particularly important in this population. In diabetics, cereal-based ORT preparations can generally be used much the same as in nondiabetics because they are very effective and unlikely to influence glucose metabolism. However, the diabetic traveler should not be dissuaded from using glucose-containing oral rehydration solutions if they are more easily available. A study of diabetic patients with diarrhea in Bangladesh showed no difference in blood glucose levels, stool output, or duration of recovery in patients receiving standard WHO ORS formulation versus those receiving rice powder- or glycine-containing rehydration solutions.[38]

Prophylactic antibiotics to prevent travelers' diarrhea would in general be considered appropriate under the same situations that they would be for the healthy traveler. Empiric antibiotics for self treatment would also be similar, with the caveat being that the fluoroquinolones have lately been shown to have some dysglycemic effects. Gatifloxacin in particular has been associated with episodes of difficult to control hyperglycemia and should be avoided. Levofloxacin and ciprofloxacin appear to be less likely to cause hyperglycemia but rarely may cause hypoglycemia.[39,40] All diabetics should be prepared to monitor their blood glucose conscientiously while traveling.

INFLAMMATORY BOWEL DISEASE

Inflammatory bowel disease (IBD), may be either unmasked following an episode of travelers' diarrhea[41] or exacerbated following an acute intestinal infection, but there is no published evidence that travelers with IBD are at higher risk of or suffer from a more severe or prolonged diarrheal illness. However, an infection with an invasive pathogen would be a significant risk factor for an exacerbating quiescent IBD. On these grounds it would be reasonable to consider prescribing chemoprophylaxis for travelers with IBD in certain cases, recognizing and discussing the small but important risk of precipitating *C. difficile* colitis.

TRAVELERS RECEIVING IMMUNOSUPPRESSIVE THERAPY

Patients under treatment for malignancy are likely to have some degree of immune compromise due to both the underlying disease and the therapy. There are little data on this group of travelers; most concerns have focused on the advisability of giving live vaccines rather than diarrhea. However, it can generally be predicted that such travelers will have relatively fragile health, and every effort should be made to prevent travelers' diarrhea and to respond rapidly should it occur.

Persons who have received transplants, whether solid-organ or bone marrow transplants, are most definitely including travel in their plans, and travel to more exotic destinations. A recent study in Canada showed that 35.6% of solid-organ recipients had traveled in the previous year outside of Canada and the US. Most had sought pretravel advice only from their transplant physician, and only 18% reported that they carried antibiotics for self treatment of travelers' diarrhea.[42] No published data suggest an increased risk of travelers' diarrhea in persons with solid-organ transplants. However, transplant recipients, like AIDS patients, are at risk for a variety of opportunistic pathogens, in particular the coccidian parasites, microsporidia, and Giardia. Bacterial agents of travelers' diarrhea such as *Salmonella* may also become persistent or invasive. The use of broad-spectrum antibiotics, not infrequent in this group of travelers, is associated with an increased risk of *C. difficile* colitis, which is also a common pathogen in transplant recipients in general.[43] Other causes of infection in transplant patients include *Cryptosporidium* and enteroviruses. Noninfectious diarrhea is also frequent and may include graft versus host reaction. Unusual pathogens such as Cytomegalovirus can be expected in these immunosuppressed travelers, especially in persons on high dose corticosteroids, and may be unrelated to travel.

Tumor necrosis factor (TNF) inhibitors (ie, infliximab, certolizumab, etanercept, and adalimumab) are a class of drugs that are being used with greater frequency and have now been clearly associated with an increased incidence of infections, most typically the granulomatous mycobacterial and fungal diseases. Tuberculosis, histoplasmosis, and coccidiomycosis have all been described as diseases associated with travel, and the patient on TNF antagonists should be counseled about possible exposures. Diarrheal disease has not been specifically noted; however, the systemic granulomatous diseases can sometimes present with GI manifestations and should be considered should any patient taking these medications presents with diarrhea.

PREVENTION AND EMPIRIC THERAPY

All immunocompromised travelers should be counseled to follow scrupulous food and water precautions. The consequences of dehydration while taking some of the antirejection drugs such as cycolosporin and tacrolimus can be severe, especially as many transplant patients may have some underlying renal insufficiency even at baseline. Oral rehydration solution should be carried by all such travelers. A plan for self treatment of travelers' diarrhea with antibiotics is mandatory, and in certain cases prophylactic antibiotics may be appropriate. The flouroquinolones in general should cause no difficulties with the usual antirejection medications; however, azithromycin, frequently recommended as empiric travelers' diarrhea therapy in areas where *Campylobacter* is prevalent, can increase levels of cyclosporin and tacrolimus. The potential use of a short treatment course should be discussed with the transplant care provider. Rifaximin is an option for both treatment of travelers' diarrhea due to ETEC and (as an off-label use) for prophylaxis; because it is not absorbed, drug interactions are not expected to be a problem.

DIAGNOSTIC APPROACH

As is the case with the HIV-infected patient, empiric therapy for bacterial travelers' diarrhea is appropriate for other immunocompromised travelers. If a diagnosis is not made promptly with basic studies, an empiric trial of antiparasitic therapy is not unreasonable, but a more extensive diagnostic workup should not be delayed. When possible, reduction or cessation of the immunosuppressive regimen may be necessary to control some infections. Noninfectious causes of diarrhea, including graft versus host disease and drug side effects, should remain in the differential.

Conclusion

With advances in medical technology, HIV treatment, and immune-modulating therapies, an increasing number of people with immune deficits are enjoying a quality of life that allows travel to be a realistic consideration. Nonetheless, these travelers still carry certain risks, and special preparation and precautions are important to reduce the possibility of travel-related infections and illness, including travelers' diarrhea. In all cases, the traveler will benefit from good advance preparation and should be stabilized on his or her medical regimen. He or she should be well advised on avoidance of risk, and prepared to deal with travelers' diarrhea if it occurs. Should diarrhea become chronic, the health care provider must be prepared to embark upon a thorough

Table 1 Traveler's Diarrhea in HIV-Infected Travelers, Travelers with decreased Gastric Acid, Diabetic Travelers, and Travelers on Immunosuppressive Regimens: Summary of Recommendations for Evaluation, Diagnosis, and Management as Compared to Healthy, Immunocompetent Adults (based on multiple sources referenced in the text)

Special Host Group:	Risk of TD as Compared to Normal Adults	Morbidity from TD as Compared to Normal Adults	Common Etiologies of TD	Use of Antibiotics for TD Prophylaxis	Empiric Antibiotic Therapies for TD	Use of Oral Rehydration for TD	Use of Nonantimicrobial Drugs for TD
HIV-Infected Travelers	Increased when CD4 count is low, similar if CD4 count is normal	Greater risk of prolonged or severe diarrhea with certain pathogens (if CD4 is low), or development of systemic disease	Pathogens common in normal adults and other opportunistic infections (*Cryptosporidium, Cyclospora, Giardia*)	Consider if CD4 count is low and traveler is visiting areas with poor sanitation; fluoroquinolones or rifaximin are effective and have been studied in prophylaxis; azithromycin is a consideration but prophylaxis dose is uncertain	As in normal adults, fluoroquinolones, azithromycin, or rifaximin* could be used (do not use same family of drugs used for prophylaxis); suggest lab evaluation for bacterial and parasitic agents and consider empiric metronidazole if TD is refractory to routine antibiotic therapy	Recommended with WHO or low-osmolarity solutions	BSS and antimotility agents may be used as in normal adults
Travelers with Decreased Gastric Acid	Increased, likely due to increased survival of pathogens transiting stomach	Similar	Pathogens common in normal adults, documented increased susceptibility to ETEC and cholera	Similar to other adults; if possible, suspend use of agents reducing gastric acidity	Similar to other adults	Recommended with WHO or low-osmolarity solutions	BSS and antimotility agents may be used as in normal adults
Diabetic Travelers	Little data on increased risk of infectious diarrhea; high rates of gastrointestinal disorders and diarrhea at baseline	Increased risk of consequences of nausea and dehydration; loss of glycemic control, worsening of renal dysfunction	Little data; presumably pathogens common in normal adults	Similar to other adults; however, potential for dysglycemic effects on fluoroquinolones not studied in travelers diarrhea; avoid gatifloxacin	Similar to other adults; however, potential for dysglycemic effects on fluoroquinolones not studied in travelers diarrhea; avoid gatifloxacin	Recommended with WHO or low-osmolarity solutions	BSS and antimotility agents may be used as in normal adults; however, in traveler with renal insufficiency, risk is increased for salicylate toxicity from BSS

Table 1 Continued

Special Host Group:	Risk of TD as Compared to Normal Adults	Morbidity from TD as Compared to Normal Adults	Common Etiologies of TD	Use of Antibiotics for TD Prophylaxis	Empiric Antibiotic Therapies for TD	Use of Oral Rehydration for TD	Use of Nonantimicrobial Drugs for TD
Transplant Recipients and Other Travelers on Immunosuppressive Regimens	No data, but can assume higher risk, increasing with more potent immunosuppressive regimen	Greater risk of prolonged or severe diarrhea with certain pathogens or development of systemic disease; may have increased risk of consequences of dehydration	Pathogens common in normal adults, *Clostridium difficile,* and other opportunistic infections (*Cryptosporidium, Cyclospora, Giardia*)	Consider if traveler is visiting areas with poor sanitation; fluoroquinolones or rifaximin are effective and have been studied in prophylaxis; azithromycin is a consideration but prophylaxis dose is uncertain and there may be drug interactions with azithromycin	As in normal adults, fluoroquinolones, azithromycin, or rifaximin* could be used (do not use same family of drugs used for prophylaxis); suggest lab evaluation for bacterial and parasitic agents and consider empiric metronidazole if TD is refractory to routine antibiotic therapy	Recommended with WHO or low-osmolarity solutions	BSS and antimotility agents may be used as in normal adults; however, in traveler with renal insufficiency, risk is increased for salicylate toxicity from BSS

BSS = bismuth subsalicylate; HIV = human immunodeficiency virus; TD = travelers' diarrhea; WHO = World Health Organization.
*Rifaximin is not approved for use in treating diarrhea caused by invasive pathogens, so caution must be exercised in its use in immunocompromised patients.

workup, with consideration of specific risks according to the traveler's underlying condition, and keeping causes unrelated to travel in mind.

A summary of these special considerations for immunocompromised travelers is presented in Table 1.

References

1. Valdez H, Connick E, Smith KY, et al. Limited immune restoration after 3 years' suppression of HIV-1 replication in patients with moderately advanced disease. Aids 2002;16: 1859–66.
2. Hunt PW, Martin JN, Sinclair E, et al. T-cell activation is associated with lower CD4+ T-cell gains in human immunodeficiency virus-infected patients with sustained viral suppression during antiretroviral therapy. J Infect Dis 2003;187:1534–43.
3. Bushen OY, Davenport JA, Lima AB, et al. Diarrhea and reduced levels of antiretroviral drugs: improvement with glutamine or alanyl-glutamine in a randomized controlled trial in northeast Brazil. Clin Infect Dis 2004;38:1764–70.
4. Brantley RK, Williams KR, Silva TMJ, et al. AIDS-associated diarrhea and wasting in northeast Brazil is associated with subtherapeutic plasma levels of antiretroviral medications and with both bovine and human subtypes of Cryptosporidium parvum. Braz J Infect Dis 2003;7:1622.
5. Weinberg WG. Nevirapine absorbed well despite chronic diarrhea. AIDS Res Hum Retroviruses 2005;21:597.
6. Trout H, Mentre F, Panhard X, et al. Enhanced saquinavir exposure in human immunodeficiency virus type 1-infected patients with diarrhea and/or wasting syndrome. Antimicrob Agents Chemoth., 2004;48:538–45.
7. Clerinx J, Bogaerts J, Taelman H, et al. Chronic diarrhea among adults in Kigali, Rwanda: association with bacterial enteropathogens, rectocolonic inflammation, and human immunodeficiency virus infection. Clin Infect Dis 1995;21: 1282–4.
8. Orenstein JM, Kotler DP. Diarrheogenic bacterial enteritis in acquired immune deficiency syndrome: a light and electron microscopy study of 52 cases. Human Pathol 1995; 26:481–92.
9. Baer JT, Vugia DJ, Reingold AL, et al. HIV infection as a risk factor for shigellosis. Emerg Infect Dis 1999;5:820–3.
10. Sorvillo FJ, Lieb LE, Waterman SH. Incidence of campylobacteriosis among patients with AIDS in Los Angeles County. J Acquir Immune Defic Syndr Hum Retrovirol 1991;4:598–602.
11. Celum CL, Chaisson RE, Rutherford GW, et al. Incidence of salmonellosis in patients with AIDS. J Infect Dis 1987; 156:998–1002.
12. Attia A, Huet C, Anglaret X, et al. HIV-1-related morbidity in adults, Abidjan, Cote d'Ivoire: a nidus for bacterial diseases. J Acq Immun Defic Synd 2001;28:478–86.
13. Vincent D, Petit JC, Pradalier A, et al. Manifestation of AIDS by recurrent Salmonella infection. [French] [Letter] An Med Interna 1989;140:215–7.

14. Tocalli L, Nardi G, Mammino A, et al. Salmonellosis diagnosed by the laboratory of the 'L. Sacco' Hospital of Milan (Italy) in patients with HIV disease. Europ J Epidemiol 1991;7:690–5.

15. Lindsay DS, Dubey JP, Blagburn BL. Biology of Isospora spp. from humans, nonhuman primates, and domestic animals. Clin Microbiol Rev 1997;10:19–34.

16. Lebbad M, Norrgren H, Naucler A, et al. Intestinal parasites in HIV-2 associated AIDS cases with chronic diarrhoea in Guinea-Bissau. Acta Tropica 2001;80:45–9.

17. Maiga I, Doumbo O, Dembele M, et al. Human intestinal microsporidiosis in Bamako (Mali): the presence of Enterocytozoon bieneusi in HIV seropositive patients. [French] Sante 1997;7:257–62.

18. Garcia C, Rodriguez E, Do N, et al. Intestinal parasitosis in patients with HIV-AIDS. [Spanish] Revista de Gastroenterologia del Peru 2006;26:21–4.

19. Rogelio López-VélezM. Carmen TurrientesCarla GarrónPedro MontillaRaquel NavajasSoledad Fenoy-Carmen del AguilaMicrosporidiosis in travelers with diarrhea. Tropics Journal of Travel Medicine , 6:223–7.

20. Masuda G, Ajisawa A, Imamura A, et al. Cyclosporiasis: four case reports with a review of the literature. [Japanese] Kansenshogaku Zasshi. J Japan Assoc Infect Dis 2002;76: 416–24.

21. Chacin-Bonilla L, Estevez J, Monsalve F, Quijada L. Cyclospora cayetanensis infections among diarrheal patients from Venezuela. Am J Trop Med Hyg 2001;65:351–4.

22. Junod C. Comparative results of coprological tests for the detection of intestinal amebae and flagellates in 200 male homosexuals. An appraisal of the risk of amebiasis. [French] Bull Soc Pathol Exot Filiales 1983;76(5 Pt 2): 805–17.

23. Lucas SB. Missing infections in AIDS. Trans Roy Soc Trop Med Hyg 1990;84Suppl 1:34–8.

24. Feitosa G, Bandeira AC, Sampaio DP, et al. High prevalence of giardiasis and stronglyloidiasis among HIV-infected patients in Bahia, Brazil. Brazil J Infect Dis 2001;5: 339–44.

25. Dias RM, Mangini AC, Torres DM, et al. Occurrence of strongyloides stercoralis in patients with acquired immunodeficiency syndrome (AIDS)]. [Portuguese] Rev Instit Med Trop Sao Paulo 1992;34:15–7.

26. Plourde PJ. Interactions between HIV and helminthic diseases. In: Ronald AR, editor. Opportunistic complications of HIV: classical tropical diseases 5, no. 4. Bala Cynwyd, PA, Meniscus Health Care Communications, 1997, p 93.

27. Anonoymous. Statement Statement on travellers and HIV/ AIDS. Canad Med Assoc J 1995;152:379–80.

28. Ericsson CD. Travelers' diarrhea. In: Freedman DO, editor. Infect Dis Clin N Amer 1998;12:285–303.

29. Engberg J, Aarestrup FM, Taylor DE, et al. Quinolone and macrolide resistance in Campylobacter jejuni and C. coli: resistance mechanisms and trends in human isolates. Emerg Infect Dis 2001;7:24–34.

30. Dionisio D, Sterrantino G, Meli M, et al. Treatment of isosporiasis with combined albendazole and ornidazole in patients with AIDS. [Letter] AIDS 1996;10:1301–2.

31. Zulu I, Kelly P, Njobvu L, et al. Nitazoxanide for persistent diarrhoea in Zambian acquired immune deficiency syndrome patients: a randomized-controlled trial. Aliment Pharmacol Ther 2005;21:757–63.

32. Larner AJ, Hamilton MI. Review article: infective complications of therapeutic gastric acid inhibition. Aliment Pharmacol Ther 1994;8:579–84.

33. Giannella RA, Broitman SA, Zamcheck N. Influence of gastric acidity on bacterial and parasitic enteric infections: a perspective. Ann Intern Med 1973;78:271–6.

34. Evans CA, Gilman RH, Rabbani GH, et al. Gastric acid secretion and enteric infection in Bangladesh. Trans R Soc Trop Med Hyg 1997;91:681–5.

35. Cobelens FG, Leentvaar-Kuijpers A, Kleijnen J, Coutinho RA. Incidence and risk factors of diarrhoea in Dutch travellers: consequences for priorities in pre-travel health advice. Trop Med Int Health 1998;3:896–903.

36. Bytzer P, Talley NJ, Leemon M, et al. Prevalence of gastrointestinal symptoms associated with diabetes mellitus: a population-based survey of 15,000 adults. Arch Int Med 2001;161:1989–96.

37. Lysy J, Israeli E, Goldin E. The prevalence of chronic diarrhea among diabetic patients. Am J Gastroent 1999;94: 2165–70.

38. Haider R, Azad Khan AK, Roy SK, et al. Management of acute diarrhoea in diabetic patients using oral rehydration solutions containing glucose, rice, or glycine. BMJ 1994; 308:624–6.

39. Park-Wyllie LY, Juurlink DN, Kopp A, et al. Outpatient gatifloxacin therapy and dysglycemia in older adults. N Engl J Med 2006;354:1352–61.

40. Kanbay M, Aydogan T, Bozalan R, et al. A rare but serious side effect of levofloxacin: hypoglycemia in a geriatric patient. Diabetes Care 2006;29:1716–7.

41. Yanai-Kopelman D, Paz A, Rippel D, Potasman I. Inflammatory bowel disease in returning travelers. J Travel Med 2000;7:333–5.

42. Boggild AK, Sano M, Humar A, et al. Travel patterns and risk behavior in solid organ transplant recipients. J Travel Med 2004;11:37–43.

43. Philip M, Ginsburg, Paul J. Thuluvath. Diarrhea in liver transplant recipients: etiology and management. Liver Transpl 2005;11:881–90.

CHAPTER 12

DIARRHEA IN EXPATRIATES

DAVID R. SHLIM, MD

PRATIVA PANDEY, MD

Introduction

Expatriates face the same issues as all travelers in terms of the risk of traveler's diarrhea (TD), with the additional concerns of confronting a constant risk of TD over time, and determining whether immunity eventually plays a role in decreasing either the frequency or severity of diarrhea.

The term "expatriate," for the purposes of this chapter, is meant to include any person from a developed country who takes up residence in a developing country. Expatriates live differently within a foreign country than most short-term travelers. They usually have their own homes and kitchens and are exposed to restaurant food less often. However, because some expatriates may have official roles, either as diplomats, aid workers, or business people, they may be required to eat out more often at official functions, and in local homes.

Few studies have focused on the etiology and risk factors for diarrhea in expatriates, but the studies that have been done, especially in Nepal, have shed some light on the issues mentioned above.

The Risk of Diarrhea in Expatriates

Most studies of the incidence of TD are done on populations of short-term travelers.[1] Thus, we obtain a glimpse of the risk of TD in a limited period of time, usually 2 weeks or less. Since the incidence of TD in these studies is often 30 to 70%, one could calculate very high annual rates of TD if this incidence was consistent.[2] If a traveler runs a 30% risk of TD in a 2-week period, this would predict an annual incidence of 7 episodes per person per year.

A 2-year study of 36 Peace Corps volunteers in Guatemala found that the incidence of diarrhea was 4.7 episodes of diarrhea per person per year, but that the risk decreased over the 2-year period. The rate was 6.1 for the first 6-month period, but had dropped to 3.6 by the start of the second year in country.[2]

In Nepal, the rate of diarrhea was addressed in two ways. In one study, 70 expatriates were approached, outside of the clinic setting, who had resided in Nepal between 2 and 23 months (median 10 months). Forty-nine percent recalled having an episode of diarrhea in the past month, and 74% recalled having diarrhea in the past 3 months. This latter figure would predict an annual incidence of 3 episodes of diarrhea per person per year.[3]

In the second Nepal study, a cohort of 77 expatriates in Kathmandu, who had moved to Nepal within the past year, were recruited. They were asked to submit a stool sample every time they had a new episode of TD, and they were contacted by telephone every 2 weeks to see if an episode had been missed. Using the conservative numerator of episodes for which stool samples were actually obtained, the annual incidence of TD in this cohort was 3.3 episodes per person per year.[4]

The figure of 3.3 episodes of diarrhea per person per year is remarkably comparable to most studies that have been done on children under the age of 5 years in developing countries, including Nepal, where the annual incidence is 4.2 episodes of diarrhea per child per year.[5] This means that despite pretravel counseling and the efforts that almost all expatriates make to avoid drinking tap water and eating unwashed vegetables, the annual rate of diarrhea is no different than a child born in that same country.

Etiology of Diarrhea in Expatriates

The etiology of TD in multiple studies of travelers around the world has been remarkably consistent.[2] Enterotoxigenic *E coli* (ETEC) is always the most frequently isolated pathogen (17 to 70%), followed by *Campylobacter* spp (1 to 39%) and *Shigella* spp (0 to 30%).[2] Additional pathogens found include *Salmonella* spp (1 to 33%), and a handful of other bacterial pathogens that are usually found in less than 5% of samples. Intestinal viral pathogens are usually found in less than 8% of samples.[6] Protozoal pathogens are relatively uncommon in short-term travelers with diarrhea.

In longitudinal studies of expatriates, the order in which bacterial pathogens are acquired does not appear to be random. ETEC is usually the first pathogen to be acquired, and the incidence drops off dramatically after the first year. In a study of American Embassy personnel in Egypt, ETEC was rarely detected in longer-term expatriates.[7] This was also true for a cohort of US citizens residing in Lima, Peru.[8] In Nepal, the risk of ETEC infection was double in the first 2 months of residence compared to the next 3 months.[9] The risk of *Shigella* and *Campylobacter* infections remained stable over a 1-year period in Nepal, but in Thailand, the risk of *Campylobacter* decreased in a population of expatriates in their second year.[10,11]

Protozoal pathogens become more important with continual exposure over time. In a Peace Corps study in Guatemala, the median length of time in the country until infection by the first protozoal pathogen was over 8 months.[11] Overall, *G. lamblia* was found in 12% of Peace Corps volunteers, and *Entamoeba histolytica* or *E. dispar* was found in about 5% of volunteers. In a study of protozoal pathogens among 251 expatriates followed for a year in Bangladesh, the incidence of *G. lamblia* was 11.8%, and the incidence of *E. histolytica* or *E. dispar* was 8.6%.[12] These figures are similar to *G. lamblia* and *E. histolytica* or *E. dispar* infection rates among expatriates in Nepal.[13]

A pathogen that still causes consternation when found in the stool is *Blastocystis hominis.* This organism has been studied for over 80 years, but it is still unresolved as to whether it is pathogenic. The organism is commonly found in Nepal. In a case-control study among 301 foreigners in Nepal, *B. hominis* was found in 30% of 189 diarrhea cases and in 36% of 112 asymptomatic controls.[14] There was no significant difference between the numbers of *B. hominis* found in the stools of case subjects and control subjects, when *B. hominis* was the only pathogen found in the stools. In addition, the presence of *B. hominis* in the stool exam of the diarrhea cases did not make it less likely that another pathogen would be found in the same stool. Efforts to eradicate *B. hominis* have not lead to conclusive results. The patient may become asymptomatic while *B. hominis* persists in the stool, or *B. hominis* might be eliminated with no clinical improvement in the patient. It appears to be safe to ignore *B. hominis* as a pathogen, and continue to look for and treat other causes of diarrhea when *B. hominis* is present in the stool exam.

Cryptosporidium is a rare pathogen among expatriates in Nepal, with fewer than five cases per year. This finding is consistent with other studies of diarrhea in travelers.[2] Unlike *C. cayetanensis*, there was no seasonal pattern to the few *Cryptosporidium* infections in Nepal.

One final pathogen that occasionally causes persistent low-grade diarrhea in expatriates is *Dientamoeba fragilis.* This organism is actually a flagellate without flagellae, and can be mistaken on the stool exam for an amebic trophozoite. The symptoms associated with *D. fragilis* tend to consist of low-grade, intermittent loose stools, with mildly increased gas, and mild fatigue. Treatment with 250 mg tetracycline qid for 10 days results in resolution of these symptoms and eradication of the organism.

Helminths

Intestinal helminths rarely cause any symptoms in expatriates, although there is widespread awareness and concern about infestations. The passage of a visible adult worm often causes great consternation. Some expatriates regularly "de-worm" themselves and their families every 6 to 12 months with mebendazole. A study in Peace Corps volunteers in Nepal found that only 4% of stool exams were positive for any of three helminths. Cumulatively, however, 19% of volunteers became infested with a helminth during their 2-year tour of duty.[15]

The three main types of worms that are found most often in expatriates are the roundworm, *Ascaris lumbricoides*, the whipworm, *Trichuris trichiura*, and the hookworms, *Necator americanus* and *Ancylostoma duodenale.* None of these species are capable of reproducing within the intestinal tract, so the load of expatriate infection is generally extremely small. Worm eggs, when found, are usually an incidental finding during a stool exam for an acute diarrheal episode. Treatment with mebendazole or albendazole is then appropriate. The beef and pork tapeworms, *Taenia saginata* and *Taenia solium*, are very rare in expatriates in Nepal, but are occasionally found. Found slightly more often than the pork and beef tapeworms is the dwarf tapeworm, *Hymenolepsis nana.* None of the tapeworms appeared to cause any distress in the expatriates we treated. *Taenia solium* pose a risk of cysticercosis, so infection with either tapeworm (the species cannot be differentiated at the egg level) should be treated promptly.

Rarely, expatriates become infected with *Strongyloides stercoralis*, which can complete its life cycle within the intestine, and lead to persistent infections that can last indefinitely.[16] In addition, when the host becomes immunocompromised for some season, the worms can migrate out of the intestine, causing severe problems. Unlike the other intestinal helminths, *Strongyloides* can occasionally present with low-grade symptoms. In routine blood screening, *Strongyloides* is the one worm out of the group mentioned here that should be considered when eosinophilia is noted.

Risk Factors for Diarrhea in Expatriates

The traditionally listed risk factors for acquiring diarrhea in developing countries have always included uncooked vegetables, unpeeled fruits, and untreated water.[17] However, epidemiologic evidence is lacking over the fact that travelers who make greater efforts to avoid eating contaminated foods are protected from TD. [18] There are a number of studies that noted an increased risk of diarrhea based on the locale where food is obtained. [19,20] In all of these studies, the risk of diarrhea is least in one's own home, greater in restaurants, and greatest in food stalls on the street. In a study in Kathmandu, eating in a restaurant just four times in the week prior to coming to the clinic significantly predicted that the person would enter the study as a diarrhea patient, rather than a control.[4]

Younger expatriates were more likely to present with TD than older expatriates in the Nepal case-control study, and the length of time that one had resided in Nepal was inversely proportional to the risk of diarrhea (Table 1).

Expatriates have control over their home kitchen environments, and can take measures to safeguard their food chain. Foods sold in markets in developing countries are likely to be contaminated with potential enteropathogens, but proper handling in the expatriate kitchen can minimize the risk.[23] Water can be boiled and stored for drinking in clean dispensers. Counters and utensils can be regularly cleaned, and staff can be taught the need for hand-washing. Vegetables and fruits can be disinfected by soaking in iodine solutions. When these rules are followed, illness acquired at home is uncommon. In addition to being able to afford refrigerators and freezers, expatriates can often afford back-up generators or battery systems to supply power during inevitable power cuts.

However, expatriates will always want to eat out in restaurants, both for the chance to eat local and varied cuisine, and to fulfill social obligations. In addition, expatriates may be invited to attend local feasts and celebrations, which may be particularly high risk for diarrhea. Rather than urge expatriates to avoid these activities, it is important to make sure that they have a method for diagnosing and treating diarrheal illness when it occurs.

Diagnosis and Treatment of Expatriate Diarrhea

The risk of acquiring TD in an expatriate may exceed 100% in the first months of their stay. Thus, there will always be a need to be able to diagnose and treat inevitable illness. If a reliable expatriate clinic is available, then the person can obtain reliable stool examination and advice, and eventually develop the skills of self-diagnosis and treatment in the country. If there is only local medical care available, the quality and availability of the care will vary widely, both between countries and within the same country. Some aid workers work in remote, inaccessible areas, while others are in the capital cities.

Local medical care has not proven itself to be reliable in most countries for the diagnosis and treatment of TD. The local laboratories have a tendency to both mis-diagnose and overdiagnose protozoal pathogens. The treatment approach tends toward a shotgun rather than a pistol, with multiple medications prescribed for a single episode. For these reasons, many expatriates may have better results with self-diagnosis and treatment.

In order for self-diagnosis and treatment to be effective, the main etiology of the diarrhea should be

Table 1 Risk Factors for Expatriate Diarrhea from a Case-Control Study in Nepal

Risk Factor	Resident Cases (n=69)	Resident Controls (n=87)	p-Value
Drank untreated water	9%	9%	NS
Ate unpeeled fruit	39%	37%	NS
Ate raw vegetables	38%	32%	NS
Took ice in drink	9%	12%	NS
Ate at least one meal in restaurant during week	96%	83%	.013
Ate quiche or lasagna	22%	7%	.007
Drank blended fruit and yogurt drink	32%	9%	.004
Median age in years (IQR)	33 (27–43)	40 (32–46)	.003
Mean duration living in Nepal in months (IQR)	9 (4.5–19.5)	23 (8–67)	$<.0001$

NS, not significant; IQR, interquartile range.

known, there should be a definable clinical syndrome, and treatment should be simple to apply. In the case of TD, the etiology is almost 80% bacterial. The clinical syndrome associated with bacterial diarrhea can be defined as "the sudden onset of relatively uncomfortable diarrhea." This is in contrast to protozoal diarrhea, which is usually more gradual in onset and not as severe. The treatment of most bacterial pathogens is a fluoroquinolone antibiotic for 1 to 2 days. In areas where resistance to fluoroquinolones is known to be higher than usual, azithromycin can be used.[21]

By using an antibiotic to treat episodes of diarrhea that have acute onset and are relatively uncomfortable, most expatriates will be able to manage most of their diarrheal episodes at home. If the symptoms are less severe, but more persistent, then a protozoal pathogen can be suspected. The use of tinidazole, available in most countries, and now available in the United States through selected pharmacies, simplifies the empiric treatment of suspected *G. lamblia* or *E. histolytica* infections. If the person's symptoms consist of a gradual onset of four to five loose stools per day with increased intestinal "churning," and gas, along with mild to moderate fatigue, then *G. lamblia* infections can be suspected. If the symptoms consist of bouts of crampy diarrhea for 1 day interspersed with 1 to 2 days of no diarrhea, along with fatigue and gradual weight loss, then an *E. histolytica* infection can be suspected.

If a reliable medical resource is available, the expatriate can seek medical evaluation before treatment. But if the person is living in a remote area, or in a country where reliable medical care is not available, then there is a role for empiric self-treatment. Treatment will either cure the problem or it will not. Complications from failed empiric treatment are extremely rare. If the problem is not cured, then further evaluation is warranted.

In Nepal, Haiti, Peru, and Guatemala, *C. cayetanensis* has been shown to be a recurrent, seasonal risk.[22] The symptoms of *C. cayetanensis* are distinctive. The onset of diarrhea is sudden, and often severe, with multiple crampy watery stools. Fever is present during the first 1 to 3 days of onset in 30% of patients.[23] This initial severe bout of diarrhea subsides spontaneously, evolving into a syndrome of intermittent diarrhea, nausea, and persistent fatigue and anorexia. Untreated, the mean length of illness is 6 weeks, with a range of 2 to 12 weeks.[27] The organism is effectively treated with cotrimoxazole, double-strength, bid for 7 days.[24] For patients who may be allergic to a component of cotrimoxazole, there is no reliable alternative. Many other drugs have been tried unsuccessfully.[25] The report of success using ciprofloxacin against *C. cayetanensis* in patients in Haiti has not been replicated in Nepal (Prativa Pandey, MD, personal communication).[29]

For the expatriate with persistent diarrhea, fatigue, and weight loss, who does not respond to empiric treatment, the person should be evaluated for malabsorption. Tropical sprue is an illness that is characterized by gradual damage to the upper intestinal mucosa, leading to malabsorption with consequent diarrhea and weight loss. The nonmetabolizable sugar D-xylose, is readily absorbed by a functioning intestinal mucosa. The D-xylose absorption test can be used to determine intestinal integrity. A decrease in absorption suggests the possibility of tropical sprue. If biopsy is not readily available, a trial of treatment can be undertaken with tetracycline and folic acid. A simplified schedule of 500 mg tetracycline twice a day (instead of 250 mg qid) can be used. Folic acid is given as 5 mg twice a day. The response to treatment is dramatic—the person begins to improve within days. Treatment is then continued for 6 weeks, as shorter treatments have been associated with relapse.

One of the key points in evaluating someone with a complaint of persistent diarrhea is to get a detailed history. Often, patients will connect a series of isolated episodes of diarrhea into one long illness. A patient may present with a chief complaint of diarrhea for 1 month. The history might be as follows: "I had diarrhea for 2 days, 4 weeks ago. I got better, but then it recurred 10 days later. I took some antibiotics, and felt better for 2 weeks, but it came back last night." Acute episodes of diarrhea that resolve for at least 5 days do not usually recur. The patient in the example has experienced three unrelated episodes of diarrhea, not persistent diarrhea for a month. The doctor can focus on the episode that began the night before.

It should be noted that many expatriates living in high-risk countries for TD will not have completely normal stools during the majority of their overseas stay. Repeated insults to the intestine may alter the functioning for an extended period of time, leading to looser than normal stools, floating stools, or increased gas. If the person is otherwise functioning well, without fatigue or weight loss, it is not usually fruitful to pursue these symptoms. Reassurance has worked well for this patient population in Nepal.

It should also be borne in mind, however, that expatriates often spend their entire working career in developing countries. As they age, they are also susceptible to noninfectious related diseases, such as colon cancer, or the development of celiac sprue. The treating physician needs to exercise judgment as to when to continue the work-up for weight loss and fatigue beyond the investigation for enteric pathogens. For example, blood in the stool unassociated with acute dysentery symptoms should always be investigated for cancer, using the same criteria that one would for a patient who was not overseas.

Antibiotic Resistance

The issue of antibiotic resistance among enteric pathogens may ultimately be more important to long-term expatriates. From a practical point of view, if the bacteria are becoming resistant over time, empiric antibiotic therapy may need to be changed to achieve the same results.[26] Resistance to cotrimoxazole, once the drug of choice for TD, is now greater than 90% among *Shigella* strains in Thailand. [27] *Campylobacter* isolates went from zero resistance to ciprofloxacin before 1991 to 84% resistant in 1995. Fifteen percent of ETEC isolates were resistant to azithromycin by 1995.[32] Even protozoal pathogens are beginning to show resistance to long available treatments, with several case reports of giardiasis resistant to both metronidazole and albendazole.[28.29]

Expatriates living and working in remote areas may only infrequently seek prophylactic medical advice, unlike tourists who may see a travel health practitioner prior to each trip. Thus, expatriates may continue to rely on older antibiotics out of habit.

The use by expatriates of antibiotics to treat enteric pathogens probably does not help induce resistance in the pathogens. Expatriates comprise tiny proportions of the population in a developing country, and could not be expected to change the available bacterial pool for that country. Only when the antibiotics used to treat enteropathogens are in widespread use within a given country does antibiotic resistance become problematic.

Seasonality of Diarrhea Risk

The risk of diarrhea is not consistent throughout the calendar year in many developing countries in which seasonality has been studied. The highest-risk time of year is usually the dry season, right before the monsoon rains in Asian countries. The dry season was also associated with higher diarrhea risk among expatriates in Ethiopia.[30]

In Nepal, the seasonal difference in risk is striking, with a doubling of risk in the second quarter of the year, April to June.[4] This increased risk of enteric pathogens in the spring was also true for *Salmonella typhi*, *Salmonella paratyphi*, and hepatitis A infections. Thus, some expatriates who move to Nepal in September or October will have relatively few incidents of diarrhea until the following spring. The hot, dry seasons in several countries, including Nepal, coincide with the time of maximum fly populations. The role of flies as vectors of diarrheal disease is recently being re-evaluated. [31,32] Efforts to exclude flies from kitchen environments may be an effective way to decrease diarrheal disease during the high-risk season.

The coccidian pathogen *C. cayetanensis* is the only pathogen in Nepal (besides *Vibrio cholerae*, which has not proven to be a risk for expatriates) that disappears completely from the environment for several months a year. [33] The risk of *C. cayetanensis* begins in late April, peaks in mid-June through mid-July, and then drops off rapidly, with the last few cases usually diagnosed in October or November. The risk of *C. cayetanensis*, however, for newly arrived expatriates, was highly significant, outstripping the risk of ETEC in the months in which *C. cayetanensis* was prevalent. Overall, 32% of the expatriate cohort studied in Nepal had a *C. cayetanensis* infection in their first year, surpassed only by ETEC (at 42%), which has a year-round risk.[5]

Evidence for Immunity in Expatriates

One of the worst events in the life of an expatriate is the sudden onset of severe gastrointestinal symptoms, including fever, vomiting, abdominal cramps, and profuse watery diarrhea. The symptoms can be so uncontrollable that patients may have to sit on a toilet for hours, vomiting into a waste basket, wracked by abdominal cramps, shaking with fever, and growing faint with dehydration.

It became evident, after a number of years working in Nepal, that longer-term residents were no longer at risk for such severe bouts of gastroenteritis. The correlation of decreased risk of severe symptoms with a longer stay in the country suggests that partial immunity is playing a role.

Antibodies are known to be generated by diarrheal pathogens.[38-40] The questions that are unanswered are how quickly one begins to show a protective effect of immunity, how long the protection may last, and how much cross-protection there may be between serotypes of the same organism.

The Peace Corps study in Guatemala demonstrated that the incidence of diarrhea was highest in the first 6-month period (6.1 episodes of diarrhea per person), less in the second 6-month period (5.2 episodes of diarrhea per person), and then stabilized at 3.6 episodes of diarrhea per person.[3] Haneveld reported that the annual rates for diarrhea in US troops in the Mediterranean area, from 1942 to 1945, declined from a high of 196 per 1,000 to 79 per 1,000 in the fourth year. [34] ETEC infections were much less common in a cohort of American expatriates who lived in Lima, Peru.[10]

A study in Mexico calculated the odds ratio (OR) of diarrhea for students who had been living in Mexico for a year or longer, compared to newly arriving students, to be 0.37 (95% CI 0.18 to 0.77).[35] For expatriates who had lived in Nepal for at least 1 year, the OR for their risk of diarrhea was nearly identical at 0.36 (95% CI, 0.18 to 0.74).[5]

Figure 1 shows the likely influence of immunity on the OR of appearing as a diarrhea case at a clinic in Kathmandu during a case-control study. Expatriates who presented to the clinic with diarrhea were enrolled as cases and compared to patients who presented to the clinic with a complaint other than diarrhea (and had not had diarrhea for at least 2 weeks). The graph shows the decreasing likelihood of enrolling a person as a case the longer that they had lived in Nepal, a decrease that continued to be evident for up to 6 years of residence.[4] In practice, expatriates become less fearful about diarrhea and appear to suffer less severe consequences over a residence period of several years. Although not clear, there may be evidence that expatriates who move between developing countries may not bring all of their immunity with them and therefore be at risk of infection in the country they move to. Someone who moves to Nepal after several years in Kenya, for example, may be exposed to specific serotypes and strains that were not circulating in Kenya. In addition, they may face specific pathogens, like *C. cayetanensis*, that were not a risk in their previous posting.

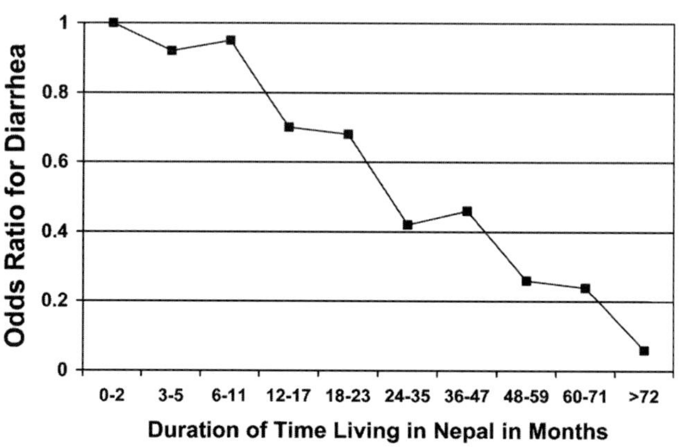

Figure 1 Decrease in odds ratio for diarrhea (relative to baseline) for increasing duration of time living in Nepal among 69 expatriate residents with diarrhea compared with 87 asymptomatic expatriate resident controls.

Summary

Expatriates, unlike short-term tourists, face a continued risk of diarrheal disease over a prolonged period of time. The risk may vary seasonally. Maintaining a clean home kitchen environment may be one of the best protective measures against TD. Restaurant eating is the main risk factor for diarrhea in expatriates. Since diarrhea appears to be unavoidable, despite the best efforts of the expatriate, a strategy for diagnosis and treatment needs to be available, whether this entails access to adequate medical care, or self-diagnosis and treatment. Immunity does occur, but is acquired slowly with continuous exposure. One of the major benefits of immunity is decreased severity of disease when it does occur.

References

1. Peltola H, Gorbach SL. Travelers' diarrhea: epidemiology and clinical aspects. In: DuPont HL, Steffen R, editors. Textbook of travel medicine and health, 2nd ed. Hamilton (ON): BC Decker Inc.; 2001.
2. Herwaldt BL, de Arroyave KR, Roberts JM, Juranek DD. A multiyear prospective study of the risk factors for and incidence of diarrheal illness in a cohort of Peace Corps Volunteers in Guatemala. Ann Intern Med 2000;132:982–8.
3. Hoge CW, Shlim DR, Echeverria P, et al. Epidemiology of diarrhea among expatriate residents living in a highly endemic environment. J Am Med Assoc 1996;275:533–8.
4. Shlim DR, Hoge CW, Rajah R, et al. Persistent high risk of diarrhea among foreigners in Nepal during the first two years of residence. Clin Infect Dis 1999;29:613–6.
5. Ministry of Health. Nepal fertility, family planning, and health survey (NFHS, 1991) 1993. Kathmandu, Nepal: His Majesty's Government, Ministry of Health; 1993.
6. Taylor DN, Houston R, Shlim DR, et al. Etiology of diarrhea among travelers and foreign residents in Nepal. J Am Med Assoc 1988;260:1245–8.
7. Haberberger RL, Lissner CR, Podgore JK, et al. Etiology of acute diarrhea among United States Embassy personnel and dependents in Cairo, Egypt. Am J Trop Med Hyg 1994; 51:870–4.
8. Pazzaglia G, Escamilla J, Batchelor R. The etiology of diarrhea among American adults living in Peru. Military Medicine 1991;156:484–7.
9. Shlim DR. Traveler's diarrhea. Wilderness Environ Med 1999;10:165–70.
10. Gaudio PA, Echeverria P, Hoge CW, et al. Diarrhea among expatriate residents in Thailand: correlation between reduced *Campylobacter* prevalence and longer duration of stay. J Travel Med 1996;3:77–9.
11. Herwaldt BL, de Arroyave KR, Wahlquist SP, et al. Multiyear prospective study of intestinal parasitism in a

cohort of Peace Corps Volunteers in Guatemala. J Clin Microbiol 2001;39:34–42.

12. Speelman P, Ljungstrom I. Protozoal enteric infections among expatriates in Bangladesh. Am J Trop Med Hyg 1986;35:1140–5.
13. Taylor DN, Houston R, Shlim DR, et al. Etiology of diarrhea among travelers and foreign residents in Nepal. J Am Med Assoc 1988;260:1245–8.
14. Shlim DR, Hoge C, Rajah R, et al. Is *Blastocystis hominis* a cause of diarrhea in travelers? A prospective controlled study in Nepal. Clin Infect Dis 1995;21:97–101.
15. Houston R, Schwartz E. Helminithic infections among Peace Corps Volunteers in Nepal. J Am Med Assoc 1990; 263:373–4.
16. Gill GV, Bell DR. *Strongyloides stercoralis* infection in former Far East prisoners of war. Br Med J 1979;12:572–4.
17. Kozicki M, Steffen R, Schar M. "Boil it, cook it, peel it, or forget it": does this rule prevent travellers' diarrhoea? Int J Epidemiol 1985;14:169–72.
18. Steffen R, van der Linde F, Byr K, Schar M. Epidemiology of diarrhea in travelers. J Am Med Assoc 1983;249:1176–80.
19. Tjoa WS, DuPont HL, Sullivan P, et al. Location of food consumption and travelers' diarrhea. Am J Epidemiol 1977; 106:61–6.
20. Ericsson CD, Pickering LK, Sullivan P. The role of location of food consumption in the prevention of travelers' diarrhea in Mexico. Gastroenterology 1980;79:812–6.
21. Kuschner RA, Trofa AF, Thomas RJ, et al. Use of azithromycin for the treatment of *Campylobacter* enteritis in travelers to Thailand, an area where ciprofloxacin resistance is prevalent. Clin Infect Dis 1995;21:536–41.
22. Herwaldt BL. *C. cayetanensis* cayetanensis: a review, focusing on the outbreaks of cyclosporiasis in the 1990s. Clin Infect Dis 2000;31:1040–57.
23. Shlim DR, Cohen MT, Eaton M, et al. An alga-like organism associated with an outbreak of prolonged diarrhea among foreigners in Nepal. Am J Trop Med Hyg 1991;45:383–9.
24. Hoge CW, Shlim DR, Ghimire M, et al. Placebo-controlled trial of co-trimoxazole for the treatment of *C.* cayetanensis, infections among travelers and foreign residents in Nepal. Lancet, 1995;345:691–3.
25. Shlim DR, Pandey P, Rabold JG, et al. An open trial of trimethoprim versus *C. cayetanensis* infections. J Travel Med 1997;4:44–5.
26. Isenbarger DW, Hoge CW, Srijan A, et al. Comparative antibiotic resistance of diarrheal pathogens from Vietnam and Thailand, 1996–1999. Emerg Infect Dis 2002;8:175–80.
27. Hoge CW, Gambel JM, Srijan A, et al. Trends in antibiotic resistance among diarrheal pathogens isolated in Thailand over 15 years. Clin Infect Dis 1998;26:341–5.
28. Nash TE, Ohl CA, Subramanian G, et al. Treatment of patients with refractory giardiasis. Clin Infect Dis 2001;33: 22–8.
29. Abboud P, Lemee V, Gargala G, et al. Successful treatment of metronidazole- and albendazole-resistant giardiasis with nitazoxanide in a patient with acquired immunodeficiency syndrome. Clin Infect Dis 2001;32:1792–4.
30. Brickfield FX, Gebreegzi M, Beyenne A. Incidence of protozoal diarrheal disease in an expatriate community in Addis Ababa. Ethiop Med J 1996;34:107–17.
31. Cohen D, Green M, Block C, et al. Reduction of transmission of shigellosis by control of houseflies (*Musca domestica*). Lancet 1991;337:993–7.
32. Chavasse DC, Shier RP, Murphy OA, et al. Impact of fly control on childhood diarrhoea in Pakistan: community-randomised trial. Lancet 1999;353:22–5.
33. Hoge CW, Shlim DR, Rajah R, et al. The epidemiology of diarrheal illness associated with a coccidian-like organism among travelers and foreign residents in Nepal. Lancet 1993;341:1175–9.
34. Haneveld GT. Some epidemiologic aspects of "travellers' diarrhoea" in Lebanon. Trop Geogr Med 1960;12:339–44.
35. DuPont HL, Haynes GA, Pickering LK, et al. Diarrhea in travelers to Mexico: relative susceptibility of United States and Latin American students attending a Mexican university. Am J Epidemiol 1977;105:37–41.

CHAPTER 13

DIARRHEAL OUTBREAKS ASSOCIATED WITH AIRLINE TRAVEL

ERICA N. JOHNSON, MD

LYNN L. HORVATH, MD

CLAUDE THIBEAULT, MD

Since the first regular passenger air travel began in 1919, air travel has grown into a massive industry, with passenger traffic reaching the two billion mark in 2005.[1,2] As travel becomes more streamlined and new routes are added, the airline industry continues to break down the barriers of time and geography. But with this convenience comes increasing concern and awareness over the risks associated with air travel, including the transmission of infectious diseases.

Any time groups of people are fed at the same time (eg, banquets, picnics, and airline flights), the possibility of food-related illness is real. Unfortunately, airline passengers do not share the commonalities of the banquets and picnic attendees; that is, they are less likely to know each other.[3] This is possibly one of the reasons that reported outbreaks of diarrheal illness associated with airline travel have been limited in number. Since 1947, when the first outbreak was investigated, there have been only 45 diarrheal outbreaks associated with airline travel reported in the literature.[1,4,5] The source is often contaminated food, and the most commonly implicated pathogens are *Salmonella* spp., *Staphylococcus* spp., and *Vibrio* spp.[1] These outbreaks, although few in number, can be potentially devastating if the onset of symptoms occur during a flight, when medical resources may be limited, or if the outbreak affects crew members, especially the cockpit personnel. The duration of flights, particularly international flights, the disparity in sanitation practices in origin and destination countries, and the limited food storage capabilities on aircraft have historically played a role in many of these outbreaks. Additionally, the time between preparation and consumption can sometimes be quite long because of frequent irregular operations (delayed flights) in the airline industry. Other factors include close quarters within the cabin and small restroom facilities that may be difficult to keep sanitized in flight.

Outbreaks on Aircraft

MODES OF TRANSMISSION

There are four routes of infectious disease transmission: airborne, contact, common vehicle, and vector-borne.[4] Of these, contact (including contact with contaminated droplets or infected fomites) and common vehicle (which includes both foodborne and waterborne transmission) are the most likely means of spreading the agents of acute infectious gastroenteritis on an aircraft. While it is clear that contaminated food or water served in flight may result in the rapid dissemination of infection among passengers, the risk of disease associated with contact transmission while traveling in an aircraft cabin is difficult to assess, at best.[4]

Of the 45 outbreaks of gastroenteritis associated with air travel that have been reported (Table 1), a food source was identified (or deemed the most probable means of transmission) in 41 cases. In-flight food service began with the first charter flights between London and Paris in 1919, and has been customary since, resulting in the rapid expansion of the airline catering industry over the years.[1] But this rapid growth magnified the risks associated with improper food handling and storage. Early air travel was particularly susceptible to these outbreaks due to the nature of food catering practices and the limitations of food refrigeration on many aircraft.

IN-FLIGHT CATERING

Many major airlines operate their own flight kitchens at their home airport, but often rely on contracts with other flight kitchens or caterers when away from their hub.[6] On international flights, airlines may use caterers able to provide cuisine with a regional influence. Thus, it is the airline's responsibility to elect caterers whose standards of sanitation and hygiene meet the expectations of the airline itself as well as the aviation industry's standards.

Table 1. Diarrheal Outbreaks Associated with Airline Travel 1947–2006*

No.	Year	Agent	Food Item	No. Infected	Reference
1	1947	*Salmonella typhi*	Sandwiches	4	9
2	1961	*Staphylococcus aureus*	Chicken	13	36
3	1965	*S. aureus*	Turkey	4	37
4	1966	*Salmonella, Staphylococcus*	Chicken	3	37
5	1966	*S. aureus*	Trifle dessert	15	37
6	1967	*Escherichia coli*	Oysters	1	22
7	1967	*Salmonella enteritidis*	Mayonnaise	380	37
8	1969	*Multiple agents*	Unknown	21	1
9	1969	*Multiple agents*	Unknown	24	29, 30
10	1970	*Clostridium perfringens*	Turkey	3	1
11	1971	*Unknown*	Seafood salad	23	38
12	1971	*Shigella sonnei*	Unknown	219	38
13	1971	*S. sonnei*	Seafood cocktail	78	39
14	1972	*Vibrio parahaemolyticus*	Seafood appetizer	9	40
15	1972	*Vibrio cholerae 01*	Appetizer	47	17
16	1973	*V. cholerae non 01*	Appetizer with egg	64	41
17	1973	*S. aureus*	Custard	247	1
18	1973	*Salmonella thompson*	Breakfast	17	1
19	1974	*Clostridium botulinum*	Unknown	15	42
20	1975	*S. aureus*	Ham	196	15
21	1975	*Salmonella oranienburg*	Unknown	23	37
22	1976	*Salmonella typhimurium*	Cold salads	1,800	43
23	1976	*Salmonella brandenburg*	Cold dishes	232	44
24	1976	*S. aureus*	Éclair	28	45
25	1976	*S. typhi*	Tourist class menu	13	1
26	1976	*V. parahaemolyticus*	Unknown	28	46
27	1978	*V. cholerae* non 01	Chicken sandwich	61	46
28	1978	*Salmonella typhimurium*	Unknown	11	42
29	1981	*V. parahaemolyticus*	Unknown	42	42
27	1982	*S. aureus*	Custard	6	1
28	1983	*S. enteritidis*	Swiss steak	12	1
29	1983	*Shigella*	Unknown	42	1
30	1984	*S. enteritidis*	Appetizer	631	1
31	1985	*S. enteritidis*	Mousse	30	47
32	1986	*Salmonella infantis*	Multiple	91	12
33	1988	*S. sonnei*	Cold dish	240	8
34	1989	*S. enteritidis*	Unknown	80	5
35	1990	*Salmonella ohio*	Ham	5	5
36	1991	*Salmonella*	Unknown	415	48
37	1991	*S. aureus*	Chocolate cake	25	49
38	1991	Norovirus	Orange juice	3,053	25
39	1992	*V. cholerae* 01	Seafood salad	80	18
40	1993	Enterotoxigenic *E. coli*	Unknown	56	23
41	1997	*S. enteritidis*	Chocolate éclair	455	5
42	2002	Norovirus	N/A	8	26

*Table adapted in part from Tauxe et al.[1]

In one study reviewing in-flight catering and the occurrence of *Salmonella* in meals served on flights between 1989 and 1992, over 2,000 samples were reviewed from multiple flight kitchens in 29 countries.[7] The samples included both hot and cold food items. *Salmonella* spp. were isolated from six samples from three countries, which represented less than 1% of all samples. Five of the contaminated food samples were hot dishes. Only one dish, the cold food item, was connected to an outbreak of salmonellosis on a flight from Bangkok, Thailand to Helsinki, Finland in 1990. Five passengers became infected with *S. enterica* serovar *Ohio* believed to be associated with the consumption of a ham dish served in flight.[7] The fact that only two airline-associated diarrheal outbreaks have been reported in the past decade may be attributable to the increased use of prepackaged frozen meals and better food-handling practices, decreasing the potential risks of using in-flight catering services, but under-reporting cannot be excluded.[4]

LIMITATIONS OF OUTBREAK INVESTIGATION

Although 45 outbreaks have been documented in the literature, this likely represents only a small number of the cases of true airline-associated transmission of acute infectious gastroenteritis. The recognition of outbreaks depends on a number of factors, including high attack rates, short incubations periods, a group of people knowing each other, and the occurrence of an illness that is likely to be reported to public health officials, thus leading to the initiation of an investigation.[8] Even after an outbreak is suspected, airline and public health officials often have difficulty locating passengers, particularly when multiple flights to more than one country are involved.[1] The investigation requires swift and seamless cooperation among multiple agencies to obtain necessary data such as food samples from the flight kitchen and biologic specimens from affected passengers.[1] If the reported exposures of passengers are similar and a great number of passengers report symptoms consistent with gastroenteritis, it becomes quite difficult to implicate a single food item as the vector for transmission.[1]

Review of Outbreaks by Pathogen

SALMONELLA

Salmonella has been implicated in the most outbreaks connected with airline travel, with sixteen reported outbreaks since 1947. It is estimated that over 4,000 people have been affected, including seven fatalities.[1,4,5] A food item served onboard was the source of the outbreak in the majority of these cases.

The earliest reported outbreak occurred in 1947, in which four passengers became ill after eating sandwiches onboard a flight; *Salmonella typhi* was later identified as the causative agent.[1,9]

The largest reported outbreak of *Salmonella* infection on a commercial airline occurred in February 1976 on a series of flights to various European cities. At least 1,800 of the nearly 2,500 passengers on these flights developed symptoms of gastroenteritis and six later died; mayonnaise infected with *Salmonella enterica* serovar *Typhimurium* that originated in a kitchen in Las Palmas, Spain and was served on at least 11 flights was identified as the source of the outbreak.[10]

Another large outbreak occurred in 1984, when 631 people worldwide (including 11 US cities) developed a diarrheal illness following travel on one of 29 flights originating in London. An epidemiologic investigation into the outbreak led to the identification of *S. enterica* serovar *Enteritidis* in stool specimens of affected individuals. Although a single food item was never linked to the outbreak, *Salmonella* was isolated from seafood cocktails prepared in the kitchen that serviced each of the 29 flights. [1] Another report of that incident showed that although the introduction of the causative agent (*Salmonella*) into the food chain proved to be a key factor, the scale of the outbreak was the result of an interaction of other factors.[11]

One outbreak in Finland affected multiple aspects of the transportation industry.[12] In 1986, 91 airline passengers, 107 railway passengers, and 28 food service employees developed symptoms of gastroenteritis; stool samples isolated *S. enterica* serovar *Infantis*. The outbreak was later traced to the food establishment kitchen that serviced both the airline and the train company. The epidemiologic investigation could not conclusively link the outbreak to a symptom-free *S. infantis* carrier who likely acquired the infection during any of a series of outbreaks of *Salmonella* in Finland in 1986.

There has not been a reported outbreak of *Salmonella* on an aircraft since 1997. This is likely related to improved food handling by airline catering industry. Better surveillance by the regulators may also be another factor; for instance, a routine inspection (microbiological sampling) by the US Department of Agriculture in 2003 led to the recall of a salad contaminated by *Salmonella*. This salad was normally used by a major airline caterer. It is therefore quite possible that an outbreak was avoided.[13]

STAPHYLOCOCCUS AUREUS

Staphylococcal food poisoning is the second most common reported cause of outbreaks of gastroenteritis associated with airline travel, with a total nine outbreaks reported. The largest occurred in 1973, when *S. aureus* was found in a custard dessert served to passengers on three flights originating in Italy with stops in Lisbon, Portugal before arrival in the US. 247 of the 440 passengers on these flights reported symptoms, and analysis of patient samples matched the *S. aureus* found in the dessert.[1,5,14]

The second largest outbreak occurred 2 years later in 1975.[15,16] 196 of the 343 passengers and one crew member on a single flight from Tokyo, Japan to Copenhagen, Denmark developed gastroenteritis, with diarrhea and vomiting, within hours of reaching the flight's destination. 143 victims required hospitalization, although all recovered. *S. aureus* and enterotoxin was found in leftover ham served on the flight. Phage-typing analysis matched that of stool and vomitus specimens of ill passengers. *S. aureus* of an identical phage-type was also isolated from hand lesions found on one of the cooks in the catering kitchen in Anchorage, Alaska that serviced the flight. This cook was directly involved in the preparation of the ham and was considered the source of the outbreak. The investigation also revealed that the ham had been stored at room temperature for 6 hours, refrigerated overnight, then kept at room temperature again for 8 hours while in-flight, conditions which allow more than enough time for *S. aureus* to grow and produce enterotoxin.

VIBRIO

Four outbreaks of *Vibrio cholerae* and three outbreaks of *Vibrio parahaemolyticus* connected to airline travel have been reported. In 1972, 47 passengers on two airline flights between London and Sydney, with stops in Bahrain and Singapore, were affected by an outbreak of *V. cholerae* O1 (El Tor, serotype Inaba) attributed to contaminated food served during the flight.[17] Bahrain was experiencing a cholera epidemic at the time. During the epidemiological investigation that followed, a food item from a hors d'oeuvres tray was identified as the most likely source of the outbreak. These trays were prepared in a flight kitchen in Bahrain by food service employees, of whom two were found to be asymptomatic carriers of the same strain of cholera found in fecal samples of affected passengers. It is theorized that the food was contaminated during preparation, although there was no direct evidence of this.

Air travel during the outbreak of epidemic cholera in Latin America that began in January 1991 permitted the spread of cholera to other countries including the United States. The Centers for Disease Control and Prevention began to receive reports from the Los Angeles County Health Department in early 1992 of *V. cholerae* O1 isolated from stool specimens of several patients with diarrhea.[18,19] These patients all traveled on the same airline flight, which originated in Buenos Aires, Argentina and stopped in Lima, Peru before reaching its destination in Los Angeles. Overall, 80 people were affected, including one who died; infection was strongly associated with a cold seafood salad served during the flight between Lima and Los Angeles, although the exact mechanism of contamination was never identified.[20]

SHIGELLA

There have been four reported outbreaks of *Shigella* infection associated with airline flights. The earliest was in 1971, involving flights from the Canary Islands to Sweden. Seafood cocktail contaminated with *Shigella sonnei* served during the flight was associated with the development of diarrhea in 19 passengers.[5]

The most widely investigated *Shigella* outbreak tied with air travel was a 1988 outbreak of *Shigella sonnei* infection among 21 players and staff of a Minnesota football team several days following an airline flight from Miami, FL to Minneapolis, MN.[8] This incident reinforces the notion that outbreak recognition is much more likely if it involves a group of people who know each other. Further investigation identified a total of 240 cases of probable or confirmed Shigellosis internationally, associated with 219 flights. A single flight kitchen serviced these flights, between September and October 2002, and development of illness was strongly associated with the consumption of cold food items prepared in this kitchen and served on the flights. An identical strain of *S. sonnei* was isolated from fecal samples provided by ill team members and other passengers. Two food handlers working in the kitchen preparing cold food items at the time of the outbreak had elevated IgG antibody titers to *S. sonnei* lipopolysaccharide. Although an identical strain of *S. sonnei* was never isolated from remaining food samples served by the kitchen, it was hypothesized that contamination of the food occurred during preparation by asymptomatic carriers working in the kitchen.

Another suspected incident of *Shigella* contamination that was never published in the scientific literature involved a major airline caterer in 2004. A state epidemiologist narrowed the likely source to carrots contained in salads. A warning letter to the airline caterer as a result of an inspection in early 2005 revealed so many gross violations that it would not be surprising that food poisoning had resulted from such a situation.[21] This incident also emphasizes the need for routine inspection.

ESCHERICHIA COLI

There have been only two airline outbreaks attributed to *E. coli*. In the first, oysters contaminated with *E. coli* caused symptoms of diarrhea in 23 crewmembers on a single flight in 1967.[1,22] It is not clear from the investigation performed at the time if other pathogens may have been involved. In 1993, 56 passengers on multiple flights developed gastroenteritis associated with consuming a salad contaminated with enterotoxigenic *E. coli*.[23]

NOROVIRUS

Although norovirus transmission has been well documented on other types of transportation,[24] there have only been two reported cases of probable norovirus infection transmitted in flight. The first and largest occurred in 1991, when over 3,000 passengers on several flights originating in Melbourne, Australia developed gastroenteritis with norovirus later detected from stool samples provided by some of the ill passengers.[25] During the investigation that followed, the risk of infection was highest (nearly 100%) among those who consumed orange juice provided in flight, although norovirus was never detected from juice samples. The orange juice was produced from a single supplier but served from multiple kitchens.

The second case of norovirus transmission occurred on an 8-hour flight from Philadelphia, Pennsylvania to London, England in 2002.[26] An investigation was started when 8 of 14 crew members developed gastroenteritis after the plane reached its destination in London. Norovirus was identified via reverse transcriptase PCR in the stool samples of the ill crew members. This led to further investigation into the in-flight exposures and occurrence of symptoms consistent with gastroenteritis among passengers. Overall, there were five passengers identified during the investigation who met the case definition for probable norovirus. Frequency of bathroom visits was the only statistically significant risk exposure. Unlike the other outbreaks, no food item was implicated, which is not surprising due to the high transmissibility of norovirus via airborne and waterborne droplets.[26]

Other Pathogens

Several other enteric pathogens have also been implicated in outbreaks of diarrheal illness on commercial airlines. These pathogens include *Clostridium perfringens* and *Plesiomonas shigelloides*.[1,5] The flight affected by contamination of a hot food item containing turkey with *C. perfringens* was notable in that 22 of 62 crewmembers were affected, compared with only 3 passengers.[27,28] Plesiomonas shigelloides was actually one of multiple pathogens including several *Salmonella* serotypes and noncholera *Vibrio* isolated from fecal specimens during an outbreak of gastroenteritis among two American charter flights to Asia in 1969.[29,30]

To date, there have been no reported outbreaks of Hepatitis A virus associated with food served during an airline flight.

Airline Safety Practices to Reduce Transmission

Multiple government agencies regulate catering companies within the United States that service the airline industry. These include the United States Drug Administration, Environmental Protection agency, the Food and Drug Administration (FDA), and state boards of health. In particular, the FDA, through its Interstate Travel Sanitation Program is given authority to enforce Title 21 of the Code of Federal Regulations (CFR), parts 1,240 and 1,250, which address food safety and control of infectious disease transmission on airlines, respectively. These regulations offer general guidance on food preparation and storage as well as the proper sanitation of lavatory facilities. Airline catering firms must conform to these regulations as well as those outlined in the FDA Food Service Sanitation Manual. Domestic firms are also subject to routine inspections by the FDA, in accordance with these regulations.[31]

These regulations apply only to US airlines and do not apply to other international airlines at this time. Many countries do follow similar regulations, but there is no means for universal enforcement.

There are also no international regulations for airline catering companies. However, the World Health Organization (WHO) has published a very comprehensive "Guide to hygiene and sanitation in aviation" that covers all aspects of airline catering.[32] Even though this book was published in 1977, most of the information is still appropriate. Unfortunately, the guide is out of print, but the WHO has plans to publish an updated version in the near future, as it is needed for the new International Health Regulations (IHR) that will come into effect in June 2007.

Because outbreaks of diarrheal illness can have such a major impact on airline operations, from a business as well as a safety standpoint, many airlines have taken a very proactive approach.[11] Although there are no statutory or policy requirements for the pilot and the copilot to consume different meals or the same meal at different times, a large number of airlines have procedures requiring the flight crew to eat different meals before and during the flight to prevent simultaneous incapacitation.[3] Furthermore, the International Air Transport Association (IATA) has recently created an IATA International Catering Quality Assurance Program (ICQA).[33] The ICQA is partly based on the HACCP

(Hazard Analysis and Critical Control Point) concept. Although the HACCP concept has been developed many years ago and is very sound, it needs to be integrated into a program with clearly defined, applicable and measurable standards to make a difference such as been instituted with ICQA. The program is offered to airline companies as a third party audit for their current or future caterer. Although the program is voluntary, several airlines are already participating and many more are expected to follow suit. It has been proposed that participation in this program should be mandatory for all IATA members. The IATA has also innovated self-regulation with its IATA Operation Safety Audit. Since regulations in the international arena are very difficult to enforce and frequently nonexistent, self regulation is the most commercially viable alternative and airlines are moving proactively in that direction.

Reporting Suspected Outbreaks

Under title 21 of the CFR, part 1240.45, US airlines are required to report any suspected case of infectious disease to the local health authority as soon as possible, to follow the agency's guidance in efforts to contain the outbreak, and to cooperate with the epidemiological investigation.[31] As above, these regulations only apply to US airlines and though many countries do follow similar regulations, there is no means for universal enforcement.

A WHO working group is currently developing procedures for the IHR that will come into effect in June 2007. One of the procedures will require the aircraft captain to radio ahead to the destination if there is a suspected case of a communicable disease onboard so that the public health authorities can be notified before the arrival of the aircraft. This procedure will also be matched by the requirements of the International Civil Aviation Organization Annex 9. In 2005, the IATA had already developed guidelines for cabin crew for suspected cases of a communicable disease.[33] Furthermore, several airlines now have specific protocols for suspected cases of food poisoning so that evidence can be appropriately collected. As with everything else in life, the risk of food poisoning will never be zero; however, important steps are being taken to bring the risk to as low a level as possible, and at least to a much lower level than the average traveler is willing to accept at many travel destinations.

Advice to Travelers

In general, the risk of diarrheal illness associated with airline travel is likely significantly lower than the risk of diarrheal illness in a high-risk travel destination. Risk has been further reduced as many airlines have decreased food service on shorter domestic flights to prepackaged snacks with long shelf lives and no temperature requirements for storage. However, on longer flights, particularly international flights, where several meals and snacks may be served, it would be prudent to advise patients to follow the same practices as they would in the destination country, especially because the airline may rely on local catering services. This means that the adage "boil it, cook it, peel it, or forget it" would generally apply to meals served in flight.[34] This is particularly true for travel to higher-risk areas where the most stringent food hygiene practices and safe water sources are not as readily applied or available.[35]

The opinions or assertions contained herein are the private views of the authors and are not to be construed as official or reflecting the views of the Department of Defense or the government.

References

1. Tauxe RV, Tormey MP, Mascola L, et al. Salmonellosis outbreak on transatlantic flights; foodborne illness on aircraft: 1947–1984. Am J Epidemiol 1987;125:150–7.
2. International Civil Aviation Organization. http/icao.int (accessed November 3, 2006).
3. Thibeault C. The impact of the Aerospace Industry on environment and public health. In: DeHart, Davis, editors. Fundamentals of Aerospace Medicine. 3rd ed, 2002;30:645–68.
4. Mangili A, Gendreau MA. Transmission of infectious diseases during commercial air travel. Lancet 2005;365: 989–95.
5. Hatakka M. Hygienic quality of foods served on aircraft. Helsinki: University of Helsinki, Oct 27, 2000. http://ethesis.helsinki.fi/julkaisut/ela/elint/vk/hatakka/index.html (accessed October 23, 2006).
6. Kelly M. Control of infection in an international airline. Occup Med 1993;43:91–4.
7. Hatakka M, Asplund K. The occurrence of *Salmonella* in airline meals. Acta Vet Scand 1993;34:391–6.
8. Hedberg CW, William CL, White KE, et al. An international foodborne outbreak of shigellosis associated with a commercial airline. JAMA 1992;268:3208–12.
9. William RB, Morley LA, Kohler M. Foodborne typhoid outbreak of with rapid dissemination of cases through air transportation. Northwest Med 1950;49:686–9.
10. Back E, Romanus V, Sjoberg L, et al. An epidemic of *Salmonella typhimurium* infection among aircraft passengers. Scand J Infect Dis 1977;9:175–9.
11. Burslem CD, Kelly MJ, Preston FS. Food poisoning—a major threat to airline operations. J Soc Occup Med 1990; 40:97–100.
12. Hatakka M. *Salmonella* outbreak among railway and airline passengers. Acta Vet Scand 1992;33:253–60.

13. Food safety and inspection services, USDA: Washington DC, Recall release FSIS-RC-059-2003.

14. Centers for Disease Control and Prevention. Staphylococcal food poisoning aloft. MMWR 1973;22:381–2.

15. Eisenberg M, Gaarsley K, Brown W, et al. Staphylococcal food poisoning aboard a commercial aircraft. Lancet 1975; 2:595–9.

16. Effersoe P, Kjerulf K. Clinical aspects of outbreak of Staphylococcal food poisoning during air travel. Lancet 2: 599–600.

17. Sutton RG. An outbreak of cholera in Australia due to food served in flight on an international aircraft. J Hyg Camb 1974;72:441–51.

18. Eberhart-Phillips J, Besser RE, Tormey MP, et al. An outbreak of cholera from food served on an international flight. Epidemiol Infect 1996;116:9–13.

19. Centers for Disease Control and Prevention. Cholera associated with an international airline flight. JAMA 1992;267:1444.

20. Centers for Disease Control and Prevention. Update: Cholera—Western Hemisphere and recommendations for treatment of cholera. MMWR 1991;40:562–5.

21. US Food and Drug Administration. Warning Letter, Reference Number 2940020, April 21, 2005.

22. Preston FS. An outbreak of gastroenteritis in aircrew. Aerospace Med 1968;18:150.

23. Centers for Disease Control and Prevention. Foodborne outbreaks of enterotoxigenic *Escherichia coli*—Rhode island and New Hampshire, 1993. MMWR 1994;43:81–9.

24. Widdowson M-A, Cramer EH, Hadley L, et al. Outbreaks of acute gastroenteritis on cruise ships and on land: identification of a predominant circulating strain of norovirus— United States 2002. J Infect Dis 2004;190:27–36.

25. Lester R, Stewart T, Carnie J, et al. Air travel-associated gastroenteritis outbreak, August 1991. Communicable Dis Intelligence 1991;15:292–3.

26. Widdowson M-A, Glass R, Monroe S, et al. Probable transmission of norovirus on an airplane. JAMA 2005;293: 1859–60.

27. World Health Organization. Gastroenteritis aboard planes. Weekly Epidemiol Record 1971;46:149.

28. Bryan FL. Time temperature observations of food and equipment in airline catering operations. J Food Protect 1978;41:80–92.

29. Centers for Disease Control and Prevention. An outbreak of acute gastroenteritis during a tour of the Orient. MMWR 1969;18:150.

30. Centers for Disease Control and Prevention. Acute gastroenteritis among tour groups to the Orient—United States. MMWR 1969;18:301–2.

31. Code of Federal Regulations. http://www.gpo.access.gov/cfr/index.html (accessed October 23, 2006).

32. Bailey J. Guide to hygiene and sanitation in aviation. World Health Organization, Geneva 1977.

33. International Air Transport Association (IATA) Catering Quality Assurance Programme (IQAP). www.iata.org (accessed November 3, 2006).

34. Kozicki M, Steffen R, Schar M. "Boil it, cook it, peel it or forget it": does this rule prevent travelers' diarrhea? Int J Epidemiol 1985;14:169–72.

35. Ericsson CD, DuPont HL. Prevention and treatment of traveler's diarrhea. New Engl J Med 1993;328:1821–7.

36. Centers for Disease Control and Prevention. Staphylococcal food poisoning on a trans-Pacific airline. MMWR 1961;10:8.

37. Munce BA. Microbiological hazards of airline catering. Food technol Australia 1978:470–6.

38. Mossel DA, Hoogendoorn J. Prevention of food-borne diseases in civil aviation. Ind Med 1971;40:25–6.

39. Centers for Disease Control and Prevention. Shigellosis related to an airplane meal— Northeastern United States. MMWR 1971;20:397–402.

40. Peffers AS, Bailey J, Barrow GI, et al. *Vibrio parahaemolyticus* gastroenteritis and international air travel. Lancet 1973;1:143–5.

41. Dakin WP, Howell DJ, Sutton RG, et al. Gastroenteritis due to non-agglutinable (non-cholera) vibrios. Med J Aust 1974;2:487–90.

42. Steffen R, Somaini B, Gubser A. Incidents of epidemiological significance at intercontinental airports. Trav Med Intl 1985;3:9–12.

43. World Health Organization. *Salmonella typhimurium* foodborne outbreak. Weekly Epidemiol Rec 1976;51:117–8.

44. World Health Organization. Foodborne *Salmonella* infections contracted on aircraft. Weekly Epidemiol Rec 1976; 51:256–66.

45. Centers for Disease Control and Prevention. Outbreak of staphylococcal food poisoning aboard an aircraft. MMWR 1976;25:1–3.

46. Desmarchelier P. *Vibrio* outbreaks from airline food and water. Food Technol Aust 1978;2:477–81.

47. World Health Organization. Food safety microbiological quality of airline meals. Weekly Epidemiol Rec 1989;42: 324–7.

48. Lambiri M, Mavridou A, Papadakis JA. The application of hazard analysis critical control point (HACCP) in a flight catering establishment improved the bacteriological quality of meals. J Roy Soc Health 1995:26–30.

49. Socket P, Ries A, Wieneke AA. Food poisoning associated with in-flight meals. Communicable Dis Rep 1993;3:103–4.

CHAPTER 14

ACUTE GASTROENTERITIS AT SEA AND OUTBREAKS ASSOCIATED WITH CRUISES

NEBOJŠA NIKOLIĆ, MD

EILIF DAHL, MD, PhD

ROISIN ROONEY, MS

CHIARA DEBERNARDIS, MD

All forms of travel have elements of risk. Cruising is considered a pleasant and relatively safe way to see exotic areas, but although cruise ships offer the comfortable familiarity of home, they can not entirely remove the risks of international travel. In 2000, 10 million people traveled on cruise ships, which represents an increase of over 1,000% the last few decades. This figure is expected to double by the year 2010.[1] Cruise itineraries include all continents and areas, including regions not easily accessible by other means of travel. The average duration of a cruise is about 7 days, with three to five ports of call, but cruise voyages can last from several hours to several months (eg, around-the-world cruises).

In general, the kinds of diseases seen on ships mirror those on land. The main differences are high population density aboard, high turnover of passengers, and the large number of countries from which the crew and passengers originate. These issues are significant in the transmission of infectious diseases on the cruise ships, as ships are isolated communities with crowded living accommodation, shared sanitary facilities, and common water and food supplies.[2] Some vessels carry over 5,000 passengers and crew per sailing. On many ships the majority of the passengers are elderly, and a growing number are immunosuppressed because of various infections and therapies. These people are at increased risk of foodborne and waterborne diseases, which may not present a major problem in the general population, but can have devastating consequences for vulnerable subgroups.[3,4] The cruise ships' rapid movement from one port to another, where there may be differences in sanitation standards and exposure risks, can introduce sightseeing and embarking passengers and crew to communicable diseases, which may result in outbreaks aboard. Shipboard conditions facilitate person-to-person spread of infectious diseases at sea, and disembarking passengers and crew might then contaminate their home communities.

A World Health Organization (WHO) literature review has identified over 100 disease outbreaks associated with ships between 1970 and 2000.[5] Such outbreaks are of concern because they can have serious health consequences and can result in high costs to an industry relying heavily on tourism. (Outbreaks of measles, rubella, varicella, meningococcal meningitis, hepatitis A, Legionnaires' disease, influenza, and gastroenteritis among ship travelers have been reported. The magnitude of outbreaks and sporadic cases of infection around the world is unknown because surveillance systems are very variable in collection of data and reporting of results. However, reported clusters of infection associated with ships demonstrate that passengers, and sometimes crew, are potential groups of susceptible persons at risk of disease.[6]

Travelers' diarrhea has been a frequent problem in the early cruises.[7] The first systematic investigations took place between 1972 and 1973.[8] Over 100 outbreaks of infectious diseases, particularly gastrointestinal disease, were reported to be associated with ships between 1970 and 2000.[9–13] In recent years, influenza and norovirus (Norwalk-like virus) outbreaks have been public health challenges for the cruise industry. Thirteen outbreaks of norovirus, spread mainly by person to person, were reported to be associated with ships between 1970 and 2000.[9]

During the summer 2002 there was an increase in outbreaks of gastroenteritis on cruise ships and shore locations worldwide. Norovirus was the primary cause for the increase.[14] That year the US Centers for Disease Control and Prevention (CDC) investigated 21 outbreaks of acute gastroenteritis on 17 cruise ships. Nine of these outbreaks were confirmed by laboratory analysis of stool specimens to be associated with norovirus.[4] Such outbreaks have continued to occur, and several ships have had to stop operations and cancel cruises in order to decontaminate the vessels.[15]

Between January 1 and July 5, 2006, 42 reported outbreaks of gastroenteritis on 13 different cruise ships sailing in European waters were confirmed or suspected to be caused by norovirus. Almost 1,500 cases of gastroenteritis were reported, but no common source has been determined. Two new norovirus variants were identified through the microbiological analysis of patient and environmental samples during these outbreaks. Based on previous years' experience, it was considered likely that the emergence of new norovirus strains coincided with increased virus activity in the community, which in turn reflected an increased activity on cruise ships.[16] The outbreak investigation was coordinated by the European Union (EU) funded surveillance network Divine-net, in collaboration with European Centre for Disease Prevention and Control (ECDC).[17]

Epidemiology of Acute Gastroenteritis at Sea

A cruise ship's population is ever changing and its stores are constantly being replenished with local food and water. If joining passengers and crew are infected or the food and water supplies are contaminated, an infection can spread rapidly throughout an entire community. Most of the detected gastrointestinal disease outbreaks associated with cruise ships before 2000 were linked to food or water consumed onboard ship.[9] Factors contributing to outbreaks included contaminated bunkered water; inadequate disinfection of potable water; potable water contaminated by sewage on ship; poor design and construction of potable water storage tanks; deficiencies in food handling, preparation, and cooking; and use of seawater in the galley.

Table 1 lists the pathogens and toxins in outbreaks of foodborne disease associated with ships.[9] The importance of water as a vehicle for infectious disease transmission on ships has been clearly documented.[9] Waterborne transmission on board ships, by ingestion of the pathogens listed in Table 2, has been confirmed by epidemiologic evidence.[9] Waterborne illnesses result either from ingestion of contaminated water or ice, contact with water (eg, bathing, wading, swimming, ocular exposure), or inhalation of aerosols generated from water that contains etiologic agents.[18] However, chemical outbreaks of water poisoning have also occurred on ships, and in some waterborne outbreaks, no known agents were identified.[9]

Noroviruses are now the most common cause of outbreaks of viral gastroenteritis on cruise ships. The number of outbreaks is increasing in parallel with the

Table 1. Foodborne Disease Outbreaks Associated with Ships

Organism/Toxin Bacteria	No. of Outbreaks
Salmonella species	14
Shigella species	8
Escherichia species	9
Vibrio species	6
Staphylococcus aureus	2
Clostridium perfringens	1
Parasites	
Cyclospora	1
Trichinella	1
Viruses	
Norwalk-like virus	6
Chemical food poisoning	
Ciguatera fish poisoning	2
Unknown	3
Total	53

Table 2. Pathogens/Toxins in Outbreaks of Waterborne Disease

Associated with Ships	
Organism/Toxin Bacteria	No. of Outbreaks
Salmonella species	2
Shigella species	1
Escherichia species	7
Parasites	
Cryptosporidium	1
Giardia	1
Viruses	
Norwalk-like virus	4
Chemical food poisoning	1
Unknown	5
Total	22

increase in norovirus infections on land. Symptoms often start with sudden onset of vomiting and/or diarrhea. There may be fever, abdominal cramps and malaise.[19] Gastroenteritis caused by norovirus is very contagious, and although outbreaks may begin as foodborne or waterborne disease, the virus is easily transmitted by person-to-person contact.[20,21] Norovirus illness is difficult to diagnose because the symptoms are similar to those caused by other types of gastroenteritis, and presently there is no fast and sufficiently reliable diagnostic test to distinguish norovirus from other pathogens on board. Outbreaks often affect both passengers and crew, sometimes with very high attack rates. Recurrences of infection on successive cruises are common. Outbreaks may continue because groups of new susceptible passengers are introduced on a regular basis, so that rather than running its course, the outbreak continues over a period of several cruises. Bridging between groups may occur by a reservoir of illness in the crew or by failure to decontaminate the environment.

Statutory Provisions for Outbreak Prevention and Control

INTERNATIONAL REGULATIONS

A ship is basically an isolated international community, and one should not expect the same level of medical service as ashore. There are no internationally accepted standards of care for the cruise ships, but fortunately many have medical facilities staffed and equipped in accordance with the guidance provided by the American College of Emergency Physicians (ACEP) or the International Council of Cruise Lines (ICCL). They are capable to provide reasonable emergency care on board, serving passengers and crew 24 hours a day.[22,23]

The only fully international regulations are supervised by the International Labour Organization (ILO) and WHO. According to Article 8 of the ILO Convention (No. 164) "Concerning Health Protection and Medical Care for Seafarers, 1987," vessels carrying over 100 crew members on an international voyage of 3 days or greater must provide a physician for care of the crew. Nothing is said about passengers or quality of care.[22] Some other international regulations and recommendations, like the revised International Health Regulations (IHR), address health requirements for ship operations and construction.[24] There are global standards regarding ship and port sanitation, disease surveillance, as well as response to infectious diseases. Guidance is given for provision of safe water, food, vector and rodent control, and waste disposal. Although control of persistent infectious agents is not specifically covered in IHR, there is a general overview of responsibilities for responding to and managing suspected or confirmed disease outbreaks on ships. Framework for policy making and local decision making can be found in the WHO Guide for Ship Sanitation, the global reference on health requirements for ship construction and operation.[25] It was first published in 1967, referenced under the International Health Regulations, and the next revised edition is expected to be published by the end of 2006. Regarding containment of patients, its 2005 draft version simply states at 7.5.1.: "Symptomatic passengers or crew are best advised to stay in cabin."

REGIONAL REGULATIONS

Ships have to follow international regulations and the rules of their flag states, but regarding sanitation they also have to adhere to public health regulations of the ports they are visiting. As the North American market covers two-thirds of the global cruise volume,[1] cooperation with US authorities is particularly important for the cruise industry.

The US CDC established the Vessel Sanitation Program (VSP) in the 1970s as a cooperative activity with the cruise ship industry.[26] The program assists the cruise ship industry in fulfilling its responsibility for developing and implementing comprehensive sanitation programs in order to minimize the risk of gastrointestinal diseases. Every vessel that has a foreign (non-US) itinerary and carries 13 or more passengers is subject to twice-yearly inspections and, when necessary, re-inspection. The VSP operated continuously at all major US ports from the early 1970s through 1986, when CDC terminated portions of the program. Industry and public pressures resulted in the US Congress directing CDC to resume the VSP, and a user fee based on the vessel's size is charged for inspections to reimburse the US government for costs. To assist the cruise ship industry in educating shipboard personnel, a *VSP Operations Manual* based partly on the WHO's *Guide to Ship Sanitation* was published in 1989 and last updated in 2005.[27]

Medical staff on cruise ships visiting US ports will need to familiarize themselves thoroughly with this manual, but the points below are crucial for cooperation with CDC to prevent and control outbreaks aboard.[27]

VSP defines a reportable case of gastrointestinal illness as: 1) diarrhea (three or more episodes of loose stools in a 24-hour period); or 2) vomiting and one additional symptom including one or more episodes of loose stools in a 24-hour period, or abdominal cramps, or headache, or muscle aches, or fever (temperature of ≥ 38 °C = 100.4 °F).

VSP furthermore states:

- Antidiarrheal medications shall not be sold or dispensed to passengers or crew except by designated medical staff.
- A standardized gastrointestinal illness surveillance log for each cruise shall be maintained daily and shall list: 1) all reportable cases of gastrointestinal illness; 2) all passengers and crew members who are dispensed antidiarrheal medication from the vessel.
- The gastrointestinal illness surveillance log entry for each passenger or crew member shall contain the following information: 1) the first date of report to staff of illness; 2) the person's name, age, and gender; 3) a designation as passenger or crew; 4) crew member position or job on the vessel, if applicable; 5) cabin number; 6) meal seating information; 7) date and time of illness onset; 8) illness symptoms, including the presence of the following selected signs and symptoms: numbers of episodes each of diarrhea and vomiting per day, bloody stools, fever, recorded temperature, abdominal cramps, headaches and muscle aches; 9) notation on whether or not a stool specimen was requested and received; 10) use of antidiarrheal medication; and 11) the presence of underlying medical conditions that may affect interpretation of acute gastrointestinal illness, for example diabetic diarrhea, inflammatory bowel disease, gastrectomy, or others.
- Questionnaires detailing activities and meal locations for the 72 hours before illness onset shall be distributed to all passengers and crew members who are gastrointestinal illness cases.
- The medical log, gastrointestinal illness log and the 72-hour self-administered questionnaires shall be maintained on the vessel for 12 months.
- The master of a vessel destined for a US port from a foreign port shall submit at least one standardized gastrointestinal illness report (by telephone, facsimile, or preferably electronically) based on the number of reportable cases in the gastrointestinal illness log, even if the number is 0, to the VSP 24 to 36 hours before the vessel's expected arrival at the US port.
- If the number of cases changes after submission of the initial report, an updated report shall be submitted no less than 4 hours before the vessel's arrival at the US port.
- The master shall also submit a special report at any time during a cruise when the cumulative percentage of reportable cases entered in the gastrointestinal illness surveillance log reaches 2% among passengers or 2% among crew and the vessel is within 15 days of expected arrival at a US port.
- The medical staff will be responsible for maintaining a supply of at least 10 clinical specimen-collection containers for both viral and bacterial agents (10 for each), as well as the proper shipping containers and labels for same. When a vessel reaches 2% reportable gastrointestinal illness in passengers or crew members, the medical staff will begin collecting whole stool specimens for viral analysis, unless it is clear from clinical and epidemiological data that the causative agent is of bacterial or parasitic aetiology.

The VSP requirements for isolating symptomatic and primary contacts of crew and passengers with acute gastroenteritis are:[27]

- Food-handling employees are to be isolated until symptom-free for a minimum of 48 hours, and other crew for 24 hours. Follow-up with and approval by medical personnel is required before returning isolated crew to work. Medical or supervisory staff shall conduct a verbal interview with asymptomatic cabin mates and immediate contacts of symptomatic crew (immediately and then daily until 48 hours after onset of the ill crew members symptoms began) to confirm their condition, advise them of the hygiene and hand washing facts, and to instruct them to report immediately to medical staff if they develop illness symptoms.
- Ill passengers should be advised to remain isolated in cabin until well for a minimum of 24 hours after symptom resolution. Follow-up by medical personnel is advised, including hand washing tips and personal hygiene information sheet provided by ship.

In an attempt to avoid outbreaks, some ships have company directives that exceed the CDC and ICCL recommendations and isolate food handling crew for 72 hours and other crew and passengers for 48 hours after their last symptom, while asymptomatic contacts of ill crew and passengers are isolated for 24 hours for observation.[28]

Enforced isolation puts a heavy strain on the doctor-patient relationship from the beginning, and the doctor's unwanted role of warden demands superior diplomatic and psychological skills to ensure compliance and avoid confrontations.

Isolation itself has its own dangers, like various degrees of depression and impaired conditions for clinical and laboratory follow-up. Furthermore, fear of getting isolated may keep patients from seeking prompt medical attention, thus delaying diagnosis and treatment of life-threatening illnesses, like peritonitis following appendicitis.[28]

In an attempt to avoid isolation, many experienced travellers have their own physicians prescribe antibiotics and antidiarrheal medication to take if gastroenteritis symptoms occur during their cruise. Believing that they already have the best treatment available, a passenger with viral gastroenteritis will then spread norovirus around the ship for days while taking a useless antibiotic.

Despite good performance on environmental health sanitation inspections by cruise ships, outbreaks of gastroenteritis per 1,000 cruises increased almost tenfold from 2001 to 2004, and the increase was most likely attributable to norovirus.[29]

Companies that believe that their ships are not able or willing to maintain the VSP standard, keep their ships out of US ports, but should know that other countries, like Canada and Australia, have their own strict sanitation programs, and an expert panel of the ECDC recently announced coordinated European actions to prevent and control norovirus outbreaks on cruise ships, including development of practical and standardized guidelines based on best practices identified from previous experience.[30]

GENERAL SANITARY MEASURES

Based on the cruise lines' experience, according to ICCL, the most effective means of preventing the spread of norovirus, include, in addition to patient isolation:[31]

- An aggressive communications effort on board ships encourages passengers to thoroughly wash their hands frequently (every hour or two) to help avoid unknowingly spreading the virus.
- Aboard ship, staterooms and public areas are cleaned and disinfected daily.
- Cleaning procedures include the use of disinfectants on areas including, but not limited to, counters, bathroom surfaces, door handles, railings and grab bars, exercise equipment, video arcade equipment, vanities, and TV remote controls.
- Cleaning measures go as far as disinfecting the Scrabble game tiles, poker chips, and anything that a passenger might touch.
- Other measures include disposing of playing cards after each evening in the casino, not shaking hands at cocktail parties to reduce the risk of spreading the virus, and the elimination of all self-serve buffets (passengers point to the food they would like and staff will serve them).
- Areas where people are or have been sick are immediately and thoroughly cleaned, and sanitized/disinfected.
- On turnaround days, extra crew may be brought on board to disinfect the ship with the CDC-recommended disinfectants from top to bottom before additional passengers board.
- Passengers with obvious symptoms of illness upon embarkation may be refused boarding.

FOOD HANDLING SANITARY MEASURES

The continuing problem of foodborne gastrointestinal disease in cruise ships underscores the need for basic hygienic control for food handlers and food preparation areas. Other important factors in the prevention of foodborne disease are

- Time and temperature control
- Control of cross-contamination
- Adequate heat treatment
- Safe raw ingredients from reliable sources
- Exclusion of infected food handlers from work.

The above should be supported by the implementation of a Hazard Analysis Critical Control Point (HACCP) system.[32] Such a system should be used as a tool to help determine critical control points specific to a particular menu; that is, the stages in the preparation and cooking of food, which must be controlled to ensure the safety of the food. Once identified, a monitoring system can be set up for each critical control point to ensure that correct procedures are maintained and action taken if control point criteria are not achieved. The chief advantage of HACCP is that it is proactive; it aims to prevent problems from occurring.

The principles of HACCP have been described by Codex15 and are summarized in Table 3.[32] Additional information is available from publications by the International Commission for Microbiological Specifications for Food, the National Advisory Committee on Microbiological Criteria for Foods, International Life Sciences Institute Europe, and others.[32–34]

WATER SAFETY SANITARY MEASURES

The traditional approach to assuring the safety of water on board ships relied on sampling the end product. However, Water Safety Plans (WSPs) are a tool that could help ship operators manage water safety aboard and prevent future outbreaks.

WSPs can cover both design (materials and construction) and operation. They comprise three essential

Table 3. Principles of HACCP

	Subject	Action
1	Hazard analysis	Construct a flow diagram of the process stages Identify and list all of the potential hazards
2	Identification of the CCPs	Identify the CCPs using a decision tree Specify the systems of control
3	Establishing critical limits	Target values and critical limits must be set for each CCP
4	Monitoring	Continual or regular registering at each CCP to verify maintenance of control
5	Correction	Establish protocols for: i) when a CCP is moving toward loss of control ii) when a CCP is already out of control
6	Verification	Establish systems to confirm the correct functioning of HACCP
7	Documentation	Establish documentation regarding all of the procedures and records necessary for the implementation and operation of the above principles

Adapted from Kirby R. HACCP in practice. Food Control 1994;5(4):230–5.
CCP = critical control points; HACCP = Hazard Analysis Critical Control Point Principle.

actions, which are the responsibility of the ship owner and master to ensure that drinking water is safe:

- A system assessment
- Effective monitoring
- Management

This approach builds on the HACCP system, which has gained the approval of the food industry for controlling food quality.

The purpose of system assessment is to determine whether a system has control measures in place that would ensure water quality is consistently maintained on the ship. This assessment involves understanding the characteristics of the drinking water system, what hazards may arise, how these create risks, and the processes and practices that affect drinking water quality. These hazards should be monitored on a routine basis. Management includes control measures, corrective action, and verification. Control measures are actions, activities, and processes applied to prevent or minimize hazards from occurring or to reduce them.

WSPs should include the following:

- Assessment of source water loaded onto the ship for the prevention or reduction of pathogen contamination.
- If source water is contaminated, the selection and operation of treatment processes that are controlled by monitoring parameters that are critical to achieving the target level of pathogen reduction.
- The prevention of contamination by pathogens in the storage and distribution system.
- The prevention of contamination during production (desalination).

SANITARY MEASURES FOR PREVENTING OUTBREAKS OF VIRAL GASTROENTERITIS

Consecutive and prolonged outbreaks on ships suggest that norovirus survive well in this environment. An effective cleaning and disinfection program is essential to control outbreaks. Objects that are frequently handled, such as taps, door handles, and toilet or bath rails, should be thoroughly cleaned and disinfected. Contaminated hard surfaces should be washed with detergent and hot water, using disposable cloths, and then disinfected with 0.1% hypochlorite solution. Cloths should be disposed of as clinical waste.[35] Other control measures on cruise ships may include removing the ship for 7 to 10 days from service for aggressive cleaning, quarantine of ill crew members and passengers until symptom-free for 72 hours, and reinforcement of water and food sanitation practices.[4]

Hypochlorite is not generally recommended for disinfecting carpets and soft furnishings because prolonged contact is required and many such items are not bleach resistant. Steam cleaning may be used for carpets and soft furnishings, provided they are heat tolerant (some carpets are "bonded" to the underlying floor with heat-sensitive materials). However, in-use tests with steam cleaners have shown failure to achieve temperatures of 60°C within carpets. Vacuum cleaning carpets and buffing floors have the potential to recirculate norovirus and are not recommended. Nondisposable mop heads should be laundered as a hot wash. Contaminated carpets should be cleaned with detergent and hot water and then disinfected with hypochlorite (if bleach resistant) or steam cleaned.[36]

PERSONAL PREVENTIVE MEASURES

For most passengers, cruising possesses few health risks that can be minimized by sensible planning and a few precautions before, during, and after the voyage. By buying a ticket for the cruise, the passengers enters a contract with the cruise company with the distinct obligation to notify the cruise company of any medical condition that can impact the health and safety of the passenger, or make him or her unfit to travel. Those travelers should be advised to carry a summary of medical records with them on board. Fitness to travel is an important part of the contract with the cruise company, to the level that embarkation can be denied. In cases of contagious disease posing a threat to other persons aboard, the master can deny embarkation, enforce isolation, or order medical debarkation of passengers and crew.

Guidelines on the implementation of prevention and control measures need to be simple and practical, based on best practices identified from previous experience. The HACCP program used on cruise ships was originally designed to monitor NASA (National Aeronautics and Space Administration) astronaut's food and water from source to consumption and have been effectively used on board ships, but strict control of hygiene in shore-side restaurants visited by passengers is more difficult.[37] Eating and drinking ashore increase the risk of gastrointestinal disease, therefore general advice on food and hygiene precautions should be followed carefully. Hand washing frequently with soap and water, rubbing hands together vigorously for 20 or more seconds, is strongly recommended for cruise passengers. Antibacterial and antiviral solutions may be useful alternatives if provided aboard. Passengers should also verify in advance that their travel insurance makes it possible for them to change their cruise dates if they present with symptoms of gastroenteritis before their trip begins.

Conclusions

Repeated gastrointestinal and respiratory tract outbreaks on cruise ships have resulted in programs to improve prevention, detection, and control and to improve and maintain a high level of sanitation. Each company has issued very detailed operational directives on how to deal with every aspect of shipboard sanitation: under normal circumstances, when there is a threat of an outbreak, and during an outbreak.

On cruises lasting from 3 days to 2 weeks and having at least 100 passengers, gastrointestinal illness outbreaks investigated by the CDC decreased from 8.1 to 3.0 per 10 million passenger days between 1975 to 1979 and 1980 to 1993, respectively.[12] In addition, the percentage of ships with acceptable levels of sanitation has increased dramatically.[38] But despite good performance on health inspections, outbreaks of gastroenteritis per 1,000 cruises increased almost tenfold from 2001 to 2004. The increase is likely attributable to noroviruses and highlights the inability of environmental programs to fully predict and prevent risk factors common to person-to-person and fomite spread of disease.[28]

The fact that the ports and the ships have a common interest in limiting and containing norovirus outbreaks, there is an opportunity for a mutually beneficial partnership between the public health sector and the cruise industry. Close collaboration between the different stakeholders is therefore a priority. Because of the rapidly growing cruise industry, continuing efforts are needed to guarantee superior sanitary measures on ships and to safeguard the health of travelers and crew, as well as to prevent the spread of infections from one country to another.

References

1. Crye JM. Testimony before the Subcommittee on Commerce, Trade and Consumer Protection. House Energy and Commerce Committee, October 17th 2001. http://www.iccl.org/pressroom/testimony101701.pdf (accessed October 29, 2006).
2. Gascon J, Ruiz L, Canela J, et al. Epidemiology of travelers' diarrhea in Spanish tourists traveling in developing countries. Med Clin 1993;100:365–7.
3. De Louvois J, Dadswell J. Emerging pathogens and drinking water supply. London: Public Health Laboratory Services; 1998.
4. Cramer EH, Forney D, Dannenberg MD, et al. Outbreaks of gastroenteritis associated with Noroviruses on cruise ships—United States. Morb Mortal Wkly Rep 2002;51: 1112–5.
5. World Health Organization. Sustainable development and healthy environments. Sanitation on ships. Compendium of outbreaks of foodborne and waterborne disease and Legionnaires' disease associated with ships, 1970–2000. WHO/SDE/WSH/01.4. 2001.
6. Minooee A, Rickman LS. Infectious diseases on cruise ships. Clin Infect Dis 1999;29:737–44.
7. De Las Casas C, Adachi J, DuPont H. Travelers' diarrhoea [review]. Aliment Pharmacol Ther 1999;13:1373–8.
8. Merson MH, Hughes JM, Wood BT, et al. Gastrointestinal illness on passenger cruise ships. J Am Med Assoc 1975;231: 723–5.
9. WHO. Sanitation on ships. Compendium of outbreaks of foodborne and waterborne and Legionnaires' disease associated with ships, 1970–2000. WHO/WSH/01.4; 2001.

10. Dannenberg AL, Yashuk JC, Filedman RA. Gastrointestinal illness on passenger cruise ships, 1975–1978. Am J Public Health 1982;72:484–8.

11. Addis DG, Yashuk JC, Clapp DE, Blake PA. Outbreaks of diarrhoeal illness on passenger cruise ships, 1975–85. Epidemiol Infect 1989;103:63–72.

12. Koo D, Maloney K, Taux R. Epidemiology of diarrhoeal disease outbreaks on cruise ships 1986 through 1993. JAMA 1996;275:545–7.

13. DiGiovanna T, Rosen T, Forsett R, et al. Shipboard medicine. A new niche for emergency medicine. Ann Emerg Med 1993;22:1639.

14. Widdowson MA, Cramer EH, Hadley L, et al. Outbreaks of acute gastroenteritis on cruise ships and on land: identification of a predominant circulating strain of norovirus—United States, 2002. J Infect Dis 2004;190:27–36.

15. CDC Cruise Ship Outbreaks by Year (1994–2004). www.cdc.gov/nceh/vsp/surv/outbreakslist.pdf (accessed September 20, 2004).

16. Lopman B, Vennema H, Kohli E, et al. Increase in viral gastroenteritis outbreaks in Europe and epidemic spread of new norovirus variant. Lancet 2004;363:682–8.

17. Koopmans M, Harris J, Verhoef L, et al. European investigation into recent norovirus outbreaks on cruise ships: update. Euro Surveill 2006;11:E060706.5.

18. International Association of Milk, Food and Environmental Sanitarians, Inc. Procedures to investigate waterborne illness. 5th ed. Iowa: IAMFES; 1996. p. 6.

19. Kaplan JE, Gary GW, Baron RC, et al. Epidemiology of Norwalk gastroenteritis and the role of Norwalk virus in outbreaks of acute, nonbacterial gastroenteritis. Ann Intern Med 1982;96:756–61.

20. Lawrence DN. Outbreaks of gastrointestinal diseases on cruise ships: Lessons from three decades of progress. Curr Infect Dis Rep 2004;6:115–23.

21. Centers for Disease Control and Prevention. Norwalk-like viruses: public health consequences and out-break management. MMWR Morb Mortal Wkly Rep 2001;50(No. RR-9).

22. Dahl E. Cruise medicine: call for an international standard. Internat Marit Health 2001;52:24–6.

23. American College of Emergency Physicians. Guidelines of care for cruise ship medical facilities. Ann Emerg Med 1996;27:846.

24. International Health Regulations. Geneva: WHO; 1969. (Revised 2005). http://www.who.int/csr/ihr/en/ (accessed October 29, 2006).

25. Guide to ship sanitation. Geneva: WHO; 1967. Reprinted with amendments in 1987. (Revised 2005) http://www.who.int/water_sanitation_health/hygiene/ships/en/guidetoshipsanitation.pdf) (accessed October 29, 2006).

26. Korcok M. Sick at sea: outbreaks prompt reinstatement of cruise ship inspections. Can Med Assoc J 1987;136:1298–300.

27. CDC Vessel Sanitation Program Operations Manual 2005. www.cdc.gov/nceh/vsp (accessed October 29, 2006).

28. Dahl E. Dealing with gastrointestinal illness on a cruise ship—Part 1: description of sanitation measures Part 2: an isolation study. Internat Marit Health 2004;55:19–29.

29. Cramer EH, Blanton CJ, Blanton LH, et al. Epidemiology of gastroenteritis on cruise ships, 2001–2004. Am J Prev Med 2006;30:252–7.

30. Depoortere E, Takkinen J. Coordinated European actions to prevent and control norovirus outbreaks on cruise ships. Eurosurveillance weekly releases 2006;11:3–5, http://www.eurosurveillance.org/ew/2006/061018.asp#2 (accessed October 29, 2006).

31. International Council of Cruise Lines. Norovirus—Policies, procedures and prevention. http://www.iccl.org/policies/norovirus.cfm (accessed October 29, 2006).

32. International Commission for Microbiological Specifications for Food. Microorganisms in foods. 4. Application of the hazard analysis critical control point (HACCP) system to ensure microbiological safety and quality. Oxford: Blackwell Scientific Publications; 1988. p. 12.

33. National Advisory Committee on Microbiological Criteria for Foods. Hazard analysis and critical control point system. Report of the National Advisory Committee on microbiological criteria for food. USDA; 1992.

34. ILSI Europe. A simple guide to understanding and applying the hazard analysis critical control point. Washington: Concept ILSI Press; 1993.

35. Chadwick PR, Beards G, Brown D, et al. Management of hospital outbreaks of gastro-enteritis due to SRSV. J Hosp Infect 2000;45:1–10.

36. Ho MS, Glass RI, Monroe SS, et al. Viral gastroenteritis aboard a cruise ship. Lancet 1989;2:961–4.

37. Smith A. Cruise ship medicine. In: Dawood R, editor. Traveller's Health. Oxford: Oxford University Press; 2002. p. 227–89.

38. Nguyen CH. A cost-effectiveness analysis of the vessel sanitation program. US Department of Health and Human Services Document. Centers for Disease Control and Prevention; 1997.

CHAPTER 15

DIARRHEA IN MILITARY POPULATIONS: FROM HISTORICAL CONSIDERATIONS UNTIL MODERN TIMES

C. KENNETH MCALLISTER, MD

MARK S. RIDDLE, MD, MPH&TM

When physicians use the term "travelers' diarrhea," they are generally referring to an attack of "Montezuma's Revenge" that has suddenly ruined a vacation in a tropical destination. However, travelers' diarrhea can be a serious illness. It does not selectively afflict those on a holiday as a mere inconvenience. In fact, military personnel have frequently been victims of travelers' diarrhea throughout both historical and modern times, with sometimes devastating consequences. No one has more eloquently stated the enormous impact of diarrhea on military populations than Sir William Osler: "Dysentery has been more fatal to armies than powder and shot."[1]

Historical Considerations

Though it remains a formidable foe in modern times, diarrhea has had devastating effects on soldiers throughout military history. Diarrhea and dysentery have been major causes of morbidity and mortality in every military campaign. The effects of diarrhea are noted as early as biblical times, where a diarrheal illness is described in David's lament from Psalms 22:15 (Bible: King James Version): "I am poured out like water, and all my bones are out of joint; my heart is like wax; it is melted in the midst of my bowels."

Throughout the history of war, infections have taken more lives than battlefield injuries during times of war. The ratio of soldiers killed by infectious diseases to those killed by battle wounds was 8:1 during the Napoleonic Wars, and 3:1 during the Crimean War 50 years later.[2] Once basic sanitation principles were embraced during the American Civil War, the infections to battle wounds mortality ration was reduced to 2:1. Nevertheless, over 500,000 soldiers died secondary to infectious disease during the Civil War. Of these deaths, diarrhea accounted for 21,000, while typhoid fever resulted in 35,000 deaths.[2] Typhoid fever also felled such notables as Stephan Douglas and the Hero of Little Round Top, Joshua L. Chamberlain[3]

Early military physicians perceived the role of dietary changes in precipitating diarrhea, calling it "the bloody flux." Diarrhea was also thought to be secondary to cold exposure, dampness, and even unsuitable food. The seasonal production of vectors like flies was also recognized as an important cause of diarrhea.[4]

John Pringle, the father of military hygiene, defined dysentery as diarrhea with blood in the stool. He steered physicians away from "purging and bleeding" to prevention through field sanitation.[4] During the 1860s, Jonathan Letterman and the US Sanitary Commission propagated sanitation during the American Civil War, by directing appropriate sanitation, quarantines in camp, and Letterman's triage system, ultimately saving countless patient lives.[5] During Letterman's tenure as the Chief Medical Officer of the Army of the Potomac, the ratio of deaths from disease to those from battle improved over that of prior wars.

Great military leaders of the past and present have realized that diarrhea often makes victory most elusive: "Dysentery of this Arabian coast used to fall like a hammer blow and crush its victims...and left men curiously tired."[6] T. E. Lawrence (Lawrence of Arabia)

Diarrhea during Modern Warfare

In World War II, diarrheal illness contributed to a major allied victory—a turning point in the war. During the campaign for El Alamein, 50% of German soldiers suffered from dysentery. Ultimately, a combination of dysentery and Field Marshall Montgomery's strategy produced a victory.

The wars of the post-1940 era have also revealed ongoing problems with diarrhea. Fifty-five percent of American soldiers in the Korean War developed diarrhea upon arriving in the theater.[7] The prevalence of diarrhea in American troops in Vietnam approached 30%. During the Vietnam War, diarrhea exceeded even malaria as the most common cause of hospitalization for US soldiers.[8]

Another modern war experience has further chronicled diarrhea's debilitating role. The Russian-Afghanistan War data reveal that little effort was given to field sanitation among Russian soldiers. The prevalence of diarrhea was overall 30% during this campaign and increased to 70% during the summer months.[9]

While diarrhea remained a problem during the Persian Gulf War, for perhaps the first time in military history, there was not a major loss of manpower—a finding most likely attributable to the vastly improved sanitation and attention to personal hygiene. The Persian Gulf War provided an ideal opportunity to analyze the incidence, risk factors, and pathogens associated with infectious diarrhea in modern military campaigns. Hyams and colleagues surveyed 2,022 US soldiers deployed to the Persian Gulf from 1990 to 1991.[10] Fifty-seven percent of the troops reported at least one episode of diarrhea. Contaminated water, which was so often implicated as the cause of diarrhea in past wars, was an unlikely etiology. Supplies of potable water were plentiful either from bottled sources or reverse-osmosis units. Fresh produce and dairy products were highly desired by troops, but difficult to provide. Supplies of these products generally came from local producers in the Middle East or Asia, and ensuring the safety of these items was not fully possible. Eating raw vegetables, especially salad, was associated with the highest risk of developing diarrhea. Enterotoxigenic *E. coli* (ETEC) was isolated from the culture of lettuce in one military food preparation facility.[10]

In 1990, Wasserman and colleagues reviewed the charts of 6,772 sick-call visits.[11] One unit reported a less than 3% incidence of diarrhea. This was likely attributable to the fact that the unit provided its troops with no raw vegetables and enforced strict hand-washing near the latrines and the dining facilities. However, one squadron was noted to have an isolated outbreak of diarrheal illness. It was later determined that this squadron was the only one to eat raw vegetables during a special Christmas dinner.[11]

Although bacteria compose the majority of diarrheal pathogens in soldiers, it is important to recognize that viral etiologies may also play a role in diarrhea among military populations. During the Persian Gulf War, paired sera from 404 US military personnel were tested for serologic evidence of Norwalk virus. At least a fourfold increase in antibody was detected in 23% of patients with vomiting, 12% of patients with diarrhea and vomiting, and 6.5% of patients with diarrhea alone.[12]

Diarrhea and Wars in Afghanistan and Iraq

Despite the knowledge of infectious diarrhea's impact on centuries of military campaigns, diarrhea continues to afflict troops around the world, particularly in deployments in the Middle East region. The multinational military campaign in Afghanistan initiated in 2001 is not without exception. A group of British soldiers became acutely ill with fever accompanied by severe diarrhea and vomiting in May of 2002. The gastroenteritis was quite severe, necessitating hospitalization in all afflicted, as well as ventilatory support for two patients. Eleven soldiers were ultimately evacuated out of Afghanistan to England, but not before three health care providers were also exposed. The British field hospital was temporarily closed to all but those with gastroenteritis in order to contain the outbreak. Analysis of stool specimens was performed in England, and Norovirus (NV) was detected. NV is a particular problem among military personnel because it is extremely contagious, has a prolonged asymptomatic shedding period, and is relatively resistant to chlorination and environmental conditions. Twenty-nine soldiers and health care workers were ultimately affected. All of the patients rapidly recovered;[13] however, this small outbreak essentially incapacitated the unit's ability to operate and cost the British government an extraordinary amount of money in order to quarantine, evacuate, treat, and investigate the illness.

Reports of acute gastroenteritis attributable to NV were noted during the initial invasion period among both British and US forces and usually characterized as causing outbreaks among particular combat units[14,15] Although these illnesses are neither life threatening nor of long duration, these outbreaks can affect and incapacitate large numbers of personnel in a unit. The potential to impact military operations and readiness was put very clearly by DO Matson, who writes, "I expect that our imaginations cannot fathom the problems attendant from the absolute urgency for relief from explosive vomiting and diarrhea when experienced within an armored vehicle under fire and at ambient temperature of 140°F."[16] The impact of diarrhea was further substantiated by a study of deployed troops who had one or more episodes of diarrhea: 32% experienced fecal incontinence when they were unable to access a latrine in time.[17]

While acute gastroenteritis epidemics have not been reported since the early phases of the war (though likely due to lack of enhanced surveillance, rather than absence of events), sporadic diarrhea has continued to be a problem and has been described in a number of epidemiologic studies. Data collected in the in the winter of 2003/2004 from 4,348 troops on deployment to Iraq or Afghanistan (median time in country: 8 months Iraq, 6.7 months Afghanistan) found that 76% of responders had at least one episode of diarrhea and more than half reported multiple episodes.[18] A monthly incidence of ~29% was estimated, with significant reports of decreased days of performance (45% reporting for median of 3 days), days lost due to illness (17%, median 2 days) and health care utilization. A follow-on study among 15,459 persons surveyed that monthly minimum incidence rates (does not include multiple episodes) for diarrhea doubled from the precombat operations period (6%) to the combat operations period (12%) and then significantly dropped off in the postcombat operation period (1%) (Figure 1).[17] For diarrheal illness, this finding closely paralleled the soldier's perception of availability of safe food and water during these combat operation phases. It was also noted that the incidence of diarrhea was higher in Iraq compared to Afghanistan, and 3 to 4 times higher compared to incidence of acute respiratory illness and nonbattle injury. Time spent off base and local food consumption are contributing risk factors to differential country-specific disease rates.[19]

As with previous conflicts, disease and nonbattle injury (DNBI) continue to be important health concerns to deployed troops, resulting in medical use and individual work impact. During October 2003 to June 2004, a medical unit located outside of Baghdad with a catchment population of about 6,000 reported that while infectious gastrointestinal illness accounted for approximately 8% of all DNBI initial visits, nearly 1 in 5 hospitalizations could be attributable to these illnesses.[20] Furthermore, 14% of troops reported decreased unit effectiveness due to diarrheal illness during combat operations compared to respiratory illness (9%) and nonbattle injury (10%).[17] Prevention of diarrhea during the critical combat operations period is most important, but also most challenging and calls for continued efforts to develop effective primary preventive strategies.

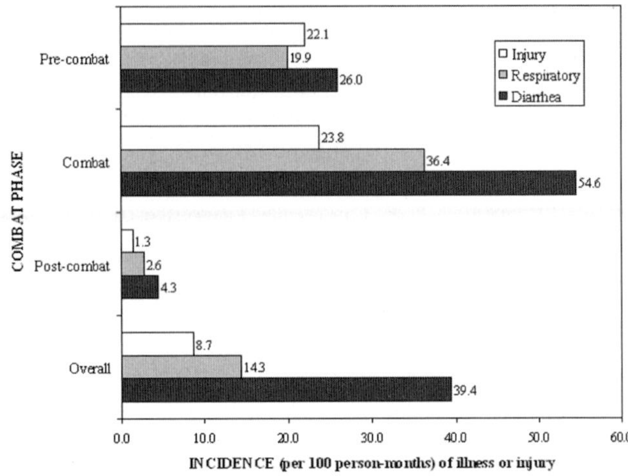

Figure 1 Incidence of common illnesses and non-battle injury among US military personnel deployed to Iraq or Afghanistan by phase of combat operations, 2003–2004. Adapted from Sanders JW.[17]

In addition to diarrhea incidence and impact surveillance, two studies have reported on the etiology of diarrhea in the region. A study in the Anbar province of Iraq during the summer of 2004 enrolled 123 subjects with acute diarrhea describes diarrheagenic *E. coli* (ETEC 23%, enteroaggregative E. *coli* [EAEC] 12.5%) as the predominate etiolgy.[21] As opposed to earlier reports, *Shigella* spp. and norovirus were less common (0.8% and 2.5% respectively). Diarrheagenic *E. coli* predominance was also noted in an observational study during the same year where 109 subjects with acute diarrhea from the region who traveled to Doha, Qatar for 4 days of leave were enrolled and provided stool specimens for testing.[22] In thirty-five (32%) cases, ETEC was identified and 13 (12%) grew EAEC, though 7% of asymptomatic individuals also grew EAEC in their stools. An additional finding these two studies had in common was a 7 to 20% prevalence of protozoan organisms (commensal and pathogenic), further emphasizing the need to consider a thorough evaluation for chronic diarrhea in deployed troops and continued preventive medicine efforts to assure safe food and water availability and consumption.

Diarrhea during Peacekeeping Missions and Exercises

Over the past 50 years, the United Nations (UN) has had a great impact on the role of a soldier. The UN essentially created the "Peacekeeping Soldier," and with this role came many of the risks of war, including infectious diarrhea. Sanchez and colleagues reported the incidence of diarrhea among US troops during 11 overseas peacekeeping missions from 1981 to 1990.[23] During that time, the incidence of diarrhea varied widely, affecting between 1 and 52% of deployed troops. Factors associated with increased risk of diarrhea included location of deployment, food, and beverages, particularly ice. US troops deployed to Beirut, Lebanon in 1982 also suffered from a tremendous amount of diarrheal illness. Diarrhea accounted for 96.5% of the infectious diseases presenting to the clinic from the thirty-second Marine Amphibious Unit.[24]

Peacekeeping missions followed in Somalia from 1992 to 1994. Multiple nations participated in Operation Restore Hope, and diarrhea spared no one. Italian soldiers reported 55% were affected by at least one episode of diarrhea.[25] During Operation Restore Hope, less than 15% of US troops experienced one episode of diarrhea. However, severe diarrheal illness represented 16% (61 of 381) of all hospital admissions.[26]

A recent systematic review of the literature describing regional estimates of pathogen-specific prevalence and incidence associated with diarrhea among deployed US military and similar populations living for longer durations overseas.[27] Between January 1990 to June 2005, 52 studies fulfilled inclusion criteria. A majority of the studies were conducted among US Military populations (63%) with foreign military, expatriate (including NGOs and Embassy populations) and student populations each consisting of about 12% included studies. Overall, 37% were from the Middle East, 31% from Southeast Asia, 24% from Latin America/Caribbean, and 6% from sub-Saharan Africa. Median duration of travel was 1.5 months (IQR 1 to 3 months). Similar to short-term traveler studies, ETEC, *Campylobacter* spp. and *Shigella* spp. were identified as causing 38 to 45% of diarrhea with regional and population differences (Table 1). Incidence based on self-report was higher than studies using passive surveillance or clinical-based methods (29 versus 7 versus 6 episodes per 100 person-months, respectively) without regional differences.

Diarrhea on Shipboard Environments

With their tight quarters and frequent port calls, outbreaks of acute gastroenteritis aboard US Navy ships have increasingly gained recognition as a potential threat to mission capacity and operational readiness. Although these illnesses are neither life threatening nor of long duration, these outbreaks can affect and incapacitate large numbers of personnel in a unit. The explosive nature of these outbreaks on ships may be related to the multiple modes of transmission. This includes consumption of contaminated food or water, direct person-to-person, airborne droplets of vomitus, and contaminated environmental surfaces.[28,29] In addition to the multiple modes of transmission, low infectious dose and the large reservoir of susceptible persons (due to the short-lived immunity and multiple strain types) make these outbreaks particularly difficult to control in these settings.[30] It appears that crowding and communal toileting may also serve as risk factors for epidemic shipboard gastroenteritis.[31–33]

While descriptions of acute gastroenteritis outbreaks on single US Navy vessels have been published,[32–35] with many anecdotes of real mission impact, epidemiologic data on rates and burden of these outbreaks is currently lacking. The Centers for Disease Control and Prevention

Table 1. Incidence of Diarrhea and Prevalence of Pathogens Among US Military and Other Long-Term Travelers Overall and From Select Geographic Regions

	Geographic Region (number of studies)			
Pathogen	Latin America & Caribbean (7)	Middle East & N. Africa (13)	Southeast Asia (12)	Summary Estimate (99% CI)
ETEC	29	28	13	22 (17 - 28)
EAEC	6	17	12	13 (8 - 19)
Campylobacter	3	1	24	10 (5 - 15)
Norovirus	9	7	9	8 (4 - 13)
Shigella	6	7	4	7 (3 - 10)
Salmonella	3	1	11	5 (3 - 7)
Rotavirus	6	2	3	4 (2 - 6)
Incidence (per 100 person-months)	30*	24	37	29 (16 - 42)

*Based on five studies.
EAEC = enteroaggregative E. *coli*; ETEC = enterotoxigenic *E. coli*.
Adapted from Riddle MS.[27]

(CDC) under Vessel Sanitation Program has established an outbreak identification threshold of $\geq$ 3% of the shipboard passengers developing AGE symptoms during a single cruise, no similar threshold has been established for the US Naval Fleet. This cutoff, developed by the CDC, was based on previous data of ship-associated outbreaks where the incidence of gastrointestinal illness was found to be $\leq$ 1% of 92% of cruises and $\geq$ 3% on 3% of cruises.[36] Riddle and colleagues conducted a retrospective cohort analysis of compiled DNBI health data collected in 2000 to 2001 from 44 US Navy ships deployed to the Persian Gulf region, and discovered 11 possible AGE outbreaks with an overall incidence of 3.3 outbreaks per 100 ship-weeks.[37] While using a different definition compared to the CDC (though not overly sensitive), these rates are 5 to 9 times as high as those reported from cruise ship data. A trend towards a higher incidence for the larger ships (> 1,000 persons on board) with 6.6 outbreaks per 100 ship-weeks compared with smaller ships, which had 2.6 outbreaks per 100 ship-weeks was found (Poisson regression, p = .08). Morbidity, represented by days lost due to personnel being placed on sick-in-quarters status, was higher during outbreak weeks compared to nonoutbreak weeks (p = .002). While this study could not attribute specific etiology to each of the outbreaks, viral etiology was suspected due to the epidemic curves, and of the several shipboard outbreaks that have been studied, most have been found to be caused by norovirus.[38] Clearly, whatever the causes of these possible shipboard outbreaks, the epidemic potential, combined with the associated morbidity, suggests an immediate need for epidemiologic research, development of rapid identification assays, outbreak intervention strategies, and prophylaxis and treatment modalities.

Diarrhea at Home

Military populations are at risk for infectious diarrhea even when not at war. By virtue of living in close quarters, recruits are at increased risk for outbreaks of infectious diarrhea. An outbreak of gastroenteritis was reported from a military training facility in El Paso, Texas, during 1998.[39] The outbreak resulted in hospitalization of 99 of 835 (12%) soldiers from one unit. Norwalk-like virus was ultimately determined to be the cause of this outbreak of gastroenteritis.

Prevention of Diarrhea in Military Deployments

Employment of preventative measures is extremely effective in decreasing infectious diarrhea rates during deployment. Hygiene may be the most effective method of diarrhea prevention. However, hand washing, reliable sources of potable water, and sanitation are often simply not compatible with the austere environment of soldiers on the battlefield. Therefore, military physicians have attempted to improve hygiene measures as well as develop other methods to prevent diarrhea. Bismuth preparations were the first prophylactic medications employed. The preparations are only marginally effective. Furthermore, they are cumbersome to take with liquid formulations and dosing schedules of up to four times daily, limiting the usefulness of these compounds in mobile military populations.

Doxycycline and trimethoprim–sulfamethoxazole (TMP–SMX) have both been demonstrated to have a role in diarrhea prevention. A direct comparison of these two agents was conducted in 1990 among naval personnel during a port call in Rio de Janeiro, Brazil. The participants were instructed to start their respective prophylactic therapy the night before and throughout the duration of the port call for a total of 6 days. Doxycycline and TMP–SMX were both found to be equally effective in diarrhea prevention. Side effects were minimal, with none reported in the doxycycline group and 3% with minor side effects in the TMP–SMX group.[40]

Along the Thai-Myanmar border, doxycycline potentially has dual benefits because it may be used for both malaria and diarrhea prophylaxis. A cautionary letter was published in 1988 by Taylor and colleagues, who noted their observations in military populations stationed in the region.[41] Fifty percent (14/28) of the US soldiers who developed diarrhea while using doxycycline for malaria prophylaxis ultimately grew *C. jejuni.* The group theorized that the use of doxycycline malaria prophylaxis may actually be increasing the likelihood of developing diarrhea with resistant *Campylobacter* spp. This observation led to a double-blind study performed at the Armed Forces Research Institute of Medical Sciences in Bangkok, Thailand. Diarrhea incidence was monitored in 253 US soldiers using either doxycycline or mefloquine malaria prophylaxis. There was no significant difference in the incidence of diarrhea in either group, with 49% in the doxycycline group and 48% in the mefloquine group reporting at least one episode of diarrhea by the end of the 5-week trial. However, the percentage of multidrug-resistant pathogenic bacteria isolated from the participants in the doxycycline group increased to 93%.[42] As drug resistance increases, the role for both doxycycline and TMP–SMX will be less useful in travelers' diarrhea prophylaxis.

Fluoroquinolone prophylaxis of travelers' diarrhea has had the best results over the past decade in both civilian and military populations. One of the first studies to illustrate the use of norfloxacin in diarrhea prophylaxis was published in 1990, in which 222 US military personnel in Egypt took part in a double-blinded randomized trial comparing the effectiveness of diarrhea prophylaxis with norfloxacin and placebo. Acute diarrhea was noted in only 2% (2/105) of those using norfloxacin prophylaxis, but in 26% (30/117) taking a placebo.[43]

A combination of hygiene measures and antibiotic prophylaxis has a potentially useful role in short-term military missions. This is demonstrated quite well by a real life scenario of British and Australian medical teams involved in Operation Safe Haven in 1991 in Northern Iraq, immediately following the Persian Gulf War. Thirty-six British and 72 Australian soldiers all had similar vaccinations and shared the same living area, food, and water. However, the Australian soldiers also took doxycycline 100 mg daily and enforced strict hand-washing and plate-washing. Over a 5-week period, the incidence of diarrhea between the two groups was noted to be markedly different. Sixty-nine percent of the British soldiers experienced at least one episode of diarrhea versus 36% of the Australian soldiers. In addition, the British soldiers had significantly more stools per day, longer duration of diarrhea, and more total days of incapacitation.[44]

One wonders which had the greater impact—doxycycline or hygiene measures? A study of 432 stool specimens collected during the Persian Gulf War may shed light on this question. Less than 50% of the specimens grew a bacterial pathogen, potentially indicating a greater incidence of viral etiologies. The bacterial pathogens isolated were most commonly ETEC, followed by *Shigella* spp. In this study, 63% of ETEC and 68% of *Shigella* spp. were resistant to tetracycline.[10] It seems clear that strict enforcement of hygiene measures were likely the biggest factor in preventing disease amongst the Australian troops. Although antibiotic prophylaxis may be helpful in some select settings, in prolonged military deployments, daily antibiotics for diarrhea prophylaxis may be difficult to adhere to and cost prohibitive.

Vaccinations for travelers' diarrhea would be highly advantageous for both travelers and military populations. Ideally, physicians would provide one vaccine to prevent all future episodes of travelers' diarrhea. Unfortunately, vaccines for travelers' diarrhea pose a developmental challenge: a separate vaccine is needed for each virus, bacteria, and even each serotype in many cases. The cholera and typhoid fever vaccines are currently the only diarrhea vaccines available; two rotavirus vaccine are licensed, but rotavirus is not typically a pathogen of concern to deployed military populations. There is, however, hope on the horizon. The military currently has active research programs dedicated to the development of *Campylobacter* spp., ETEC, and *Shigella* spp. predeployment vaccines. The ETEC, *Campylobacter jejuni*, *Shigella flexneri*, and *Shigella sonnei* vaccines are all in Phase I trials. It is hopeful there will be several predeployment vaccines available for routine use within the next decade (Stephan Savarino, private communication, October 2006).

Treatment of Diarrhea in Military Deployments

Measures to prevent diarrhea are not 100% effective, and diarrhea will most certainly occur in the military setting. Effective therapies are still needed. Oral rehydration remains the cornerstone of diarrhea therapy. The glucose-electrolyte solution, developed throughout a lifetime of research and dedication by Captain Robert Allan Phillips, has saved millions of lives worldwide.[45] Although initially developed to combat cholera, oral rehydration therapy can be used to treat all causes of diarrhea. Antimotility agents, such as loperamide, have a role in controlling the symptomatology of mild, noninvasive diarrhea. Viral etiologies of diarrhea may be quite easily treated with a combination of both antimotility agents and oral rehydration.

Therapy of invasive bacterial diarrhea is more complicated and may require antibiotics to shorten the duration of the illness. Of the bacterial etiologies of diarrhea, ETEC, EAEC, *Campylobacter* spp., and *Shigella* spp. are most commonly isolated in military populations.[27] Invasive bacterial diarrhea is often associated with fever, abdominal pain, and more than four episodes of bloody diarrhea per day. Doxycycline and TMP–SMX were once reliable therapies for these organisms, but increasing resistance has made these drugs less optimal choices over the past decade. A reasonable first line choice of therapy in a patient with this constellation of symptoms is 1 to 3 days of fluoroquinolone therapy. Many clinicians currently recommend a combination of a fluoroquinolone adjuvanted with antimotility agent because this regimen has been consistently more efficacious than antibiotic therapy alone, resulting in an average duration of diarrhea of less than half a day.

The most recent treatment trial among US Military personnel was a randomized, double-blind trial conducted at Incirlik Air Base, Turkey from June 2003 through August 2004 where a total of 207 US adults with noninflammatory diarrhea were randomized to receive a single dose of azithromycin (1,000 mg; 105 persons) or levofloxacin (500 mg; 100 persons) plus loperamide (4 mg initially and then as needed).[46] ETEC (43%) and *Campylobacter* spp. (7%) were as the most common pathogens without difference between the treatment groups. The median time between initiation of therapy and passage of the last diarrheal stool (azithromycin group, 13 hours; levofloxacin group 3 hours), resolution of associated symptoms (2 days), and additional loperamide after the initial dose (azithromycin group, 39%; levofloxacin group, 34%) were similar. Azithromycin was associated with more nausea in the 30 minutes post-dosing (azithromycin group, 8%; levofloxacin group, 1%, p = .004), but there was no vomiting or other adverse events noted in either group. This study further supports the use of loperamide adjuvanted antibiotic regimens for treatment of ambulatory diarrhea in deployed US troops to quickly return soldiers back to work in good health.

However, there is concern over antibiotic resistance, particularly evident in Asia, where *Campylobacter* spp. are often more commonly isolated than either ETEC or *Shigella* spp. *Campylobacter* spp. have demonstrated a marked increase in resistance to fluoroquinolones. Therefore, current experts recommend azithromycin for therapy in geographic areas where *Campylobacter* spp. diarrheal infections predominate.[9]

While effective regimens are available and relatively inexpensive, there appears to be a gap in use of best practices for infectious diarrhea among deployed troops. An important difference between civilian and military travel medicine is that empiric standby therapy is not usually provided to those troops who deploy. If a troop develops diarrhea, he or she will usually consult a field medic or corpsman that can provide nonprescription therapies (loperamide or bismuth subsalycilate). Alternatively, an individual could seek treatment (at "sick call") at their nearest medical treatment facility where they could be evaluated and provided antibiotic therapy if indicated. It appears that a majority (60 to 80%) of those who develop diarrhea while deployed, do not go to sick call for their illness.[17,19,27] Based on self-report data, about 50% will see their medic and only about 20% will use any form of self-treatment (medications brought from home).[19] Of those who sought care from a medic or sick call, 15% were given fluids only, 37% were provided loperamide, and 27% were treated with antibiotics (17% given intravenous rehydration). The probability of treatment with combination therapy was not reported. A single pilot study has been conducted on this subject among forward deployed US military health care providers (mostly physician assistants) attending a Professional Development and Trauma Management Conference in Doha, Qatar in 2004.[47] The survey was administered at the beginning of the conference and 58 of the 76 attendees participated by completing a questionnaire. Respondents were aware of the standard definition of travelers' diarrhea; however, their knowledge about the epidemiology and management of travelers' diarrhea was low. Less than one-third correctly answered questions on etiology, and more than two-thirds made incorrect management choices in treatment of mild-moderate watery diarrhea and dysentery.

It may be impracticable to issue every soldier, sailor, airman, and marine who is about to deploy a treatment course (or courses) of antibiotics and loperamide for the likely episode of diarrhea he or she will have. However, from these data, there is obviously an important burden of disease that is not being treated at all or is not being treated appropriately. Translational activities aimed at informing the troops on the availability and effectiveness of therapies, and giving frontline providers the knowledge and skills to appropriately manage diarrhea in the deployed setting, are clearly needed.

Summary

The modern soldier has to fight a battle far different from his ancestors, but in many ways, life on the battlefield is improved. Clean water and food supplies accompanied by proper hygiene have truly helped decrease, but not eradicate, the incidence of infectious diarrhea in military populations in recent times. However, the increase in drug-resistant organisms may make the pathogens that are able to cause disease much more difficult to treat in the future. Military strategists can only hope that effective vaccines will be available before widespread antibiotic resistance develops in diarrheal pathogens.

References

1. Osler W. The principles and practice of medicine (Appleton, New York, 1892).
2. Sartin JS. Infectious diseases during the Civil War: the triumph of the "Third Army". Clin Infect Dis 1993;16:580–4.
3. McAllister CK. Fire, blood, and the lion of the Union: Joshua Chamberlain's Civil War ailments. Pharos Alpha Omega Alpha Honor Med Soc 1998;61:40–1.
4. Cook GC. Influence of diarrhoeal disease on military and naval campaigns. J R Soc Med 2001;94:95–7.
5. Bollet A. Tuscan: Galen Press, Ltd.; 2001. p. 283–386.
6. Lawrence TE. Seven pillars of wisdom. Hants, England: Castle Hill Press; 1926. p. 23–5.
7. Kilpatrick ME. Diarrhoeal disease: current concepts and future challenges. Diarrhoeal disease—a military perspective. Trans R Soc Trop Med Hyg 1993;87Suppl 3:47–8.

8. Sheehy TW. Digestive disease as a national problem. VI. Enteric disease among United States troops in Vietnam. Gastroenterology 1968;55:105–12.

9. Wallace MR, et al. Endemic infectious diseases of Afghanistan. Clin Infect Dis 2002;34:S171–207.

10. Hyams KC, et al. Diarrheal disease during Operation Desert Shield. N Engl J Med 1991;325:1423–8.

11. Wasserman GM, et al. A survey of outpatient visits in a United States Army forward unit during Operation Desert Shield. Mil Med 1997;162:374–9.

12. Hyams KC, et al. Norwalk virus infection among Desert Storm troops. J Infect Dis 1993;167:986–7.

13. Brown D, Gray J, MacDonald P, et al. Outbreak of acute gastroenteritis associated with Norwalk-like viruses among British military personnel: Afghanistan, May 2002. MMWR Morb Mortal Wkly Rep 2002. p. 477–9.

14. Thornton SA, et al. Gastroenteritis in US Marines during Operation Iraqi Freedom. Clin Infect Dis 2005;40:519–25.

15. Bailey MS, et al. Gastroenteritis outbreak in British troops, Iraq. Emerg Infect Dis 2005;11:1625–8.

16. Matson DO. Norovirus gastroenteritis in US Marines in Iraq. Clin Infect Dis 2005;40:526–7.

17. Sanders JW, et al. Impact of illness and non-combat injury during Operations Iraqi Freedom and Enduring Freedom (Afghanistan). Am J Trop Med Hyg 2005;73:713–9.

18. Sanders JW, Putnam SD, Riddle MS, Tribble DR. Military importance of diarrhea: lessons from the Middle East. Curr Opin Gastroenterol 2005;21:9–14.

19. Putnam SD, et al. Self-reported description of diarrhea among military populations in operations Iraqi freedom and enduring freedom. J Travel Med 2006;13:92–9.

20. Murray CK, et al. Spectrum of care provided at an echelon II Medical Unit during Operation Iraqi Freedom. Mil Med 2005;170:516–20.

21. Sanders JW, Putnam SD, Antosek LE, et al. Annual Meeting of the American Society of Tropical Medicine and Hygiene (American Society of Tropical Medicine and Hygiene, Washington, DC, 2005).

22. Monteville MR, et al. Incidence, etiology, and impact of diarrhea among deployed US military personnel in support of operation Iraqi freedom and Operation Enduring Freedom. Am J Trop Med Hyg 2006;75:762–7.

23. Sanchez JL, Gelnett J, Petruccelli BP, et al. Diarrheal disease incidence and morbidity among United States military personnel during short-term missions overseas. Am J Trop Med Hyg 1998;58:299–304.

24. Daniell FD, Crafton LD, Walz SE, Bolton HT. Field preventive medicine and epidemiological surveillance: the Beirut, Lebanon experience, 1982. Mil Med 1985;150:171–6.

25. Cali G. The Italian Army Medical Corps in the United Nations "peace-keeping" operations: Somalia and Mozambique, December 1992–December 1994. Med Trop 1996;56:400–3.

26. Sharp TW, et al. Diarrheal disease among military personnel during Operation Restore Hope, Somalia, 1992–1993. Am J Trop Med Hyg 1995;52:188–93.

27. Riddle MS, Sanders JW, Putnam SD, Tribble DR. Incidence, etiology, and impact of diarrhea among long-term travelers (US military and similar populations): a systematic review. Am J Trop Med Hyg 2006;74:891–900.

28. Glass RI, et al. Gastroenteritis viruses: an overview. Novartis Found Symp 2001;238:5–19.

29. Lopman BA, Reacher MH, Vipond IB, Sarangi J, Brown DW. Clinical manifestation of norovirus gastroenteritis in health care settings. Clin Infect Dis 2004;39:318–24.

30. Bresee JS, Widdowson MA, Monroe SS, Glass RI. Foodborne viral gastroenteritis: challenges and opportunities. Clin Infect Dis 2002;35:748–53.

31. Foote F. Navy Medicine. https://navymedicine.med.navy.mil/Files/Media/ecm/sitedata/93E9008D-802E-D019-ABBA0925B2764081/library/Issuefinalrevised21705.pdf (accessed 14 May 2005).

32. Sharp TW, et al. Epidemiology of Norwalk virus during an outbreak of acute gastroenteritis aboard a US aircraft carrier. J Med Virol 1995;45:61–7.

33. Thornton S, et al. Detection of Norwalk-like virus infection aboard two U.S. Navy ships. Mil Med 2002;167:826–30.

34. Whittaker DR, Campbell JT, McCarten MD. Viral gastroenteritis: the USS THEODORE ROOSEVELT experience. Mil Med 2004;169:747–50.

35. Oyofo BA, et al. Norwalk-like virus and bacterial pathogens associated with cases of gastroenteritis onboard a US Navy ship. Am J Trop Med Hyg 1999;61:904–8.

36. Merson MH, Hughes JM, Wood BT, Yashuk JC, Wells JG. Gastrointestinal illness on passenger cruise ships. Jama 1975;231:723–7.

37. Riddle MS, et al. Epidemic infectious gastrointestinal illness aboard U.S. Navy ships deployed to the Middle East during peacetime operations—2000–2001. BMC Gastroenterol 2006;6:9.

38. DOD-GEIS. Viral gastroenteritis surveillance and diagnosis aboard U.S. Navy vessels. http://www.geis.fhp.osd.mil/GEIS/aboutGEIS/annualreports.asp (accessed 1993).

39. Arness M, Canham M, Geighner B, et al. Norwalk-like viral gastroenteritis in U.S. Army Trainees—Texas, 1998. Morb Mortal Wkly Rep 1999;225–7.

40. Hipskind JE. A prophylactic program to prevent traveler's diarrhea in United States Naval personnel comparing

doxycycline and trimethoprim-sulfamethoxazole. Mil Med 1993;158:141–4.

41. Taylor DN, Pitarangsi C, Echeverria P, Diniega BM. Campylobacter enteritis during doxycycline prophylaxis for malaria in Thailand [letter]. Lancet 1988;2:578–9.

42. Arthur JD, et al. A comparative study of gastrointestinal infections in United States soldiers receiving doxycycline or mefloquine for malaria prophylaxis. Am J Trop Med Hyg 1990;43:608–13.

43. Scott DA, Haberberger RL, Thornton SA, Hyams KC. Norfloxacin for the prophylaxis of travelers' diarrhea in U.S. military personnel. Am J Trop Med Hyg 1990;42:160–4.

44. Rudland S, Little M, Kemp P, et al. The enemy within: diarrheal rates among British and Australian troops in Iraq. Mil Med 1996;161:728–31.

45. Savarino SJ. A legacy in 20th-century medicine: Robert Allan Phillips and the taming of cholera. Clin Infect Dis 2002;35:713–20.

46. Sanders JW, et al. Annual Meeting of the Infectious Diseases Society of America (San Francisco: 2005).

47. Riddle MS, et al. Knowledge, attitudes, and practices regarding epidemiology and management of travelers' diarrhea: a survey of front-line providers in Iraq and Afghanistan. Mil Med 2005;170:492–5.

PART THREE

CLINICAL FEATURES

CHAPTER 16

GENETIC SUSCEPTIBILITY TO ENTERIC INFECTIONS: IMPLICATIONS FOR ENDEMIC AND TRAVELERS' DIARRHEA

PABLO C. OKHUYSEN, MD

STEPHANIE A. LEE, MD

RICHARD L. GUERRANT, MD

Susceptibility to gastrointestinal infection is determined by the complex interplay of environmental, host, and pathogen factors. In the past, our approach to understanding infectious diseases focused on the study of each one of these contributors individually, with emphasis predominantly on the environment and the specific microorganisms while the role of the host was limited to studies on pathogenesis and the immune response. Until a few decades ago, our knowledge on the contribution of genetics to susceptibility to infectious diseases was limited to a few well-characterized familial syndromes with clearly defined phenotypes. Although long suspected, genetics was also thought to contribute to the variability in individual response to common and uncommon infections. The advent of the genomic era has revolutionized our understanding of the genetic basis for host susceptibility to infection.

Examples on the impact that polymorphisms in the human genome have on infection are numerous. The strongest associations being with infectious diseases that are parasitic and or chronic in nature such as Leishmaniasis,[1] tuberculosis,[2] leprosy,[3] malaria[4] and human immunodeficiency virus (HIV) infection among others. Associations have been made between single nucleotide polymorphisms (SNPs) in the mannose binding lectin gene and its promoter with acute bacterial diseases such as meningococcemia,[5] infections in neutropenic patients[6] and more recently in recipients of stem cell transplants.[7] Gene polymorphisms in Toll-like receptors (TLR), which are vital in the recognition of infectious agents, have been described in the setting of bacterial infections[8] and variants in tumor necrosis alpha (TNFα) have been implicated in an unfavorable prognosis in the setting of sepsis and pneumonia.[9,10] It follows that genetic polymorphisms are of relevance in gastrointestinal infections since the gastrointestinal tract is the largest contact surface with the environment and potential pathogens and home to the largest proportion of immune effector cells.

Every year, over 70 million adults and children from developed nations travel to tropical and semitropical areas of the world.[11] At-risk adults typically lack specific immunity to the agents of travelers' diarrhea and become infected pathogens that are commonly identified in infants and children of endemic regions. It is estimated that approximately 40% of individuals at risk will develop diarrhea.[12] The syndrome of travelers' diarrhea is an important cause of morbidity in military troops during deployment[13,14] and can decrease military performance by temporarily disabling 1 of every 5 soldiers.[15] Bacterial enteropathogens account for up to 85% of cases. Enterotoxigenic *E. coli*, enteroaggregative *E. coli*

(EAEC), *Shigella* species, *Campylobacter jejuni,* and *Salmonella* species account for the majority of cases, while *Aeromonas* species, *Plesiomonas* species, and non-*cholerae Vibrio* species are isolated infrequently. Within the remainder 15%, a subset of individuals respond to antibiotic therapy, suggesting that these cases are also due to bacterial agents that are yet to be characterized or that current diagnostic techniques are not sensitive enough to detect small numbers of enteropathogens. Although the relative proportions of enteric pathogens causing diarrhea vary according to the season and region of the world studied, the relative proportions of cases remain fairly constant from year to year when similar at-risk populations are studied in the same season and geographical locale over time. This suggests that in an environment where food and water are frequently contaminated,[16] individual host factors determine susceptibility to infection. In this chapter we review emerging data on host genetic susceptibility to infection with agents of diarrhea and its implications in travelers' diarrhea. Examples are provided on how polymorphisms in genes of the innate immunity, those that mediate the initial adherence and colonization by enteropathogens, respond with inflammation during injury or process electrolyte exchange or antigens are important in determining outcomes after infection.

Host Variation in Innate Immunity

The innate immune system is a complex group of molecules that represent the first line of defense against enteric pathogens and is composed of collectins, defensins, and components of the complement cascade and toll-like receptors, among others. Genetic defects in the innate immune system can lead to increased susceptibility to infection by failing to recognize signals from pathogens and are of particular relevance in subjects in whom other components of the immune system may be compromised. This can be seen for instance with cryptosporidiosis and HIV co-infection.

Cryptosporidium parvum and *C. hominis* are the predominant species of *Cryptosporidium* that infect humans. The low infectious dose and hardiness of this protozoan parasite favors waterborne and person to person transmission through fecal-oral routes. Infections with *Cryptosporidium* are responsible for a self-limited infection in immunocompetent individuals; however in immunocompromised patients, particularly in advanced AIDS, it can cause incapacitating disease that is sometimes fatal. Cell-mediated immunity is critical in controlling the infection; however, some patients with advanced HIV disease can sometimes spontaneously control the infection[17] presumably via the innate immune system.

Mannose-binding lectin (MBL) is able to activate the complement system in an antibody independent fashion and is an important mediator of innate immunity to many agents. Mutations in MBL have been associated with an increased risk of infection.[18] MBL polymorphisms that result in low or dysfunctional MBL levels have been studied in HIV infected Zambian patients with persistent diarrhea due to cryptosporidiosis[19] There are at least two patients reported in the literature who developed persistent diarrhea with cryptosporidium whose only known immunodeficiency was homozygosity for MBL mutation,[20] additionally low levels of MBL have also been associated with cryptosporidiosis in Haitian children with diarrhea.[21]

Host Variation in Molecules that Facilitate Pathogen Adhesion or Colonization

Enteric pathogens frequently co-opt host molecules as their specific receptors; examples include the cystic fibrosis conductance regulator in the case of some species of *Salmonella,*[22] blood group antigens and secretor antigens for the case of norovirus, CD55 for a subset of diffusely adhering *E. coli.* Thus, variation in the genes of proteins that serve as receptors may be associated with variable degrees of susceptibility

A prototypic agent that co-opts a host molecule as a receptor is Norwalk virus, which was originally identified in stools collected from a winter time acute gastroenteritis outbreak in an elementary school in Norwalk, Ohio in 1968.[23] It is now recognized as a calicivirus that, with other noroviruses, is the most common cause of nonbacterial acute gastroenteritis in the US and is a major cause of epidemics and sporadic disease worldwide. The infectious dose for this agent is very small and can be transmitted via fecal oral transmission. Crowded environments, contaminated food, and water frequently lead to outbreaks of gastroenteritis in communities, cruise ships, nursing homes, as well as in the military. Norwalk-like viruses are increasingly becoming recognized as important agents of travelers' diarrhea.

In challenge studies done with Norwalk virus on volunteers in the 1970s, it was noted that a group of participants was resistant to infection. Parrino and colleagues[24] found that of 12 subjects challenged, only 6 became ill, and that when the subjects were rechallenged 1 to 2 years later, only those who had become ill with the first challenge became ill a second time. It was also noted that serum antibodies to the virus measured prior to the initial challenge predicted susceptibility to infection instead of immunity, and the authors suggested that a genetic factor, perhaps a receptor, might explain their results. It was then recognized that O type and few type B red blood cells can be agglutinate in the presence by Norovirus.[25,26] Hutson and colleagues hypothesized that uninfected volunteers who were challenged with Norwalk virus would express the type B antigen. Data from 51 volunteers showed that persons with type O phenotype were significantly more likely to become infected with Norwalk virus, and that individuals expressing type B antigen had a decreased risk of developing symptomatic disease.[27]

The molecular basis for the A, B, and O blood group phenotypes is determined by the presence or absence of specific carbohydrate antigens on glycolipids and glycoproteins. These glycoproteins were originally identified in red blood cells but can also be found on the surface of mucosal epithelial cells. The finding of decreased susceptibility to Norwalk virus infection with type B antigen would suggest that the presence of a terminal alpha-galactose could modify the ability for Norwalk virus binding.[27] However, this finding did not completely explain the susceptibility because it did not account for the individuals of the A and O phenotypes who remained uninfected.

The cloning and expression of the Norwalk virus capsid protein was of use in understanding this interaction further. Through self assembly, this protein can form virus-like particles (VLPs). We now know that VLPs bind to the H type-1 glycoprotein in the gastroduodenal epithelial cells of the so called secretors, but not to cells from nonsecretors.[28] The secretor status phenotype is determined by the *FUT2* gene, which encodes an enzyme required for the synthesis of carbohydrate H type-1determinant found on epithelial cells and mucosal secretions.[20] This gene is inactivated by a G428 nonsense mutation that is found in approximately 20% of Europeans,[29] and at least five other inactivating mutations have also been described. Lindesmith and colleagues analyzed saliva samples in volunteers challenged with Norwalk virus and found that secretor status is an important predictor of susceptibility. Norwalk VLPs bound to saliva from group O and A secretors, but much less to group B secretors, whereas it did not bind to any of the saliva from nonsecretors.[28] However, this binding specificity is not general to all noroviruses. Recent publications[30,31] suggest that within the different noroviruses there is variable binding to the ABO and secretor schema, and that some, like Snow Mountain Virus, use receptors that are different to the H type determinants.

VIBRIO CHOLERAE

Although an unusual cause of diarrhea in travelers, the factors associated with host susceptibility to infection with *Vibrio cholerae* are probably the best studied and provide some insights associated with other agents.

Over 30 years ago it was recognized that cholera patients were more likely to be of the blood group O.[32] This was later demonstrated in volunteer challenge studies, where individuals with group O had more severe clinical manifestations.[33] Although first thought to be related to infection with *Vibrio cholerae* O1 and the El Tor biotype, the connection has also been shown to exist with the non-O1 *V. cholerae* serogroup O139.[34] However, recent epidemiologic studies in Bangladesh have shown that subjects with blood group O are less susceptible to infection with *V cholerae O1* but when infected are more likely to have severe illness, suggesting that the relevance of the blood group is more likely to be at a later stage of infection and the effects of cholera toxin than with the early colonization or adherence of the enteropathogen.

This association is proving to be important in determining cholera vaccine efficacy. Inactivated oral cholera vaccines do not protect persons of blood group O as well as the other groups.[35] Conversely, the attenuated live cholera vaccine strain CVD 103-HgR appeared to elicit a stronger response in those with blood group O and confers better protection for these individuals.[36] Similar correlates will be relevant in the development of new vaccines.

Host Variability in Inflammatory Response

EAEC is a common cause of diarrhea worldwide. Initially, this *E. coli* pathotype was described in children of developing countries with acute and persistent diarrhea and later in adults from developed countries traveling to undeveloped regions of the world as well as in patients co-infected with HIV. Recent studies suggest that it is also an important pathogen in children with diarrhea in the US.[37]

Studies looking at the natural history of EAEC infection in healthy students traveling to Mexico have suggested that some individuals are more susceptible than others to infection[16] and that asymptomatic colonization with EAEC is common. When symptomatic, EAEC can cause secretory or inflammatory diarrhea with fecal leukocytes, and elevated lactoferrin levels. EAEC carrying the *aggR* regulon are more likely to produce inflammatory diarrhea and elevated levels of fecal interleukin (IL)-8, a pro-inflammatory chemokine.[38] The differences in clinical manifestations with EAEC are partially explained by host genetic variability in inflammatory response. Subjects with the AA polymorphism in the promoter region (-251) of the IL-8 gene produce higher levels of IL-8. A study in US travelers showed that subjects with EAEC diarrhea were more likely to belong to the high IL-8 producer genotype[39] whereas those with asymptomatic infection or with pathogen negative diarrhea belonged to the low IL-8 producer genotype.

Host Variability in Antigen Processing

Entamoeba histolytica is an intestinal protozoan parasite that can cause amebic colitis, amebic liver abscess, and extra-intestinal disease. It is an infection commonly seen among children in the developing world and can result in lethal dysentery. Careful epidemiologic studies in endemic areas suggest that only 1 in every 5 infections with *E. histolytica* resulted in symptoms, and that a lack of serum antiparasite IgG is associated with resistance to infection. Further analysis demonstrated that this phenomena was noted to be clustered in families,[40] and it has been hypothesized that children who lack serum anti-amebic IgG have a more robust innate immune response, preventing parasite invasion into the intestinal epithelium and thereby preventing a systemic IgG immune response. Human leukocyte antigen (HLA) studies have demonstrated a protective association of the HLA class II allele DQB1*0601 and the heterozygous haplotype DQB1*0601/DRB1*1501.[41]

Genetic Determinants of the Impact of Early Childhood Diarrhea

Not only are specific infections determined by host genetics, but the long-term impact of common early childhood diarrhea in highly endemic areas may also have important host genetic determinants. Data over recent years are increasingly showing that common diarrheal illnesses in the first 2 formative years of life in areas lacking adequate water and sanitation may have substantial lasting consequences for physical and cognitive development.[42–46] Furthermore, heritable traits appear to determine significant portions of the variance in endemic diarrhea rates,[47] much as they do Ascaris worm burdens.[48,49] As an example, the apolipoprotein allele ApoE4 that is associated with increased risk of Alzheimer's and cardiovascular disease in later life appears to actually protect children in impoverished areas against the cognitive impairment seen with heavy diarrhea burdens in their early childhood[50] In addition to ApoE4, the understanding of other genetic traits, which regulate body index and energy balance, host immune and inflammatory responses, critical to the recovery from infection and catch-up growth, will help elucidate potential therapeutic and preventive approaches, especially in children in developing areas. Hence host genetics influence not only the susceptibility to enteric infections, but also their acute manifestations and longer-term developmental consequences.

Conclusions and Future Directions

Our understanding of the contribution that genetics has on enteric infections and their complications is in its infancy. Only few studies are published and have been conducted for the most part in developing countries where diarrheal diseases are endemic. The relevance of host genetics and the pathways associated with infection may differ in travelers from developed countries, and additional studies are needed in both settings. It is likely that variability in host receptors mediating adherence and colonization, the cytokines and effector molecules of the innate and acquired immune systems will dictate not only susceptibility but also the intensity of the host response and the clinical manifestations associated with infection. Furthermore, in a redundant and complicated system such as the gut-associated lymphoid tissue system, the genetic contribution will be likely be multigenic with strong environmental-, geographical-, and pathogen-specific determinants. Unraveling the complex role host genetics play in vulnerability to both the cognitive and physical long-term consequences of diarrheal diseases among children will further elucidate ways to interrupt the cycle of enteric infections and their consequences in developing areas around the world. Similar studies in travelers will assist with not only decreasing the risk for travelers' diarrhea but also its long-term consequences, such as postinfectious irritable bowel and reactive arthritis. Future studies in large populations with genome-wide approaches will be of use in developing more accurate, risk modeling optimized strategies for prevention of travelers' diarrhea through chemoprevention or vaccines and could result in the identification of new microbial targets for pharmacological therapy.

References

1. Blackwell JM. Tumour necrosis factor alpha and mucocutaneous leishmaniasis. Parasitology Today 1999;15:73–5.
2. Bellamy R. Identifying genetic susceptibility factors for tuberculosis in Africans: a combined approach using a candidate gene study and a genome-wide screen. Clin Sci 2000;98:245–50.
3. Greiner J, Weber FJ, Mauff G, Baur M. Genetic polymorphisms of properdin factor B(Bf), the second

component (C2), and the fourth component (C4) of complement in leprosy patients and healthy controls from Thailand. Immunobiology 1980;158(1–2):134–8.

4. Luty AJ, Kun JF, Kremsner PG. Mannose-binding lectin plasma levels and gene polymorphisms in Plasmodium falciparum malaria. J Infect Dis 1998;178:1221–4.
5. Bax WA, Cluysenaer OJ, Bartelink AK, et al. Association of familial deficiency of mannose-binding lectin and meningococcal disease. Lancet 1999;354:1094–5.
6. Ezekowitz RA. Mannose-binding lectin in prediction of susceptibility to infection. [letter; comment]. Lancet 2001; 358:598–9.
7. Mullighan CG, Heatley S, Doherty K, et al. Mannose-binding lectin gene polymorphisms are associated with major infection following allogeneic hemopoietic stem cell transplantation. Blood 2002;99:3524–9.
8. Read RC, Pullin J, Gregory S, et al. A functional polymorphism of toll-like receptor 4 is not associated with likelihood or severity of meningococcal disease. J Infect Dis 2001;184:640–2.
9. Majetschak M, Flohe S, Obertacke U, et al. Relation of a TNF gene polymorphism to severe sepsis in trauma patients. Ann Surg 1999;230:207–14.
10. Shimazu T, Shimaoka M, Sugimoto H, Taenaka N, Hasegawa T. Does blood type B protect against haemolytic uraemic syndrome? An analysis of the 1996 Sakai outbreak of Escherichia coli O157:H7 (VTEC O157) infection. The Osaka HUS Critical Care Study Group. J Infect 2000;41:45–9.
11. Keystone J, Steffen R, Kozarsky P. Health advice for international travel in tropical infectious diseases: principles, pathogens and practice. 2nd ed. Philadelphia: Churchill Livingstone, Elsevier; 2006.
12. Ramzan NN. Traveler's diarrhea. Gastroenterol Clin North Am 2001;30:665–78.
13. Sharp TW, Thornton SA, Wallace MR, et al. Diarrheal disease among military personnel during Operation Restore Hope, Somalia, 1992–1993. Am J Tropical Medicine & Hygiene 1995;52(2):188–93.
14. Sanchez JL, Gelnett J, Petruccelli BP, Defraites RF, Taylor DN. Diarrheal disease incidence and morbidity among United States military personnel during short-term missions overseas. Am J Trop Med Hyg 1998;58:299–304.
15. Hyams KC, Bourgeois AL, Merrell BR, et al. Diarrheal disease during Operation Desert Shield. [see comments.]. N Eng J Med 1991;325:1423–8.
16. Adachi JA, Ericsson CD, Jiang ZD, et al. Natural history of enteroaggregative and enterotoxigenic Escherichia coli infection among US travelers to Guadalajara, Mexico. J Infect Dis 2002;185:1681–3.
17. Hewitt RG, Yiannoutsos CT, Higgs ES, et al. Paromomycin: no more effective than placebo for treatment of cryptosporidiosis in patients with advanced human immunodeficiency virus infection. AIDS Clinical Trial Group. Clin Infect Dis 2000;31:1084–92.
18. Summerfield JA, Sumiya M, Levin M, Turner MW. Association of mutations in mannose binding protein gene with childhood infection in consecutive hospital series. [see comments]. BMJ 1997;314:1229–32.
19. Kelly P, Jack DL, Naeem A, et al. Mannose-binding lectin is a component of innate mucosal defense against Cryptosporidium parvum in AIDS. Gastroenterology 2000;119:1236–42.
20. Rouquier S, Lowe JB, Kelly RJ, et al. Molecular cloning of a human genomic region containing the H blood group alpha(1,2)fucosyltransferase gene and two H locus-related DNA restriction fragments. Isolation of a candidate for the human Secretor blood group locus. J Biol Chem 1995;270: 4632–9.
21. Kirkpatrick BD, Huston CD, Wagner D, et al. Serum mannose-binding lectin deficiency is associated with cryptosporidiosis in young Haitian children. Clin Infect Dis 2006;43:289–94.
22. Pier GB, Grout M, Zaidi T, et al. Salmonella typhi uses CFTR to enter intestinal epithelial cells. Nature 1998;393:79–82.
23. Adler JL, Zickl R. Winter vomiting disease. J Infect Dis 1969;119:668–73.
24. Parrino TA, Schreiber DS, Trier JS, et al. Clinical immunity in acute gastroenteritis caused by Norwalk agent. N Engl J Med 1977;297:86–9.
25. Green KY, Lew JF, Jiang X, et al. Comparison of the reactivities of baculovirus-expressed recombinant Norwalk virus capsid antigen with those of the native Norwalk virus antigen in serologic assays and some epidemiologic observations. J Clin Microbiol 1993;31:2185–91.
26. Prasad BV, Hardy ME, Dokland T, et al. X-ray crystallographic structure of the Norwalk virus capsid. Science 1999;286:287–90.
27. Hutson AM, Atmar RL, Graham DY, Estes MK. Norwalk virus infection and disease is associated with ABO histo-blood group type. J Infect Dis 2002;185:1335–7.
28. Lindesmith L, Moe C, Marionneau S, et al. Human susceptibility and resistance to Norwalk virus infection. Nat Med 2003;9:548–53.
29. Marionneau S, Ruvoen N, Le Moullac-Vaidye B, et al. Norwalk virus binds to histo-blood group antigens present on gastroduodenal epithelial cells of secretor individuals. Gastroenterology 2002;122:1967–77.
30. Rockx BH, Vennema H, Hoebe CJ, et al. Association of histo-blood group antigens and susceptibility to norovirus infections. J Infect Dis 2005;191:749–54.
31. Lindesmith L, Moe C, Lependu J, et al. Cellular and humoral immunity following Snow Mountain virus challenge. J Virol 2005;79:2900–9.

32. Barua D, Paguio AS. ABO blood groups and cholera. Ann Hum Biol 1977;4:489–92.

33. Levine MM, Nalin DR, Rennels MB, et al. Genetic susceptibility to cholera. Ann Hum Biol 1979;6:369–74.

34. Faruque AS, Mahalanabis D, Hoque SS, Albert MJ. The relationship between ABO blood groups and susceptibility to diarrhea due to Vibrio cholerae 0139. Clin Infect Dis 1994;18:827–8.

35. Clemens JD, Sack DA, Harris JR, et al. ABO blood groups and cholera: new observations on specificity of risk and modification of vaccine efficacy. J Infect Dis 1989;159:770–3.

36. Lagos R, Avendano A, Prado V, et al. Attenuated live cholera vaccine strain CVD 103-HgR elicits significantly higher serum vibriocidal antibody titers in persons of blood group O. Infect Immun 1995;63:707–9.

37. Cohen MB, Nataro JP, Bernstein DI, et al. Prevalence of diarrheagenic Escherichia coli in acute childhood enteritis: a prospective controlled study. J Pediatr 2005;146:54–61.

38. Jiang ZD, Greenberg D, Nataro JP, et al. Rate of occurrence and pathogenic effect of enteroaggregative Escherichia coli virulence factors in international travelers. J Clin Microbiol 2002;40:4185–90.

39. Jiang ZD, Okhuysen PC, Guo DC, et al. Genetic susceptibility to enteroaggregative Escherichia coli diarrhea: polymorphism in the interleukin-8 promotor region. J Infect Dis 2003;188:506–11.

40. Haque R, Duggal P, Ali IM, et al. Innate and acquired resistance to amebiasis in Bangladeshi children. J Infect Dis 2002;186:547–52.

41. Duggal P, Haque R, Roy S, et al. Influence of human leukocyte antigen class II alleles on susceptibility to Entamoeba histolytica infection in Bangladeshi children. J Infect Dis 2004;189:520–6.

42. Guerrant DI, Moore SR, Lima AA, et al. Association of early childhood diarrhea and cryptosporidiosis with impaired physical fitness and cognitive function four-seven years later in a poor urban community in northeast Brazil. Am J Trop Med Hyg 1999;61:707–13.

43. Niehaus MD, Moore SR, Patrick PD, et al. Early childhood diarrhea is associated with diminished cognitive function 4 to 7 years later in children in a northeast Brazilian shantytown. Am J Trop Med Hyg 2002;66:590–3.

44. Patrick PD, Oria RB, Madhavan V, et al. Limitations in verbal fluency following heavy burdens of early childhood diarrhea in Brazilian shantytown children. Child Neuropsychol 2005;11:233–44.

45. Lorntz B, Soares AM, Moore SR, et al. Early childhood diarrhea predicts impaired school performance. Pediatr Infect Dis J 2006;25:513–20.

46. Checkley W, Epstein LD, Gilman RH, et al. Effects of acute diarrhea on linear growth in Peruvian children. Am J Epidemiol 2003;157:166–75.

47. Pinkerton R, Williams-Blangero S, Lima AA, Guerrant RL. Heritability as a major determinant of early childhood diarrhea. Amer J Trop Med Hyg 2007; submitted.

48. Williams-Blangero S, VandeBerg JL, Subedi J, et al. Genes on chromosomes 1 and 13 have significant effects on Ascaris infection. Proc Natl Acad Sci U S A 2002;99:5533–8.

49. Williams-Blangero S, Subedi J, Upadhayay RP, et al. Genetic analysis of susceptibility to infection with Ascaris lumbricoides. Am J Trop Med Hyg 1999;60:921–6.

50. Oria RB, Patrick PD, Zhang H, et al. APOE4 protects the cognitive development in children with heavy diarrhea burdens in Northeast Brazil. Pediatr Res 2005; 57:310–6.

CHAPTER 17

TRAVELERS' DIARRHEA: CLINICAL FEATURES AND SYNDROMES

GILBERT R. KAUFMANN, MD

LEENA MATTILA, MD, PhD

NIKLAUS GYR, MD, MPH, TM

An infectious etiology for travelers' diarrhea (TD) was confirmed in the 1970s. The discovery of important enteropathogens such as *Campylobacter* and *Rotavirus*, the development of new laboratory methods, and the understanding of the mechanisms of action of cholera toxin led to investigations that demonstrated the existence of enterotoxins in *Escherichia (E.) coli* and other bacteria.[1–3]

TD is defined as the occurrence of three or more watery or unformed stools per day during a journey, or any number of such stools, if accompanied by fever, abdominal cramps, nausea, tenesmus, vomiting, or chills.[4–6] It is usually an acute diarrhea characterized by a short duration of 3 to 4 days and uncommonly meets the criteria of persistent diarrhea that lasts for longer than 14 days. Symptoms are prolonged for more than 7 days in 8 to 15% of cases. Two percent of patients even develop chronic diarrhea lasting at least 1 month.[7] Small children are more prone to severe, long-lasting illness and can show multiple relapses. The symptoms are the consequence of bacterial colonization, the production of enterotoxins, and intestinal inflammation.

Bacteria are responsible for the majority of TD cases, but viruses and parasites are important as well. In 8 to 20% of cases, two or more pathogens are responsible for symptoms of TD. However, the reason for TD remains unknown in 10 to 30% of cases. The incidence of TD is not the same throughout the year and may vary according to the season. The principal agents in high-risk areas are, in decreasing order of importance, enterotoxigenic *E. coli* (ETEC), *Salmonella enterica*, *Shigella* spp., *Campylobacter* spp. and *Aeromonas* spp.[8] The symptoms associated with different etiologic agents are very similar, especially within the first days. The clinician has usually a difficult task to predict the etiology of TD.[9]

Acute infectious diarrhea can be roughly classified according to whether an obvious inflammation or an invasive process is present or not. However, the classification is not clear-cut, and overlapping syndromes exist. The syndromes can be classified into noninflammatory or secretory diarrhea and into inflammatory or dysenteric diarrhea. *Vibrio cholerae* and ETEC cause a secretory diarrhea with voluminous watery stools (Table 1). These pathogens produce enterotoxins that affect the intestinal water balance and fluxes of electrolytes. Typically, this mechanism is not associated with an inflammation or invasion of the pathogen. On the other hand, *Shigella* spp. are typical pathogens causing mucosal damage, ulcers, and an acute inflammation of the lamina propria by invasion. The consequence is a dysentery syndrome with multiple, usually 10 to 30, small-volume bloody and purulent stools. This form of diarrhea is typically accompanied by abdominal cramps, fever, tenesmus, and fecal urgency. For many years *Shigella* spp. were thought to be the only bacteria that cause dysentery, but it is now clear that dysenteric diarrhea may be caused by enteroinvasive *E. coli* (EIEC), enterohemorrhagic *E. coli* (EHEC), some *Campylobacter* spp., most Salmonella serovars, *Entamoeba histolytica* and *Vibrio parahemolyticus*. However, a mixed picture of secretory and dysentery syndrome is frequently observed. The reason for this observation is that many invasive organisms causing dysentery also produce enterotoxins. Representative examples include *Campylobacter jejuni*, *Salmonella* spp., *Yersinia (Y.) enterocolitica*, EIEC, and EHEC (Table 2). Bacteria causing classic toxin-related food poisoning, such as *Staphylococcus aureus*, *Clostridium perfringens* and *Bacillus cereus* may also be a reason for TD. The possibility of histamine poisoning should be particularly considered if patients suffer from

Table 1 Characteristics of the Cholera-Like Secretory Syndrome and the Dysentery Syndrome

	Dysentery Syndrome	Secretory Syndrome
Clinical Characteristics		
Stool volume	Small	Large
Stool Characteristics	Bloody, purulent	Watery
Pain	Left lower abdominal quadrant	Periumbilical
Vomitus	Rare	Common
Tenesmus	Common	Absent
Fever	Common	Occasionally
Anatomic site	Colon, ileum	Small bowel

headache, palpitations, and skin symptoms in addition to the typical gastrointestinal complaints.

Noninflammatory or Secretory Diarrhea

ETEC

The most frequent pathogen in travelers causing a secretory syndrome is ETEC. The organism passes the acid barrier of the stomach and colonizes the mucosa of the small bowel. It acts through its heat-labile (LT) and heat-stable (ST) enterotoxins, but it does not cause any damage to the mucosa, nor is it associated with bacteremia or a systemic illness.[10] The incubation period ranges from 24 to 48 hours. The clinical picture is characterized by a distress of the upper intestinal tract, followed by watery diarrhea. Symptoms can be mild with only a few loose stools, but can also reach the severity of cholera, causing life-threatening dehydration, particularly in children. ETEC infections are usually self limited, lasting for 3 days.[9]

Table 2 Pathogens Causing Infectious Diarrhea

	Watery Diarrhea	Dysentery
Viruses		
Rotavirus	+	-
Norwalk virus	+	-
Bacteria		
V. cholerae	+	-
V. parahaemolyticus	+	+
Aeromonas spp	+	-
ETEC	+	-
EPEC	+	-
EIEC	+	+
EHEC	+	+
Shigella spp	+	+
Salmonella spp	+	+
Campylobacter spp	+	+
Yersinia enterocolitica	+	+
Plesiomonas shigelloides	+	+
Protozoa		
Giardia lamblia	+	+
Cryptosporidium parvum	+	+
Microsporidia	+	+
Isospora belli	+	+
Cyclospora cayetanensis	+	+
Entamoeba histolytica	+	+

VIBRIO CHOLERAE

Vibrio cholerae is not a frequent agent of TD, but is a classical example of a pathogen causing watery, secretory diarrhea. Infections with *Vibrio* bacteria are acquired after ingestion of contaminated water, fish, and shellfish. In addition, they are frequently found in conditions of poor sanitation, although outbreaks of cholera have been reported in environments without pollution. The incubation period ranges from several hours to 5 days and depends on the inoculum size. The onset of cholera caused by *Vibrio cholerae* O1 and 0139 is generally rapid with painless watery diarrhea. The diarrhea may continue for 1 to 5 days. The stool contains flecks of mucus, known as rice water stool that is associated with a high mortality of 50% in untreated individuals. Mild fever may occur, but signs of septicemia are absent.

The major complication of cholera is a rapid and extensive dehydration as a result of the massive loss of intestinal fluid. The maximum volume of stool is excreted after 24 hours, which can easily reach 500 to 1,000 mL per hour, resulting in a daily fluid loss of 15 to 20 liters. As a consequence, electrolyte disturbances, hypokalemia, and metabolic acidosis may develop. The clinical signs of severe dehydration include a reduced skin turgor, hoarseness, sunken bulbi, dry mucous membranes, washerwomen's hands, missing pulses, cold extremities, hypothermia, hypovolemic shock, impaired renal function, and change of consciousness (Figure 1).

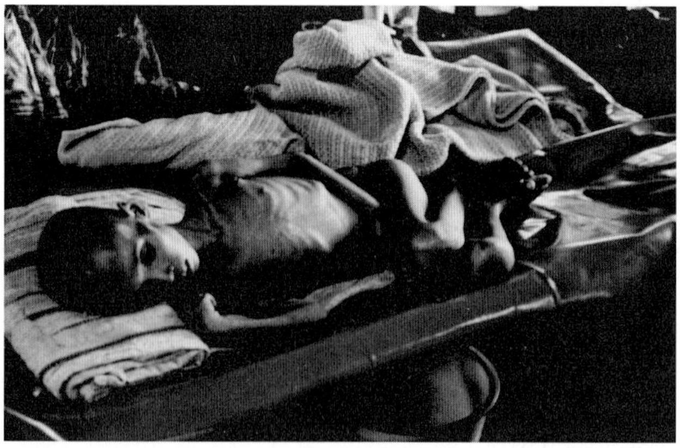

Figure 1 Child suffering from cholera with severe symptoms of dehydration.

Inflammatory or Dysenteric Diarrhea

SHIGELLOSIS

The classical Shigella enterocolitis causes a dysentery syndrome and has been reported all over the world. In general, the most common species in developed countries is *S. sonnei*, whereas the least common one is *S. dysenteriae*. *S. flexneri*, *S. boydii*, and *S. dysenteriae* account for most isolates from developing countries. The mode of transmission of Shigellosis is the direct person-to-person contact or an indirect fecal-oral transmission from symptomatic patients. The incubation period ranges from 36 to 72 hours.

The clinical picture can vary from mild to severe forms of dysentery with systemic toxicity. The initial phase is characterized by fatigue, anorexia, watery diarrhea, and abdominal cramps. In 40% of cases, the body temperature is elevated, reaching 38° to 40°C. Within 24 hours, the abdominal pain wanders to the lower quadrants and the characteristics of diarrhea changes to multiple small-volume bowel movements. Before and after bowel movements, strong tenesmus occurs. One-third of affected individuals show the typical dysentery stool.[11,12] The infection is primarily located in the colon, but may spread to the terminal ileum. Endoscopically, the lamina propria of affected areas shows scattered ulcers. The average duration of symptoms is 7 days, but more severe cases can remain symptomatic for 3 to 4 weeks and are more likely to show a relapse of the infection. Malnutrition and *S. dysenteriae* type I infections have both been associated with a more severe course of the disease. Mortality is particularly high in young children in developing countries. However, Shigella infections are rare in travelers, occurring in 0 to 7%. Fecal excretion of Shigella for more than 3 months has been observed in less than 1% of patients and permanent Shigella carriers are very rare.

Shigellosis may be complicated by toxic megacolon, colonic perforation, and large intestinal loss of protein. The major histocompatibility antigen (HLA) B 27 positive subjects tend to have more severe symptoms. Extraintestinal complications in patients with Shigella infection include erythema nodosum, conjunctivitis, and reactive arthritis, occurring in 7% of patients. *S. flexneri*, *S. sonnei*, and *S. dysenteriae* can also trigger reactive arthritis.[13] Other extraintestinal manifestations include respiratory symptoms such as cough, coryza, and hypoglycemia in children. In 18 to 45% of cases, neurological symptoms develop such as encephalitis, lethargy, and seizures. The hemolytic uremic syndrome and thrombotic thrombocytopenic purpura (Moschkowitz Syndrome) are rare complications of Shigella dysenteriae serotype 1, one of the most virulent Shigella strains.[14]

EIEC

EIEC infections resemble Shigella infections in their mechanism and clinical picture. EIEC infection begins with fever, severe abdominal cramps, and watery diarrhea followed by dysentery with frequent scanty stools of mucus and blood.

EHEC

EHEC infections have been associated with the ingestion of contaminated hamburgers, milk, water, fruit, and vegetables.[15,16] However, person-to-person transmission is also possible. EHEC infection begins with abdominal pain and cramps and occasionally short-term fever. Within 1 to 2 days watery diarrhea ensues. In around 10% of cases, diarrhea is watery without blood. Endoscopy usually reveals an inflamed mucosa with patchy erythema and submucosal edema in the ascending and transverse colon. The duration of uncomplicated illness ranges from 1 to 12 days. The development of fever, leukocytosis, and the decline in platelet count indicates the emergence of complications such as the hemolytic uremic syndrome (HUS) or thrombotic-thrombocytopenic purpura. HUS complicates 2 to 7% of EHEC infections, affecting mainly children younger than 5 years and elderly individuals. It was first described in two separate outbreaks in Michigan and Oregon in 1982 and has been associated with *E. coli* serotype O157:H7.[17] HUS manifests itself 2 to 16 days after onset of gastrointestinal symptoms and is initially characterized by severe abdominal cramps and nonbloody diarrhea, which may become grossly bloody by the second or third day of illness. Half of the patients suffer from nausea and vomiting. In addition, low-grade fever may be present. The characteristic findings in the laboratory are microangiopathic hemolytic anemia, thrombocytopenia, and renal failure.[18] In addition, neurologic complications develop in one-quarter of patients, including seizures, coma, and hemiparesis. Half of the patients require dialysis due to progressive renal failure. In 75% of affected individuals, hemolysis reaches a level of severity that causes a rapid decline in hematocrit of more than 10% within 24 hours, urging the need for red cell transfusions. Usually hyperkalemia does not evolve because of the concomitant gastrointestinal loss of potassium. The mortality reaches 3 to 5%, but higher rates of 16 to 35% have been reported in specific populations such as individuals in nursing homes.

SALMONELLOSIS

Salmonella enterica includes almost all serotypes associated with human infections, such as *S. enteritidis*, *S. typhimurium*, *S. infantis*, *S. hadar*, and *S. virchow*. *S. Typhi* causes the typhoid fever and will be discussed elsewhere. Salmonella serotypes vary markedly in their virulence. Salmonella infections are acquired after ingestion of contaminated water or food, especially meat, poultry, eggs, and dairy products. Patients receiving corticosteroid therapy or suffering from acquired immune deficiency syndrome (AIDS), sickle cell anemia, malaria, leukemia, lymphomas, and other malignancy are at particular risk for Salmonella infections.

NONTYPHOID SALMONELLOSIS

Many salmonella strains produce cytotoxin and enterotoxins, but their role in the pathogenesis remains unresolved. The incubation period of nontyphoid salmonellosis ranges normally from 6 to 48 hours. The symptoms are nausea and vomiting, followed by periumbilical abdominal pain, cramps in the right lower quadrant, and watery diarrhea. However, in 50% of cases severe dysentery with bloody and purulent feces develops, which is usually accompanied by fever. The diarrhea usually disappears after 2 to 5 days, but tends to last longer if the colon is affected, persisting for up to 3 weeks.[19] In 5 to 6% of patients, Salmonella bacteremia is observed.

Proctoscopy reveals hyperemia, mild edema, granularity, friability, and ulcerations of the mucosa. Potential complications include intestinal bleedings, septicemia, and toxic megacolon.[20,21] Persistent fever usually suggests metastatic organ infection, such as meningitis, arteriitis, endo/pericarditis, liver or spleen abscess, cholecystitis, osteomyelitis, spondylodiscitis, and septic arthritis. Reactive arthritis has been reported to develop in 10% of patients with symptomatic or asymptomatic Salmonella infections.[23,24] Extraintestinal manifestations have been associated with a high mortality of up to 50%.[22] Excretion of Salmonella in stool for weeks is quite common, but a chronic carrier state is rare affecting only 1 to 4%. Newborns, children, and patients older than 60 years are more likely to become chronic carriers.

Y. ENTEROCOLITICA

Y. enterocolitica is a pathogen found in freshwater streams as well as in lakes. In addition, it has been isolated from a number of animals including dogs, cats, cows, chickens, and horses. *Y. enterocolitica* infections have been found after ingestion of contaminated ice cream, milk, meat, and shellfish. In addition, person-to-person transmission has been reported. *Y. enterocolitica* invades the mucosa of the terminal ileum, followed by ulcerations. Most isolates of *Y. enterocolitica* produce a heat-stabile enterotoxin of the ST type. Moreover, some *Yersinia* strains contain a virulence plasmid. The clinical course and the severity depend on the age of the patient and concomitant medical conditions. Only some biotypes and serotypes of *Y. enterocolitica* (1B to 5) can cause diarrhea, while biotype/serotype 1A seems to be mainly apathogenic. 75% of affected patients are children, in which life-threatening septicemia can occur. The incubation period is 4 to 6 days. Prodromal symptoms include anorexia and headache. The subsequent symptoms of acute enterocolitis are the most common manifestations and are found in two-thirds of patients. Typical symptoms include abdominal cramps, watery or bloody diarrhea, fever, nausea, and vomiting.[25–27] In older children and young adults, aphtous mouth ulcers, mesenteric adenitis, and terminal ileitis are common, often mimicking acute appendicitis. Symptoms usually disappear after 1 to 4 weeks, but can occasionally last for longer time periods.

Postinfectious complications occur in 1 to 5% of patients and include myocarditis, glomerulonephritis, erythema nodosum, and ankylosing spondylitis. Reactive arthritis or Reiter's syndrome is found in 2 to 6% of cases. Severe cases are associated with the major histocompatibility antigen HLA-B27. *Yersinia* bacteremia is uncommon, but may occasionally occur in patients with neoplasia, diabetes, anemia, or chronic liver disease. Metastatic infections have also been noted, including osteomyelitis, endocarditis, meningitis, cutaneous infections, arthritis, pneumonia, and abscesses of the liver, kidney, spleen, and lung.

Y. PSEUDOTUBERCULOSIS

Y. pseudotuberculosis can cause a syndrome that resembles appendicitis. The characteristics include fever, abdominal pain, tenderness of the right lower quadrant, and leukocytosis. The infection often causes mesenteric lymphadenitis and terminal ileitis. The syndrome is more common in older children and young adults. *Y. pseudotuberculosis*, especially serotype O:3 infection, is frequently associated with reactive arthritis and a severe clinical picture.[28]

VIBRIO PARAHAEMOLYTICUS

Vibrio parahaemolyticus is a common pathogen in countries where raw and undercooked seafood is consumed. In 90% of cases, explosive watery diarrhea is the cardinal symptom, which is accompanied by abdominal cramps, nausea, vomiting, and headache. Fever and chills occur in 25% of patients. Occasionally, patients present with a dysentery syndrome. Although hypotension and shock have been reported, these complications are rare and less severe than in patients with cholera. The duration of illness is short, ranging from 2 hours to 10 days. A carrier state is unknown.

VIBRIO VULNIFICUS

Vibrio vulnificus is usually not a problem for healthy persons, but can cause fever and general discomfort in susceptible patients. In particular, persons with human immunodeficiency virus (HIV)-1 infection, diabetes mellitus, hemachromatosis, and liver diseases are susceptible to systemic infection. In these cases, immediate medical attention is advised because of the high mortality.

Overlap Syndrome

Many pathogens such as *Campylobacter jejuni* are responsible for dysentery as well as secretory diarrhea, producing an overlap syndrome. Also, other pathogens such as *Salmonella enterica* and *Shigella* spp. may produce toxins.

CAMPYLOBACTER JEJUNI

Campylobacter jejuni infections are acquired after ingestion of contaminated eggs, poultry, milk, or water. Direct contamination from infected animals has also been reported. Infants and patients with immunodeficiency appear to be particularly susceptible to this infection. A wide spectrum of symptoms is possible, ranging from asymptomatic infection to watery diarrhea or even dysentery.[29] The prodromes include malaise, anorexia, headache, and myalgia. After an incubation period of 2 to 4 days, diarrhea and fever are found in 90% of affected individuals, while 70% experience abdominal pain and 50% have bloody stools. The fever can be low grade or even reach 40°C. In addition, vomiting may accompany the cardinal symptoms.[2,30,31] The duration of illness usually does not exceed 7 days, but in up to 20% of cases, symptoms may persist for up to 3 weeks.[30] In 16%, a prolonged carrier state is observed, lasting for 2 to 10 weeks. Possible complications include gastrointestinal hemorrhage, toxic megacolon, pancreatitis, cholecystitis, mesenteric adenitis, and appendicitis. Extraintestinal manifestations are rare and include osteomyelitis, hemolytic uremic syndrome, meningitis, septic arthritis, or radiculitis such as Guillain-Barré syndrome, which is usually observed 1 to 3 weeks after onset of symptoms. Moreover, a mild reactive arthritis can occur in 7 to 10% of patients with Campylobacter infection.[32] Cardiac complications such as myocarditis, pericarditis, or atrial fibrillation during or after Campylobacter infections are rare.[29] Recurrent infections of Campylobacter gastroenteritis are not uncommon.

Other Pathogens Causing Acute Diarrhea

ENTEROAGGREGATIVE *E. COLI*

Enteroaggregative *E. coli* (EAEC) is increasingly recognized as a pathogen of traveler's diarrhea. It can cause acute or chronic nonbloody diarrhea without invasion or inflammation.

ENTEROPATHOGENIC *E. COLI*

Enteropathogenic *E. coli* (EPEC) causes a watery diarrhea associated with fever similar to ETEC infections. In addition, it can cause outbreaks of diarrhea in newborns in nurseries. However, ST and LT toxins are not produced by EPEC.

AEROMONAS

Aeromonas spp. have been isolated from water, including chlorinated supplies. Only certain *Aeromonas* spp. has been found in TD; however, the causative role of those species is still unclear.[33] The most common finding is a mild, self-limiting watery diarrhea of short duration. However, in a small proportion of patients, other clinical features like bloody or mucoid stools, abdominal cramps, fever, and vomiting are possible.

VIRAL GASTROENTERITIS

An incubation period of more than 14 hours and a duration of illness of fewer than 72 hours suggests a viral etiology of gastroenteritis.[34] The most important viruses causing TD are rotavirus, noro viruses, sapo viruses, astroviruses, enteric adenoviruses, and enteroviruses.

Viral gastroenteritis predominantly causes vomiting and watery diarrhea as a result of the disruption of the mucosal structure and villous atrophy. In addition, malabsorption may occur and have an additional osmotic effect, contributing to the development of diarrhea. However, the exact pathogenesis of viral gastroenteritis is not known in detail. *Rotavirus* infections are usually observed in young children aged 3 to 15 months. They are highly contagious and the main reason of death in young children in developing countries. *Rotavirus* can also become a major problem in child care centers and children's hospitals all over the world. Adults can acquire the infection from children, but usually show milder forms. Travelers may be affected in up to 10% by *Rotavirus* infection.[35,36] Large numbers of virus particles are shed into stool of patients in the acute phase, but prolonged excretion is unusual. The infectious dose of *Rotavirus* is small and the incubation period ranges from 1 to 3 days. The clinical picture is characterized by an abrupt onset of nausea and abdominal cramps followed by watery diarrhea and vomiting. Low-grade fever develops in about half of affected individuals. The duration of symptoms ranges between 5 and 7 days.

Norovirus are members of the caliciviruses and affect all age groups. They are responsible for more than 90% of epidemic nonbacterial gastroenteritis. Transmission is fecal-oral and very similar to *Rotavirus*. Symptoms usually begin after 24 to 48 hours, mainly consisting of watery diarrhea in travelers after ingestion of contaminated water, salads, clams, and oysters.[37] Other typical symptoms include diarrhea, nausea, abdominal cramps, vomiting, and muscle aches. In addition, headache and symptoms of the upper respiratory tract are common. However, the duration of illness usually does not exceed 1 to 2 days.

ENTERIC FEVER (TYPHOID FEVER)

Enteric fever is a severe and prolonged systemic illness and the result of *S. typhi* infection. The clinical picture is completely different from *Salmonella enteritidis* infections. The incubation period ranges from 7 to 14 days. Diarrhea is usually brief and not a major symptom. The classical clinical course lasts for 4 weeks. In the first stage, patients suffer from unspecific symptoms such as low-grade fever, arthralgia, and headache. The second stage indicates systemic infection. The body temperature rises, reaching up to 40°C. The headache becomes more intense and patients suffer from abdominal pain in the right upper quadrant. Frequently, a relative bradycardia of less than 100 beats per minute is observed despite the high body temperature of 40°C. The abdominal skin may show the classic rash, characterized by light red, pinhead sized nonpruritic spots, known as rose spots. Bowel habits change in 50% of affected individuals. However, constipation is more common than diarrhea. The size of lymphoid organs such as the spleen and lymph nodes increases due to hyperplasia of the reticuloendothelial system. In severe cases, the patient may enter the typhoidal state, which is characterized by fatigue, apathy, and anorexia. The third stage is characterized by more frequent bowel movements, declining body temperature, but more intense abdominal pain in the ileocecal region. During this time, the stool resembles a greenish pea soup. Peyer's patches are hyperplastic and may ulcerate. As a consequence, the bowel wall becomes thinner, which occasionally results in colonic perforation. After 6 weeks, 50% of affected individuals still harbor Salmonella in stool. Although this proportion declines to 5 to 10% at 3 to 6 months, 1 to 3% remain chronic carriers of Salmonella.[38]

Common intestinal complications include bleeding (20 to 25% of cases) and perforation (5%), both of which are usually noted in the third week. Systemic complications of typhoid fever include pneumonia, pleuritis, pyelonephritis, bone and joint infections, brain abscesses, necrotic cholecystitis, thromboembolic events, endocarditis, arteriitis, and liver abscesses.

Chronic Diarrhea and Parasites

Chronic infectious diarrhea affects 0 to 12% of subjects with travelers' diarrhea and is mainly the result of parasitic infection. The pathogens most commonly detected are *Giardia lamblia*, *Entamoeba histolytica*, and *Microsporidia*. The main features are soft stools or watery diarrhea. A dysentery-like syndrome is occasionally observed in individuals with Entamoeba histolytica infections.

GIARDIA LAMBLIA

Giardia lamblia infection can be passed through ingestion of any infested water source. It is easily passed from person to person through poor hygiene and also infects animals. The ingestion of a small number of 10 to 100 cysts can either result in asymptomatic infection, in an acute self-limited diarrhea, or in a long-lasting intermittent diarrhea. After an incubation period of 1 to 2 weeks, a non-watery, greasy, foul-smelling diarrhea without blood, abdominal cramps, nausea, vomiting, low-grade fever, and malaise are observed. Although acute symptoms disappear within 1 to 2 weeks, milder symptoms such as irregular bowel movements, soft stools, and flatulence can persist. In addition, malabsorption, fatigue, anorexia, nausea, weight loss, and large amounts of greasy stool are common. Extraintestinal manifestations are rare and may include maculopapular rash, urticaria, polyarthritis, aphthous ulceration, and eosinophilia.

ENTAMOEBA HISTOLYTICA

Entamoeba (E.) histolytica infections are highly prevalent in Mexico, India, Africa, Central America, and South America. Individuals at highest risk are migrant workers in developing countries. The major routes of transmission are the consumption of contaminated water and food as well as direct fecal-oral contact. In addition, *E. histolytica* can be transmitted sexually. *E. histolytica*, to be distinguished from the similarly looking *E. dispar*, are symptomatic in 4 to 10% of cases and usually cause mild symptoms.[39] The incubation period is variable and ranges from 1 to 3 weeks. The number of bowel movements can be normal or can reach six or more stools per day. In addition, abdominal cramps in the right or left lower abdominal quadrant occur independently of bowel movements. Two to 20% of affected individuals show an invasive form of the disease and suffer from severe dysentery with frequent small volumes of bloody mucoid stool. Endoscopy can reveal ulcerations of the mucosa of the colon and typical flask-shaped abscesses. Occasionally, the formation of an inflammatory mass of the intestinal wall, called ameboma, can be found. Liver abscess is a typical complication of E. histolytica infection. Signs of liver involvement include anemia, fatigue, abdominal pain, jaundice, fever, and elevated liver function tests. Other complications include splenic abscesses, brain abscesses, empyema, and pericarditis.[40] Individuals treated with corticosteroids are at increased risk for intestinal complications such as toxic megacolon and bowel perforation.

CRYPTOSPORIDIA

Cryptosporidium parvum is a protozoan parasite transmitted via the fecal-oral route, close contacts to animals or pets, and the ingestion of contaminated drinking water or food.[41,42] A small number of 10 oocysts is sufficient for symptomatic infection in humans. After a short incubation period of 1 to 2 weeks, watery stools, abdominal pain and cramps, vomiting, fatigue, flatulence, general malaise, anorexia, nausea, and weight loss are observed. Fever is uncommon. Extraintestinal manifestations include acalculous cholecystitis and cholangitis. The illness is usually self limited, but can last for 1 to 2 weeks. Cryptosporidium species have a more severe outcome in HIV-1 infected subjects.

ISOSPORA BELLI

Isospora (I.) belli is endemic in tropical and subtropical areas. Transmission most likely occurs via contaminated water. The clinical features of *I. belli* infections include abdominal cramps, nausea, watery diarrhea, steatorrhea, headache, fever, malaise, vomiting, and occasionally eosinophilia. In the immunodeficient host, prolonged diarrhea, the dissemination of bacteria to mesenteric lymph nodes, and acalculous cholecystitis have been reported. The illness is usually self limited.

MICROSPORIDIA

Microsporidia have sporadically been reported to be responsible for chronic diarrhea in travelers. *Microsporidia* are small intracellular parasites and are more commonly detected in immunodeficient individuals, particularly in HIV-1 infected patients. In humans, two species are associated with enteric infection, including *Enterocytozoon (E.) bieneusi* and *E. intestinalis*. *E. bieneusi* infects enterocytes of the proximal jejunum and occasionally migrates to the biliary tract. *E. intestinalis* is located in enterocytes, macrophages, and fibroblasts, and is found in kidneys and mesenteric lymph nodes. The symptoms consist of watery diarrhea without abdominal pain, malabsorption, and weight loss. Complications of *Microsporidia* infections are keratoconjunctivitis, sinusitis, peribronchitis, and myositis.

CYCLOSPORA CAYETANENSIS

Cyclospora cayetanensis was previously referred to as Cyanobacteria-like pathogen. The transmission occurs via contaminated water and food that contain viable sporulated oocysts.[43] Outbreaks have also been traced back to the ingestion of raspberries.[44] Cyclospora needs days or sometimes weeks to become infectious. After an average incubation period of 7 days, affected individuals suffer from watery diarrhea, abdominal cramps, weight loss, nausea, vomiting, fatigue, muscle aches, and occasionally low-grade fever. Generally, the infection is self limited, but can last for up to 6 to 12 weeks.[45]

CLOSTRIDIUM DIFFICILE

Clostridium (C.) difficile is a major cause of antibiotic-associated diarrhea in hospitals and occasionally affects travelers. Antibiotics disrupt the normal bacterial flora and allow an overgrowth with *C. difficile*, which may in rare cases result in pseudomembranous colitis. Signs of pseudomembranous colitis are usually observed 4 to 9 days after the initiation of antibiotics.[46,47] The clinical symptoms vary from mild to severe diarrhea with more than 20 bowel movements per day.[48] The stool is profuse, watery and may occasionally contain blood and mucus.[49] In addition, abdominal cramps and signs of systemic toxicity such as fever, anorexia, and malaise are observed.[48,50] Proctoscopically, small 1 to 5 mm raised, whitish-yellow plaques or "pseudomembranes" are found without evidence of ulcers or erosions. Fulminant colitis develops in 1 to 3% of patients and may be complicated by toxic megacolon, bowel perforation, or death.[51] Extraintestinal spread is rare, but can result in bacteremia, septic arthritis, and splenic abscesses.

Food Poisoning

Occasionally, travelers suffer from classical food poisoning, which is characterized by a short incubation period of 1 to 6 hours and a rapid onset of nausea and vomiting that occur after ingestion of preformed neurotoxins.[52] If the toxin needs to be produced after ingestion, the incubation period is usually longer, reaching 8 to 16 hours. Vomiting is less prominent and fever is usually

Table 3 Characteristics of Food Poisoning

Incubation Period *(h)*		Duration *(h)*	Clinical Symptoms
Staphylococcus aureus	1–6h	< 24	Vomiting, diarrhea, fever
Clostridium perfringens	8–16h	< 24	Diarrhea, abdominal cramps, nausea
Bacillus cereus	1–6h	< 24	Vomiting, nausea, abdominal cramps

absent, but abdominal cramps are frequent. The pathogens responsible for these symptoms are *Staphylococcus aureus*, *Clostridium perfringens*, and *Bacillus cereus*. Common to all forms of classical food poisoning is the short duration of illness, usually lasting for fewer than 24 hours (Table 3). Consumption of food containing histamine, most often fish such as tuna, mackerel, dolphin, and blue fish, can cause food poisoning with rapidly appearing symptoms. The possibility of histamine poisoning should be considered if patients suffer from headache, palpitations, and symptoms of the skin in addition to the gastrointestinal symptoms.

SPECIAL CONSIDERATIONS

The normal enteric microflora plays an important role in reducing the number of intestinal pathogens. Alterations of the normal microflora allow an overgrowth with pathogenic organisms. Infant botulism, nosocomial salmonellosis, and EPEC occur with increased frequency in newborns who have not yet acquired the normal enteric microflora. Whether a person acquires a gastrointestinal infection largely depends on the inoculum size. A number of 100,000 to 100,000,000 pathogens are usually necessary to defeat the gastric barrier and the host's immune response. However, *Shigella*, *Rotavirus* and certain parasites such as *Cryptosporidia* can cause gastrointestinal infection after transmission of a small number of 10 to 100 organisms. The neutralization of gastric acid with antacids or proton blocking agents drastically reduces the number of organisms required for gastrointestinal infection.[53] The reduction in gut motility increases the risk of bacterial overgrowth and toxic megacolon. Salmonella bacteremia is more likely to develop in patients who are treated with opiates.[1] The use of antimotility drugs has also been associated with prolonged fever, reduced effectiveness of antibiotics, and a longer bacterial shedding in patients with *Shigella* infections.[54] In addition, several case reports suggest that complications of *Campylobacter* and *C. difficile* infections occur more frequently when using antimotility agents.[55] These drugs also appear to favor the development of HUS in patients with EHEC infections.[3] Alterations of the immune system increase the risk of gastrointestinal infections. The lack of a sufficient number of neutrophils is associated with a defect in phagocytic activity, increasing the likelihood of gram-negative infections.[56] Patients with advanced HIV infection are particularly susceptible to *Salmonella*, *Shigella*, *Cryptosporidia*, *Microsporidia*, and *Isospora belli* infections. The host's genotype may also be of importance. Individuals with blood group O appear to be more susceptible to cholera. In contrast, persons with blood group A are more likely to acquire *G. lamblia* infections.[57,58] Young and old age represent further risk factors. *Rotavirus* infection and EPEC predominantly affect young children, probably due to differences in gut mucus, cell-surface factors, microbial flora, and the expression of intestinal receptors for bacteria. Lew and colleagues reviewed 28,538 deaths due to infectious diarrhea and found that 51% were older than 74 years, indicating that elderly patients are more susceptible to serious complications of infectious diarrhea.[59] The post-diarrhea irritable bowel syndrome (IBS) has been found to be common in travelers with diarrhea. In one study, a prevalence of 11% has been reported in students in the United States returning from Mexico.[60]

Differential Diagnosis

A number of noninfectious causes of diarrhea have to be considered in the differential diagnosis, including IBS, inflammatory and ischemic bowel disease, laxative abuse, Whipple's disease, diverticulitis, appendicitis, adnexitis, celiac sprue, malabsorption, and diabetes. Some cases may be caused by food intolerance, high intakes of fatty foods or alcohol, which may result in loose bowel movements. Especially in elderly subjects, the reason for diarrhea may be conditions like diverticulosis, carcinoma, or inflammatory bowel disease. In travelers returning from tropical areas, other systemic infections such as malaria should also be considered in the differential diagnosis.

References

1. Sprinz H. Pathogenesis of intestinal infections. Arch Pathol 1969;87:556–62.
2. Blaser MJ, Wells JG, Feldman RA, et al. Campylobacter enteritis in the United States. A multicenter study. Ann Intern Med 1983;98:360–5.

3. Slutsker L, Ries AA, Greene KD, et al. Escherichia coli O157:H7 diarrhea in the United States: clinical and epidemiologic features. Ann Intern Med 1997;126:505–13.
4. Merson MH, Morris GK, Sack DA, et al. Travelers' diarrhea in Mexico. A prospective study of physicians and family members attending a congress. N Engl J Med 1976;294: 1299–305.
5. Sack RB. The epidemiology of diarrhea due to enterotoxigenic Escherichia coli. J Infect Dis 1978;137:639–40.
6. Baqui AH, Black RE, Yunus M, et al. Methodological issues in diarrhoeal diseases epidemiology: definition of diarrhoeal episodes. Int J Epidemiol 1991;20:1057–63.
7. Ericsson CD, DuPont HL. Travelers' diarrhea: approaches to prevention and treatment. Clin Infect Dis 1993;16:616–24.
8. Mattila L, Siitonen A, Kyronseppa H, et al. Seasonal variation in etiology of travelers' diarrhea. Finnish-Moroccan Study Group. J Infect Dis 1992;165:385–8.
9. Mattila L. Clinical features and duration of traveler's diarrhea in relation to its etiology. Clin Infect Dis 1994;19: 728–34.
10. Levine MM, Ferreccio C, Prado V, et al. Epidemiologic studies of Escherichia coli diarrheal infections in a low socioeconomic level peri-urban community in Santiago, Chile. Am J Epidemiol 1993;138:849–69.
11. Gots RE, Formal SB, Giannella RA. Indomethacin inhibition of Salmonella typhimurium, Shigella flexneri, and cholera-mediated rabbit ileal secretion. J Infect Dis 1974; 130:280–4.
12. DuPont HL, Hornick RB, Dawkins AT, et al. The response of man to virulent Shigella flexneri 2a. J Infect Dis 1969; 119:296–9.
13. Hannu T, Mattila L, Siitonen A, Leirisalo-Repo M. Reactive arthritis attributable to Shigella infection: a clinical and epidemiological nationwide study. Ann Rheum Dis 2005; 64:594–8.
14. Barrett-Connor E, Connor JD. Extraintestinal manifestations of shigellosis. Am J Gastroenterol 1970;53:234–45.
15. Swerdlow DL, Woodruff BA, Brady RC, et al. A waterborne outbreak in Missouri of Escherichia coli O157:H7 associated with bloody diarrhea and death. Ann Intern Med 1992;117:812–9.
16. Spika JS, Parsons JE, Nordenberg D, et al. Hemolytic uremic syndrome and diarrhea associated with Escherichia coli 0157:H7 in a day care center. J Pediatr 1986;109:287–91.
17. Riley LW, Remis RS, Helgerson SD, et al. Hemorrhagic colitis associated with a rare Escherichia coli serotype. N Engl J Med 1983;308:681–5.
18. Neill MA, Tarr PI, Clausen CR, et al. Escherichia coli O157:H7 as the predominant pathogen associated with the hemolytic uremic syndrome: a prospective study in the Pacific Northwest. Pediatrics 1987;80:37–40.
19. Mandal BK, Mani V. Colonic involvement in salmonellosis. Lancet 1976;1:887–8.
20. Bellary SV, Isaacs P. Toxic megacolon (TM) due to Salmonella. J Clin Gastroenterol 1990;12:605–7.
21. Deppisch LM, Crans CA. Salmonellosis: a cause of toxic megacolon. J Clin Gastroenterol 1990;12:483–5.
22. Cohen JI, Bartlett JA, Corey GR. Extra-intestinal manifestations of salmonella infections. Medicine (Baltimore) 1987;66:349–88.
23. Mattila L, Leirisalo-Repo M, Koskimies S, et al. Reactive arthritis following an outbreak of Salmonella infection in Finland. Br J Rheumatol 1994;33:1136–41.
24. Mattila L, Leirisalo-Repo M, Pelkonen P, et al. Reactive arthritis following an outbreak of Salmonella Bovismorbificans infection. J Infect 1998;36:289–95.
25. Lee LA, Gerber AR, Lonsway DR, et al. Yersinia enterocolitica O:3 infections in infants and children, associated with the household preparation of chitterlings. N Engl J Med 1990;322:984–7.
26. Vantrappen G, Ponette E, Geboes K, Bertrand P. Yersinia enteritis and enterocolitis: gastroenterological aspects. Gastroenterology 1977;72:220–7.
27. Vantrappen G, Geboes K, Ponette E. Yersinia enteritis. Med Clin North Am 1982;66:639–53.
28. Hannu T, Mattila L, Nuorti JP, et al. Reactive arthritis after an outbreak of Yersinia pseudotuberculosis serotype O:3 infection. Ann Rheum Dis 2003;62:866–9.
29. Allos BM, Blaser MJ. Campylobacter jejuni and the expanding spectrum of related infections. Clin Infect Dis 1995;20:1092–9.
30. Blaser MJ, Berkowitz ID, LaForce FM, et al. Campylobacter enteritis: clinical and epidemiologic features. Ann Intern Med 1979;91:179–85.
31. Lambert ME, Schofield PF, Ironside AG, Mandal BK. Campylobacter colitis. Br Med J 1979;1:857–9.
32. Hannu T, Mattila L, Rautelin H, et al. Campylobacter-triggered reactive arthritis: a population-based study. Rheumatology (Oxford) 2002;41:312–8.
33. Hanninen ML, Salmi S, Mattila L, et al. Association of Aeromonas spp. with travellers' diarrhoea in Finland. J Med Microbiol 1995;42:26–31.
34. DuPont HL. Guidelines on acute infectious diarrhea in adults. The Practice Parameters Committee of the American College of Gastroenterology. Am J Gastroenterol 1997;92:1962–75.
35. DuPont HL, Ericsson CD. Prevention and treatment of traveler's diarrhea. N Engl J Med 1993;328:1821–7.
36. Ryder RW, Oquist CA, Greenberg H, et al. Travelers' diarrhea in panamanian tourists in Mexico. J Infect Dis 1981;144:442–8.

37. Johnson PC, Hoy J, Mathewson JJ, et al. Occurrence of Norwalk virus infections among adults in Mexico. J Infect Dis 1990;162:389–93.

38. Kaye D, Merselis JG Jr, Connolly S, Hook EW. Treatment of chronic enteric carriers of Salmonella typhosa with ampicillin. Ann N Y Acad Sci 1967;145:429–35.

39. Weinke T, Friedrich-Janicke B, Hopp P, Janitschke K. Prevalence and clinical importance of Entamoeba histolytica in two high-risk groups: travelers returning from the tropics and male homosexuals. J Infect Dis 1990;161:1029–31.

40. Petri WA Jr. Recent advances in amebiasis. Crit Rev Clin Lab Sci 1996;33:1–37.

41. Outbreak of cryptosporidiosis associated with a water sprinkler fountain—Minnesota, 1997. MMWR Morb Mortal Wkly Rep 1998;47:856–60.

42. Foodborne outbreak of cryptosporidiosis—Spokane, Washington, 1997. MMWR Morb Mortal Wkly Rep 1998;47:565–7.

43. Sturbaum GD, Ortega YR, Gilman RH, et al. Detection of Cyclospora cayetanensis in wastewater. Appl Environ Microbiol 1998;64:2284–6.

44. Herwaldt BL, Beach MJ. The return of Cyclospora in 1997: another outbreak of cyclosporiasis in North America associated with imported raspberries. Cyclospora Working Group. Ann Intern Med 1999;130:210–20.

45. Huang P, Weber JT, Sosin DM, et al. The first reported outbreak of diarrheal illness associated with Cyclospora in the United States. Ann Intern Med 1995;123:409–14.

46. Samore MH, DeGirolami PC, Tlucko A, et al. Clostridium difficile colonization and diarrhea at a tertiary care hospital. Clin Infect Dis 1994;18:181–7.

47. Johnson S, Clabots CR, Linn FV, et al. Nosocomial Clostridium difficile colonisation and disease. Lancet 1990;336:97–100.

48. Kelly CP, Pothoulakis C, LaMont JT. Clostridium difficile colitis. N Engl J Med 1994;330:257–62.

49. Spencer RC. The role of antimicrobial agents in the aetiology of Clostridium difficile-associated disease. J Antimicrob Chemother 1998;41 Suppl C:21–7.

50. Gerding DN, Olson MM, Peterson LR, et al. Clostridium difficile-associated diarrhea and colitis in adults. A prospective case-controlled epidemiologic study. Arch Intern Med 1986;146:95–100.

51. Fekety R, Silva J, Kauffman C, et al. Treatment of antibiotic-associated Clostridium difficile colitis with oral vancomycin: comparison of two dosage regimens. Am J Med 1989;86:15–9.

52. Sugiyama H, Hayama T. Abdominal viscera as site of emetic action for staphylococcal enterotoxin in the monkey. J Infect Dis 1965;115:330–6.

53. Hornick RB, Music SI, Wenzel R, et al. The Broad Street pump revisited: response of volunteers to ingested cholera vibrios. Bull N Y Acad Med 1971;47:1181–91.

54. DuPont HL, Hornick RB. Adverse effect of lomotil therapy in shigellosis. JAMA 1973;226:1525–8.

55. Smith GS, Blaser MJ. Fatalities associated with Campylobacter jejuni infections. JAMA 1985;253:2873–5.

56. Bodey GP, Buckley M, Sathe YS, Freireich EJ. Quantitative relationships between circulating leukocytes and infection in patients with acute leukemia. Ann Intern Med 1966;64:328–40.

57. Levine MM, Nalin DR, Rennels MB, et al. Genetic susceptibility to cholera. Ann Hum Biol 1979;6:369–74.

58. Zisman M. Blood-group A and giardiasis. Lancet 1977;2:1285.

59. Lew JF, Glass RI, Gangarosa RE, et al. Diarrheal deaths in the United States, 1979 through 1987. A special problem for the elderly. JAMA 1991;265:3280–4.

60. Okhuysen PC, Jiang ZD, Carlin L, et al. Post-diarrhea chronic intestinal symptoms and irritable bowel syndrome in North American travelers to Mexico. Am J Gastroenterol 2004;99:1774–8.

CHAPTER 18

POSTINFECTIOUS IRRITABLE BOWEL SYNDROME

ANDREW W. DUPONT, MD, MSPH

ROBIN C. SPILLER, MD, MSC, FRCP

Irritable bowel syndrome (IBS), broadly defined as a chronic episodic medical condition associated with abdominal pain or discomfort and altered bowel habits, affects many individuals with a prevalence in general ranging from 10.3 (Manning criteria) to 6.7% (Rome II criteria) and up to 14.1% of individuals in western societies meeting any diagnostic criteria when evaluated by telephone survey.[1] A unifying pathophysiology has not been identified; however, a subset of those with IBS have been shown to develop their symptoms after an episode of acute infectious gastroenteritis. In fact, a large epidemiologic study has identified infectious gastroenteritis as the most significant environmental risk factor in the development of IBS.[2] Postinfectious irritable bowel syndrome (PI-IBS), which subsequently develops in 4 to 31% of those with bacterial gastroenteritis,[3] appears to be a nonspecific response to infection being observed after infection with a wide range of bacteria, including *Campylobacter*, *Salmonella*, *Escherichia coli*, and *Shigella*.[4–6] PI-IBS has typically been defined by the acute onset of IBS diagnostic criteria (Rome III criteria being the most recently defined: Table 1 [7] with 2 or more of the following: fever, vomiting, diarrhea, and positive stool culture.[8] Although PI-IBS was first observed 45 years ago,[9] it was not until recently that prospective evaluations have been completed. In contrast to the long-held belief that patients with IBS have no structural abnormalities, mechanistic studies in recent years have documented subtle mucosal abnormalities in IBS. These recent studies have demonstrated the importance of low-grade inflammation and its association with symptoms in IBS. The majority of research on PI-IBS has not focused on travelers; thus, data must be extrapolated to this subset of PI-IBS patients. Also, due to lack of treatment studies in PI-IBS, therapy for the most part is typically similar for PI-IBS and those with IBS without preceding infection. The role of acute infection and the mechanism of persistent inflammation with associated symptoms in PI-IBS are the focus of this chapter.

Epidemiology

INCIDENCE

Chaudhary and Truelove[9] in 1962 evaluated 130 cases of "irritable colon syndrome," of which 26% dated their onset of IBS symptoms to an episode of dysentery.

In contrast to those who developed symptoms without preceding infection, these authors reported less psychological disturbances and a better prognosis in those with PI-IBS. Over recent years, acute gastroenteritis as a risk factor for subsequent IBS has been substantiated

Table 1 Rome III Diagnostic Criteria* for Irritable Bowel Syndrome

Recurrent abdominal pain or discomfort** at least 3 days per month in the last 3 months associated with two or more of the following:
1. Improvement with defecation
2. Onset associated with a change in frequency of stool
3. Onset associated with a change in form (appearance) of stool

*Criteria fulfilled for the last 3 months with symptom onset at least 6 months prior to diagnosis.
**Discomfort means an uncomfortable sensation not described as pain. Adapted from Longstreth GF et al.[7]

by several other researchers. The first of these studies included a small retrospective series of 38 patients admitted with Salmonellosis in which 31% were found to have persistent PI-IBS when assessed at 1 year after the outbreak.[10] In this analysis, female gender and increased severity of initial infection were associated with the development of PI-IBS. Two years later a similar frequency of PI-IBS was reported in a prospective analysis of patients admitted with clinically diagnosed gastroenteritis, in which 26% where found to have IBS at 6 months after infection.[11] The following year, a large (n=357) community-based study[12] evaluated subjects 6 months after proven bacterial gastroenteritis and found 25% had persistent bowel symptoms. In this study, however, only 7% met Rome I criteria for IBS. The comparatively low rate of PI-IBS in this study may be due to overall less severe symptoms of initial illness as reflected by the fact that 90% of these individuals were managed as outpatients.

These studies, however, lacked control groups that would have made it possible to compare the normal incidence of IBS in the absence of acute infection in these populations. Two prospective studies have included control groups.[2,13] In this first case-control study, Rodriguez and Ruigomez,[2] using the General Practice Research Database in the United Kingdom, found 4% (12 of 318) of patients with documented bacterial gastroenteritis were diagnosed with IBS during a 12-month follow-up period compared to 0.35% (2027 of 584,308) of uninfected controls. The adjusted relative risk of developing IBS in those with bacterial infections was 11.9 (95% confidence interval [CI], 6.7 to 21) compared to the control population. Of note, the incidence rate seen in the control population was less than the 1% incidence rate reported in a more recent population study.[14] The comparatively lower incidence rates in both cases and controls in this study may at least partially reflect a decreased inclination of general practitioners to diagnose IBS. Also, infrequent evaluation of stool cultures, which has been reported to be obtained in only 10% of cases of gastroenteritis,[15] may underestimate the frequency of infection and subsequently decrease the incidence of PI-IBS. In contrast to this first case-control study, Parry and colleagues,[13] using the Rome II criteria for IBS, reported an incidence of PI-IBS at 6 months of 16.7% (18/108) compared to 1.9% of controls (4/206) developing new IBS giving an odds ratio of 10.1 (95% CI, 3 to 31). Recently, in a meta-analysis in which eight studies were included, Halvorson and colleagues[16] reported a mean prevalence of IBS in those with a history of infectious gastroenteritis of 9.8% compared to a 1.2% prevalence of IBS in controls with a pooled odds ratio of 7.3% (95% CI, 4.7 to 11.1). In addition, subgroup analysis revealed clinical/laboratory confirmed gastroenteritis to have twice the odds of PI-IBS as self-reported gastroenteritis with pooled odds ratio estimates of 10.9 (95%, CI 6.7 to 17.7) and 5.3% (95%, CI 3.0 to 9.3), respectively.

Two studies have specifically evaluated the risk of PI-IBS in those with travelers' diarrhea (TD).[17,18] Ilnyckyj and colleagues[17] prospectively followed 109 healthy adults who were traveling outside Canada or the United States with the majority of travel destinations listed as developing countries. Consistent with expected attack rates, 44% developed TD. Surprisingly, only 4.2% (2/48) who had an episode of TD subsequently were found to have IBS (Rome I criteria) at 3-month follow-up. By contrast, the incidence of IBS in those who remained healthy was 1.6% (1/61). Possibly due to the small study size, there was no significant difference in incidence of IBS between the two groups (relative risk = 2.5, 95% CI = 0.2 to 27.2, p = .41). Okhuysen and colleagues[18] evaluated 97 healthy US college students who developed TD while studying in Mexico for 5 weeks and reported 10% had newly diagnosed IBS by Rome II criteria 6 months after returning from Mexico. Of note, 17% of those with acute diarrheal illness during their time in Mexico had chronic gastrointestinal (GI) symptoms (eg, abdominal pain, loose stools) at 6 months. The incidence of PI-IBS reported in these two studies is lower than typically reported for nontravelers who develop bacterial gastroenteritis. In part, this may be explained by smaller patient populations in these two studies. However, another potential explanation might be the specific bacteria with associated sequelae and virulence properties. The most common identified causes of diarrhea among North American travelers to Mexico are diarrheagenic *E. coli*, which are less virulent compared to *Campylobacter*, *Salmonella*, or *Shigella* reported in other studies. Viral gastroenteritis typically produces short-lived symptoms with little residual injury and might be predicted to cause less PI-IBS than bacterial infections. There is only one abstract, but this suggests the incidence of IBS 6 months after viral gastroenteritis is not increased compared to controls.[19]

RISK FACTORS FOR POSTINFECTIOUS IBS

Several factors, both host and pathogen related, have been associated with the subsequent development of PI-IBS. The presence of preexisting psychological abnormalities has repeatedly been shown to be associated with an increased risk of PI-IBS.[20,21] Gwee and colleagues[21] reported an increased risk with high hypochondriasis scores and adverse life events. Although psychiatric comorbidities appear to increase the risk of subsequent PI-IBS, a lifetime history of anxiety or depression has been shown to be less common among patients with PI-IBS compared to those with IBS without an infectious onset (26% versus 54%).[22] Possibly the strongest risk factor for the development of PI-IBS is the duration of initial infection. Those with initial illness lasting longer than 3 weeks are 11 times more likely to develop PI-IBS compared with individuals with illness limited to 1 week or less.[12] Similar to IBS patients overall, female gender has been associated with an increased risk of developing PI-IBS. Women have been shown to be more than 3 times more likely then males to subsequently develop PI-IBS.[12,21,23] However, in multivariate analysis by Gwee and colleagues[21] when psychological variables were included, female gender was no longer a significant risk factor, suggesting female predisposition may be due to psychological factors.[23] Other reported factors that may increase the risk of PI-IBS include younger age,[12, 24] vegetarian diet,[23] and smoking.[24] Vomiting with initial infection appears protective,[12] possibly due to a decrease in pathogen load. Although vomiting may decrease the risk of PI-IBS, it has recently been associated with an increased risk of postinfectious dyspepsia,[25] suggesting the phenotype of persistent postinfectious complications may be due to the predominant site of involvement of initial illness.

Pathophysiology

EFFECT OF SEROTONIN

Increases in serotonin-containing enterochromaffin (EC) cells have been documented in animal models of colitis,[26,27] as well as in humans with celiac disease and after Campylobacter infection,[4] which may signify a nonspecific response to mucosal injury and inflammation. Dunlop and colleagues[8] reported a 25% increase in rectal EC cells in those with PI-IBS compared to non-PI-IBS and controls (Figure 1). EC cells are responsible for synthesizing and storing approximately 85% of the body's serotonin (5-hydroxytryptamine [5-HT)]), which affects GI motility, secretion, and sensation.[28] Dunlop and colleagues[20] also documented significant increases in both EC cells and lymphocytes in rectal biopsies from those who developed PI-IBS compared to age and sex-matched individuals who recovered from their initial illness without postinfectious complications. These authors have also reported an increase in postprandial plasma levels of serotonin in PI-IBS patients compared to healthy controls and patients with constipation-predominant IBS (C-IBS) without infectious onset.[29] In fact, the group with C-IBS had significantly depressed

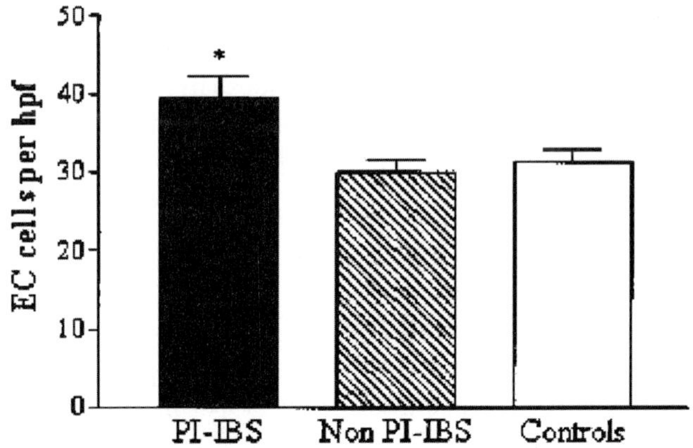

Figure 1 Number of enterochromaffin (EC) cells in clinical subtypes of irritable bowel syndrome and control subjects. Mean EC cell counts are shown for each high power field (hpf). *p = .02 vs. controls.[22]

postprandial plasma serotonin, which corresponded to slowed colonic transit. This same study demonstrated a decreased ratio of rectal mucosal 5-hydroxyindoleacetic acid (5-HIAA)/5-hydroxytryptophan (5-HT) in patients with C-IBS. 5-HIAA/5-HT ratio is used as an index of 5-HT turnover because 5-HT released from EC cells is taken up by enterocytes and one of its metabolites is 5-HIAA produced by intracellular monoamine oxidases. Reduced 5-HIAA/5-HT in C-IBS is consistent with decreased 5-HT release and turnover. Interestingly, despite an enhanced release of 5-HT, patients with PI-IBS were also found to have depressed ratios of 5-HIAA/5-HT compared to healthy controls without IBS. One possible explanation for this paradoxical decrease in 5-HIAA/5-HT is an impaired serotonin reuptake by enterocytes. Enterocytes possess the serotonin transporter (SERT), which enables them to take up and terminate the action of 5-HT after its release from EC cells. A decreased SERT activity would be expected to decrease 5-HT uptake by enterocytes and would result in a decrease in mucosal 5-HIAA/5-HT. The level of SERT has been reported to be decreased in females with either diarrhea- or C-IBS by immunofluorescence and messenger ribonucleic acid (mRNA) analysis.[30] Decreased SERT may be acquired, possibly through the effects of inflammation, or may be influenced by genetic factors. Interleukin (IL)-4 , an inflammatory cytokine, has been shown to down-regulate SERT.[31] Also, SERT has been shown to be decreased in ulcerative colitis,[28] and studies in a colitis model have documented down-regulation of SERT with decreased mRNA and expression of SERT by immunofluorescence staining.[32] These results add to the hypothesis that symptoms of PI-IBS are perpetuated by low-grade inflammation. There also may be a genetic component to the development of impaired SERT function. Yeo and colleagues[30] reported an increase in those who were homozygous for the short form (ss) SERT polymorphism in females with diarrhea-predominant IBS (D-IBS). However, data on SERT polymorphisms have been inconsistent as others have documented an excess of ss homozygotes in C-IBS. This polymorphism's potential role in PI-IBS, and whether it predisposes to all subtypes of IBS, remains unknown at this time.[33]

INTESTINAL INFLAMMATION

There is growing evidence to suggest that symptoms of PI-IBS initially result from and may be maintained by immunologic factors. Unlike inflammatory bowel disease (IBD), macroscopic evidence of inflammation does not exist in IBS; however, subtle microscopic changes have been documented in the GI tract of patients with PI-IBS. Patients with PI-IBS have been found to have increased intraepithelial lymphocytes (IEL) and lamina propria lymphocytes that have persisted at least 1 year after infection and have been associated with increased intestinal permeability.[4] Although rectal biopsies by conventional criteria have been shown to be normal in patients with PI-IBS, Dunlop and colleagues[8] showed that patients with PI-IBS and non-PI-IBS had elevated (18% increase) lamina propria T lymphocytes compared to controls. Despite similar levels of increased lamina propria lymphocytes in the PI-IBS and non-PI-IBS individuals, those with PI-IBS were the only group in this study to show an increase in EC count.

Recently, studies evaluating cytokine profiles have also given support to the argument that inflammation plays a role in PI-IBS. Two recent studies have reported increased expression of IL-1β in PI-IBS.[5,6] Gwee and colleagues, [5] reported higher IL-1β expression in rectal biopsies in patients with infectious enteritis who subsequently developed IBS compared to individuals who did not develop subsequent PI-IBS. Levels of IL-1β remained elevated at 3 months in PI-IBS patients, while those who did not develop IBS had similar levels to healthy controls. Wang and colleagues[6] endoscopically evaluated the entire colon and terminal ileum in patients with *Shigella* infection and found increased IL-1β mRNA expression in both the rectosigmoid region and ileum in PI-IBS patients, in contrast to normal levels seen in patients with IBS without an infectious onset of symptoms. Increased levels of the proinflammatory cytokine IL-1β in PI-IBS lends further support for the concept of ineffective down regulation of the inflammatory response seen after acute infectious enteritis. Tumor necrosis factor-α (TNF-α) is another proinflammatory cytokine, which has been associated with macrophage production stimulated by enteric pathogens such as *Campylobacter jejuni*, *Salmonella*, and *Shigella*.[34] Secretion of TNF-α is enhanced in individuals with a single nucleotide polymorphism (SNP) in the promoter region of the TNF-α gene (GA substitution at position -308). van der Veek and colleagues found an increased portion of genotype A (A/A or A/G) in IBS (41%) compared to controls (30%). A subgroup analysis found the A allele in 48% PI-IBS compared to 40% of non-PI-IBS; however, this did not reach statistical significance owing to inadequate numbers ($p = .49$).[35] Likewise, production of the counter-inflammatory cytokine IL-10 is associated with SNPs at positions -1082 (GA) and -819 (CT). Gonsalkorale and colleagues[36] found that IBS patients had significantly reduced frequencies of the high producer genotype for IL-10 (G/G for the -1082) compared to healthy, ethnically matched controls (21% versus 32%; $p < .05$) though a subsequent study failed to replicate this.[35] These findings may suggest individuals with this polymorphism (-1082A) might produce lesser amounts of IL-10 and would be more likely to develop IBS after an episode of acute infectious gastroenteritis due to an inappropriate inflammatory response. It appears immunologic dysregulation is not a specific finding for IBS with an infectious onset. This was reinforced in a study by Chadwick and colleagues[37] who evaluated 77 IBS patients (55% diarrhea predominant) by colonic biopsies that had a history of insidious onset of symptoms without preceding infection and found 49% had normal conventional histology and 40% had evidence of microscopic inflammation with increased lamina propria cellularity, frequently with focal neutrophilic infiltration (8% met diagnostic criteria for lymphocytic colitis). However, among patients with normal histology, immunohistochemistry revealed increased intraepithelial lymphocytes in addition to increased $CD3^+$ and $CD25^+$ cells, and therefore all showed evidence of immune activation. There is growing evidence IBS is a heterogeneous entity with at least a subset of patients demonstrating a persistent immunological response to either enteric pathogens, normal commensal bacteria, or possibly other antigens contained in the diet.

MAST CELLS

One of the most intriguing cell types noted to be increased in the mucosa of patients with IBS is the mast cell, which gives further support to the idea that inflammation is a factor in the pathogenesis of IBS. Mast cell degranulation in an animal model has been shown to influence muscle contraction and enteric nerve excitability as well as pain behavior in response to colorectal distention.[38] Mast cells have been found to be increased in the mucosa of the terminal ileum in both PI-IBS and non-PI-IBS,[6] whereas at least two studies have reported a lack of increased mast cells from rectal biopsies.[6,8] Increased mast cells have also been identified in colonic mucosal biopsies in unselected IBS patients compared to controls,[39–41] and an association between mast cells and enteric nerves has also been demonstrated. In a report by Barbara and colleagues,[40] patients with IBS compared to controls had a threefold increase in mast cells located within 5μm of nerve fibers, and this finding correlated significantly with the severity and frequency of abdominal pain. This study also demonstrated enhanced mucosal mast cell release of tryptase, an enzyme that appears important in somatic and visceral pain,[42,43] in addition to increased release of histamine, which is capable of sensitizing nociceptors[44] and may increase intestinal permeability,[45] a finding that has been documented in PI-IBS.[4,46] In a waterborne outbreak of acute gastroenteritis due to *Campylobacter jejuni* and *Escherichia coli* 0157:H7, Marshall and colleagues[46] reported an increase in intestinal permeability defined by a lactulose/mannitol ratio of > 0.020 in 35% of new IBS cases compared to 13% in non-IBS controls ($p = .03$). Increased intestinal permeability resulting in a breakdown of the mucosal barrier could enhance neuromuscular exposure to luminal bacteria and may be a mechanism for chronic inflammatory dysregulation.

Diagnosis

The diagnosis of postinfectious IBS should be considered in individuals with a clear history of acute onset symptoms and persistent abdominal discomfort or pain and altered bowel habits. The diagnosis of acute gastroenteritis should be based on the presence of at least two of the following: fever, vomiting, diarrhea, or positive stool culture.[23] Patients should not meet diagnostic criteria for IBS (see Table 1) prior to onset of acute illness. Symptoms other than abdominal discomfort/pain and altered bowel habits typically resolve, with the predominant bowel alteration in PI-IBS typically being diarrhea,[22,47,48] whereas individuals with IBS without infectious onset appear to be more likely to have alternating diarrhea and constipation.[1] In the presence of persistent systemic complaints, such as weight loss or fever, or other alarm symptoms (eg, anemia or gross bleeding, significant nocturnal symptoms, elevated sedimentation rate), other diagnoses should be considered. In the past IBS was considered a diagnosis of exclusion; however, Vanner and colleagues[49] reported a nearly 100% positive predictive value in individuals who met diagnostic criteria for IBS without alarm symptoms when they were followed for a period of 2 years. A published summary of the available literature by Cash and colleagues[50] reported the pretest probability of IBD, colon cancer, lactose malabsorption, and thyroid dysfunction in patients with unspecified IBS was similar to the prevalence of these disorders in the general population. The only organic GI disorder reported to occur at an increased frequency in this IBS population was celiac disease, which has been found to have a pretest probability 10 times greater in patients with suspected IBS compared with the estimated prevalence of celiac disease in the general population.[50] Therefore, it is reasonable to evaluate IBS patients with antibody testing for celiac disease (antiendomysial or tissue transglutaminase), at least in those with diarrhea- predominant IBS. However, the prevalence of celiac disease in PI-IBS patients and the cost-effectiveness of antibody testing in this subpopulation of IBS patients have not been evaluated. In those individuals with persistent or recurrent symptoms after acute infectious gastroenteritis, specific organic diseases that need to be considered in the differential diagnosis would include IBD and microscopic colitis. A recent, large prospective study evaluating cases of acute gastroenteritis, either diagnosed by positive stool culture or clinical criteria, reported the estimated incidence rate of IBD at 68.4 per 100,000 person-years after an episode of gastroenteritis and 29.7 per 100,000 person-years in the control cohort without a history of gastroenteritis when followed for a mean duration of 3.5 years.[51] Microscopic colitis (MC), which includes lymphocytic colitis and collagenous colitis, and requires colonic mucosal biopsies for diagnosis, should also be considered in the differential diagnosis in the appropriate clinical setting. MC has been shown to occur in 10% of all individuals referred with nonbloody diarrhea and in 20% of those > 70 years of age with watery diarrhea.[52] Up to 47% of those with MC will have abdominal pain,[53,54] and therefore they may have symptoms consistent with D-IBS. MC, however, tends to have an older age of onset relative to IBS and is more likely to present with other complaints, such as weight loss, nocturnal symptoms, and electrolyte disturbances in the setting of more severe diarrhea. It should also be kept in mind that approximately 40% of patients with MC have a sudden onset of symptoms, which is seen in PI-IBS.[54] Also of note, a case of microscopic colitis has been reported after *Campylobacter jejuni* infection.[55]

Bile salt malabsorption has been described developing after acute infectious gastroenteritis including Salmonellosis.[56] This can be diagnosed by the 7-day retention of a labeled bile salt Selenium[75] Homocholic acid taurine (SeCHT). Those with levels $< 5\%$ uniformly respond to cholestryramine.[57] Important clinical markers include abrupt onset, voluminous stools, and nocturnal defecation.[58]

Management

DIET AND BULKING AGENTS

Overall, there is no therapy specifically designed for PI-IBS, and efficacy of treatments must be extrapolated from studies involving IBS patients in general with therapy typically targeted at individual symptoms. If patients are able to identify specific exacerbating foods, these should be avoided. Elimination diets may be beneficial in IBS; however, they are frequently difficult to maintain and not all identified offending food items prove to cause symptoms under double-blind testing.[59] Certain dietary substances, such as fatty foods, sorbitol, fructose, caffeine, alcohol, gas-producing vegetables, grains and lactose in lactase-deficient patients may aggravate symptoms in some individuals. However, patients more frequently complain of symptoms with ingestion of any food and care should be taken to avoid unnecessary restrictive diets.[60] Although well documented in the pediatric population,[61] postinfectious lactose intolerance appears much less common in adults. In a small study from the UK, there were no cases of lactose intolerance by breath testing among 16 patients with PI-IBS following bacterial gastroenteritis.[62] It appears dietary fiber and fiber supplementation improves constipation associated with IBS through the addition of bulk and water to stools with an acceleration of gut transit; however, bloating, discomfort, and diarrhea may worsen.[63–65]

ANTIDIARRHEAL AGENTS

Opiates are effective for the treatment of diarrhea through prolongation of intestinal transit, which leads to inhibition of intestinal secretion and electrolyte absorption. Loperamide, a peripherally-acting μ-receptor agonist with a more rapid onset and duration of action without sedating effects, is generally preferred over codeine or diphenoxylate.[66] Loperamide has been shown to be superior to placebo for the treatment of diarrhea but not abdominal pain in IBS.[67–70] Frequently, other agents such as Simethicone and/or antispasmodics are prescribed for bloating and abdominal discomfort, although there are no proper trials demonstrating efficacy. Loperamide may be particularly helpful in preventing postprandial urgency and can be scheduled 30 minutes before meals.

ANTISPASMODIC AGENTS

Antispasmodics such as dicyclomine (bentyl) and hyoscyamine (levsin), despite limited evidence of efficacy in controlled trials, are frequently used in the clinical management of IBS.[71] Antispasmodics, which are thought to act through a decrease in spontaneous activity of intestinal smooth muscle,[72] may lead to improvement of global symptoms in IBS; [73–75] however, adverse events, such as constipation, dry mouth, and urinary retention are not uncommon, especially at higher doses.[75]

ANTIDEPRESSANTS

Tricyclic antidepressants (TCAs) and selective serotonin re-uptake inhibitors (SSRIs), through their effects on nociception, have been used to treat chronic abdominal pain in IBS and are generally given in lower doses compared to doses used for treatment of depression. In addition to neuromodulatory and analgesic properties, antidepressants have been shown to affect intestinal transit.[76,77] For example, TCAs appear to prolong orocecal and whole gut transit times, likely through anticholinergic properties.[78] On the other hand, SSRIs reduce orocecal transit time without alteration of whole gut transit.[79] Results from two meta-analyses suggest TCAs are more effective at improving abdominal pain and patients' well being compared to placebo.[80,81]

SEROTONERGIC AGENTS

After identifying the importance of serotonin in the pathophysiology of IBS, serotonergic agents have been shown to be effective for the management of IBS. The 5-HT_3 antagonist alosetron reduces visceral pain, enhances small intestinal absorption, slows colonic transit, and has been shown to be effective in females with D-IBS.[82–84] Unfortunately, alosetron was withdrawn from the US market several months after initial approval due to side-effects of severe constipation, ischemic colitis, and bowel perforation.[85] It has subsequently been reapproved through a restricted prescribing program for females with severe D-IBS who have failed to respond to other therapies.[86] Cilansetron, another 5-HT_3 antagonist, has also been shown to be effective in D-IBS,[87] and in a subset analysis, unlike alosetron, was shown to be effective for males with D-IBS.[88] Unfortunately, the side-effect profile of cilansetron appears similar to alosetron,[87,88] and cilansetron has not yet been approved for use in the US and Europe. Ondansetron, also a 5-HT_3 antagonist, has been widely used for many years as an antinauseant and has been shown to slow gut transit. One small study showed efficacy in IBS with improvement in stool consistency[89] but this has not been repeated.

Tegaserod, a selective partial 5-HT_4 agonist, has been shown to accelerate orocecal transit,[90] increase the frequency and softness of bowel movements,[91] and improve abdominal pain by reducing visceral afferent firing.[92] Tegaserod has consistently shown statistically-significant improvement of constipation, abdominal pain/discomfort, bloating, and global relief in women with C-IBS.[81] Due to limited male enrollment in clinical trials of Tegaserod, which parallels gender predominance seen in clinical practice, no definitive conclusions can be made for men with C-IBS. The lack of approval of tegaserod for men with C-IBS is generally thought to be a statistical rather than a clinical issue.

PROBIOTICS AND ANTIBIOTICS

Due to the inflammatory infiltration of the intestinal mucosa in PI-IBS and other IBS patients, probiotics have been used in an attempt to improve the barrier function and intestinal permeability by strengthening the intestinal immunologic defense. Probiotics are suspected to exert anti-inflammatory effects and have shown variable, but for the most part positive, results in unspecified IBS patients.[93] Two recently evaluated probiotics, *Lactobacillus salivaris* and *Bifidobacterium infantis*, have been shown to have an anti-inflammatory effect in IL-10 knockout mice.[94] In a recent probiotic trial in humans with nonspecific IBS,[95] patients were found to have lower baseline ratios of IL-10/IL-12 indicative of a proinflammatory state. In this study, patients were randomized to receive 8 weeks of *L. salvaris*, *B. infantis*, or placebo. Only patients who received *B. infantis* were found to have improved composite symptom scores as well as abdominal pain, bloating, and distention. Also, this symptomatic response was associated with normalization of the ratio of anti-inflammatory to proinflammatory cytokine levels.

The role of probiotics in the management of IBS has yet to be fully determined. Also, to date no trials have been conducted in PI-IBS, although their relative safety and potential anti-inflammatory properties make probiotics an intriguing option for management of these patients. Unfortunately, high-dose steroids (prednisolone 30 mg/day) for 3 weeks has showed no effect in a randomized, double-blind, placebo-controlled trial involving 29 patients with PI-IBS following *Campylobacter jejuni* enteritis.[96] Insufficient duration of treatment is one possible explanation for this negative result. Probiotics, however, might offer a safer alternative for the long-term treatment of this population.

Antibiotics have been reported to benefit IBS patients diagnosed with small intestinal bacterial overgrowth (SIBO) by lactulose breath testing.[97] The prevalence of SIBO in PI-IBS has yet to be evaluated; however, antibiotics should be considered in those patients with positive breath tests.

Prognosis

In an early prognostic evaluation of IBS patients followed for at least 5 years, those with an acute onset of symptoms had higher remission rates compared to those with an insidious onset of IBS.[98] More recently, in a 6-year prospective analysis, Neal and colleagues[99] reported only a slightly improved recovery rate in PI-IBS compared to pre-existing IBS (43% versus 31%). Similarly, a poor prognosis was reported by McKendrick,[100] in which 80% of patients with PI-IBS after *Salmonella* infection had persistent symptoms after 5 years. Long-term remission rates appear to be inversely related to psychiatric comorbidities,[9,99] a finding that is seen in unspecified IBS as well.[101] In general, patients with PI-IBS have a similar prognosis compared to those with IBS without an infectious onset and most effected individuals can expect to have chronic episodic symptoms.

References

1. Hungin APS, Chang L, Locke GR, et al. Irritable bowel syndrome in the United States: prevalence, symptom patterns and impact. Aliment Pharmacol Ther 2005;21: 1365–75.
2. Rodriguez LA, Ruigomez A. Increased risk of irritable bowel syndrome after bacterial gastroenteritis: cohort study. Br Med J 1999;318:565–6.
3. Spiller RC, Campbell E. Post-infectious irritable bowel syndrome. Curr Opin Gastroenterol 2006;22:13–7.
4. Spiller RC, Jenkins D, Thornley JP, et al. Increased rectal mucosal enteroendocrine cells, T lymphocytes and increased gut permeability following acute *Campylobacter* enteritis and in post-dysenteric irritable bowel syndrome. Gut 2000;47:804–11.
5. Gwee KA, Collins SM, Read NW. Increased rectal mucosal expression of interleukin 1beta in recently acquired postinfectious irritable bowel syndrome. Gut 2003;52: 523–6.
6. Wang LH, Fang XC, Pan GZ. Bacillary dysentery as a causative factor of irritable bowel syndrome and its pathogenesis. Gut 2004;53:1096–101.
7. Longstreth GF, Thompson WG, Chey WD, et al. Functional bowel disorders. Gastroenterol 2006;130: 1480–91.
8. Dunlop SP, Jenkins D, Spiller RC. Distinctive histological patterns of chronic inflammatory cells in rectal biopsies of patients with different clinical subtypes of IBS. Gastroenterol 2002;122(Suppl 1):A60.
9. Chaudhary NA, Truelove SC. The irritable colon syndrome: a study of the clinical features, predisposing

causes, and prognosis in 130 cases. Q J Med 1962;123: 307–22.

10. McKendrick MW, Read NW. Irritable bowel syndrome—post Salmonella infection. J Infect 1994;29:1–3.

11. Gwee KA, Graham JC, McKendrick MW, et al. Psychometric scores and persistence of irritable bowel after infectious diarrhoea. Lancet 1996;347:150–3.

12. Neal KR, Hebden J, Spiller R. Prevalence of gastrointestinal symptoms six months after bacterial gastroenteritis and risk factors for development of the irritable bowel syndrome: postal survey of patients. Br Med J 1997;314: 779–82.

13. Parry SD, Stansfield R, Jelley D, et al. Does bacterial gastroenteritis predispose people to functional gastrointestinal disorders? A prospective, community-based, case-control study. Am J Gastroenterol 2003;98:1970–5.

14. Locke GR, Yawn BP, Woolan PC, Lydick E. The incidence of clinically diagnosed irritable bowel syndrome in the community [Abstract]. Gastroenterol 1999;116:A76.

15. Wheeler JG, Sethi D, Cowden JM, et al. Study of infectious intestinal disease in England: rates in the community, presenting to general practice, and reported to national surveillance. The Infectious Intestinal Disease Study Executive. Br Med J 1999;318:1046–50.

16. Halvorson HA, Schlett CD, Riddle MS. Post-infectious irritable bowel syndrome: a meta analysis. Am J Gastroenterol 2006;101:1894–9.

17. Ilnyckyj A, Balachandra B, Elliott L, et al. Post-traveler's diarrhea irritable bowel syndrome: a prospective study. Am J Gastroenterol 2003;98:596–9.

18. Okhuysen PC, Jiang SD, Carlin L, et al. Post-diarrhea chronic intestinal symptoms and irritable bowel syndrome in North American travelers to Mexico. Am J Gastroenterol 2004;99:1774–8.

19. James C, Thabane M, Borgaonkar MR, Marshall JK. Post infectious irritable bowel syndrome (PI-IBS) is transient following a foodborne outbreak of acute gastroenteritis attributed to a viral pathogen. Gastroenterol 2004;126: A53.

20. Dunlop SP, Jenkins D, Neal KR, et al. Relative importance of enterochromaffin cell hyperplasia, anxiety, and depression in postinfectious IBS. Gastroenterology 2003;125: 1651–9.

21. Gwee KA, Leong YL, Graham C, et al. The role of psychological and biological factors in postinfective gut dysfunction. Gut 1999;44:400–6.

22. Dunlop SP, Jenkins D, Spiller RC. Distinctive clinical, psychological, and histological features of postinfective irritable bowel syndrome. Am J Gastroenterol 2003;98: 1578–83.

23. Spiller RC. Postinfectious irritable bowel syndrome. Gastroenterol 2003;124:1662–71.

24. Parry SD, Barton JR, Welfare MR. Factors associated with the development of post-infectious functional gastrointestinal diseases: does smoking play a role? Eur J Gastroenterol & Hep 2005;17:1071–5.

25. Mearin F, Perez-Oliveras M, Perello A, et al. Dyspepsia and irritable bowel syndrome after a Salmonella gastroenteritis outbreak: one-year follow-up cohort study. Gastroenterol 2005;129:98–104.

26. Linden DR, Sharkey KA, Mawe GM. Inflammation is associated with an increased availability of serotonin from enterochromaffin cells in the guinea pig distal colon. FASEB J 2002;16:A890.

27. Wheatcroft J, Wakelin D, Jenkins D, Spiller RC. Increased enteroendocrine cells numbers in the *Trichinella spiralis* infected mouse model of post-infectious bowel dysfunction. Gastroenterol 2002;122(Suppl 1): A162.

28. Coates MD, Mahoney CR, Linden DR, et al. Molecular defects in mucosal serotonin content and decreased serotonin reuptake transporter in ulcerative colitis and irritable bowel syndrome. Gastroenterol 2004;126:1657–64.

29. Dunlop SP, Coleman NS, Blackshaw E, et al. Abnormalities of 5-hydroxytryptamine metabolism in irritable bowel syndrome. Clin Gastroenterol Hepatol 2005;3:349–57.

30. Yeo A, Boyd P, Lumsden S, et al. Association between a functional polymorphism in the serotonin transporter gene and diarrhoea predominant irritable bowel syndrome in women. Gut 2004;53:1452–8.

31. Mossner R, Daniel S, Schmitt A, et al. Modulation of serotonin transporter function by interleukin-4. Life Sci 2001;68:873–80.

32. Linden DR, Chen JX, Gershon MD, et al. Serotonin availability is increased in mucosa of guinea pigs with TNBS-induced colitis. Am J Physiol 2003;285: G207–16.

33. Pata C, Erdal ME, Derici E, et al. Serotonin transporter gene polymorphism in irritable bowel syndrome. Am J Gastroenterol 2002;97:1780–4.

34. Jones MA, Totemeyer S, Maskell DJ, et al. Introduction of proinflammatory responses in the human monocytic cell line THP-1 by *Campylobacter jejuni*. Infect Immun 2003; 71:2626–33.

35. van der Veek PP, van den Berg M, de Kroon YE, et al. Role of tumor necrosis factor-alpha and interleukin-10 gene polymorphisms in irritable bowel syndrome. Am J Gastroenterol 2005;100:2510–6.

36. Gonsalkorale WM, Perrey C, Pravica V, et al. Interleukin 10 genotypes in irritable bowel syndrome: evidence for an inflammatory component? Gut 2003;52: 91–3.

37. Chadwick VS, Chen W, Shu D, et al. Activation of the mucosal immune system in irritable bowel syndrome. Gastroenterol 2002;122:1778–83.

38. Barbara G, Vallance BA, Collins SM. Persistent intestinal neuromuscular dysfunction after acute nematode infection in mice. Gastroenterol 1997;113:1224–32.

39. O'Sullivan M, Clayton N, Breslin NP, et al. Increased mast cells in the irritable bowel syndrome. Neurogastroenterol Motil 2000;12:449–57.

40. Barbara G, Stanghellini V, De Giorgio R, et al. Activated mast cells in proximity to colonic nerves correlate with abdominal pain in irritable bowel syndrome. Gastroenterol 2004;126:693–702.

41. Park CH, Joo YE, Choi SK, et al. Activated mast cells infiltrate in close proximity to enteric nerves in diarrhea-predominant irritable bowel syndrome. J Korean Med Sci 2003;18:204–10.

42. Coelho AM, Vergnolle N, Guiard B, et al. Proteinases and proteinase-activated receptor 2: a possible role to promote visceral hyperalgesia in rats. Gastroenterol 2002;122:1035–47.

43. Hoogerwerf WA, Zou L, Shenoy M, et al. The proteinase-activated receptor 2 is involved in nociception. J Neuroscience 2001;21:9036–42.

44. Fu LW, Pan HL, Longhurst JC. Endogenous histamine stimulate ischemically sensitive abdominal visceral afferents through H1 receptors. Am J Physiol 1997;273: H2726–37.

45. Dunlop SP, Hebden J, Campbell E, et al. Abnormal intestinal permeability in subgroups of diarrhea-predominant irritable bowel syndrome. Am J Gastroenterol 2006;101:1288–94.

46. Marshall JK, Thabane M, Garg AX, et al. Intestinal permeability in patients with irritable bowel syndrome after a waterborne outbreak of acute gastroenteritis in Walkerton, Ontario. Aliment Pharmacol Ther 2004;20: 1317–22.

47. Kapoor KK, Nigam P, Rastogi CK, et al. Clinical profile of irritable bowel syndrome. Indian J Gastroenterol 1985;4: 15–6.

48. Wei X, Chen M, Wang J. The epidemiology of irritable bowel syndrome and functional constipation of Guangzhou residents. Zhonghua Nei Ke Za Zhi 2001;40: 517–20.

49. Vanner SJ, Depew WT, Paterson WG, et al. Predictive value of the Rome criteria for diagnosing the irritable bowel syndrome. Am J Gastroenterol 1999;94: 2912–7.

50. Cash BD, Schoenfeld P, Chey WD. The utility of diagnostic tests in irritable bowel syndrome patients: a systematic review. Am J Gastroenterol 2002;97:2812–9.

51. Rodríguez L, Ruigómez A, Panés J. Acute Gastroenteritis is followed by an increased risk of inflammatory bowel disease. Gastroenterol 2006;130:1588–94.

52. Olesen M, Eriksson S, Bohr J, et al. Microscopic colitis: a common diarrhoeal disease. An epidemiological study in Orebro, Sweden, 1993–1998. Gut 2004;53:346–50.

53. Olesen M, Eriksson S, Bohr J, et al. Lymphocytic colitis: a retrospective clinical study of 199 Swedish patients. Gut 2004;53:536–41.

54. Bohr J, Tysk C, Eriksson S, et al. Collagenous colitis: a retrospective study of clinical presentation and treatment in 163 patients. Gut 1996;39:846–51.

55. Perk G, Ackerman Z, Cohen P, Eliakim R. Lymphocytic colitis: a clue to an infectious trigger. Scand J Gastroenterol 1999;34:110–2.

56. Niaz SK, Sandrasegaran K, Renny FH, Jones BJ. Postinfective diarrhoea and bile acid malabsorption. J R Coll Physicians Lond 1997;31:53–6.

57. Williams AJK, Merrick MV, Eastwood MA. Idiopathic bile acid malabsorption—a review of clinical presentation, diagnosis, and response to treatment. Gut 1991;32: 1004–6.

58. Sinha L, Liston R, Testa HJ, Moriarty KJ. Idiopathic bile acid malabsorption: qualitative and quantitative clinical features and response to cholestyramine. Aliment Pharmacol Ther 1998;12:839–44.

59. Jones J, Boorman J, Cann P, et al. British Society of Gastroenterology guidelines for the management of the irritable bowel syndrome. Gut 2000;47(Suppl II):ii1–ii19.

60. Drossman DA, Camilleri M, Mayer EA, Whitehead WE. AGA technical review on irritable bowel syndrome. Gastroenterol 2002;123:2108–31.

61. Szajewska H, Kantecki M, Albrecht P, Antoniewicz J. Carbohydrate intolerance after acute gastroenteritis—a disappearing problem in Polish children. Acta Paediatr 1997;86:347–50.

62. Parry SD, Barton JR, Welfare MR. Is lactose intolerance implicated in the development of post-infectious irritable bowel syndrome or functional diarrhoea in previously asymptomatic people? Eur J Gastroenterol Hepatol 2002; 14:1225–30.

63. Manning AP, Heaton KW, Harvey RF. Wheat fibre and irritable bowel syndrome. A controlled trial. Lancet 1977; ii:417–8.

64. Cann PA, Read NWH, Holdsworth CD. What is the benefit of coarse bran in patients with irritable bowel syndrome? Gut 1984;25:168–71.

65. Lucey MR, Clark ML, Lowndes JO, Dawson AM. Is bran efficacious in irritable bowel syndrome? A double-blind placebo controlled crossover study. Gut 1987;28: 221–5.

66. Tack J. Irritable bowel syndrome. In: Wolfe MM, Davis GL, Farraye FF, et al, editors. Therapy of digestive disorders—a companion to Sleisenger and Fordtran's gastrointestinal and liver disease 2nd edition. Philadelphia: W.B. Saunders; 2006;705.

67. Cann PA, Read NW, Holdsworth CD, Barends D. Role of loperamide and placebo in management of irritable bowel syndrome. Dig Dis Sci 1984;29:239–47.

68. Hovdenak N. Loperamide treatment of the irritable bowel syndrome. Scand J Gastroenterol Suppl 1987;130: 81–4.

69. Lavo B, Stenstam M, Nielsen A-L. Loperamide in treatment of irritable bowel syndrome—a double-blind placebo controlled study. Scand J Gastroenterol Suppl 1987;130:77–80.

70. Efskind PS, Bernklev T, Vatn MH. A double-blind placebo-controlled trial with loperamide in irritable bowel syndrome. Scand J Gastroenterol 1996;31:463–8.

71. Talley N, Spiller RC. Irritable bowel syndrome: a little understood organic bowel disease? Lancet 2002;360:555–64.

72. Brandt LJ, Bjorkman D, Fennerty MB, et al. Systematic review on the management of irritable bowel syndrome in North America. Am J Gastroenterol 2002;97(Suppl 11): S7–26.

73. Wheatley D. Irritable colon syndrome treated with an antispasmodic drug. The Practitioner 1976;217:276–80.

74. Ritchie JA, Truelove SC. Treatment of irritable bowel syndrome with lorazepam, hyoscine butylbromide, and ispaghula husk. BMJ 1979;10:376–8.

75. Page J, Dirnberger GM. Treatment of the irritable bowel syndrome with bentyl (dicyclomine hydrochloride). J Clin Gastroenterol 1981;3:153–6.

76. Clouse RE. Antidepressants for irritable bowel syndrome. Gut 2003;52:598–9.

77. Kilkens TO, Honig A, Rozendaal N, et al. Systematic review: serotonergic modulators in the treatment of irritable bowel syndrome—influence on psychiatric and gastrointestinal symptoms. Aliment Pharmacol Ther 2003; 17:43–51.

78. Gorard DA, Libby GW, Farthing MJ. Influence of antidepressants on whole gut and orocaecal transit times in health and irritable bowel syndrome. Aliment Pharmacol Ther 1994;8:159–66.

79. Gorard DA, Libby GW, Farthing MJ. 5-Hydroxytryptamine and human small intestinal motility: effect of inhibiting 5-hydroxytryptamine reuptake. Gut 1994;35:496–500.

80. Jackson JL, O'Malley PG, Tomkins G, et al. Treatment of functional gastrointestinal disorders with antidepressant medications: a meta-analysis. Am J Med 2000;108:65–72.

81. Lesbros-Pantoflickova D, Michetti P, Fried M, et al. Meta-analysis: the treatment of irritable bowel syndrome. Aliment Pharmacol Ther 2004;20:1253–69.

82. Houghton LA, Foster JM, Whorwell PJ. Alosetron, a 5-HT3 receptor antagonist, delays colonic transit in patients with irritable bowel syndrome and healthy volunteers. Aliment Pharmacol Ther 2000;14:775–82.

83. De Ponti F, Tonini M. Irritable bowel syndrome: new agents targeting serotonin receptor subtypes. Drugs 2001; 61:317–32.

84. Clemens CH, Samsom M, Van Berge Henegouwen GP, et al. Effect of alosetron on left colonic motility in non-constipated patients with irritable bowel syndrome and healthy volunteers. Aliment Pharmacol Ther 2002;16:993–1002.

85. Anonymous. Glaxo Welcome withdraws irritable bowel syndrome medication. FDA Consum 2001;35:3.

86. McCarthy M. FDA allows controversial bowel drug back on market. Lancet 2002;359:2095.

87. Bradette M, Moennikes H, Carter F, et al. Cilansetron in irritable bowel syndrome with diarrhea predominance (IBS-D): efficacy and safety in 6-month global study. Gastroenterol 2004;126 (4 Suppl. 2):351.

88. Coremans G, Clouse RE, Carter F, et al. Cilansetron, a novel 5-HT3 antagonist, demonstrated efficacy in males with irritable bowel syndrome with diarrhea-predominance (IBS-D). Gastroenterol 2004;126(4 Suppl. 2): W1471.

89. Maxton DG, Morris J, Whorwell PJ. Selective 5-hydroxytryptamine antagonism: a role in irritable bowel syndrome and functional dyspepsia? Aliment Pharmacol Ther 1996;10:595–9.

90. Prather CM, Camilleri M, Zinsmeister AR, et al. Tegaserod accelerates orocecal transit in patients with constipation-predominant irritable bowel syndrome. Gastroenterol 2000;228:463–8.

91. Muller-Lissner SA, Fumagalli I, Bardhan KD, et al. Tegaserod, a 5-HT(4) receptor partial agonist, relieves symptoms in irritable bowel syndrome patients with abdominal pain, bloating and constipation. Aliment Pharmacol Ther 2001;15:1655–66.

92. Coffin B, Farmachidi JP, Rueegg P, et al. Tegaserod, a 5-HT4 receptor partial agonist, decreases sensitivity to rectal distention in healthy subjects. Aliment Pharmacol Ther 2003;17:577–85.

93. Floch MH. Use of diet and probiotic therapy in the irritable bowel syndrome: analysis of the literature. J Clin Gastroenterol 2005;39(5 Suppl):S243–6.

94. McCarthy J, O'Mahony L, O'Callaghan L, et al. Double blind, placebo controlled trial of two probiotic strains in interleukin 10 knockout mice and mechanistic like with cytokine balance. Gut 2003;52:975–80.

PART FOUR

PREVENTION

CHAPTER 19

DIET AND EDUCATION ABOUT RISKS

DAVID R. HILL, MD, DTM&H, FRCP

EDWARD T. RYAN, MD, DTM&H

"Boil it, cook it, peel it, or forget it." This is the mantra of travel medicine specialists and others who advise travelers about trying to avoid diarrhea during travel.[1–3] Of the three potential modes of prevention, namely dietary avoidance measures, chemoprophylaxis (either antibiotics or nonantimicrobial products), and immunoprophylaxis, care in food and liquid selection is considered a cornerstone in the prevention of travelers' diarrhea (TD).[4] Antibiotic prophylaxis is not recommended for most travelers, and except for some cross protection with the oral whole cell-inactivated cholera vaccine against heat-labile (LT) toxin-producing *Escherichia coli*,[5] immunoprophylaxis against the syndrome of TD is not currently available.[1,4]

Although most people agree upon the importance of exercising care in diet during travel, others, including some health care providers, feel that sampling the local foods is part of the enjoyment of international travel. There is also the increasing realization that being careful in what a traveler eats and drinks may not always protect them against diarrhea.[6] Each traveler will need to decide how motivated or able he or she is to follow the recommendations outlined in this chapter. This decision is likely to be based upon their willingness to accept a risk of diarrhea and how much their underlying health or travel plans will be affected by a diarrheal illness.

Diet is not the only determinate for acquiring TD; several other risk factors are discussed in other chapters of this book. These include the age and host characteristics of the traveler; the destination, duration, and season of travel; type of accommodation and eating establishment; and a history of previous travel or residence in developing regions. This chapter will focus on the role of diet in causing TD. Three essential questions arise when considering diet and education:

- Which foods and liquids are a risk?
- Does avoidance of these items decrease the risk of diarrhea?
- Do (can) travelers comply with avoidance measures?

The Risk From Food and Liquids

It was not until the early to mid-1970s, after enterotoxin-producing *Escherichia coli* were associated with diarrhea in travelers to Mexico, that excellent epidemiologic studies on risk items and behavior were initiated.[7–9] Some risk items have been identified by formal epidemiologic studies, some by culture, and others because of the pervasive opinion that poor sanitation in developing regions leads to near universal contamination of foods and water with enteric flora. The focus has also been on items that carry the most frequently implicated agents associated with TD: enterotoxigenic (ETEC), enteroaggregative, and other *E. coli*; *Shigella*; *Salmonella*; *Campylobacter*; enteric viruses such as norovirus and rotavirus; and the protozoan parasites *Giardia*, *Cryptosporidium*, and *Cyclospora*. Measures taken to avoid these organisms will also help prevent other less common but enterically transmitted microbes such as hepatitis A and E, *Salmonella enterica* serotype Typhi and Paratyphi, *Brucella*, intestinal nematodes such as ascaris and whipworm (*Trichuris trichiura*), tissue nematodes (eg, *Trichinella*), adult tapeworm infections (eg, *Taenia solium* and *saginata*), and the larval cestode infection, cysticercosis. Therefore, care in food and liquid selection should help to maintain the overall health of travelers. Table 1 lists items that have been implicated as a risk for TD.

FOOD

There are several stages during which food can become contaminated with enteric organisms of human or animal origin. Contamination may occur when leafy

Table 1 Dietary Items that have been Associated with Travelers' Diarrhea and Other Infectious Processes

Raw or undercooked meats, fish, or seafood
Raw, ground-grown vegetables and leafy greens (salads)
Unpasteurized dairy products such as milk, custard, cream, ice cream, butter, cheese
Foods containing raw or undercooked eggs
Tap water and ice
Noncarbonated bottled water
Fruits that have been peeled (not by the traveler)
Fruit juices
Cold sauces and toppings such as mayonnaise, guacamole, spicy sauces
Buffet food that has sat at room temperature for several hours
Food that requires cold storage and then reheating
Food that is served by street vendors

greens and vegetables are fertilized with "night soil" or when crops are watered with polluted water. Fruits such as strawberries and raspberries may be especially difficult to wash if they become contaminated, and others such as melons may have been injected with contaminated water to increase their weight.[10] Products that are sold in a market can become contaminated if they lie on the market floor, are exposed to flies, or are handled by unsanitary fingers. Improper storage (ie, inadequate refrigeration) can lead to bacterial overgrowth in contaminated foods.[11] Some sauces and toppings that use eggs or cream may not be pasteurized. If foods are insufficiently cooked or reheated prior to serving, any previous contamination will not be eliminated. Finally, foods may become contaminated if prepared by infected food handlers.

Other agents are not strictly associated with TD; nevertheless, they are acquired following ingestion of undercooked fish, crustaceans, and meats. These foods may carry the intermediate lifecycle forms of *Diphyllobothrium*, *Paragonimus*, *Clonorchis*, *Taenia*, *Trichinella*, or the dormant cysts of *Toxoplasma gondii*. Shellfish may be contaminated with hepatitis A virus or vibrios if it has been harvested from polluted waters. Although ciguatera toxin poisoning is not an infectious disease, it is acquired through ingestion of large reef fish (eg, barracuda, snapper, amberjack, sea bass, and grouper) in the Caribbean and South Pacific regions. Cooking will not destroy the heat-stable toxin; therefore, travelers should be aware of the potential risk from these fish. Other seafood toxins (eg, scromboid and puffer fish) may also be a risk.

Food is most frequently implicated in the transmission of bacterial pathogens.[12–14] A large body of literature that describes the risk, pathogens, and pattern of diarrhea came from the study of travelers to Mexico in the mid and late 1970s. Although much of the early epidemiologic work defining this risk was done in Mexico, the findings from these studies are applicable throughout developing regions, although the predominant organisms may differ. In addition, regardless of whether a particular region is designated as high, moderate, or low risk for TD, nearly every country in the world will have areas where food and liquid sanitation may pose a risk to the traveler. The experience with foodborne outbreaks of enteric illness in the United States involving *Listeria*,[15] Shiga toxin-producing *E. coli*,[16] enterotoxigenic *E. coli*,[17] hepatitis A, and *Cyclospora* emphasizes this point.[18,19] Therefore, all travelers should be thoroughly educated about food and liquid hygiene.

A hierarchy has been established for the risk of diarrhea from eating in different settings. Tjoa and colleagues studied students newly arrived in Mexico and demonstrated that eating from street vendors carried the highest risk.[13] In Guatemala, street vendor food and liquids were implicated in contributing to the spread of cholera in the early 1990s.[20] In the study by Tjoa and colleagues, the next level of risk was eating in public restaurants and/or a school cafeteria; the lowest risk for diarrhea was eating in private homes. Eating out in restaurants also correlated with an increased risk of diarrhea for expatriates living in Kathmandu, Nepal.[11] Examination of some of these restaurants revealed multiple opportunities for contamination of food items, an inability to adequately refrigerate stored foods, and no sinks for employees to wash hands or to clean food preparation surfaces.[21] In the home, there may be a better chance of preparing food properly. Nevertheless, depending upon the setting, foods taken in private homes may still be a source of diarrhea-producing organisms, and eating from street vendors may not always increase risk.[14,22]

In Mexico, food items that have cultured positive for enteric pathogens included watermelons (possibly injected with contaminated water), hamburger, mushrooms, dairy products, and ice that had been stored in an open market.[13] Even cooked foods that may not have been served promptly after cooking, properly refrigerated, or sufficiently reheated were positive on culture. These data on risk were confirmed in a subsequent study, also carried out with students in Guadalajara, Mexico.[23]

In a prospective study of Peace Corps volunteers in Guatemala, there were several actions that correlated with an increased risk of diarrhea. These included eating in the home of a native resident or in a small restaurant, eating fruit already peeled (not by the volunteer), eating ice cream, drinking water from an unknown source, and drinking iced beverages.[24] For expatriates in Nepal, risk factors included eating in restaurants, eating restaurant take-out food that required reheating (such as quiche,

lasagna, or casseroles), and drinking blended fruit drinks.[11] Other food items that were implicated were salads, raw vegetables, and popular hot sauces (guacamole, green and red sauces) used in restaurants.[9,25] In the study of Adachi and colleagues, even a low pH did not inhibit growth of diarrhea-producing *E. coli.*[25]

Environmental sources may contribute to diarrhea when there are conditions of crowding or high population densities and extensive contamination. This has occurred on cruise ships, as highlighted by recurrent outbreaks of norovirus infection.[26, 27] In these cases, it is important to exercise strict hand washing to prevent acquisition of the virus from environmental sources.

Water and Other Liquids

Although food has been documented to be the major source of pathogenic enteric organisms, water has also been suggested or implicated.[24, 28–30] It is likely that water is less frequently a vehicle for typical TD because many of the common bacterial pathogens, such as ETEC and *Salmonella*, require a large inoculum to establish infection. Unless the water is heavily contaminated, or has been contaminated with a small number of bacteria and left standing, such as in a holding tank or a homemade storage vessel, there will usually be dilution of the inoculum. Also, if a traveler has normal gastric acid, then the risk of a small inoculum, as may occur during teeth brushing, is often not enough to establish infection. If the water is frozen, the bacteria may be preserved, but there will not be additional multiplication prior to ingestion.

The most common causes of waterborne outbreaks of diarrheal illness in the United States (from water either intended for drinking or for recreation) are *Giardia*, *Cryptosporidium*, *Shigella*, *E. coli* O157:H7 (Shiga toxin-producing), and norovirus.[31,32] Common to these agents is that they require a much lower inoculum to establish infection (often only 10 to 100 organisms), and for the parasites and enteric viruses, they are relatively resistant to halogenation. In addition, *Giardia* cysts can survive in cold water for weeks.[33]

In areas such as Mexico, where ETEC predominates in the summer months, water was not seen to be an additional risk factor in early studies.[9] Nevertheless, water has been associated with diarrhea in other studies, and if one shifts the focus of study from the summer season in Mexico to the winter months, then water has been associated with risk.[24,29,30,34] In the study by Ericsson and colleagues, it was postulated that enteric viruses contributed to diarrhea and were waterborne.[29] This would be consistent with the finding of decreased clearance of enteric viruses by water treatment plants and the more frequent contamination of samples during the winter months in Guadalajara.[35]

Water may be contaminated at its source, particularly if surface water is used. Municipal water supplies are often adequately chlorinated, but the water becomes contaminated following distribution and storage. This was found to be the case with water used by street vendors for making various drinks and fruit beverages; it was generally coliform-free at the source, but became contaminated as it was handled to prepare the drinks.[36]

Water can be a source of diarrhea on cruise ships that obtain water in foreign ports and do not adequately purify it.[37] During the rainy season in many countries, flooding may wash ground contamination into surface water supplies or flood wells, leading to an increased incidence of diarrhea. The rainy season is also the period when diseases that require contact with contaminated water, such as leptospirosis, can be seen.[38] The relative chlorine resistance of *Cryptosporidium* and *Giardia* can lead to diarrhea acquired during recreational activities such as swimming in fecally contaminated swimming pools or freshwater lakes.[32]

In addition to microbial contamination, water may contain chemical or other inorganic and organic substances such as arsenic, lead, and benzene, or herbicides and pesticides that might not be removed by routine treatment methods.[31]

Pathogenic enteric bacteria (ETEC, *Salmonella*, and *Shigella*) can survive in ice and multiply if the ice is placed in drinks with less than 80 proof alcohol.[39] The viability of the bacteria declines if the ice remains frozen for more than 24 hours. If the ice has surface contamination, as may occur when a block has been left standing outside a restaurant, it can be a direct vehicle for transmission of enteric agents.

What about bottled water and other beverages? The standards for purification of bottled water are not uniform, and thus noncarbonated bottled water, even if sealed, could potentially be contaminated.[40] One investigation even documented Norwalk-like viral sequences in three brands of European mineral water for up to 1 year following bottling.[41] The act of carbonation, probably by lowering the pH, should render carbonated bottled water safe. When a large inoculum of *Salmonella*, *Shigella*, or *E. coli* (2×10^6 organisms/mL) was added to different beverages (sour mix, cola, and beer) with an acidic pH, they survived poorly at 48 hours.[42] It appeared that the low pH was the common factor for poor survival because none of the bacteria would multiply in growth medium that had been rendered acidic. There were no bacteria recovered at 4 hours in wine. Milk and water supported growth.

Despite the fact that alcohol in drinks can kill infectious pathogens, the offer of free alcoholic beverages to travelers may lead to higher rates of diarrhea,[43] and excessive alcohol ingestion itself has been associated with TD. Male travelers who consumed more than five drinks per day in Mexico were at high risk for TD (79%),[44] suggesting that educational efforts aimed to minimize excessive alcohol consumption among young male travelers could lower the incidence of TD.

Water Purification

The provision of potable water, or water that can be drunk with a minimal risk for microbial contamination, is a universal goal. For the traveler, there are several ways to prepare water so that it is potable.[45] Although bottled water is often safe, it may not be reliably so in developing regions. Therefore, it may be prudent to drink carbonated bottled water because of the added antibacterial effect of a lower pH and the reassurance that if the water remains carbonated at the time of opening, it is likely to have been prepared properly.

To render surface or tap water safe for drinking, there are three standard methods that are comprehensively reviewed by Backer, and are outlined in Table 2.[46] These methods are heat, filtration, and halogenation. Heat is the most reliable and will kill all bacterial, viral, and parasitic pathogens. However, it will not always be easy for the traveler to heat water. An electric heating element may be needed, and if the traveler is in a wilderness or rural setting, there has to be a source of fuel. In order to conserve resources, it is only necessary to bring water to a boil. The higher the temperature, the shorter the period of time it takes to kill enteric organisms. Because most enterics are killed at 70°C, when they are maintained at this temperature for < 1 minute to 10 minutes, the process and time that it takes to bring water to a boil (100°C) is sufficient to kill them.[47–51] This is the concept behind pasteurization: the maintenance of a dietary product at a temperature below 100°C (usually 65° to 70°C) for a sufficient period of time to kill microbes. Tap water that is too hot to touch (60°C or cooler) may not be hot enough to render it potable.[47,48] The Centers for Disease Control and Prevention have taken a more conservative view and recommend boiling for 1 minute.[52]

Filtration, using a filter of an absolute micron size of 0.2 to 1 μm, will remove bacteria and parasitic cysts and ova because of their size.[46] However, enteric viruses will not be reliably eliminated because they are too small to be filtered. Although some filters claim to remove viruses by viral adherence to the filter itself, this may not be the case for all products.[53] In areas where water is a low risk for enteric viruses, such as in remote wilderness areas where the watershed is not contaminated with human waste, it may be possible to use filtration alone to purify water for drinking. For travel to all other developing regions, an additional purification process will be necessary. This process is usually halogenation.

Halogenation can be performed before or after filtration, and once complete, the water may be passed through a carbon filter or have citric acid crystals added to render the taste more palatable. There is a hierarchy of susceptibility of organisms to halogenation: bacteria are the most sensitive (killed by a concentration of 0.1 to 1.0 mg/L), then viruses (0.5 to 5.0 mg/L), and finally parasitic cysts and ova (1 to ≥ 50 mg/L).[46] While *Giardia* may be killed with a sufficient concentration of halogen over time, *Cryptosporidium* is highly resistant, and other agents such as *Cyclospora* and parasitic eggs are likely to be equally resistant.[49, 54–57] The efficacy of halogenation is also dependent upon temperature, contact time, turbidity, and pH, although iodine preparations are less subject to these factors compared with chlorine preparations. Thus, if the water is particularly cold, the contact time should be increased, or if it is turbid, the concentration should be increased. Filters with iodine resins are not reliably effective and should not be used.

Table 2 Water Disinfection

Technique	Bacteria	Viruses	Giardia	Cryptosporidium
Heat*	+	+	+	+
Filtration†	+	–	+	+
Halogenation‡	+	+	+**	–

*Water should be brought to a boil (100°C). Water held for several minutes at temperatures of 70°C or higher should be potable.
† The filter size should be ≤ 0.2 μm for bacteria and ≤ 1 μm for parasites.
‡ Concentrations of the halogen should be 1 to 10 mg/L for 30 to 60 minutes. There are several options: iodine tablets (tetraglycine hydroperiodide; eg, Globaline, Potable Aqua; tincture of iodine at 2%, 5 drops/L; chlorine tablets; or chlorine bleach at 5 to 6%, 2 to 4 drops/L. The activity of chlorine varies more with changes in pH, turbidity, and temperature than iodine-based methods.
**Giardia usually requires 5 to 8 mg/L of halogen and a longer contact time to be killed.
Abbreviations: +: susceptible; –: not susceptible.
Adapted from Backer.[46]

Water that has been rendered potable should be stored in a clean vessel that can be sealed against contamination. There should also be residual halogen so that bacteria that have not been eliminated will not multiply during storage. Use of iodine for short periods should not be problematic; however, some pregnant women and individuals with thyroid disease should not use iodine.[58]

Do Avoidance Measures Decrease Risk?

It makes intuitive sense that being careful about food and liquids during travel should decrease the incidence of diarrhea. Several studies on TD have examined this directly or indirectly, and concluded that avoidance measures are not always associated with decreased risk.[12,22,59–64] However, many of these studies are retrospective and rely upon recall of behavior rather than prospective recording of actions taken during travel. In one of the earliest studies to address this question, individuals who attended a congress in Mexico City, and who avoided salads, raw vegetables, peeled fruit, or untreated water, had the same incidence of diarrhea as those who did not practice any precautions.[59] In another study from Mexico, only the ingestion of salads with raw vegetables was associated with diarrhea, and drinking untreated water or eating unpeeled fruits was not a risk for infection.[9] For Finnish travelers to Morocco who made frequent dietary mistakes, there was a similar number of travelers with and without diarrhea who made the same errors.[61] In a study of more than 16,000 predominantly Swiss travelers who visited multiple destinations, those who took at least three of the standard precautions actually had a slightly increased risk of diarrhea.[62] Visitors to Jamaica who ate meals outside of their tourist hotel had the same risk of diarrhea compared with those who took their meals in the hotels.[63] Thirty-four percent of nearly 800 American travelers to many world destinations, who were provided both verbal and written pretravel information on avoidance measures, had moderate to severe TD, and another 11% had mild diarrhea.[64]

Steffen and colleagues recently analyzed the epidemiology of TD in Mombasa, Kenya; Goa, India; Montego Bay, Jamaica; and Fortaleza, Brazil.[43] Over a 12-month period, more than 73,000 short-term travelers completed an airport departure lounge questionnaire that evaluated the incidence, risk factors, and impact of diarrhea. Travelers were asked whether they had ingested 12 food or beverage products classically considered high risk for TD (eg, tap water, ice cubes, rare meats, hamburgers, raw oysters, lobster, shrimp, salad, creamy dressing, street vendor products, ice cream). Individuals were scored at 0 if they never ingested them, 1 if they occasionally ingested them, and 2 if they ingested them daily. The total attack rate of diarrhea ranged from a low of 14% in Fortaleza to higher than 54% in Mombasa, with a 14-day incidence rate varying between 20 and 66%. Although a breakdown by individual ingestion was not provided, in aggregate, there was no difference between the mean food score in travelers with or without diarrhea among all four geographic locations.

On the other hand, a prospective study of charter holiday tourists to Sri Lanka and East or West Africa, who recorded in detail their dietary habits for the first few days of travel, documented that the more dietary mistakes committed, the higher the incidence of diarrhea.[65] In a prospective study of Peace Corps volunteers that covered their entire time of service in Guatemala, several dietary errors were independently associated with an increased risk of diarrheal illness: water from an unknown source, eating in the home of a Guatemalan friend or family, eating in a small restaurant, eating peeled fruit, drinking iced beverages, eating ice cream, and traveling (and presumably eating) outside the area of residence.[24] Therefore, if one was able to avoid the risk behavior, one had a lower incidence of diarrhea. Visitors to Jamaica, who stayed with family and friends and ate in their homes had less diarrhea compared with other visitors to the island.[63] Students in Mexico, who were careful about water and ice consumption, had lower rates of diarrhea compared to newly arrived students who did not exercise these precautions.[29]

HAND WASHING

Except for a few notable exceptions of infection following ingestion of very small inocula (*Shigella*, Shiga-toxin producing *E. coli*, *cryptosporidium*, and viruses), it would be anticipated that hand washing immediately prior to eating would not have a major effect on the risk of TD. However, in a different setting, hand washing following defecation was associated with a decreased incidence of diarrhea among wilderness hikers in the United States.[66] Many travelers eat their meals "on the road" and may not have access to hygienic facilities for hand washing. Alcohol-based solutions have been shown to be equivalent to or superior to hand washing with soap and water,[67] so it is possible that the use of alcohol-based hand sanitizers may alter the risk of TD. They might be predicted to have their highest efficacy in preventing ingestion of small infecting inocula, such as that associated with norovirus that can be contained on fomites. Norovirus was recently found in up to 10% of travelers with diarrhea after travel to Mexico.[68] One retrospective study preliminarily addressed the role of alcohol-based hand sanitizers among travelers. In a study

of 155 returned US travelers, Horvath and colleagues stratified them via a post-trip telephone interview into those who said they always used alcohol-based hand sanitizer (n=41) versus those who never used alcohol-based hand sanitizer (n=44) before eating during travel.[69] Although the use of the alcohol-based hand sanitizer was associated with a decreased risk of developing diarrhea (decreased from 31% to 23%) and respiratory infection (decreased from 19% to 11%), neither of these differences achieved statistical significance. Nevertheless, the role of alcohol-based hand sanitizers may warrant further evaluation.

Do (Can) Travelers Practice Avoidance Measures During Travel?

The information on whether or not travelers practice avoidance measures during travel is less encouraging. Whether intentionally or not, most travelers find it difficult to meticulously follow these measures. In the previously quoted study on charter tourists to Sri Lanka or East or West Africa, 98% made at least one error in the first 72 hours.[65] It was not known how many of these travelers had been counseled in care about foods and liquids. In a multicenter study of approximately 67,000 travelers to India, Kenya, Jamaica, and Brazil, more than 96% did not completely follow preventive measures.[70] However, travelers to areas considered a higher risk for TD (eg, Kenya and India) did practice more preventive measures than those who traveled to areas perceived as a lower risk (eg, Jamaica and Brazil). Even travelers to Jamaica who received health advice did not always practice avoidance measures.[63]

Ninety-five percent of Finnish travelers to Morocco made a dietary error.[61] In this same group, if a person had traveled overseas before, then there was an increased likelihood of eating potentially contaminated food items; those who traveled in the previous 12 months were more likely to make dietary errors than those who had not. On the other hand, in two studies of UK travelers, those who had sought pretravel advice worried more about food and liquid hygiene or practiced more preventive measures; however, their risk of diarrhea remained high.[71,72] In Horvath and colleagues' study of 155 older, well-educated and experienced travelers, the researchers found that despite detailed pretravel education, 58% used ice, 34% drank tap water, and 15% ate food from street vendors.[69] Similarly, among the subgroup of individuals who lived with locals, 66% ate raw vegetables and salad, 58% drank tap water, and 24% ate food from street vendors, underscoring the difficulty travelers have adhering to pretravel advice.

What about diarrhea in long-term travelers and expatriates? Do they need to continue to practice care in their dietary habits? There is conflicting information on whether the risk of TD decreases with increasing duration of residence in a developing region. In a study of American students in Puebla, Mexico, the incidence of diarrhea was 40% in those who were newly arrived compared with 20% in those who were living there year round.[73] Additional episodes of diarrhea were also more common in new students (15% versus 4%). This finding was confirmed in a later study of American students in Guadalajara, Mexico.[29] The decreased incidence of diarrhea suggested that partial immunity developed to the etiologic agents. In support of this was the finding of elevated titers of anti-*E. coli* LT toxin antibody in year-round students.[74] However, it may also be that long-term residents of endemic areas learn behaviors that allow them to remain well. This seemed to be the case with the follow-up study of students in Mexico, in whom a lower rate of diarrhea in the winter months correlated with decreased consumption of tap water and unsafe ice.[29]

In long-term residents of Kathmandu, Nepal, there remained a high risk of diarrhea—3.2 episodes of diarrhea per person per year.[75] This was in an area where there was a wide variety of pathogens: *E. coli* (42% of persons affected), *Cyclospora* (32%), *Giardia* (16%), *Shigella* (16%), *Campylobacter* (10%), rotavirus (≥ 10%), and *Entamoeba* (6%). Only for ETEC did the incidence decrease with increasing duration of residence. In Peace Corps volunteers in Guatemala, the risk for all episodes of diarrhea decreased slightly over time, even though risk behavior remained about the same.[24] However, the median time to acquisition of a parasite was 187 days (range, 14 to 7,452 days), indicating an ongoing risk for this type of intestinal infection with time.[76]

What is the message from the studies of long-term travelers and expatriates? There is an ongoing risk of diarrhea no matter how long one resides in a developing region. Although infection with ETEC may decrease with time, if there are multiple pathogens circulating in an area, which is the case for most areas of the world, then the traveler remains at risk for acquiring them.

Summary and Recommendations: Advice and Education

The risk of TD has persistently averaged between 20 and 60% over the last several decades, despite our increasing understanding of the causative agents of diarrhea, identification of items and behaviors that may be high risk for transmitting infectious agents, and education of travelers about these risks. This ongoing high rate is

contributed to by a number of factors, including the broad scope of contaminated food and drink items in many resource poor areas of the world, especially at many restaurants, and the inability of travelers to strictly adhere to dietary restrictions or modifications during travel. Even if the traveler is informed and careful, it is still difficult to avoid diarrhea. Although it may be that short-term travelers who receive advice about avoidance measures before their trip travel to higher-risk destinations, as documented in a retrospective study of British travelers,[71] this is not likely to explain the high rates of diarrhea for the majority of travelers.

Based on numerous epidemiologic studies, a number of dietary risk items or behaviors have been associated with TD and other infectious processes (see Table 1), although a predictive pattern of high-risk behaviors and ingestions from different geographic locations is lacking. In the pretravel session, the traveler should be advised to avoid these risk items and to try and choose food and beverages based on Table 3. Hand washing should be emphasized, especially when there may be surface or environmental contamination with enteric pathogens. The use of hand sanitizers may prove to be useful in the absence of traditional hand washing methods.

Travelers should also attempt to choose eating establishments that have a reputation for serving safe food and drink. It is increasingly clear that poor food preparation in restaurants is an important factor in the incidence of diarrhea.[6,21,77] Recognition of this fact has led tour operators and other health professionals to pursue improved public health and sanitation measures at the destinations.[78] An example of this has been the efforts of the Jamaican Ministry of Health in instituting a program in 1996 to provide education, training, and technical assistance to food and beverage staff and environmental sanitation personnel at hotels. Over a period of approximately 6 years, the risk of TD in the hotels covered through this program decreased by 72%.[79]

Developing strategies to both inform the traveler of dietary hygiene and improving their compliance are important goals in travel medicine. It has been demonstrated that straightforward, consistent education about risk and the importance of taking medication correlates with improved compliance with malaria chemoprophylaxis by travelers.[80,81] Advice should be provided both verbally and in written form. In a survey of travel clinics worldwide, 97% of clinics gave verbal advice on TD and 91% provided it in written form.[82] Knowledge provided this way can be incorporated by travelers following their visit.[83] Therefore, despite the information that many travelers do not exercise precautions in a consistent fashion, and those who do may still suffer from diarrhea, neither the traveler nor the travel health care professional should despair. The issue should be approached in a realistic fashion, understanding the potential benefits and difficulties of being careful about food and drink. It is the task of the travel medicine specialist to inform and educate and the responsibility of the traveler to act upon the information in accordance with their tolerance for becoming ill.[4]

There should also be continued emphasis on trying to get travelers to seek pretravel care from established travel medicine services, and to train travel professionals to provide consistent education. Innovative educational strategies should be developed. Compared with vaccination against vaccine-preventable disease, education may be a more cost-effective and practical way to prevent illness.[3,84,85]

Education is particularly important for those who are at high risk for complications from diarrhea: pregnant women, the elderly, the very young, diabetics, those with cardiovascular or renal disease, and those who are immunocompromised.[86] HIV/AIDS patients should be careful about their dietary habits during travel to avoid severe and chronic infection from *Salmonella*, *Cryptosporidium*, and *Toxoplasma*.[87,88] It is hoped that with improved education of travelers and improving public health conditions at many destinations, that the incidence of TD will decline over coming years.

Table 3 Dietary Items That May be Safe to Ingest

Cooked food that has been recently prepared and is steaming when served
Dry items such as breads
Fruit that can be washed off, dried, and peeled by the traveler
Bottled, carbonated beverages (with an acidic pH): beer, soda, carbonated bottled water
Coffee and tea (assumes that they have been heated above 70°C or brought to a boil)
Wine
Water brought to a boil and then properly stored
Water that has been properly treated: halogenated and filtered (see text)

References

1. Gorbach SL, Edelman R, editors. Travelers' diarrhea: National Institutes of Health Consensus Conference. Rev Infect Dis 1986;8(Suppl 2):S227–33.

2. DuPont HL, Ericsson CD. Prevention and treatment of traveler's diarrhea. N Engl J Med 1993;328:1821–7.

3. Committee to Advise on Tropical Medicine and Travel (CATMAT). Statement on travellers' diarrhea. An Advisory Committee Statement (ACS). Can Commun Dis Rep 2001; 27:3–12.

4. Hill DR, Ericsson CD, Pearson RD, et al. The practice of travel medicine: Guidelines by the Infectious Diseases Society of America. Clin Infect Dis 2006;43:1499–1539.

5. Hill DR, Ford L, Lalloo DG. Oral cholera vaccines: use in clinical practice. Lancet Infect Dis 2006;6:361–73.

6. Shlim DR. Looking for evidence that personal hygiene precautions prevent traveler's diarrhea. Clin Infect Dis 2005;41Suppl 8:S531–5.

7. Rowe B, Taylor J, Bettelheim KA. An investigation of travellers' diarrhoea. Lancet 1970;1:1–5.

8. Gorbach SL, Kean BH, Evans DG, et al. Travelers' diarrhea and toxigenic Escherichia coli. N Engl J Med 1975;292:933–6.

9. Merson MH, Morris GK, Sack DA, et al. Travelers' diarrhea in Mexico: a prospective study of physicians and family members attending a congress. N Engl J Med 1976;294: 1299–1304.

10. Herwaldt BL. Cyclospora cayetanensis: a review, focusing on the outbreaks of cyclosporiasis in the 1990s. Clin Infect Dis 2000;31:1040–57.

11. Hoge CW, Shlim DR, Echeverria P, et al. Epidemiology of diarrhea among expatriate residents living in a highly endemic environment. JAMA 1996;275:533–8.

12. Merson MH, Hughes JM, Wood BT, et al. Gastrointestinal illness on passenger cruise ships. JAMA 1975;231:723–7.

13. Tjoa WS, DuPont HL, Sullivan P, et al. Location of food consumption and travelers' diarrhea. Am J Epidemiol 1977; 106:61–6.

14. Wood LV, Ferguson LE, Hogan P, et al. Incidence of bacterial enteropathogens in foods from Mexico. Appl Environ Microbiol 1983;46:328–32.

15. Gottlieb SL, Newbern EC, Griffin PM, et al. Multistate outbreak of Listeriosis linked to turkey deli meat and subsequent changes in US regulatory policy. Clin Infect Dis 2006;42:29–36.

16. Centers for Disease Control and Prevention. Ongoing multistate outbreak of Escherichia coli serotype O157:H7 infections associated with consumption of fresh spinach—United States, September 2006. Morb Mortal Wkly Rep 2006;55:1045–6.

17. Beatty ME, Adcock PM, Smith SW, et al. Epidemic diarrhea due to enterotoxigenic Escherichia coli. Clin Infect Dis 2006;42:329–34.

18. Centers for Disease Control and Prevention. Diagnosis and management of foodborne illnesses: a primer for physicians and other health care professionals. MMWR Recomm Rep 2004;53(RR-4):1–33.

19. Lynch M, Painter J, Woodruff R, Braden C. Surveillance for foodborne-disease outbreaks—United States, 1998–2002. MMWR Surveill Summ 2006;55:1–42.

20. Koo D, Aragon A, Moscoso V, et al. Epidemic cholera in Guatemala, 1993: transmission of a newly introduced epidemic strain by street vendors. Epidemiol Infect 1996; 116:121–6.

21. Shlim DR. Update in traveler's diarrhea. Infect Dis Clin North Am 2005;19:137–49.

22. Ryder RW, Oquist CA, Greenberg H, et al. Travelers' diarrhea in Panamanian tourists in Mexico. J Infect Dis 1981;144:442–8.

23. Ericsson CD, Pickering LK, Sullivan P, DuPont HL. The role of location of food consumption in the prevention of travelers' diarrhea in Mexico. Gastroenterol 1980;79:812–6.

24. Herwaldt BL, de Arroyave KR, Roberts JM, Juranek DD. A multiyear prospective study of the risk factors for and incidence of diarrheal illness in a cohort of Peace Corps volunteers in Guatemala. Ann Intern Med 2000;132:982–8.

25. Adachi JA, Mathewson JJ, Jiang ZD, et al. Enteric pathogens in Mexican sauces of popular restaurants in Guadalajara, Mexico, and Houston, Texas. Ann Intern Med 2002;136:884–7.

26. Centers for Disease Control and Prevention. "Norwalk-like viruses:" public health consequences and outbreak management. Morb Mortal Wkly Rep 2001;50(No. RR-9):1–17.

27. Centers for Disease Control and Prevention. Outbreaks of gastroenteritis associated with noroviruses on cruise ships—United States, 2002. Morb Mortal Wkly Rep 2002; 51:1112–5.

28. Vollet JJ, Ericsson CD, Gibson G, et al. Human rotavirus in an adult population with travelers' diarrhea and its relationship to the location of food consumption. J Med Virol 1979;4:81–7.

29. Ericsson CD, DuPont HL, Mathewson JJ. Epidemiologic observations on diarrhea developing in U.S. and Mexican students living in Guadalajara, Mexico. J Travel Med 1994; 2:6–10.

30. Boccia D, Tozzi AE, Cotter B, et al. Waterborne outbreak of Norwalk-like virus gastroenteritis at a tourist resort, Italy. Emerg Infect Dis 2002;8:563–8.

31. Blackburn BG, Craun GF, Yoder JS, et al. Surveillance for waterborne-disease outbreaks associated with drinking water—United States, 2001–2002. MMWR Surveill Summ 2004;53:23–45.

32. Yoder JS, Blackburn BG, Craun GF, et al. Surveillance for waterborne-disease outbreaks associated with recreational water—United States, 2001–2002. MMWR Surveill Summ 2004;53:1–22.

33. deRegnier DP, Cole L, Schupp DG, Erlandsen SL. Viability of Giardia cysts suspended in lake, river, and tap water. Appl Environ Microbiol 1989;55:1223–9.

34. Sanchez JL, Gelnett J, Petruccelli BP, Defraites RF, Taylor DN. Diarrheal disease incidence and morbidity among United States military personnel during short-term missions overseas. Am J Trop Med Hyg 1998;58:299–304.

35. Keswick BH, Gerba CP, DuPont HL, Rose JB. Detection of enteric viruses in treated drinking water. Appl Environ Microbiol 1984;47:1290–4.

36. Sobel J, Mahon B, Mendoza CE, et al. Reduction of fecal contamination of street-vended beverages in Guatemala by a simple system for water purification and storage, handwashing, and beverage storage. Am J Trop Med Hyg 1998;59:380–7.

37. Daniels NA, Neimann J, Karpati A, et al. Traveler's diarrhea at sea: three outbreaks of waterborne enterotoxigenic Escherichia coli on cruise ships. J Infect Dis 2000;181: 1491–5.

38. Centers for Disease Control and Prevention. Outbreak of acute febrile illness among participants in EcoChallenge Sabah 2000—Malaysia, 2000. Morb Mortal Wkly Rep 2000; 49:816–7.

39. Dickens DL, DuPont HL, Johnson PC. Survival of bacterial enteropathogens in the ice of popular drinks. JAMA 1985; 253:3141–3.

40. Harris JR. Are bottled beverages safe for travelers? Am J Pub Health 1982;72:787–8.

41. Beuret C, Kohler D, Baumgartner A, Luthi TM. Norwalk-like virus sequences in mineral waters: one-year monitoring of three brands. Appl Environ Microbiol 2002;68:1925–31.

42. Sheth NK, Wisniewski TR, Franson TR. Survival of enteric pathogens in common beverages: an in vitro study. Am J Gastroenterol 1988;83:658–60.

43. Steffen R, Tornieporth N, Clemens SA, et al. Epidemiology of travelers' diarrhea: details of a global survey. J Travel Med 2004;11:231–7.

44. Huang DB, Sanchez AP, Triana E, et al. United States male students who heavily consume alcohol in Mexico are at greater risk of travelers' diarrhea than their female counterparts. J Travel Med 2004;11:143–5.

45. World Health Organization. Preventing travellers' diarrhoea: how to make drinking water safe. WHO/SDE/WSH/ 05.07 2005, World Health Organization: Geneva. p. 1–7.

46. Backer H. Water disinfection for international and wilderness travelers. Clin Infect Dis 2002;34:355–64.

47. Bandres J, Mathewson JJ, DuPont HL. Heat susceptibility of bacterial enteropathogens. Implications for the prevention of travelers' diarrhea. Arch Intern Med 1988;148:2261–3.

48. Groh CD, MacPherson DW, Groves DJ. Effect of heat on the sterilization of artificially contaminated water. J Travel Med 1996;3:11–3.

49. Ongerth JE, Johnson RL, MacDonald SC, et al. Backcountry water treatment to prevent giardiasis. Am J Pub Health 1989;79:1633–7.

50. Fayer R. Effect of high temperature on infectivity of Cryptosporidium parvum oocysts in water. Appl Environ Microbiol 1994;60:2732–5.

51. Krugman S, Giles JP, Hammond J. Hepatitis virus: effect of heat on the infectivity and antigenicity of the MS-1 and MS-2 strains. J Infect Dis 1970;122:432–6.

52. Centers for Disease Control and Prevention, Kozarsky PE, Arguin PM, Navin AW. Health Information for International Travel 2005–2006. Philadelphia: Elsevier; 2005.

53. Gerba CP, Naranjo JE. Microbiological water purification without the use of chemical disinfection. Wilderness Environ Med 2000;11:12–6.

54. Rice EW, Hoff JC, Schaefer FW 3rd. Inactivation of Giardia cysts by chlorine. Appl Environ Microbiol 1982;43:250–1.

55. Juranek DD. Cryptosporidiosis: sources of infection and guidelines for prevention. Clin Infect Dis 1995;21(Suppl 1): S57–61.

56. Centers for Disease Control and Prevention. Assessing the public health threat associated with waterborne cryptosporidiosis: report of a workshop. Morb Mortal Wkly Rep 1995;44 (No. RR-6):1–19.

57. Carpenter C, Fayer R, Trout J, Beach MJ. Chlorine disinfection of recreational water for Cryptosporidium parvum. Emerg Infect Dis 1999;5:579–84.

58. Backer H, Hollowell J. Use of iodine for water disinfection: iodine toxicity and maximum recommended dose. Environ Health Perspect 2000;108:679–84.

59. Loewenstein MS, Balows A, Gangarosa EJ. Turista at an international congress in Mexico. Lancet 1973;1:529–31.

60. Chang TW. Traveler's diarrhea (letter). Ann Intern Med 1978;89:428–9.

61. Mattila L, Siitonen A, Kyrönseppä H, et al. Risk behavior for travelers' diarrhea among Finnish travelers. J Travel Med 1995;2:77–84.

62. Steffen R, Van der Linde F, Gyr K, Schär M. Epidemiology of diarrhea in travelers. JAMA 1983;249:1176–80.

63. Steffen R, Collard F, Tornieporth N, et al. Epidemiology, etiology, and impact of traveler's diarrhea in Jamaica. JAMA 1999;281:811–7.

64. Hill DR. Occurrence and self-treatment of diarrhea in a large cohort of Americans traveling to developing countries. Am J Trop Med Hyg 2000;62:585–9.

65. Kozicki M, Steffen R, Schär M. 'Boil it, cook it, peel it or forget it': does this rule prevent travellers' diarrhoea? Int J Epidemiol 1985;14:169–72.

66. Boulware DR. Influence of hygiene on gastrointestinal illness among wilderness backpackers. J Travel Med 2004; 11:27–33.

67. Girou E, Loyeau S, Legrand P, et al. Efficacy of handrubbing with alcohol based solution versus standard handwashing with antiseptic soap: randomised clinical trial. BMJ 2002;325:362.

68. Chapin AR, Carpenter CM, Dudley WC, et al. Prevalence of norovirus among visitors from the United States to Mexico and Guatemala who experience traveler's diarrhea. J Clin Microbiol 2005;43:1112–7.

69. Horvath LL, Murray CK, Dooley DP. Effect of maximizing a travel medicine clinic's prevention strategies. J Travel Med 2005;12:332–7.

70. von Sonnenburg F, Tornieporth N, Waiyaki P, et al. Risk and aetiology of diarrhea at various tourist destinations (letter). Lancet 2000;356:133–4.

71. McIntosh IB, Reed JM, Power KG. Traveler's diarrhea and the effect of pre-travel health advice in general practice. Brit J Gen Pract 1997;47:71–5.

72. Packman CJ. A survey of notified travel-associated infections: implications for travel health advice. J Pub Health Med 1995;17:217–22.

73. DuPont HL, Haynes GA, Pickering LK, et al. Diarrhea of travelers to Mexico. Relative susceptibility of United States and Latin American students attending a Mexican University. Am J Epidemiol 1977;105:37–41.

74. Evans DJ Jr, Ruiz-Palacios G, Evans DE, et al. Humoral immune response to the heat-labile enterotoxin of Escherichia coli in naturally acquired diarrhea and antitoxin determination by passive immune hemolysis. Infect Immun 1977;16:781–8.

75. Shlim DR, Hoge CW, Rajah R, et al. Persistent high risk of diarrhea among foreigners in Nepal during the first 2 years of residence. Clin Infect Dis 1999;29:613–6.

76. Herwaldt BL, de Arroyave KR, Wahlquist SP, et al. Multiyear prospective study of intestinal parasitism in a cohort of Peace Corps volunteers in Guatemala. J Clin Microbiol 2001;39:34–42.

77. Cartwright RY. Food and waterborne infections associated with package holidays. J Appl Microbiol 2003;94 Suppl: 12S–24S.

78. Cartwright R. Gastrointestinal illnesses in tourists: whose responsibility? Euro Surveill 2004;9(3):5.

79. Ashley DV, Walters C, Dockery-Brown C, et al. Interventions to prevent and control food-borne diseases associated with a reduction in traveler's diarrhea in tourists to Jamaica. J Travel Med 2004;11:364–7.

80. Phillips-Howard PA, Blaze M, Hurn M, Bradley DJ. Malaria prophylaxis: survey of the response of British travellers to prophylactic advice. BMJ 1986;293:932–4.

81. Hill DR. Health problems in a large cohort of Americans traveling to developing countries. J Travel Med 2000;7:259–66.

82. Hill DR, Behrens RH. A survey of travel clinics throughout the world. J Travel Med 1996;3:46–51.

83. Genton B, Behrens RH. Specialized travel consultation. Part II: acquiring knowledge. J Travel Med 1994;1: 13–5.

84. Behrens RH, Roberts JA. Is travel prophylaxis worth while? Economic appraisal of prophylactic measures against malaria, hepatitis A, and typhoid in travellers. BMJ 1994; 309:918–22.

85. Committee to Advise on Tropical Medicine and Travel (CATMAT). Guidelines for the practice of travel medicine. An Advisory Committee Statement (ACS). Can Commun Dis Rep 1999;25:1–6.

86. Guerrant RL, Van Gilder T, Steiner TS, et al. Practice guidelines for the management of infectious diarrhea. Clin Infect Dis 2001;32:331–50.

87. Castelli F, Patroni A. The human immunodeficiency virus-infected traveler. Clin Infect Dis 2000;31:1403–8.

88. Suh KN, Mileno MD. Challenging scenarios in a travel clinic: advising the complex traveler. Infect Dis Clin North Am 2005;19:15–47.

CHAPTER 20

PROPHYLACTIC USE OF DRUGS

JOHN W. SANDERS, MD, MPHTM

R. BRADLEY SACK, MD, ScD

Options for the prevention of travelers' diarrhea (TD) include pretravel education with the aim of behavioral change related particularly to food and beverage selection (see Chapter 19 "Diet and Education about Risks"), immunologic protection with vaccines or immunoglobulin preparations (see Chapter 23,"Immunoprophylaxis and Immunologic Control"), and chemoprophylaxis with various drugs.[1–8] Even the best pretravel advice often fails to decrease risky behavior and the incidence of diarrhea,[9,10] and immunologic protection, while theoretically preferable, is still in the developmental stage. Furthermore, given the large number of organisms and strains that cause diarrhea, comprehensive immunoprotection will probably not be available any time in the near future.[11,12] On the other hand, several drugs have been shown to be effective for prophylaxis and will likely remain a viable option when prevention of TD is considered.

Philosophically, the use of drugs for prophylaxis with drugs must be weighed against the various options for the treatment of TD (see Chapter 25, "Nonspecific Treatment: Diet, Oral Rehydration Therapy," Chapter 26, "Symptomatic Therapy," Chapter 27, "Antimicrobial Therapy," and Chapter 29, "Approach to Prolonged Diarrhea in the Returning Traveler").[13] The treatment of TD with the combination of an antimicrobial agent and loperamide is usually very effective, often reducing symptoms to a matter of hours.[14–18] Given the excellent response to empiric therapy, many experts recommend against the use of prophylaxis. A National Institutes of Health Consensus Development Conference in 1985 concluded that the prevention of diarrhea with drugs has a very small role, if any, because TD is a self-limiting and nonfatal condition.[19] However, most agree that chemoprophylaxis should be considered in certain situations, such as for travelers with tight schedules (eg, diplomats, musicians, or lecturers), for those with a history of frequent TD, and for those with chronic medical conditions, such as chronic gastrointestinal, immunologic (including human immunodeficiency virus [HIV]), endocrinologic, and hematologic disorders.[1] Recently, a meta-analysis found an association with the development of irritable bowel syndrome (IBS) and prior infectious gastroenteritis, including TD.[20] Although it has not yet been shown that prophylaxis for TD can prevent the development of postinfectious IBS, it seems logical that it would. Determining whether to provide prophylaxis is therefore a matter of assessing a traveler's risk of illness and the importance of remaining well during the travel. The potential benefits of chemoprophylaxis should be weighed against the risks and inconvenience of disease and comparative side effects and costs of drugs for both chemoprophylaxis and self therapy.

Early History of Prophylaxis

In 1963, B. H. Kean stated in a paper describing the epidemiology of diarrhea in travelers to Mexico that "neither the cause nor the cure of TD has been discovered."[21] Despite a lack of specific evidence, the use of drugs for prevention of diarrhea was thought to be useful.[22] In fact, a study in 1957 found that more than one-third of travelers to Mexico were using antibiotic prophylaxis in an attempt to prevent diarrhea.[23] A series of studies by Kean and colleagues demonstrating the efficacy of antibacterial prophylaxis for the prevention of diarrhea provided the initial evidence that TD is primarily a result of bacterial infection and proved that antibiotic prophylaxis could be a practical option for travelers.[21,23–26] Two of the early drugs evaluated were enterovioform (iodochlorhydroxyquinoline, also called "clioquinol") and neomycin, but neither were shown to provide protection.[26] In a more controlled trial comparing neomycin sulfate and phthalylsufathiazole, both drugs were shown to provide protection (25 to 50% against any diarrhea and 60 to 70% against severe

95. O'Mahony L, McCarthy J, Kelly P, et al. Lactobacillus and bifidobacterium in irritable bowel syndrome: symptom responses and relationship to cytokine profiles. Gastroenterol 2005;128:541–51.

96. Dunlop SP, Jenkins D, Neal KR, et al. Randomized, double-blind, placebo-controlled trial of prednisolone in post-infectious irritable bowel syndrome. Aliment Pharmacol Ther 2003;18:77–84.

97. Pimentel M, Chow EJ, Lin HC. Eradication of small intestinal bacterial overgrowth reduces symptoms of irritable bowel syndrome. Am J Gastroenterol 2000;95: 3503–6.

98. Harvey RF, Mauad EC, Brown AM. Prognosis in the irritable bowel syndrome: a 5-year prospective study. Lancet 1987;1:963–5.

99. Neal KR, Barker L, Spiller RC. Prognosis in post-infective irritable bowel syndrome: a six year follow up study. Gut 2002;51:410–3.

100. McKendrick MW. Post *Salmonella* irritable bowel syndrome-5-year review. J Infect 1996;33:170–1.

101. Bennett EJ, Tennant CC, Piesse C, et al. Level of chronic life stress predicts clinical outcome in irritable bowel syndrome. Gut 1998;43:256–61.

disease).[25] In a study among British Airways personnel and their families traveling for up to 3 weeks, Turner showed that either neomycin-trisulphamide or streptotriad (ie, streptomycin, sulphadimidine, sulfadiazine, and sulfathiazole) provided low ($< 28\%$) but significant ($p < .02$) levels of protection.[22,27] Furthermore, the British Olympic team credited the use of antibiotic prophylaxis with keeping them disease free during the 1968 games in Mexico City.[28] This was also early evidence of the potential impact of developing antibiotic resistance among diarrheal pathogens because it was reported that the British use of streptomycin-sulfa drugs was more effective than the sulfonamide prophylaxis used by the US and Australian teams.[28] In 1968, Enterotoxigenic *E. coli* (ETEC) was recognized as a cause of watery diarrhea, and over the next few years was subsequently found to be the primary cause of traveler's diarrhea.[22,29] This discovery opened the door to further trials focused on prophylaxis against ETEC that are discussed later in this chapter.

The Drugs

From the time of Kean's early studies, many different drugs have been considered for prophylaxis. Because TD is caused predominantly by bacterial microorganisms, antimicrobial agents have been used most commonly, although none have been used for periods longer than 3 weeks. Nonantimicrobial agents, such as bismuth subsalicylate (BSS)-containing compounds and tannin aluminate plus ethacridine lactate, have also been recommended. Although they are not technically drugs, probiotics, such as Lactobacillus preparations have been considered attractive alternatives for prevention. Each of these alternatives will be examined in more detail in this chapter.

A variety of other agents have proven either ineffective or minimally effective in the prevention of TD, including halogenated hydroxyquinoline, activated charcoal, and polycarbophil.[30–33] Antimotility agents like loperamide, anticholinergics, and antisecretory agents such as zaldaride maleate, an intestinal calmodulin inhibitor, or racecadotril, an enkephalinase inhibitor, have no logical role in chemoprophylaxis of TD.

BSS

BSS-containing compounds (popularly marketed as Pepto-Bismol, Kaopectate, and Bismatrol) are partially effective in the prevention of TD.[34–39] The drug has antisecretory, anti-inflammatory, and antimicrobial properties.[34,37,40–42] The antimicrobial properties most likely accounts for its prophylactic efficacy.[34,42] Following ingestion, BSS undergoes acid hydrolysis and dissociates in the mouth or stomach, resulting in the release of salicylate, which is nearly completely absorbed, and numerous bismuth moieties.[3,43,44] The free salicylate appears to be responsible for the anti-secretory and anti-inflammatory activity.[3,41] The resultant insoluble bismuth salts appear to confer the antibacterial activity.[37,42,45]

BSS can provide from 41 to 65% protection from TD when dosed as two chewable tablets (262 mg of BSS per tablet) four times a day.[3,33,36,39] The liquid preparation is equally effective when dosed at 30 mL (one ounce) four times a day.[33] Protection is decreased to no better than 40% when only 1 tablet is taken four times a day and protection is no better than 35% when 2 chewable tablets are taken only twice daily.[33,38,39] If travelers are careful about what they eat, the level of protection with BSS is increased.[46]

The recommended prophylactic dose of 8 tablets daily provides the same amount of salicylate as 3 to 4 adult aspirins.[43,44] Travelers taking BSS should be cautioned about taking therapeutic doses of aspirin because of the risk of salicylate poisoning, but tinnitus is actually no more common among subjects taking BSS than among those taking placebo.[35,36] Although the salicylate does not affect anticoagulation by warfarin as strongly as acetylsalicylic acid, the use of BSS is best avoided by persons needing anticoagulation.[33] The use of BSS in areas highly endemic for Dengue fever might also be problematic. The concern is that Dengue infection concordant with aspirin use might confer a higher risk for hemorrhagic complications, but whether the same concern should be raised by use of salicylate in BSS is speculative.[30]

The bismuth salts formed during dissociation are largely insoluble and minimally absorbed, unlike bismuth gallate or citrate, from which enough bismuth can be absorbed to cause encephalopathy.[33,47] The insoluble salts are black and have been known to cause a black tongue and black stools. Developing a black tongue is a minor irritant and can be avoided by brushing the teeth and tongue and rinsing the mouth after each dose. However, black stools can be confused with melena, so patients should be counseled prior to avoid confusion.

The chewable tablet formulation of BSS has not been associated with constipation or with drug interactions. However, the vehicle of Pepto-Bismol liquid formulation contains bivalent cations (magnesium aluminum silicate), which can interfere with the absorption of doxycycline.[48] The absorption of other drugs has not been evaluated, but caution should clearly be exercised in prescribing liquid Pepto-Bismol to any traveler requiring doxycycline for malaria prophylaxis or who is on other chronic medication.[33]

There are additional limitations with BSS prophylaxis. BSS-containing products are not found in much of Europe, Australia, and New Zealand. Travelers from these regions would need to purchase the drug in the destination country. Chewing BSS tablets four times a day also requires a high level of compliance.

TANNIN ALBUMINATE PLUS ETHACRIDINE LACTATE

Adsorbents have not been shown to be effective for prophylaxis, but the adsorbent tannin albuminate, combined with the antiseptic ethacridine lactate, has been proposed as a prophylactic alternative. Raedsch and colleagues performed a placebo-controlled, randomized trial evaluating the efficacy of 500 mg of tannalbuminate and 50 mg of ethacridine lactate dosed twice daily.[31] During a 16-day cruise in Egypt, 77 Western tourists were randomized. In the placebo group, 81.4% (35 of 43 volunteers) developed diarrhea, but only 52.9% of the treatment group (18 of 34 volunteers) developed diarrhea ($p < .0125$). Furthermore, the volunteers in the treatment group who did develop diarrhea had milder symptoms than those in the placebo group. While these findings are promising, this was only a 36% protection against diarrhea. Further studies would need to be performed before this regimen could be routinely recommended.

LACTOBACILLUS AND OTHER PROBIOTIC PREPARATIONS

The concept behind probiotic prophylaxis is the intentional introduction of a preparation of an avirulent strain of either a bacteria or yeast to the gut flora in the hopes of interfering with the colonization of a pathogenic strain of bacteria that might be later introduced. The protective mechanisms at work are not clearly understood, but may include the production of antimicrobial substances, competition for adhesion receptors, competition for nutrients, antitoxin action, and stimulation of the immune system.[1,49] Several clinical studies have shown promising results for the use of probiotics for the prevention of diarrhea in select populations, such as those receiving antibiotics, but data for the prevention of TD has been less clear.[50,51] Some studies have found a reduction in TD following the use of probiotics,[52–54] but others have failed to show this benefit.[55,56] A recent randomized, double-blind trial assessed nonviable *Lactobacillus acidophilus* for the prevention of TD.[57] One hundred and seventy-four Western travelers to intermediate or high-risk areas were randomized to receive either a sachet of 10^{10} bacteria or placebo twice daily during their travel. No difference in diarrheal incidence was observed. Although this well-designed study provided clear evidence against the efficacy of *Lactobacillus acidophilus*, the investigators cautioned against generalizing the results for all probiotics. Limitations to that study may have included the use of nonviable bacteria and the choice of that species of *Lactobacillus*.[57]

There appear to be strain-specific differences in the choices of probiotics. *Lactobacillus* GG (LGG) has demonstrated bile and acid resistance, a propensity to adhere to intestinal lining better than other *Lactobacilli*, and production of an antibacterial substance.[58] It has shown promise for preventing nosocomial diarrhea,[59] and two recent meta-analyses suggest there might be a role for lactobacilli for preventing antibiotic associated diarrhea.[60,61] A large placebo-controlled study by Hilton of 245 American travelers demonstrated that LGG afforded 47% protection calculated on a per day risk of diarrhea.[53] In an accompanying editorial, DuPont noted that protection was minimal and not as effective as other drugs like BSS or antimicrobials, but that the concept was worthy of further study.[62] In a review of the subject, Ericsson pointed out that the "per day" risk of diarrhea calculation was unique for that study and makes it difficult to compare to other studies.[33] An earlier study of 756 Finnish travelers to two different sites in Turkey found only a modest 11.8% protection, but there was a large difference in the findings from the two sites that could not be explained.[52]

Meta-analyses have also suggested that *Saccharomyces boulardii* might be beneficial in preventing antibiotic-associated diarrhea, but the data for preventing TD is not clear.[60,61] Kollaritsch and colleagues performed a placebo-controlled trial among 3,000 Austrian tourists.[54] They found a clinically mild but statistically significant level of protection that was dose dependent.[54] However, they also found a regional variation in protection, with the highest benefit seen in North Africa and Turkey, that was not explained.[54]

The current findings with probiotics are inconclusive, but it does appear that some, particularly LGG, may have some benefit and the subject warrants further study. In the meantime, probiotics are safe, and if a traveler wishes to use them, the only significant risk might be complacency with proper food and beverage precautions, but the authors do not feel a recommendation for their use can be made at this time.

ANTIMICROBIAL AGENTS

Following the recognition of ETEC as the primary cause of diarrhea, it became very clear that antimicrobials could have a major impact on the prevention of TD. A series of studies by DA Sack and RB Sack and their colleagues demonstrated the benefits and limitations of doxycycline. Doxycycline was initially chosen because ETEC was generally susceptible to the drug, it had a long half-life allowing for single daily dosing, it was secreted into the small intestine (the site of ETEC colonization), it had already been shown to be effective in treating cholera, and it was considered a safe drug associated with rare adverse events.[22] When dosed at 100 mg daily, it provided 83 to 86% protection in Peace Corps volunteers in Morocco and Kenya in 1976 to 1977.[63,64] However, when dosed twice weekly in Honduras in 1978, the protection dropped to only 27% (not significant). This failure in protection was thought to be due to either the increased dosing interval or increasing doxycline resistance among ETEC.[65] A follow-on study in Honduras in 1980, using daily dosing, showed a significant level of protection (68%), but still lower than that seen in Kenya and Morocco, suggesting that resistance was playing a role in the decreased efficacy.[66] Likewise, in Thailand in 1980, where ETEC was also known to be resistant to doxycycline, the drug afforded only 59% protection (not significant).[67] Because doxycycline resistance among enteropathogens has generally risen around the world,[68–71] this drug is no longer promoted as an ideal agent for chemoprophylaxis of TD. There is still some debate as to whether doxycycline used for malaria prophylaxis might provide some protection against TD. For instance, a study among British and Australian military personnel deployed to Iraq for the Gulf War (1991) found malaria prophylaxis with doxycycline provided protection against diarrhea.[72] However, other studies have found no protection for American military personnel deployed to South East Asia, East Africa, or the Middle East.[73–75]

As resistance to doxycyline increased, other drugs were evaluated. DuPont and colleagues evaluated the efficacy of trimethoprim–sulfamethoxazole (TMP–SMX) among students from the US studying in Mexico between 1979 to 1980.[76,77] The two studies found 73 to 95% protection.[76,77] In the second study, they also evaluated trimethoprim alone, which provided 59% protection.[77] Increasing resistance rates have also diminished the efficacy of either of these drugs.[68–71] In 1981, Andremont reported 100% protection with the use of oral erythromycin in US tourists to Mexico,[78] but erythromycin itself is frequently associated with gastrointestinal (GI) side effects.[79] In 1983, Black and colleagues showed that mecillinam provided 75% protection, but it has never become routinely used and is not available in the United States.[80]

As the efficacy of TMP-SMX waned due to increasing resistance, attention became focused on the fluoroquinolones.[81–86] In a study involving 54 tourists to Tunisia, 500 mg of ciprofloxacin dosed daily provided 94% protection.[86] Even at lower doses—ciprofloxacin at 250 mg daily and norfloxacin at 400 mg daily—the fluoroquinolones provided up to 90% protection.[81,85] Heck and colleagues compared TMP–SMX with ciprofloxacin in US adult travelers to Latin America and the Caribbean and found TMP–SMX was only 51% protective, while ciprofloxacin afforded 84% protection.[84] All the currently available fluoroquinolones are considered effective for the treatment of TD,[3,4] so any of them should be efficacious in the prevention of TD, but the appropriate doses for the new quinolones have not been established. Half doses of newer fluoroquinolones given once a day or full doses given every other day are logical considerations, but these regimens would need to be studied in clinical trials before they could be recommended.[30] However, like the other antimicrobials previously tested, increasing resistance to the fluoroquinolones, especially among *Campylobacter* species, raises questions about continued efficacy. Ciprofloxacin resistance in *Campylobacter* isolated in Thailand increased from 0 in 1991 to 84% in 1995,[69] resulting in decreased efficacy of the fluoroquinolones for the treatment of TD in that region.[87] Therefore, it is not clear if the flouroquinolones are still effective for prophylaxis for South East Asia or for how long they will be effective for other regions.

Azithromycin has been shown to be effective therapy for TD[14,88] and could be effective for prophylaxis.[3] In support of this approach is one study in which epidemic dysentery was successfully prevented by use of azithromycin.[89] In a double-blind study assessing the impact of azithromycin and clarithromycin on oral and fecal flora, Matute and colleagues found no significant differences in their effect on human oropharyngeal and intestinal microflora.[90] Specifically, the use of these antibiotics was not associated with colonization by resistant, gram-positive organisms or overgrowth of opportunistic microorganisms.[90] However, azithromycin has not been studied for TD prophylaxis and can not be recommended at this time.

Conceptually, poorly absorbed antimicrobials have several advantages over systemically absorbed antimicrobials that might make them superior prophylactic agents.[91] Because they are not well absorbed, high concentrations of antibiotic can be delivered to the site of infection with little risk of systemic adverse events, toxicity, or drug interactions.[91] Because they do not apply antimicrobial pressure to bacteria outside the GI tract, they should be less likely to be associated with the development of significant antibiotic resistance in important respiratory and skin pathogens.[91] They may also be useful for certain patient groups like pregnant women, children, and those in whom the concern for drug–drug interactions is high.[30,91] Three poorly absorbed antibiotics have been evaluated in TD: bicozamycin (bicyclomycin), aztreonam, and rifaximin.[91] In a small study among US travelers to Mexico, Ericsson and colleagues found that bicozamycin provided 100% protection from TD with minimal side-effects, but the drug was never fully developed for human use.[92] In a study involving US travelers to Mexico who had already developed TD, oral aztreonam dosed at 100 mg three times daily significantly reduced the duration of symptoms,[93] but it never became commercially available and was not tested for prevention of TD.[91] Rifaximin is the best studied and most promising of the poorly absorbed antibiotics for prophylaxis.

Rifaximin is a rifamycin derivative with a broad spectrum of antibacterial coverage, negligible systemic absorption (< 0.4%), and a long history of safe use for various intestinal infections in 17 countries.[91,94] It has been shown to be as effective as ciprofloxacin and superior to placebo for the treatment of TD in diverse geographic regions,[15,95] and it was approved by the US Food and Drug Administration in May 2004 for the treatment of patients (12 years of age and older) with TD caused by noninvasive strains of *Escherichia coli.* In 2003, a double-blind, placebo-controlled trial comparing rifaximin dosed at 200 mg once, twice, or three times daily was performed involving 210 US students in Guadalajara, Mexico.[8] Each of the dosing regimens was found to be equally effective, providing 72% protection against diarrhea and 77% protection against diarrhea severe enough to require treatment.[8] Prophylaxis was associated with minimal side effects and resulted in decreased mild symptoms (abdominal pains/cramps, excessive intestinal gas) with minimal alteration of fecal flora or antimicrobial resistance.[8] While rifaximin is effective in the treatment *E. coli*-predominant TD, it has not yet been shown to be clearly effective for the treatment of invasive pathogens, such as *Campylobacter* and *Shigella,* so its utility for preventing infection with those pathogens is not clear. However, Taylor and colleagues showed that rifaximin prophylaxis, dosed at 200 mg three times daily, was effective in preventing infection with *Shigella flexneri* in a challenge study,[96] providing strong evidence that rifaximin may have broad applicability for prevention of bacterial diarrhea.

Until recently, it had been argued that the fluoroquinolones should be the primary choice for prophylaxis, preserving azithromycin and rifaximin for self-treatment (see Chapter 29, "Algorithmic Approach to Empiric Self-Treatment of Acute Travelers' Diarrhea and Management of Diarrhea in the Returning Traveler").[30] However, with the recently demonstrated success of rifaximin as a prophylactic agent combined with the theoretic benefits of using a poorly absorbed antimicrobial, rifaximin should now be considered the current agent of choice when chemoprophylaxis of TD is indicated.

The Case for Chemoprophylaxis

HOSTS AT HIGH RISK

Although TD is generally a self-limited illness usually lasting only 3 to 4 days, it can be associated with significant discomfort for a traveler and often causes alterations in travel plans, resulting in considerable economic costs for both the traveler (incurred costs associated with medication, medical services, cancelled activities, and changes in itinerary) and the destination country (loss of tourism income).[1,97] Travelers at increased risk of experiencing severe diarrhea or of developing complications from the illness include small children, pregnant women, elderly patients, and patients with immunologic disorders, or patients with chronic illnesses that could be adversely impacted by dehydration or shifts in intravascular volume (eg, heart failure, chronic kidney disease, etc.). Travelers at increased risk of acquiring TD include people with achlorhydria, including those taking potent, long-acting H2 blockers or proton pump inhibitors[98] or who have undergone gastrectomy, and patients with underlying immunodeficiencies, including malignancy, transplants, on chemotherapy, IgA deficiency, and HIV infection with CD4 counts less than 200 cells/mm3.[99,100] Travel medicine practitioners should consider offering chemoprophylaxis to travelers known to be at highest risk for TD or for developing complications from diarrhea (Table 1).[1,30,99,101]

Children of less than 6 years of age are at greater risk of acquiring diarrhea, probably because of their tendency to sample their environment with their mouths. There has been debate concerning the best way to manage diarrhea in a traveling child, but most travel medicine physicians now recommend antimicrobial treatment when diarrhea symptoms occur while traveling in developing countries typically known for high rates of TD.[102] Chemoprophylaxis for children has not been routinely recommended. Teenagers and young adults are also at higher risk of acquiring TD, likely due to adventurous behavior resulting in ingestion of larger volumes of potentially contaminated food, but prophylaxis is not routinely recommended for this age group either.[1] Elderly travelers are more likely to have chronic

Table 1 Travelers to Consider for Chemoprophylaxis of Travelers' Diarrhea with an Antimicrobial

Agent	
At special risk for acquiring travelers' diarrhea	Achlorhydria, including gastrectomy and late stage HIV/AIDS Long-acting H2 blockers and proton pump inhibitors Immunodeficiency, including: • malignancy • transplants • on chemotherapy • IgA deficiency • HIV/AIDS with CD4 counts < 200 cells/mm3
At risk of complications of diarrhea	Underlying chronic gastrointestinal disease: • Crohn's disease • Ulcerative colitis • Chronic diarrhea Elderly* Pregnancy** Small children** Extreme travel
Critical travel schedule	Subjective; examples include lecturers, musicians, and competitive athletes

*Recommendations limited by lack of data.
**Recommendations limited by lack of data and potential adverse effects of the fluoroquinolones.
AIDS = Acquired Immune Deficiency Syndrome; HIV = Human Immunodeficiency Virus.

medical problems that might make them prone to complications from diarrhea, but data on the actual risks of complications of diarrhea in the elderly, which could be used to guide the choice of chemoprophylaxis versus early self-treatment, is not available.[30]

Chemoprophylaxis has not been routinely recommended for pregnant women. The typical approach has been to advise pregnant women to postpone travel until after delivery, if possible, especially when she is contemplating travel to areas that also place her at risk of malaria.[103] To some degree, that reasoning has been dictated by a lack of good prophylactic alternatives. Fluoroquinolones are contraindicated in pregnancy. TMP-SMX could be an acceptable choice, with the exception of women late in the third trimester (risk of kernicterus), but this agent is no longer very effective. Azithromycin has not been studied for prophylaxis. Rifaximin can not currently be recommended for prophylaxis because it is currently considered Pregnancy Class C (risk can not be ruled out due to lack of evidence) and is not indicated for pregnant women in the US, but it theoretically should be very safe and it can be prescribed during pregnancy in other countries.[94]

Occasionally, travelers indicate that they intend to disregard advice on safe food and beverages in order to fully experience a new culture, or they express the desire to take prophylaxis even though they are not in a high-risk group. For these travelers, one could recommend rifaximin, but the authors prefer the recommendation of BSS, if it is available, until further data on the efficacy and potential microbial impact of rifaximin have been collected.

CRITICALITY OF TRAVEL

The concept of criticality of travel should be one of the factors considered when deciding whether or not to advise chemoprophylaxis.[3,4,6] For instance, elite athletes competing in special events, such as the Olympics, can not afford to get ill. Weighing the risks of side effects against the risk of not competing is subjective and is best accomplished in consultation with the athlete and the coaching staff, who might already have arranged a safe food and beverage supply and preparation. Participants in "extreme" travel need to remain physically fit to be able to successfully complete their tasks and return to civilization. They often have no access to medical care. Logically, such travelers might be considered for chemoprophylaxis. Should business travelers or politicians on short important trips be given prophylaxis? The opportunity cost of missed meetings due to diarrhea could be huge. Should musicians or lecturers on a tight appearance schedule be offered prophylaxis? Should the trip of a honeymooning couple be considered critical? Many people would think so. The bottom line is that criticality of a trip is a subjective decision that finally needs to be made by the informed traveler who has been thoroughly advised about the pros and cons of chemoprophylaxis.[30]

The culture of the traveler and provider probably influences the decision of whether to seek or offer chemoprophylaxis for diarrhea. For instance, North Americans typically take relatively short, 1-week vacations. Discounting a day of travel each direction and then changing or abandoning even 1 day's itinerary means giving up about 20% of their vacation at the destination.

North Americans are likely to be more interested in chemoprophylaxis than Europeans, who often take much longer vacations and in whom the fractional impact of illness is not as important.[30]

The Case Against Chemoprophylaxis

The primary argument against the routine use of chemoprophylaxis is the potential adverse effects of the drugs.[13] Mild adverse effects, such as transient rashes, vaginal candidiasis, and GI upset occur in about 3% of persons treated with antibiotics. Photosensitivity is commonly associated with doxycycline, but can also be seen with the fluoroquinolones. Major side effects, including Stevens-Johnson syndrome, which can occur in as many as 1 in 10,000 persons exposed to sulfonamide-containing products like TMP–SMX, anaphylaxis, or even death are legitimate concerns.[13,104] As mentioned previously, the poorly absorbed antimicrobials, such as rifaximin, appear to have much lower risk of systemic adverse events, toxicity, or drug interactions.[91]

The risk of these adverse events must be balanced against the potential benefits of prophylaxis. Although TD can certainly be an irritating illness associated with significant discomfort and economic impact, it is usually a self-limited illness that only results in hospitalization in less than 2% of cases and is almost never fatal.[13,105,106] If it became routine policy to provide prophylactic antimicrobial agents for up to 50 million travelers per year, a few travelers might die to prevent a self-limited illness.[13,30] This was exactly the stance adopted by the Consensus Development Conference when they decided against recommending chemoprophylaxis at all.[19] Furthermore, the risk of side effects of any prophylactic agent probably rises when use of the agent is prolonged. At a minimum, these arguments support the concept that chemoprophylaxis, if used at all, should be reserved for at-risk hosts or special circumstances, and for only short periods of time.[13,30]

ANTIMICROBIAL AGENT RESISTANCE

Another concern with the routine use of antimicrobial agents for chemoprophylaxis is increasing the burden of antimicrobial use and the risk for increasing antibiotic resistance.[13] Antimicrobial resistance is high in most developing countries, and often occurs earlier than in developed countries.[68] In countries where drugs can be bought without a prescription and used indiscriminately, widespread use of subtherapeutic doses of antimicrobials undoubtedly contributes to the level of antimicrobial resistance in a region. Compared to such widespread use by an indigenous population, a traveler's contribution to the local bacterial ecology must be minuscule.[30] However, it appears that the heavy use of antibiotics in a restricted area, such as a resort or military base, can cause a local increase in resistance,[107] a finding that could limit subsequent treatment options in that locale.

It appears that the various antibiotics can have different effects on fecal flora. When TMP–SMX was used prophylactically for 2 weeks, the concentration of gram-negative aerobic bacilli in stool was suppressed to very low levels, only to be replaced by TMP–SMX-resistant flora, with total gram-negative aerobic bacilli rising back to preprophylaxis concentrations in stool.[30,108] On the other hand, when norfloxacin was used in a similar study at the same location in Mexico, the concentration of gram-negative *aerobic bacilli* in stool was suppressed to very low levels and remained low until norfloxacin was discontinued, whereupon concentrations of gram-negative *aerobic bacilli* in stool returned to normal with norfloxacin-sensitive organisms.[30,81] The implication is that preventative antibiotic use did not foster de novo development of resistance flora but merely the acquisition from the environment of already resistant flora.[30] However, FQ-resistant *Campylobacter jejuni* has been documented to emerge with treatment of an initially sensitive strain, with relapse or failure to control symptoms.[109,110] The risk of such occurrence during chemoprophylaxis is unknown but is probably highest in Southeast Asia where the prevalence of *Campylobacter* is relatively high.[69] In DuPont's study of rifaximin, there was no difference in quantitative coliform counts between the various treatment groups and the placebo group.[111] For stool samples cultured on rifaximin containing media, 3 of 6 of the rifaximin groups showed growth of coliforms, but no growth was detected in the placebo group.[111] While the growth was low level (< 10% of growth on rifaximin free media), it is still suggestive of development of resistance while on prophylaxis. Of course, because rifaximin does not apply antimicrobial pressure to bacteria outside the GI tract, it should not be associated with the development of significant antibiotic resistance in important respiratory and skin pathogens.[91]

OVERGROWTH SYNDROMES AND SELECTION OF INVASIVE PATHOGENS

With use of absorbed antimicrobial agents, some women and men can develop oral thrush, and some women may develop *Candida* vaginitis.[3,30] Overgrowth of *Clostridium (C.) difficile* with development of colitis theoretically might occur, especially with the advent of FQ-resistant strains.[3,112] Antibiotic-associated colitis has not been reported among travelers taking antimicrobials for diarrhea prophylaxis, and when tests for *C. difficile* cytotoxin was specifically included in evaluation of persistent diarrhea after antimicrobial treatment, it was not found.[30] Nevertheless, concern for colitis invariably enters into the decision making (and cost) associated with treating a traveler who develops diarrhea despite antimicrobial prophylaxis.[30]

Use of antimicrobials might promote the development of disease by certain enteropathogens, namely *Salmonella* and *Campylobacter*. While the mechanism is not proven, it might be decreasing colonization resistance in the gut lumen that promotes invasion.[30] Early studies suggest that use of agents with substantial antianaerobic activity might be more likely to disturb colonization resistance. This concept is supported lately by the observation that acquisition of vancomycin-resistant *Enterococcus* is facilitated by use of metronidazole.[30]

DRUG–DRUG INTERACTION

BSS is known to interfere with the absorption of doxycycline.[113] If doxycycline were used for malaria prevention, regular use of BSS might lower circulating doxycycline levels and increase the risk of acquiring malaria. As a rule, the two agents should not be used together. If they must be used together, their administration should be separated by at least 2 hours.[30]

INTERFERENCE WITH NATURAL IMMUNITY

An argument might be made against chemoprophylaxis so that a traveler can be exposed to the common local enteropathogens and acquire immunity. Conceptually, this approach of intentionally allowing infection would seem to best apply to long-term travelers, such as missionaries, Peace Corps volunteers, etc., rather than short-term tourists.[30] A prospective study of US medical students in Mexico found a decline in the rate of diarrhea from 34% in the first month (August) to 5% (January) after 5 months, as compared to another group of newly arrived students whose January incidence was 28%.[114] Not all expatriates experience a drop in the incidence of diarrhea with long-term stay. In Nepal, the overall incidence of diarrhea did not appear to drop over time, but these expatriates had a relatively high incidence of protozoan parasitic disease, while diarrhea mediated by ETEC did appear to wane.[115] A more recent prospective cohort study also found no decline in diarrhea incidence among expatriates in Nepal followed for up to 1 year, and confirmed that parasites, especially *Cyclospora*, were important causes of infection.[116] Taken together, these data support the concept that an antimicrobial agent for chemoprophylaxis should be used only for short periods of time.[30]

COSTS

Reves and colleagues performed an analysis comparing the cost of chemoprophylaxis with the cost of treatment and found that prophylaxis is cost effective in short-term travelers.[104] The most important factor in establishing the cost effectiveness of prophylaxis was the cost associated with a day of incapacitation associated with illness, specifically the costs assigned to lost vacation (or business) time and the amortized costs of travel.[104] This analysis showed that chemoprophylaxis is cost-beneficial for short periods of travel.[104] Since this study, however, self-therapy with the combination of an antimicrobial agent plus loperamide has limited the duration of the average case of TD to a matter of hours, so that time lost due to diarrhea is minimal. This makes self-therapy generally more cost-beneficial than prophylaxis, except perhaps for trips of a few days. Thomson and Booth performed a more recent cost analysis comparing prophylaxis with self treatment and found all possible treatment options have a more favorable benefit-cost ratio than prophylaxis.[117]

Both of these cost analyses were designed to assess the short-term costs incurred with TD. However, evidence strongly suggests that TD is often associated with the subsequent development of IBS.[20] It appears that there is a sevenfold increase in the odds of developing IBS following TD, and that almost 10% of travelers who experience TD will develop IBS.[20] For patients with IBS, total direct cost estimates per patient per year ranged from $348 to $8,750 (US dollars calculated for year 2002) and indirect costs ranged from $355 to $3,344.[118] The average number of days off work per year because of IBS was between 8.5 and 21.6.[118] It has been suggested that symptomatic TD, rather than simply colonization with local flora, is required for this complication to occur.[4] This suggests that successful prophylaxis against TD might also be successful prophylaxis against IBS.[4] If that can be shown to be true, the cost-benefit of prophylaxis would dramatically shift to the favor of prophylaxis.

Practical Approach to Chemoprophylaxis of TD

Table 2 indicates the drugs with proven activity in the prevention of TD that can be recommended at present. Our algorithmic approach to chemoprophylaxis is shown in Figure 1. The algorithm clearly favors the use of self therapy for most travelers except those deemed by the

Table 2 Drugs Used for Chemoprophylaxis of Travelers' Diarrhea

Agent	Dose	Protective Efficacy, %	Adverse Effects	Comment
BSS	2 tablets (262 mg) or 30 ml four times per day	41–65[33]	Black tongue and stools, constipation, tinnitus, drug interactions	Limited availability in Europe, Australia, and New Zealand
Probiotics *Lactobacillus acidophilus* LGG *Saccharomyces boulardii*		0–47[53, 54]	None	LGG seems to be most promising; *Saccharomyces* has shown modest effect in North Africa and Turkey
Doxycycline	100 mg daily	Originally 59–86%[63, 66]; now minimally effective		Worldwide resistance has dramatically decreased efficacy
TMP–SMX	1 DS tab daily (160 mg TMP–800 mg SMX)	Originally 73–95%[76, 77]; now likely no better than 50%[84]	Headache, nausea, vaginitis, allergic reactions, anaphylaxis, Steven-Johnson syndrome	Efficacy may be less than that of BSS in most of the world due to increasing resistance
Fluoroquinolones Norfloxacin Ofloxacin Ciprofloxacin Levofloxacin	 400 mg QD 300 mg QD 500 mg QD 500 mg QD	80–100[1]	Infrequently nausea, gastrointestinal disturbance, central nervous system (CNS) effects, skin rash, vaginitis;	Not approved in children or pregnancy; significant resistance among *Campylobacter* in Thailand and South East Asia
Rifaximin	200 mg BID or 600 mg QD	72[8]	Gastrointestinal disturbance, headache	

BSS = bismuth subsalicylate; LGG = *Lactobacillus* GG; TMP-SMX = trimethoprim–sulfamethoxazole.

physician to be at high risk. We also recognize that some travelers on short journeys have critically important reasons for remaining well during their travel. If a traveler with no special risks or critical reasons for remaining well raises the issue of prophylaxis, or simply wants preventative medications, we still prefer to educate them about the benefits of self therapy and advise them to use this approach instead of chemoprophylaxis. When prophylaxis is indicated, our first choice is rifaximin, although there is not yet sufficient evidence for its

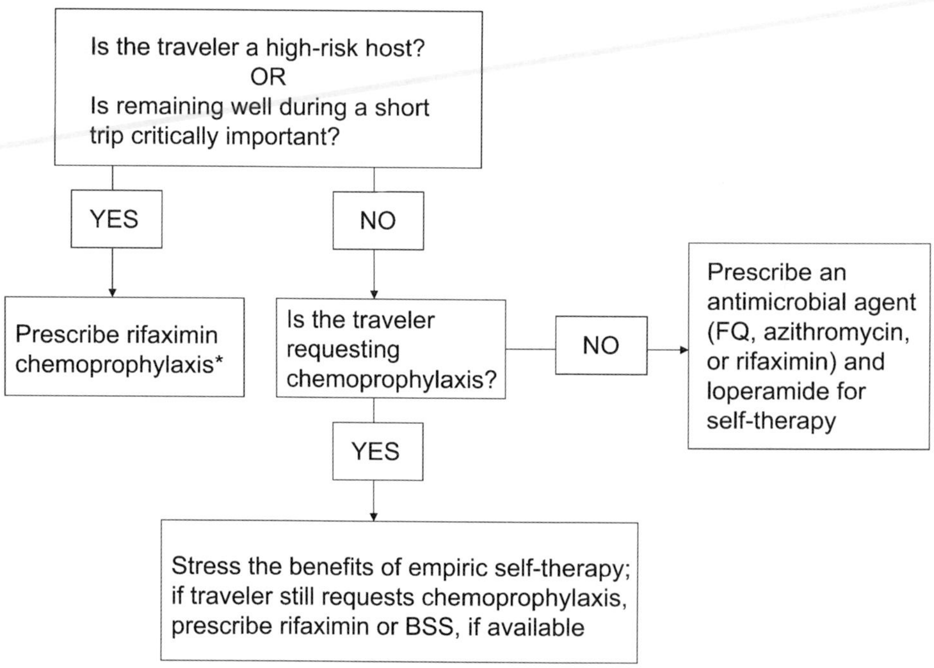

Figure 1 Algorithmic approach to chemoprophylaxis of travelers' diarrhea.
*The efficacy of rifaximin has only been documented in one trial in Mexico. Trials to determine efficacy in other regions are ongoing.

efficacy against invasive organisms. When maximal protection is a serious consideration, a fluoroquinolone should still be the primary choice. The efficacy of TMP-SMX is probably low enough in many parts of the world that it should not be recommended at all. Bismuth subsalicylate confers less protection and is not available in many regions of the world.

References

1. Rendi-Wagner P, Kollaritsch H. Drug prophylaxis for travelers' diarrhea. Clin Infect Dis 2002;34:628–33. Epub 2002 Jan 16.
2. Ericsson CD, Mattila L. Prevention of travelers' diarrhea: risk avoidance and chemoprophylaxis. In: DuPont HL, Steffen R, editors. Textbook of travel medicine and health. Hamilton (ON): BC Decker Inc.; 2000:159–64.
3. Diemert DJ. Prevention and self-treatment of traveler's diarrhea. Clin Microbiol Rev 2006;19:583–94.
4. DuPont HL. Travellers' diarrhoea: contemporary approaches to therapy and prevention. Drugs 2006;66: 303–14.
5. Castelli F, Saleri N, Tomasoni LR, Carosi G. Prevention and treatment of traveler's diarrhea. Focus on antimicrobial agents. Digestion 2006;73:109–18. Epub 2006 Feb 8.
6. DuPont HL. Travelers' diarrhea: antimicrobial therapy and chemoprevention. Nat Clin Pract Gastroenterol Hepatol 2005;2:191–8; quiz 1 p following 198.
7. Koo HL, DuPont HL. Current and future developments in travelers' diarrhea therapy. Expert Rev Anti Infect Ther 2006;4:417–27.
8. DuPont HL, Jiang ZD, Okhuysen PC, et al. A randomized, double-blind, placebo-controlled trial of rifaximin to prevent travelers' diarrhea. Ann Intern Med 2005;142: 805–12.
9. Horvath LL, Murray CK, Dooley DP. Effect of maximizing a travel medicine clinic's prevention strategies. J Travel Med 2005;12:332–7.
10. Shlim DR. Looking for evidence that personal hygiene precautions prevent traveler's diarrhea. Clin Infect Dis 2005;41Suppl 8:S531–5.
11. Boedeker EC. Vaccines for enterotoxigenic Escherichia coli: current status. Curr Opin Gastroenterol 2005;21:15–9.
12. Girard MP, Steele D, Chaignat CL, Kieny MP. A review of vaccine research and development: human enteric infections. Vaccine 2006;24:2732–50. Epub 2005 Oct 21.
13. Gorbach SL. How to hit the runs for fifty million travelers at risk. Ann Intern Med 2005;142:861–2.
14. Adachi JA, Ericsson CD, Jiang ZD, et al. Azithromycin found to be comparable to levofloxacin for the treatment of US travelers with acute diarrhea acquired in Mexico. Clin Infect Dis 2003;37:1165–71. Epub 2003 Sep 30.
15. DuPont HL, Jiang ZD, Ericsson CD, et al. Rifaximin versus ciprofloxacin for the treatment of traveler's diarrhea: a randomized, double-blind clinical trial. Clin Infect Dis 2001;33:1807–15. Epub 2001 Oct 23.
16. Ericsson CD, DuPont HL, Mathewson JJ. Single dose ofloxacin plus loperamide compared with single dose or three days of ofloxacin in the treatment of traveler's diarrhea. J Travel Med 1997;4:3–7.
17. Ericsson CD, DuPont HL, Mathewson JJ. Optimal dosing of ofloxacin with loperamide in the treatment of non-dysenteric travelers' diarrhea. J Travel Med 2001;8:207–9.
18. Ericsson CD, DuPont HL, Mathewson JJ, et al. Treatment of traveler's diarrhea with sulfamethoxazole and trimethoprim and loperamide. JAMA 1990;263:257–61.
19. Consensus panel on travelers' diarrhea: avoid prophylactic use of drugs. Am Pharm 1985;NS25:20–3.
20. Halvorson HA, Schlett CD, Riddle MS. Postinfectious irritable bowel syndrome—a meta-analysis. Am J Gastroenterol 2006;101:1894–9; quiz 1942.
21. Kean BH. The diarrhea of travelers to Mexico. Summary of a five-year study. Ann Intern Med 1963;59:605–14.
22. Sack RB. Prophylactic antimicrobials for traveler's diarrhea: an early history. Clin Infect Dis 2005;41Suppl 8: S553–6.
23. Kean BH, Waters S. The diarrhea of travelers. I. Incidence in travelers returning to the United States from Mexico. AMA Arch Ind Health 1958;18:148–50.
24. Kean BH. The diarrhea of American travelers abroad. Minn Med 1959;42:1749–51.
25. Kean BH, Schaffner W, Brennan RW. The diarrhea of travelers. V. Prophylaxis with phthalylsulfathiazole and neomycin sulphate. JAMA 1962;180:367–71.
26. Kean BH, Waters SR. The diarrhea of travelers. III. Drug prophylaxis in Mexico. N Engl J Med 1959;261:71–4.
27. Turner AC. Traveller's diarrhoea: a survey of symptoms, occurrence, and possible prophylaxis. Br Med J 1967;4: 653–4.
28. Owen JR. Diarrhoea at the Olympics. Br Med J 1968;4: 645.
29. Sack RB. Diarrhea producing factors in cultures of Escherichia coli., 4th Joint Conference, Japan–U.S. Cooperative Medical Science Program; 1968; Unzen, Nagasaki; 1968.
30. Ericsson CD, Kollaritsch H. Prophylactic use of drugs. In: Ericsson CD, DuPont HL, Steffen R, editors. Travelers' diarrhea. Vol. 1. Hamilton, Canada: B.C. Decker; 2003:160–74.
31. Raedsch R, Walter-Sack I, Galle PR, Kommerell B. Prophylaxis of traveler's diarrhea in Egypt: results of a

double blind controlled study. Klin Wochenschr 1991;69: 863–6.

32. Steffen R, Heusser R, DuPont HL. Prevention of travelers' diarrhea by nonantibiotic drugs. Rev Infect Dis 1986; 8Suppl 2:S151–9.

33. Ericsson CD. Nonantimicrobial agents in the prevention and treatment of traveler's diarrhea. Clin Infect Dis 2005; 41Suppl 8:S557–63.

34. DuPont HL, Ericsson CD, Johnson PC, de la Cabada FJ. Use of bismuth subsalicylate for the prevention of travelers' diarrhea. Rev Infect Dis 1990;12Suppl 1:S64–7.

35. DuPont HL, Sullivan P, Evans DG, et al. Prevention of traveler's diarrhea (emporiatric enteritis). Prophylactic administration of subsalicylate bismuth). JAMA 1980;243: 237–41.

36. DuPont HL, Ericsson CD, Johnson PC, et al. Prevention of travelers' diarrhea by the tablet formulation of bismuth subsalicylate. JAMA 1987;257:1347–50.

37. Ericsson CD. Bismuth subsalicylate in the treatment and chemoprophylaxis of travelers' diarrhea in adults. Drug Therapy 1990;6:31–5.

38. Steffen R. Worldwide efficacy of bismuth subsalicylate in the treatment of travelers' diarrhea. Rev Infect Dis 1990; 12Suppl 1:S80–6.

39. Steffen R, DuPont HL, Heusser R, et al. Prevention of traveler's diarrhea by the tablet form of bismuth subsalicylate. Antimicrob Agents Chemother 1986;29: 625–7.

40. Ericsson CD, Evans DG, DuPont HL, et al. Bismuth subsalicylate inhibits activity of crude toxins of Escherichia coli and Vibrio cholerae. J Infect Dis 1977; 136:693–6.

41. Ericsson CD, Tannenbaum C, Charles TT. Antisecretory and antiinflammatory properties of bismuth subsalicylate. Rev Infect Dis 1990;12Suppl 1:S16–20.

42. Cornick NA, Silva M, Gorbach SL. In vitro antibacterial activity of bismuth subsalicylate. Rev Infect Dis 1990; 12Suppl 1:S9–10.

43. Pickering LK, Feldman S, Ericsson CD, Cleary TG. Absorption of salicylate and bismuth from a bismuth subsalicylate—containing compound (Pepto-Bismol). J Pediatr 1981;99:654–6.

44. Feldman S, Chen SL, Pickering LK, et al. Salicylate absorption from a bismuth subsalicylate preparation. Clin Pharmacol Ther 1981;29:788–92.

45. Manhart MD. In vitro antimicrobial activity of bismuth subsalicylate and other bismuth salts. Rev Infect Dis 1990; 12Suppl 1:S11–5.

46. Ericsson CD, Pickering LK, Sullivan P, DuPont HL. The role of location of food consumption in the prevention of travelers' diarrhea in Mexico. Gastroenterology 1980;79: 812–6.

47. Mendelowitz PC, Hoffman RS, Weber S. Bismuth absorption and myoclonic encephalopathy during bismuth subsalicylate therapy. Ann Intern Med 1990;112:140–1.

48. Healy DP, Dansereau RJ, Dunn AB, et al. Reduced tetracycline bioavailability caused by magnesium aluminum silicate in liquid formulations of bismuth subsalicylate. Ann Pharmacother 1997;31:1460–4.

49. Gorbach SL. Probiotics and gastrointestinal health. Am J Gastroenterol 2000;95:S2–4.

50. Sazawal S, Hiremath G, Dhingra U, et al. Efficacy of probiotics in prevention of acute diarrhoea: a meta-analysis of masked, randomised, placebo-controlled trials. Lancet Infect Dis 2006;6:374–82.

51. McFarland LV. Meta-analysis of probiotics for the prevention of antibiotic associated diarrhea and the treatment of Clostridium difficile disease. Am J Gastroenterol 2006;101:812–22.

52. Oksanen PJ, Salminen S, Saxelin M, et al. Prevention of travellers' diarrhoea by Lactobacillus GG. Ann Med 1990; 22:53–6.

53. Hilton E, Kolakowski P, Singer C, Smith M. Efficacy of lactobacillus GG as a diarrheal preventive in travelers. J Travel Med 1997;4:41–43.

54. Kollaritsch H, Holst H, Grobara P, Wiedermann G. [Prevention of traveler's diarrhea with Saccharomyces boulardii. Results of a placebo controlled double-blind study]. Fortschr Med 1993;111:152–6.

55. de dios Pozo-Olano J, Warram JH Jr, Gomez RG, Cavazos MG. Effect of a lactobacilli preparation on traveler's diarrhea. A randomized, double blind clinical trial. Gastroenterology 1978;74:829–30.

56. Katelaris PH, Salam I, Farthing MJ. Lactobacilli to prevent traveler's diarrhea? N Engl J Med 1995;333:1360–1.

57. Briand V, Buffet P, Genty S, et al. Absence of efficacy of nonviable lactobacillus acidophilus for the prevention of traveler's diarrhea: a randomized, double-blind, controlled study. Clin Infect Dis 2006;43:1170–5. Epub 2006 Sep 27.

58. Silva M, Jacobus NV, Deneke C, Gorbach SL. Antimicrobial substance from a human lactobacillus strain. Antimicrob Agents Chemother 1987;31:1231–3.

59. Szajewska H, Kotowska M, Mrukowicz JZ, Armanska M, Mikolajczyk W. Efficacy of lactobacillus GG in prevention of nosocomial diarrhea in infants. J Pediatr 2001;138:361–5.

60. Szajewska H, Ruszczynski M, Radzikowski A. Probiotics in the prevention of antibiotic-associated diarrhea in children: a meta-analysis of randomized controlled trials. J Pediatr 2006;149:367–72.

61. D'Souza AL, Rajkumar C, Cooke J, Bulpitt CJ. Probiotics in prevention of antibiotic associated diarrhoea: meta-analysis. BMJ 2002;324:1361.

62. DuPont HL. Lactobacillus GG in prevention of traveler's diarrhea: an encouraging first step. J Travel Med 1997;4:1–2.

63. Sack DA, Kaminsky DC, Sack RB, et al. Prophylactic doxycycline for travelers' diarrhea. Results of a prospective double-blind study of Peace Corps volunteers in Kenya. N Engl J Med 1978;298:758–63.

64. Sack RB, Froehlich JL, Zulich AW, et al. Prophylactic doxycycline for travelers' diarrhea: results of a prospective double-blind study of Peace Corps volunteers in Morocco. Gastroenterology 1979;76:1368–73.

65. Santosham M, Sack RB, Froehlich J, et al. Biweekly prophylactic doxycycline for travelers' diarrhea. J Infect Dis 1981;143:598–602.

66. Sack RB, Santosham M, Froehlich JL, et al. Doxycycline prophylaxis of travelers' diarrhea in Honduras, an area where resistance to doxycycline is common among enterotoxigenic Escherichia coli. Am J Trop Med Hyg 1984;33:460–6.

67. Echeverria P, Sack RB, Blacklow NR, et al. Prophylactic doxycycline for travelers' diarrhea in Thailand. Further supportive evidence of Aeromonas hydrophila as an enteric pathogen. Am J Epidemiol 1984;120:912–21.

68. Sack RB, Rahman M, Yunus M, Khan EH. Antimicrobial resistance in organisms causing diarrheal disease. Clin Infect Dis 1997;24Suppl 1:S102–5.

69. Hoge CW, Gambel JM, Srijan A, et al. Trends in antibiotic resistance among diarrheal pathogens isolated in Thailand over 15 years. Clin Infect Dis 1998;26:341–5.

70. Putnam SD, Riddle MS, Wierzba TF, et al. Antimicrobial susceptibility trends among Escherichia coli and Shigella spp. isolated from rural Egyptian paediatric populations with diarrhoea between 1995 and 2000. Clin Microbiol Infect 2004;10:804–10.

71. Qadri F, Svennerholm AM, Faruque AS, Sack RB. Enterotoxigenic Escherichia coli in developing countries: epidemiology, microbiology, clinical features, treatment, and prevention. Clin Microbiol Rev 2005;18:465–83.

72. Rudland S, Little M, Kemp P, et al. The enemy within: diarrheal rates among British and Australian troops in Iraq. Mil Med 1996;161:728–31.

73. Arthur JD, Echeverria P, Shanks GD, et al. A comparative study of gastrointestinal infections in United States soldiers receiving doxycycline or mefloquine for malaria prophylaxis. Am J Trop Med Hyg 1990;43:608–13.

74. Sharp TW, Thornton SA, Wallace MR, et al. Diarrheal disease among military personnel during Operation Restore Hope, Somalia, 1992–1993. Am J Trop Med Hyg 1995;52:188–93.

75. Sanders JW, Putnam SD, Riddle MS, et al. The epidemiology of self-reported diarrhea in operations Iraqi freedom and enduring freedom. Diagn Microbiol Infect Dis 2004;50:89–93.

76. DuPont HL, Evans DG, Rios N, Cabada FJ, et al. Prevention of travelers' diarrhea with trimethoprim-sulfamethoxazole. Rev Infect Dis 1982;4:533–9.

77. DuPont HL, Galindo E, Evans DG, et al. Prevention of travelers' diarrhea with trimethoprim-sulfamethoxazole and trimethoprim alone. Gastroenterology 1983;84:75–80.

78. Andremont A, Tancrede C. Reduction of the aerobic Gram negative bacterial flora of the gastro-intestinal tract and prevention of traveller's diarrhea using oral erythromycin. Ann Microbiol (Paris) 1981;132 B:419–27.

79. Purcell BK, Dooley DP, Gray PJ, et al. Experience with directly observed prophylaxis using erythromycin in military trainees exposed to pertussis. Mil Med 2004; 169:417–20.

80. Black FT, Gaarslev K, Orskov F, et al. Mecillinam, a new prophylactic for travellers' diarrhoea. A prospective double-blind study in tourists travelling to Egypt and the Far East. Scand J Infect Dis 1983;15:189–93.

81. Johnson PC, Ericsson CD, Morgan DR, et al. Lack of emergence of resistant fecal flora during successful prophylaxis of traveler's diarrhea with norfloxacin. Antimicrob Agents Chemother 1986;30:671–4.

82. Scott DA, Haberberger RL, Thornton SA, Hyams KC. Norfloxacin for the prophylaxis of travelers' diarrhea in U.S. military personnel. Am J Trop Med Hyg 1990;42:160–4.

83. Wistrom J, Norrby SR, Burman LG, et al. Norfloxacin versus placebo for prophylaxis against travellers' diarrhoea. J Antimicrob Chemother 1987;20:563–74.

84. Heck JE, Staneck JL, Cohen MB, et al. Prevention of travelers' diarrhea: ciprofloxacin versus trimethoprim/sulfamethoxazole in adult volunteers working in Latin America and the Caribbean. J Travel Med 1994;1:136–42.

85. Parry H, Howard AJ, Galpin OP, Hassan SP. The prophylaxis of travellers' diarrhoea: a double blind placebo controlled trial of ciprofloxacin during a Himalayan expedition. J Infect 1994;28:337–8.

86. Rademaker CM, Hoepelman IM, Wolfhagen MJ, et al. Results of a double-blind placebo-controlled study using ciprofloxacin for prevention of travelers' diarrhea. Eur J Clin Microbiol Infect Dis 1989;8:690–4.

87. Sanders JW, Isenbarger DW, Walz SE, et al. An observational clinic-based study of diarrheal illness in deployed United States military personnel in Thailand: presentation and outcome of Campylobacter infection. Am J Trop Med Hyg 2002;67:533–8.

88. Kuschner RA, Trofa AF, Thomas RJ, et al. Use of azithromycin for the treatment of Campylobacter enteritis in travelers to Thailand, an area where ciprofloxacin resistance is prevalent. Clin Infect Dis 1995;21:536–41.

89. Shanks GD, Ragama OB, Aleman GM, et al. Azithromycin prophylaxis prevents epidemic dysentery. Trans R Soc Trop Med Hyg 1996;90:316.

90. Matute AJ, Schurink CA, Krijnen RM, et al. Double-blind, placebo-controlled study comparing the effect of azithromycin with clarithromycin on oropharyngeal and bowel microflora in volunteers. Eur J Clin Microbiol Infect Dis 2002;21:427–31. Epub 2002 Jun 11.

91. Taylor DN. Poorly absorbed antibiotics for the treatment of traveler's diarrhea. Clin Infect Dis 2005;41Suppl 8:S564–70.

92. Ericsson CD, DuPont HL, Galindo E, et al. Efficacy of bicozamycin in preventing traveler's diarrhea. Gastroenterology 1985;88:473–7.

93. DuPont HL, Ericsson CD, Mathewson JJ, et al. Oral aztreonam, a poorly absorbed yet effective therapy for bacterial diarrhea in US travelers to Mexico. JAMA 1992; 267:1932–5.

94. Robins GW, Wellington K. Rifaximin: a review of its use in the management of traveller's diarrhoea. Drugs 2005; 65:1697–713.

95. Taylor DN, Bourgeois AL, Ericsson CD, et al. A randomized, double-blind, multicenter study of rifaximin compared with placebo and with ciprofloxacin in the treatment of travelers' diarrhea. Am J Trop Med Hyg 2006;74:1060–6.

96. Taylor DN, McKenzie R, Durbin A, et al. Rifaximin, a nonabsorbed oral antibiotic, prevents shigellosis after experimental challenge. Clin Infect Dis 2006;42:1283–8. Epub 2006 Mar 22.

97. Steffen R, Collard F, Tornieporth N, et al. Epidemiology, etiology, and impact of traveler's diarrhea in Jamaica. JAMA 1999;281:811–7.

98. Neal KR, Scott HM, Slack RC, Logan RF. Omeprazole as a risk factor for campylobacter gastroenteritis: case-control study. BMJ 1996;312:414–5.

99. Mileno MD, Bia FJ. The compromised traveler. Infect Dis Clin North Am 1998;12:369–412.

100. Castelli F, Patroni A. The human immunodeficiency virus-infected traveler. Clin Infect Dis 2000;31:1403–8. Epub 2000 Nov 29.

101. Ericsson CD. Travellers with pre-existing medical conditions. Int J Antimicrob Agents 2003;21:181–8.

102. Mackell S. Traveler's diarrhea in the pediatric population: etiology and impact. Clin Infect Dis 2005;41Suppl 8:S547–52.

103. Cooper MC. The pregnant traveller. Travel Med Infect Dis 2006;4:196–201.

104. Reves RR, Johnson PC, Ericsson CD, DuPont HL. A cost-effectiveness comparison of the use of antimicrobial agents for treatment or prophylaxis of travelers' diarrhea. Arch Intern Med 1988;148:2421–7.

105. Steffen R. Epidemiologic studies of travelers' diarrhea, severe gastrointestinal infections, and cholera. Rev Infect Dis 1986;8Suppl 2:S122–30.

106. Steffen R, van der Linde F, Gyr K, Schar M. Epidemiology of diarrhea in travelers. JAMA 1983;249:1176–80.

107. Monteville MR, Riddle MS, Rockabrand DR, et al. Epidemiology of diarrhea among deployed military personnel in support of Operation Iraqi Freedom and Operation Enduring Freedom. American Society of Tropical Medicine and Hygiene, 54th Annual Meeting, Washington, D.C.; 2005.

108. Murray BE, Alvarado T, Kim KH, et al. Increasing resistance to trimethoprim-sulfamethoxazole among isolates of Escherichia coli in developing countries. J Infect Dis 1985;152:1107–13.

109. Segreti J, Gootz TD, Goodman LJ, et al. High-level quinolone resistance in clinical isolates of Campylobacter jejuni. J Infect Dis 1992;165:667–70.

110. Adler-Mosca H, Luthy-Hottenstein J, Martinetti Lucchini G, et al. Development of resistance to quinolones in five patients with campylobacteriosis treated with norfloxacin or ciprofloxacin. Eur J Clin Microbiol Infect Dis 1991;10:953–7.

111. DuPont HL, Jiang ZD, Okhuysen PC, et al. Antibacterial chemoprophylaxis in the prevention of traveler's diarrhea: evaluation of poorly absorbed oral rifaximin. Clin Infect Dis 2005;41Suppl 8:S571–6.

112. McDonald LC, Killgore GE, Thompson A, et al. An epidemic, toxin gene-variant strain of Clostridium difficile. N Engl J Med 2005;353:2433–41. Epub 2005 Dec 1.

113. Ericsson CD, Feldman S, Pickering LK, Cleary TG. Influence of subsalicylate bismuth on absorption of doxycycline. JAMA 1982;247:2266–7.

114. Ericsson CD, DuPont HL, Mathewson IJ. Epidemiologic observations on diarrhea developing in U.S. and Mexican students living in Guadalajara, Mexico. J Travel Med 1995;2:6–10.

115. Taylor DN, Houston R, Shlim DR, et al. Etiology of diarrhea among travelers and foreign residents in Nepal. JAMA 1988;260:1245–8.

116. Shlim DR, Hoge CW, Rajah R, et al. Persistent high risk of diarrhea among foreigners in Nepal during the first 2 years of residence. Clin Infect Dis 1999;29:613–6.

117. Thomson MA, Booth IW. Treatment of traveller's diarrhoea. Economic aspects. Pharmacoeconomics 1996; 9:382–91.

118. Maxion-Bergemann S, Thielecke F, Abel F, Bergemann R. Costs of irritable bowel syndrome in the UK and US. Pharmacoeconomics 2006;24:21–37.

Chapter 21

Probiotics in Travelers' Diarrhea

Herwig Kollaritsch, MD, PROF

Sunil Sazawal, MD, MPH, PhD

Traveler's diarrhea (TD) is a constant and fast friend of the traveler. It remains the main topic in travel medicine because this medical specialty was brought into being more than 25 years ago.

Many approaches tested out to minimize the disease burden resulting from TD. Risk minimizing by dietary recommendations, treatment, or prophylaxis with antibiotics and various nonantibiotic preparations, finally vaccines against enteropathogens—none proved to be the philosopher's stone.[1]

But travelers urge their physicians to provide help against this inevitable fate during their trip to a developing country. The prescribing doctors have then to face a difficult situation: provide a safe and effective medication that will cause no harm in the hands of a medical layperson but will be fast acting against the disease.

Probiotics are one of the potentially appealing types of medication for this purpose.

Definition and Characterization of Probiotics

One approach for the prevention and treatment of TD is the use of probiotics.[2–5] A probiotic is a "live microbial food ingredient that, when ingested in sufficient quantities, exerts health benefits on the consumer."[6]

The functionality of the intestinal immune system depends on commensal bacteria,[7] and the acting principle of probiotics is to support and restore the normal intestinal microbiota by hampering the growth of diarrheal pathogens and inducing gut-associated immune mechanisms.[8]

Probiotic strains of microorganisms must be of human origin and safe for human use,[4,9] and today a broad variety of different and unique strains are used or under investigation (Table 1).

Mechanisms of Action

Recent scientific work elucidates the health effects of probiotics more precisely, although many questions are open until today.

Potential modes of action:

- decrease the adherence of pathogenic microorganisms to the epithelial cells and by this inhibit colonization as well. This was shown for *S. typhimurium*, *C. difficile*, *E. coli*, and many other bacteria[9];
- can colonize the intestinum, competing with enteropathogens for consumption of monosaccharides and thereby slowing the growth of the pathogens[10];
- have adjuvant-like effects on intestinal and systemic immunity (for example, healthy adult volunteers who received fermented milk containing *L. acidophilus* and *Bifidobacterium* spp. for 3 weeks showed significantly higher sIgA-titers after vaccination with Ty21a live vaccine than a control group without fermented dairy products)[11];
- can influence the nonhumoral immunity (*Saccharomyces boulardii* can activate complement, *Lactobacilli* enhance capacity of blood lymphocytes to produce various cytokines (γ-Interferon (γ-IFN), Interleukin 12 (IL-12), Interleukin 18 (IL-18)), the enhanced IL-12 production may be associated with down-regulated Th2-response and

Table 1 Probiotic Strains

Species	Strain
Lactobacillus	L. johnsonii LA1
	L. acidophilus
	L. rhamnosus GG
	L. acidophilus NFCM
	L. casei Shirota
	L. bulgaricus
	L. gasseri
	L. fermentum
	L. reuteri
	L. lactis
Bifidobacterium	B. bifidum
	B. longum
	B. breve
	B. infantis
	B. adolescentis
	B. animalis
Others	**Enterococcus faecalis (SF68)**
	Streptococcus thermophilus
	Saccharomyces boulardii
	Bacillus cereus
	Propionibacterium frendsreichii subsp. shermani
	Lactococcus lacti

Bold indicates studied in prevention and/or treatment of TD
Adapted from Sazawal S et al,[3] Doron S et al,[4] Surawicz CM.[9]

giving by that way an explanation for the potential role of probiotics in allergy prevention;[9,12];
- can produce antimicrobial substances like organic acids, ammonia, fatty free acids and bacteriocins, at least in vitro; such effects were mainly demonstrated for *L. casei GG* (LGG), but also for *Bifidobacterium*; *LGG* produces four classes of bacteriocins[13] that are targeted mostly on closely related bacteria like *Lactococcus, Streptococcus, Staphylococcus, Listeria,* and *Mycobacteria*; and
- can increase the transepithelial resistance (*Lactobacilli* spp.), which may prevent an impairment of this function by pathogenic bacteria leading to a lower susceptibility of the host in case of infection.[14]

A number of other effects are possibly contributable to probiotics, particularly in elder subjects, like enhanced activity of natural killer cells[15] or a reversal of the age-related decline in cytokine production (demonstrated in mice).[16]

There is evidence too, that the immunomodulatory effects of probiotics are different to some extent in the young and in the old and in healthy subjects versus those with underlying diseases. For example, while it has been reported that probiotics have a stimulatory effect on phagocytosis in healthy subjects, probiotics cause down-regulation in patients with allergies.[12,17] Other available data suggest that the immunomodulatory effects may also depend on the immune status of the host and the dose of probiotics given, and that differences may exist between different strains.[18–22]

All these data suggest that the mechanisms of action of probiotics are complex and until today not fully understood. It is not clear which of the described features contribute to what extent in clinical disease.[23] The puzzle-like results of experimental data complicate our understanding how a probiotic will exert its beneficial effect in a person taking this kind of medication. Moreover, as a wide variety of different bacteria (see Table 1) and different preparations with different dosages are available, the effect of probiotics in general is hardly predictable in a distinct clinical case. This may be at least partially responsible for the dismissive position of many clinicians against probiotic preparations.[22]

Range of Application for Probiotics

Probiotics were tested in a broad variety of gastrointestinal (GI) diseases, allergies, dental caries, elimination of nasal colonization with potentially pathogenic bacteria, and Helicobacter pylori infections, and they are currently under investigation for their role in the treatment of rheumatoid arthritis, cancer prevention, irritable bowel syndrome (IBS), atopy, liver diseases, and treatment of graft-versus-host disease.[4]

- Probiotics have been proven to be beneficial in subjects with lactose-intolerance, leading to fewer symptoms if the milk in the diet is replaced with fermented dairy products[24]; however, strain-specific lactase activity main vary over 100-fold.[25]
- Particularly for treatment of diarrheal disease in childhood, a number of studies and meta-analyses are published.[5,26,27] Summarizing these studies, probiotics have a beneficial effect on duration and severity of infectious diarrhea caused by various etiologic agents when used as adjunct therapy to oral rehydration.[28] Most studies were performed with LGG and *Lactobacillus reuteri*, a few with *Enterococcus SF68, Bifidobacterium bifidum,* and *S. thermophilus*[27]; all studies concluded that these probiotics are beneficial for the recipient. For Rotavirus prevention and treatment, the results are controversial.[27,28]
- Since their introduction, probiotics were often used for treatment and prevention of antibiotic-associated diarrhea and for mitigation of GI side effects of antibiotics. For *Lactobacillus* and for *Enterococcus*, meta-analyses of the studies per-

formed give clear evidence that these probiotics are definitely beneficial by reducing the risk and intensity of antibiotic-associated diarrhea during treatment.[29,30]

- An interesting attribute of probiotics can be seen in their capacity to prevent and treat allergic manifestations. Atopic eczema or dermatitis could be prevented by administration of LGG to newborns, and a 6-month course with this probiotic reduced the incidence of atopic eczema to 50% versus a breastfed group of infants.[31] A trial with infants suffering from atopic eczema showed a significant improvement in skin condition 2 months after start of treatment with LGG or *Bifidobacterium lactis*.[32]
- Less effective were probiotics in preventing infections in children in daycares (respiratory or GI infections), nevertheless suggesting at least a modest reduction in incidence and severity of infections.[33]
- At least in one good study LGG was proven to have a reducing effect of the development of dental caries by reducing the counts of *S. mutans*, which is the putative cause for caries.[34]
- Only recently it could be demonstrated that fermented milk products with probiotics like LGG, *Bifidobacterium* spp. and others were able to reduce gram-positive bacteria like β-hemolytic streptococci or *S. aureus* in nasal swabs of the recipients.[35]

Other applications of probiotics seem to be quite promising. Recent studies in inflammatory bowel disease, including Crohn's disease and ulcerative colitis, necrotizing enterocolitis, or IBS exhibit conflicting results, nevertheless promising enough to intensify research in this field in the future.[4]

Future applications like the treatment of rheumatoid arthritis and the prevention of cancer remain speculative until large-scale studies give evidence for beneficial effects.

Safety Profile of Probiotics

There is consensus that probiotics are in general safe and cause only minor side effects like bloating or mild nausea. A meta-analysis[36] of probiotics for the prevention of antibiotic-associated diarrhea and the treatment of *Clostridium (C.) difficile* disease stated that in 26 clinical trials with altogether more than 2.500 subjects, not a single moderate or even severe adverse event was seen.

The most important area of concern with probiotic use is the risk of sepsis. There are some reports of sepsis with various probiotics, summarized by Boyle and colleagues.[37] There are descriptions of Bacteremia, liver abscess, and endocarditis associated with LGG and *Bacillus subtilis*; in all cases the patient had an underlying condition well known for opportunistic infections (Diabetes, neoplastic disease, short-gut syndrome, etc). It should be mentioned that most of these complications could be treated successfully.

For *Saccharomyces boulardii* Boyle and colleagues[37] counted a total of 24 documented cases of fungemia/septicemia with *S. boulardii*, with one case being fatal.[38] Again, not a single case of *S. boulardii* septicemia occurred in a healthy individual; all reported patients had severe underlying diseases.

Summarizing these data, probiotics can be considered as very safe in otherwise healthy subjects but should be used with some caution in patients with severe comorbidities. In patients with infectious diarrhea (except *C. difficile*), severe complications like sepsis or fungemia are not reported.[36,37]

Probiotics in TD

TREATMENT OF TD

TD is a short lasting, usually mild disease, causing more discomfort than real harm. It is characterized by three or more unformed stools per day, lasts for 3 to 4 days, and is accompanied by symptoms like abdominal cramps, nausea, vomiting, or fever in approximately two-thirds of cases.[39] Only about 10% of the patients experience fever, suggesting an invasive disease, and only a handful of cases of TD last for more than 14 or 30 days, fulfilling the criteria of persistent or chronic diarrhea.[39,40]

These clinical characteristics implicate that a reasonable treatment for this kind of self-limiting disease should be:

- Fast acting
- Shortening the disease
- Eradicating the etiologic agent
- Safe for self treatment

Probiotics display their therapeutic effect mainly by restoring the physiological conditions in the gut and by hindering pathogenic bacteria from causing disease.[2,4,5,8,9] They have a number of scientifically evaluated benefits and medical indications as described. However, the above described requirements for an ideal therapeutic drug for the treatment of TD make a successful application of probiotics not reliable for this disease. A medline search using the terms "traveler's diarrhea," "probiotics," and "treatment" by August 2006 did not exert a single hit for an original paper on a published study on the treatment properties of probiotics in TD. Most recent published reviews for this subject confirm the lack of controlled studies.[2,4] A few older publications uniformly state that probiotics are not able to significantly influence the clinical course of acute TD.[41]

It is, however, tempting to speculate that probiotics may have a beneficial effect as an additional or second-line treatment, particularly in cases of persistent or chronic diarrhea. Numerous studies in infectious diarrhea in children[23] verified a beneficial effect for probiotics, and a conclusion by analogy for TD seems to be acceptable.

PREVENTION OF TD

Several studies have shown in the past that travelers do not normally follow the recommendations of their physicians to avoid dangerous foods or beverages while staying abroad.[42,43] This may partly be due to the fact that dietary mistakes are "masked" by the luxurious ambiente of hotels or exotic buffets.[44] This makes it difficult for travelers to minimize their individual risk by changing their behavior unless the advice they get is very detailed.[43] Adhering very strictly to such dietary lists will make the holiday trip more difficult, less comfortable, and may be sometimes not even be applicable at all. Therefore it is understandable that travelers would strongly prefer any kind of safe and effective prevention for TD rather than a treatment after they have been struck by the disease. But as described in detail in this book and many studies during the last 25 years, etiology of TD is heterogenous, with 80% of episodes being caused by bacterial pathogens.[45–47] Less common causes include viruses like Adenoviruses, Astrovirus, or rotavirus,[48] or parasitic microorganisms like *E. histolytica* or *Giardia intestinalis,*[49] or even rarely helmithic infections.[50] At least seven bacterial species are common causes for TD,[45] among them all forms of *E. coli.*[48]

This enormous diversity of etiologic agents, all of them using at least partly different pathophysiologic mechanisms to induce diarrhea (toxins, direct cytopatic effects, invasive diseases, etc.) makes prevention by a single medication a very difficult task. Moreover, the cause remains unidentified in approximately 20% of cases of TD, adding one more problem to prevention.[45]

The concept to try to prevent TD through the use of probiotics is not new. Encouraged by a few trials with probiotics in the prevention of acute diarrhea, primarily in infant populations, these medications were also investigated with respect to their potential to prevent TD.

A meta-analysis[3] of masked, randomized, and placebo-controlled trials on the efficacy of probiotics in prevention of acute diarrhea showed that we have to differentiate to describe the effect of probiotics between TD and other forms of acute diarrhea, particularly antibiotic-associated diarrhea.

Antibiotic-associated diarrhea could be reduced by a maximum of 52% in several trials, *S. boulardii,*[51] *Bifidobacterium lactis BB12,*[52] and LGG[53] showing the highest efficacy.

To describe the beneficial effect of probiotics to prevent TD, only a few studies were published thus far in peer reviewed journals.[3] These clinical trials showed only marginal protective efficacy for such preparations (Figure 1).

In 1978, Pozo Alano and colleagues[54] described first in travelers to Mexico from the US the effect of *Lactobacilli* (Lactinex) on the incidence of TD, concluding from their data that this preparation did not exert any incidence reducing effect. However, this study included only 50 volunteers.

Oksanen and colleagues[55] indicated a protective efficacy of 11.8%, reducing the incidence of diarrhea of 46.5% in the placebo group to 41% in the group receiving LGG. However, this group reported a different protection for different destinations, reaching up to 39.5% for one destination. Similar observations were found with *S. boulardii* in a study with more than 3,000 travelers[56] going to different destinations. While in Turkey the protective efficacy was around 25%, the same preparation lacked any beneficial effect, such as in travelers going to Mexico. In this trial, a dose-dependent effect could be described as well as a direct effect of compliance with the trial medication.

More recently, a reevaluation of the prophylactic efficacy of LGG was published[57] in a study including 245 patients traveling to all continents. This study exhibited a protection rate of 47%, which was calculated by a per day risk of TD of 7.4% in the placebo group versus 3.9% in the group with *Lactobacilli.* Thus, this study confirmed a significant protective effect by LGG. Interestingly, this study did not find regional differences with respect to protection rates.

On the other hand, a fairly large study evaluated *Lactobacillus fermentum* KLD versus *L. acidophilus* versus placebo in British soldiers in Belize, with no significant effect at all.[58]

Some researchers have examined the role of nonviable probiotics preparations in preventing TD. The only study published to date found no beneficial effects of treating with nonviable *L. acidophilus* to prevent TD.

Summarizing the data on studies using probiotic prevention of TD (see Figure 1), the beneficial effect of prophylactic intake seems to be doubtful and obviously not very significant with respect to clinical relevance. There is some evidence, as described, but these effects need substantial proof. In particular, such preventive studies should be coupled with microbiological stool investigation to get deeper insight in the possible mode

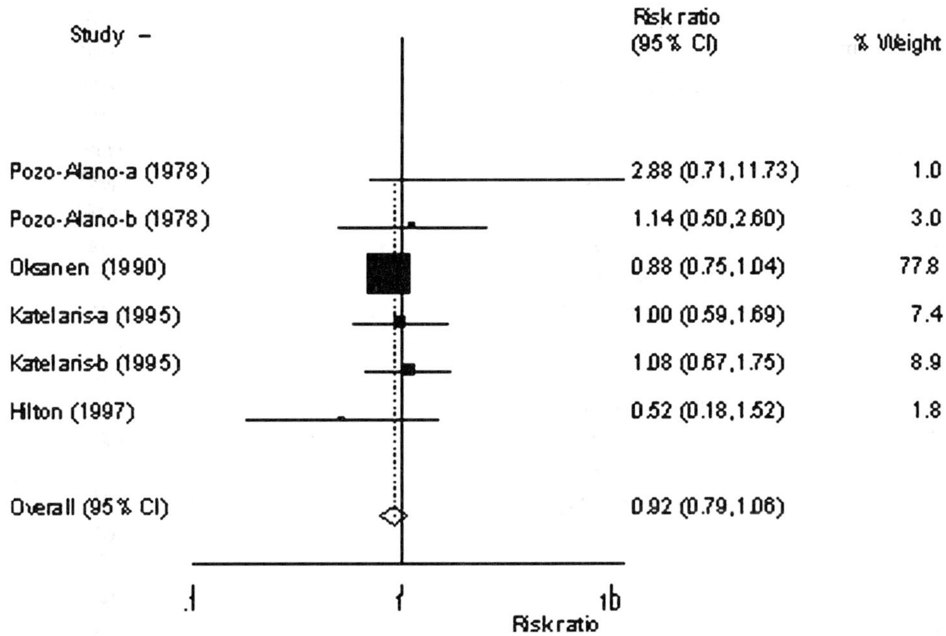

Figure 1 Clinical trials evaluating probiotics in the prevention of travelers' diarrhea.

of action of probiotics in this indication: Does a probiotic eventually inhibit only certain bacterial microorganisms to colonize in the gut while others remain untouched at all? Is there any substantial antiviral action as for example suggested—although also not proven—for treatment of rotavirus disease in childhood?[27]

There are many preparations of probiotics as well, and most of them are not evaluated with respect to their potency to inhibit TD. Moreover, because most data on the beneficial effect of probiotics derive from childhood studies,[3] dose-finding studies for adult travelers are required to find optimal prophylactic regimens.

Nevertheless it has to be conceded that we should not go too far with our expectations. The variety of etiologic agents and the variety of the epidemiology and occurrence of the different pathogens responsible for TD are certainly a limiting factor for the usefulness of probiotics.

On the other hand, the excellent safety profile of these kinds of medications predestine them for preventive intake. Their potential should therefore be investigated more thoroughly as vaccines because, even against the most common cause of TD (enterotoxic *E. coli*), probiotics are far from routine human use.[60,61]

References

1. DuPont HL, Ericsson CD, Steffen R. Historical perspective of traveler's diarrhea. In: Ericsson CD, DuPont HL, Steffen R, editors. Traveler's diarrhea 1st ed. Hamilton: BC Decker; 2003. p. 1–10.
2. Ericsson CD. Nonantimicrobial agents in the prevention and treatment of traveler's diarrhea. Clin Inf Dis 2005; 41(Suppl 8):S557–63.
3. Sazawal S, Hiremath G, Dhingra U, et al. Efficacy of probiotics in prevention of acute diarrhoea: a meta analysis of masked, randomised, placebo-controlled trials. Lancet Inf Dis 2006;6:374–82.
4. Doron S, Gorbach SL. Probiotics: their role in the treatment and prevention of disease. Expert Rev Anti Infect Ther 2006;4:261–75.
5. Szajewska H, Mrukuwicz JZ. Probiotics in the treatment and prevention of acute infectious diarrhea in infants and children: a systematic review of published randomized double-blind, placebo-controlled trials. J Ped Gatroenterol and Nutr 2001;33:S17–25.
6. Ashwell M. Concise monograph on concept of functional foods., International life sciences institute, European Commission (2002).
7. Rakoff-Nahoum S, Paglino J, Eslami-Varzaneh F, et al. Recognition of commensal microflora by toll like receptors is required for intestinal homeostasis. Cell 2004;118:229–41.
8. Surawicz CM. Probiotics, antibiotic-associated diarrhoea and Clostridium difficile diarrhoea in humans. Best Pract Res Clin Gastroenterol 2003;17:775–83.
9. Alvarez-Olmos MI, Oberhelman RA. Probiotic agents and infectious diseases: a modern perspective on a traditional therapy. Clin Inf Dis 2001;32:1567–76.
10. Lee DJ, Drongowski RA, Coran AG, Harmon CM. Evaluation of probiotic treatment in a neonatal animal model. Ped Surg Int 2000;16:237–42.

11. Link-Amster H, Rochat F, Saudan KY, et al. Modulation of a specific humoral immune response and changes in intestinal flora mediated through fermented milk intake. FEMS Immunol Med Microbiol 1994;10:55–64.
12. Shida K, Takahashi R, Iwadate E, et al. Lactobacillus casei strain Shirota suppresses serum immunoglobulin E and immunoglobulin G1 responses and systemic anaphylaxis in a food allergy model. Clin Exp Allergy 2002;32:563–70.
13. Servin AL. Antagonistic activities of lactobacilli and bifidobacteria against microbial pathogens. FEMS Microbiol Rev 2004;28:405–40.
14. Madsen K, Cornish A, Soper P, et al. Probiotic bacteria enhance murine and human intestinal epithelial barrier function. Gastroenterology 2001;121:580–91.
15. Gill HS, Cross ML, Rutherfurd KJ, Gopal PK. Dietary probiotic supplementation to enhance cellular immunity in the elderly. Br J Biomed Sci 2001;58:94–6.
16. Muscettola M, Massai L, Tanganelli C, Grasso G. Effects of lactobacilli on interferin production in young and aged mice. Ann NY Acad Sci 1994;717:403S–9S.
17. Pelto L, Isolauri E, Lilius EM, et al. Probiotic bacteria down-regulate the milk induced inflammatory response in milk-hypersensitive subjects but have an immunostimulatory effect in healthy adults. Clin Exp Allergy 1998;28: 1474–9.
18. Matsuzaki T, Chin J. Modulating immune responses with probiotic bacteria. Immun Cell Biol 2000;78:67–73.
19. Cross ML, Mortensen RR, Kudsk J, Gill HS. Dietary intake of *Lactobacillus rhamnosus* HNOO1 enhances production of both Th1 and Th2 cytokines in antigen primed mice. Med Microbiol Immunol 2002;191:49–53.
20. Gill HS, Rutherford KJ. Viability and dose response studies on the effects of the immunoenhancing lactic acid bacterium *Lactobacillus rhamnosus* in mice. Br J Nutr 2001;86:285–9.
21. Yasui H, Shida K, Matsuzaki T, Yokokura T. Immunomodulatory function of lactic acid bacteria. Ant v Leeuw 1999;76:383–9.
22. Senok AC, Ismaeel AY, Botta GA. Probiotics: facts and myths. Clin Microbiol Infect 2005;11:958–66.
23. Sullivan A, Nord CE. Probiotics and gastrointestinal diseases. J Int Med 2005;257:78–92.
24. Alm L. Effect of fermentation on lactose, glucose and galactose content in milk and suitability of fermented milk products for lactose intolerant individuals. J Dairy Sci 1982;65:346–352.
25. Fonden R, Mogensen G, Tanaka R, Salminen S. Culture containing dairy products— effect in intestinal microflora, human nutrition and health—current knowledge and future perspectives. Bulletin 2000;352–61.
26. Huang JS, Bousvaros A, Lee JW, et al. Efficacy of probiotic use in acute diarrhea in children: a meta-analysis. Dig Dis Sci 2002;47:2625–34.
27. Allen SJ, Okoko B, Martinez E, et al. Probiotics for treating infectious diarrhoea. Cochrane Database Syst Rev 2005;1.
28. Guandalini S, Pensabene L, Zikri MA, et al. Lactobacillus GG administered in oral rehydration solution to children with acute diarrhea: a multicenter European trial. J Pediatr Gastroenterol Nutr 2000;30:54–60.
29. Cremonini F, Di Caro S, Nista EC, et al. Meta-analysis: the effect of probiotic administration on antibiotic associated diarrhea. Aliment Pharmacol Ther 2002;16: 1461–7.
30. D'Souza AL, Rajkumar C, Cooke J, Bulpitt CJ. Probiotics in prevention of antibiotic associated diarrhea: meta-analysis. Br Med J 2002;324:1361.
31. Kalliomaki M, Salminen S, Arvilommi H, et al. Probiotics in primary prevention of atopic disease: a randomised placebo-controlled trial. Lancet 2001;357:1076–9.
32. Isolauri E, Arvola T, Sutas Y, et al. Probiotics in the management of atopic eczema. Clin Exp Allergy 2000;30: 1604–10.
33. Hatakka K, Savilahti E, Ponka A, et al. Effect of long-term consumption of probiotic milk on infections in children attending day care centres: double blind, randomised trial. Br Med J 2001;322:1327–33.
34. Nase L, Hatakka K, Savilahti E, et al. Effect of long-term consumption of a probiotic bacterium, Lactobacillus rhamnosus GG in milk on dental caries and caries risk in children. Caries Res 2001;35:412–20.
35. Gluck U, Gebbers JO. Ingested probiotics reduce nasal colonization with pathogenic bacteria (S. aureus, S. pneumoniae and β-hemolytic streptococci). Am J Clin Nutr 2003;77:517–20.
36. McFarland LV. Meta-analysis of probiotics for the prevention of antibiotic associated diarrhea and the treatment of Clostridium difficile disease. Am J Gastroenterol 2006;101: 812–22.
37. Boyle RJ, Robins-Browne RM, Tang MLK. Probiotic use in clinical practice: what are the risks. Am J Clin Nutr 2006; 83:1256–64.
38. Lestin F, Pertschy A, Rimek D. Fungemia after oral treatment with Saccharomyces boulardii in a patient with multiple comorbidities. Dtsch Med Wochenschr 2003;128: 2531–3.
39. Gyr N, Kaufmann G, Kozarsky P. Clinical features and syndromes. In: Ericsson CD, DuPont HL, Steffen R, editors. Traveler's diarrhea 1st ed. Hamilton: BC Decker; 2003. p. 134–46.
40. Kollaritsch H. Traveller's diarrhea among Austrian tourists to warm climate countries. II. Clinical features. Eur J Epidemiol 1989;5:335–62.

41. Kollaritsch H, Scheiner O, Kremsner G, Wiedermann G. Prevention of traveller's diarrhea: comparison of different non-antibiotic preparations for prophylaxis or treatment in double blind trials among Austrian volunteers. Travel medicine international 1989;7:9–18.

42. Hill DR, von Sonnenburg F. Diet and education about risks. In: Ericsson CD, DuPont HL, Steffen R, editors. Traveler's diarrhea 1st ed. Hamilton: BC Decker; 2003. p. 148–159.

43. Kozicki M, Steffen R, Schär M. "Boil it cook it peel it or forget it": Does this rule prevent traveler's diarrhea? Int J Epidemiol 1985;14:169–72.

44. Kollaritsch H. Traveller's diarrhea among Austrian tourists to warm climate countries: I. Epidemiology. Eur J Epidemiol 1989;5:74–81.

45. Koo HL, DuPont HL. Current and future developments in travelers' diarrhea therapy. Expert Rev Anti Infect Ther 2006;4:417–27.

46. Jiang ZD, Lowe B, Verenkar MP, et al. Prevalence of enteric pathogens among international travelers with diarrhea acquired in Kenya (Mombasa), India (Goa), or Jamaica (Montego Bay). J Infect Dis 2002;185:497–502.

47. Jiang ZD, Butzler JP, Lowe BS. The bacterial pathogens. In: Ericsson CD, DuPont HL, Steffen R, editors. Traveler's diarrhea 1st ed. Hamilton: BC Decker; 2003. p. 10–28.

48. Gascon J. Epidemiology, etiology and pathophysiology of traveler's diarrhea. Digestion 2006;73Suppl 1:102–8.

49. Okhuysen PC. Traveler's diarrhea due to intestinal protozoa. Clin Infect Dis 2001;33:110–4.

50. Hashmey R, Genta RM, White AC Jr. Parasites and diarrhea. II. Helmiths and diarrhea. J Trav Med 1997;4: 72–5.

51. Kotowska M, Albrecht P, Szajewska H. *Saccharomyces boulardii* in the prevention of antibiotic-associated diarrhoea in children: a randomized double-blind placebo-controlled trial. Aliment Pharmacol Ther 2005;21:583–90.

52. Weizman Z, Asli G, Alsheikh A. Effect of a probiotic infant formula on infections in child care centers: comparison of two probiotic agents Pediatrics 2005;115: 5–9.

53. Armuzzi A, Cremonini F, Bartolozzi F, et al. The effect of oral administration of *Lactobacillus* GG on antibiotic-associated gastrointestinal side-effects during *Helicobacter pylori* eradication therapy. Aliment Pharmacol Ther 2001; 15:163–9.

54. de dios Pozo-Olano, Warram JH Jr, Gómez RG, et al. Effect of a lactobacilli preparation on traveler's diarrhea. A randomized, double blind clinical trial. Gastroenterology 1978;74:829–30.

55. Oksanen PJ, Salminen S, Saxelin M, et al. Prevention of traveler's diarrhea by lactobacillus GG. Annals of Medicine 1990;22:53–6.

56. Kollaritsch H, Holst H, Grobara P, Wiedermann G. Prevention of traveler's diarrhea with Saccharomyces boulardii: results of a placebo-controlled double blind study (in German). Fortschr Med 1993;111:152–6.

57. Hilton E, Kolakowski P, Singer C, Smith M. Efficacy of Lactobacillus GG as diarrheal preventive in travelers. J Trav Med 1997;4:41–3.

58. Katelaris PH, Salam I, Farthing MJ. Lactobacilli to prevent travelers diarrhea? NEJM 1995;333:1360–1.

59. Briand V, Buffet P, Genty S, et al. Absence of efficacy of nonviable Lactobacillus acidophilus for the prevention of traveler's diarrhea: a randomized, double-blind, controlled study. Clin Infect Dis 2006;43:1170–5.

60. Steffen R, Castelli F, Dieter Nothdurft H, et al. Vaccination against enterotoxigenic Escherichia coli, a cause of travelers' diarrhea. J Travel Med 2005;12:102–7.

61. McKenzie R, Bourgeois AL, Engstrom F, et al. Comparative safety and immunogenicity of two attenuated enterotoxigenic Escherichia coli vaccine strains in healthy adults. Infect Immun 2006;74:994–1000.

Chapter 22

Natural Immunity with Exposure

Robin McKenzie, MD

John D. Clemens, MD

The agents that cause travelers' diarrhea are prevalent in food and water in less developed countries. Travelers with little or no natural immunity frequently become ill when they encounter these pathogens. Adults from endemic areas, on the other hand, have life-long exposure to these agents and often do not become ill when infected. Similar to travelers, young children in developing countries are immunologically susceptible to the organisms that cause travelers' diarrhea. Among children under the age of 5 years, diarrhea is the second-leading cause of death, second only to acute respiratory infections. Diarrhea causes more than two million deaths each year in children under the age of 5.[1]

Understanding natural immunity is important for developing vaccines and other forms of immunotherapy. For diarrheal illness, the economic impetus for vaccine development is often prevention of travelers' diarrhea, but a very important benefit is advancement in vaccine development for the young, very vulnerable persons who bear the massive burden of these infections.

Decreasing Rates of Diarrheal Disease with Age in Endemic Countries

In developing countries, diarrhea rates are highest in very young children and drop off sharply as children age. In a review of community-based studies, Black reported an estimated incidence of diarrheal episodes in Africa of 7 episodes per child per year under the age of 2 years and 3 episodes per year from ages 2 to 4 years. Corresponding annual rates for children less than 2 years old and children 2 to 4 years old were 6 and 2 episodes in Latin America, respectively, and 5 and 2 episodes in Asia, respectively.[2]

It is assumed that these decreasing rates of diarrheal illness are partly due to acquired immunity. Likewise, travelers may develop natural immunity over time.

Decreasing Rates of Diarrhea with Increasing Duration of Stay in Endemic Areas

Several studies have tested the hypothesis that long-term residence in endemic areas is associated with lower rates of diarrhea. International congregations of scientists and physicians are fortuitous events for diarrhea studies and specifically for comparisons of rates of diarrhea in visitors from developed countries with rates in participants from less developed countries. At the International Conference of Tropical Medicine and Malaria in Teheran in 1968, visitors from the US and northern Europe had a diarrheal attack rate of 36%, but travelers from less developed countries had an attack rate of 8%, and Iranians had only a 2% attack rate.[3] Similar findings were demonstrated at a conference in Mexico City, where 54% of US citizens had gastrointestinal illness compared to 15% of those from South America and the Far East.[4] However, the hypothesis was not supported by a study of 64 Panamanian tourists visiting Mexico, of whom 34% developed diarrhea. In this instance, the higher economic status of the Panamanians may have shielded them from extensive exposure to enteric pathogens in their native country.[5]

Among travelers to endemic areas, protection from diarrhea appears to develop over time. For over 30 years DuPont and colleagues have studied American students in Mexico. During a 1-month prospective study at the Universidad de las Americas in Cholula, Puebla, Mexico, 22 of 55 newly arrived US students (40%) developed diarrhea compared to 28 of 142 US students (20%) who had been there for 1 year or longer.[6] The rate of diarrhea in US students was higher than the rate of students from Mexico (7 of 66, 11%) and Venezuela (4 of 29, 14%) attending the same university.[6] This study implies that the US students developed some immunity from diarrhea while living in an endemic area for 1 year or longer; however, their rate of diarrhea remained higher that that of the Latin American students, who presumably acquired immunity to endemic enteric pathogens during a lifetime of exposure.

Other studies have examined the influence of visiting or residing in endemic areas on the risk of developing diarrhea. Steffen and colleagues administered questionnaires to over 73,000 travelers leaving developing countries.[7] In this large retrospective survey of generally short-term travelers, decreased rates of diarrhea were associated with previous travel to a tropical country within the preceding 6 months.[7] A prospective study of 35 Peace Corps workers in Thailand did not show a lower attack rate among the 18 volunteers with previous travel to tropical countries (67% attack rate) versus the 17 without previous travel (47% attack rate), nor was there a decrease in the attack rate during the 5 weeks of the study.[8]

These epidemiologic studies differ considerably as to the countries visited, the pathogens prevalent in these countries, and the conditions of exposure to these pathogens. Even so, the collective data suggest that immunity to the agents that cause travelers' diarrhea develops with exposure over time. Because there are numerous species and serotypes of pathogens, long-term exposure and perhaps periodic natural boosting may be important for maintenance of immune protection from the majority of these agents.

Natural Immunity to Enterotoxigenic *Escherichia coli*

Enterotoxigenic *Escherichia coli* (ETEC) are the most common bacterial cause of diarrhea in children in less developed countries, and they are the most common cause of travelers' diarrhea. In both of these groups asymptomatic carriage of toxigenic strains is frequent.

Understanding which immunogens elicit protective immune responses is crucial for vaccine development. Because there are numerous O serogroups associated with the cell wall lipopolysaccharides and H serogroups of the flagella, natural immunity to these components would require exposure to a wide number of strains. Other more conserved factors appear to be important, especially the colonization factor antigens (CFAs), which are mainly fibrillar and fimbrial proteins that mediate attachment to the small bowel wall, and the enterotoxins, heat-labile toxin (LT) and heat-stable toxin (ST). While LT is very immunogenic, ST is a nonantigenic peptide of only 18 or 19 amino acids.

The concept of naturally acquired immunity to ETEC is supported by epidemiologic studies in long-term visitors to endemic areas. In the study in Cholula, Mexico described above, ETEC was frequently isolated from US students with and without diarrhea. In newly arrived US students, 38% developed diarrhea associated with LT+ ETEC, and 13% had asymptomatic colonization with LT+ strains. Among long-term US students, 23% had diarrhea associated with LT+ ETEC, and 19% were asymptomatically colonized. In addition, ST-only strains were isolated from 8% of US students with diarrhea and 3% of those without diarrhea. In contrast, 1 of 12 ill Mexican students and 2 of 6 ill Venezuelan students, but none of 27 asymptomatic Latin American students, had isolation of LT+ ETEC from their stools.[9] In this study, ETEC infections in the US students did not become less frequent with increased stay, but they tended to become less symptomatic. In a more recent study,[10] 40 US students were enrolled within 3 days of their arrival in Guadalajara, Mexico, and followed for 4 weeks. During the first week 5% had ETEC-associated diarrhea and 7.5% had asymptomatic colonization; during week two 12.5% had ETEC illness and 11% were asymptomatically colonized; for week three 5% were ill with ETEC and none were asymptomatically colonized; and during the fourth week, no ETEC was found in stools. The 9 diarrhea-associated isolates in this study comprised 6 ST+ strains, 2 LT+ strains, and one ST+/LT+. The 7 isolates from asymptomatic subjects were 2 ST+ and 5 LT+ strains.[10]

Results from these two studies show a decrease in the incidence of ETEC illness with time spent in an endemic area. While acquired immunity may play a role, other factors such as acquired knowledge about safer eating may also be important. Because the strains in these early studies were not characterized by identification of their CFAs, we do not know whether initial infections with one strain protected against symptomatic infections with strains homologous for specific CFAs, LT, or other antigens.

In endemic areas, the incidence of ETEC illness is the greatest in children less than 2 years old and drops off sharply above the age of 5.[2] Several prospective longitudinal studies conducted among children in less developed countries examined the role of LT and CFA immunity in protecting against ETEC infection and diarrheal disease. Asymptomatic carriage of ETEC strains complicates these analyses. In a 3-year study, 397 Egyptian children under the age of 36 months were followed with semiweekly home visits. Stool specimens were collected when children had loose stools, and blood was collected every 3 months. For children under the age of 18 months, serum IgG antibody against CFA/I correlated with protection from diarrhea associated with CFA/I strains. On the other hand, serum IgG antibody against LT did not correlate with protection against diarrhea associated with LT-only strains.[11] In this setting, however, LT-only ETEC strains, most of which lacked a CFA, did not appear to be pathogenic.[12] In addition, serum IgG may not reflect mucosal immunity, which may be more important for protection against a noninvasive enteric pathogen such as ETEC. While this study suggests a protective role for CFA immunity, it does not rule out protection from LT immunity, especially in other settings. Another longitudinal study was conducted in Guinea-Bissau. Two hundred neonates were followed until the age of 2 with weekly stool cultures to see if an initial infection would protect against subsequent infection with strains homologous for CFAs or LT. Of the 11,000 stool specimens collected and analyzed for ETEC, 90% were from well children and 10% were diarrheal samples. Approximately 1,000 of the stool specimens contained ETEC, and 452 of these were positive for 1 of the 18 CFAs studied. Of the CFA-positive ETEC infections, 428 were primary infections of which 64 were symptomatic, and 24 were post-primary infections of which only 2 were symptomatic. Results showed that ETEC infections provided protection against new infections with ETEC of the same toxin and CFA profile. CFAs did not appear to contribute to this protection against infection. There were too few symptomatic post-primary infections to determine whether CFAs protected against symptomatic infection. Among the approximately 1,000 ETEC infections, 757 were LT+ ETEC infections; 21 of 163 LT+ primary infections (13%) were symptomatic, and 59 of 594 post-primary LT+ infections (10%) were symptomatic. Similar to infection with CFA+ strains, LT exposure provided no protection against subsequent infection with LT+ strains. However, LT+ infection did confer 45% protection against subsequent symptomatic LT+ infections.[13] While the results of this latter study support a role for LT immunity in protection against ETEC illness, the data are inadequate to determine whether CFA immunity protects against ETEC diarrhea.

In adults, studies with two vaccines suggest that LT and possible CFA immunity may be protective. An inactivated whole cell cholera vaccine containing the B subunit of cholera toxin, which cross-reacts with LT, protected travelers and Bangladeshi adults from LT-associated diarrhea.[14,15] A killed, whole-cell ETEC vaccine containing representative CFAs and the B subunit of cholera toxin protected travelers from moderate to severe ETEC illness, but not from mild diarrhea.[16,17] As more vaccines are tested in challenge studies and field trials, the immunologic correlates of protection will be better defined.

Natural Immunity to Enteroaggregative *E. coli*

Enteroaggregative *Escherichia coli* (EAEC), which produce a distinctive aggregative adherence pattern on HEp-2 cells, were identified as the second most common cause of travelers' diarrhea in several regions.[18] EAEC also cause chronic diarrhea in children and patients with acquired immune deficiency syndrome (AIDS).[19] Similar to ETEC, EAEC are associated with diarrheal illness and asymptomatic colonization.[20] In a study mentioned above, 40 US students who attended summer school in Guadalajara were followed for 4 weeks. During the first 2 weeks, 13 subjects were asymptomatically colonized and 14 others had EAEC-associated diarrhea (5 of the symptomatic subjects had mixed EAEC/ETEC infections and 1 had EAEC/*Salmonella* infection). During the next 2 weeks, 31 subjects were asymptomatically infected and 4 had EAEC infection with diarrhea (one was coinfected with ETEC). Plasmid deoxyribonucleic acid (DNA) analysis showed little relationship among the 60 EAEC isolates. The increase in colonization and decrease in illness suggests that immunity to disease, but not infection, may have developed.[10]

Natural Immunity to *Shigella*

Shigella are second to *Escherichia coli* (ETEC and EAEC) in frequency as causes of travelers' diarrhea. More importantly, each year in resource-poor areas, *Shigella* species cause illness in over 150 million individuals and death in over one million; 670,000 of these deaths are in children under the age of 5.[21] Rotavirus and Shigella are the most common causes of infant mortality from diarrheal illness. A recent survey of six Asian countries showed a decrease in Shigellosis after age 5 with an increase after age 40. This age distribution may be caused by the large variety of *Shigella* strains and the steady replacement of strains to which a person may be exposed.[22]

There are more than 45 O antigen serotypes and subtypes. Immunity appears to be serotype-specific; however, serologic cross-reactivity suggests that a smaller number of clinically significant strains could be represented in a vaccine.[23] In addition, *Shigella* species have virulence plasmids that encode outer membrane proteins (invasion plasmid antigens, Ipa). Among 390 Chilean children, there was an age-associated acquisition of antibodies to both lipopolysaccharide and Ipa.[24]

For children under the age of 3 years, breast-feeding protected against severe shigellosis.[25] The decrease in *Shigella*-associated illness after age 5 is likely due to naturally acquired immunity. In institutionalized children attack rates were higher for newly admitted children than for children residing there.[26]

Several studies conducted by Cohen and colleagues have prospectively followed Israeli soldiers naturally exposed during outbreaks of shigellosis.[27] These studies suggest that preexisting IgG antibodies to LPS are associated with group-specific protection,[27] but other unidentified factors also appear to be important.[28]

Natural Immunity to *Campylobacter*

Even though *Campylobacter* species are the most frequent cause of diarrhea in the US, the annual incidence of 40 to 70 cases per 100,000 persons is three logs lower than the rate of 40,000 per 100,000 among children in less developed countries.[29–32] It is surprising, therefore, that *Campylobacter* illness has received much less attention than other causes of diarrhea in developing countries. This lack of attention is due to the perception that *Campylobacter* species in less developed countries do not cause illness after the first 6 months of life. Multiple studies have shown decreasing rates of *Campylobacter*-associated diarrhea with increasing age. For instance, in a longitudinal study of 397 Egyptian children, annual rates dropped from 1.2 to 0.4 to 0.2 episodes per child for years one, two, and three of life. Of 366 episodes of diarrhea, 13% were associated with severe dehydration and 4% with bloody diarrhea.[32] Initial infections protected against diarrhea associated with subsequent infections except in infants less than 6 months old. This observation correlates with the poor serologic responses to natural infection of children under the age of 6 months in Thailand.[33]

In less developed countries, asymptomatic excretion is common among children above the age of 6 months.[34] Furthermore, the number of organisms per gram of stool and the duration of fecal excretion decrease with age.[33,35] IgA antibodies against *Campylobacter* are found in breast milk[36] and appear to be protective.[37] The antibody response to acute infection is highest in children 6 to 12 months.[33] As baseline antibodies increase with age, the rate of symptomatic infection falls.[38]

Similar to children in endemic areas, travelers may be protected by baseline immunity. Among military personnel deployed to Thailand, *Campylobacter* species have been the leading cause of diarrhea. In one study, symptomatic infection occurred in 17% of nonimmune versus 4% of immune persons.[39]

Conclusions

Children in less developed countries are severely affected by the most common causes of travelers' diarrhea. For many of these agents there is evidence of naturally acquired immunity, increasing hope that vaccines will be developed that will prevent diarrhea in travelers and lower mortality and morbidity among children in the countries visited by these travelers.

References

1. World Health Organization. Food safety and foodborne illness. Fact Sheet #237. January, 2002.
2. Black RE. Epidemiology of diarrhoeal disease: implications for control by vaccines. Vaccine 1993;11:100–6.
3. Kean BH. Turista in Teheran. Travellers' diarrhoea at the Eighth International Congresses of Tropical Medicine and Malaria. Lancet 1969;2:583–4.
4. Loewenstein MS, Balows A, Gangarosa EJ. Turista at an international congress in Mexico. Lancet 1973;1:529–31.
5. Ryder RW, Oquist CA, Greenberg H, et al. Travelers' diarrhea in Panamanian tourists in Mexico. J Infect Dis 1981;144:442–8.
6. DuPont HL, Haynes GA, Pickering LK, et al. Diarrhea of travelers to Mexico. Relative susceptibility of United States and Latin American students attending a Mexican University. Am J Epidemiol 1977;105:37–41.
7. Steffen R, Tornieporth N, Clemens SA, et al. Epidemiology of travelers' diarrhea: details of a global survey. J Travel Med 2004;11:231–7.
8. Echeverria P, Blacklow NR, Sanford LB, Cukor GG. Travelers' diarrhea among American Peace Corps volunteers in rural Thailand. J Infect Dis 1981;143:767–71.
9. DuPont HL, Olarte J, Evans DG, et al. Comparative susceptibility of Latin American and United States students to enteric pathogens. N Engl J Med 1976;295:1520–1.
10. Adachi JA, Ericsson CD, Jiang ZD, et al. Natural history of enteroaggregative and enterotoxigenic Escherichia coli infection among US travelers to Guadalajara, Mexico. J Infect Dis 2002;185:1681–3.
11. Rao MR, Wierzba TF, Savarino SJ, et al. Serologic correlates of protection against enterotoxigenic Escherichia coli diarrhea. J Infect Dis 2005;191:562–70.
12. Clemens J, Savarino S, Abu-Elyazeed R, et al. Development of pathogenicity-driven definitions of outcomes for a field trial of a killed oral vaccine against enterotoxigenic

Escherichia coli in Egypt: application of an evidence-based method. J Infect Dis 2004;189:2299–307.

13. Steinsland H, Valentiner-Branth P, Gjessing HK, et al. Protection from natural infections with enterotoxigenic Escherichia coli: longitudinal study. Lancet 2003;362:286–91.
14. Clemens JD, Sack DA, Harris JR, et al. Cross-protection by B subunit-whole cell cholera vaccine against diarrhea associated with heat-labile toxin-producing enterotoxigenic Escherichia coli: results of a large-scale field trial. J Infect Dis 1988;158:372–7.
15. Peltola H, Siitonen A, Kyronseppa H, et al. Prevention of travellers' diarrhoea by oral B-subunit/whole-cell cholera vaccine. Lancet 1991;338:1285–9.
16. Sack DA. Safety and efficacy of a killed oral vaccine for enterotoxigenic *E. coli* diarrhea in adult travelers to Guatemala and Mexico. 42nd ICAAC; 2002 Sept 27–30; San Diego, CA; 2002.
17. Bourgeois AL, Halpern J, Gustafsson B. 45th Annual ICACC; 2005 Dec 16 –19; Washington DC; 2005.
18. Adachi JA, Jiang ZD, Mathewson JJ, et al. Enteroaggregative Escherichia coli as a major etiologic agent in traveler's diarrhea in 3 regions of the world. Clin Infect Dis 2001;32:1706–9.
19. Mathewson JJ, Jiang ZD, Zumla A, et al. HEp-2 cell-adherent Escherichia coli in patients with human immunodeficiency virus-associated diarrhea. J Infect Dis 1995; 171:1636–9.
20. Okeke IN, Lamikanra A, Czeczulin J, et al. Heterogeneous virulence of enteroaggregative Escherichia coli strains isolated from children in Southwest Nigeria. J Infect Dis 2000;181:252–60.
21. Kotloff KL, Winickoff JP, Ivanoff B, et al. Global burden of Shigella infections: implications for vaccine development and implementation of control strategies. Bull W H O 1999;77:651–67.
22. von Seidlein L, Kim DR, Ali M, et al. A multicentre study of Shigella diarrhoea in six Asian countries: disease burden, clinical manifestations, and microbiology. PLoS Med 2006; 3:e353.
23. Noriega FR, Liao FM, Maneval DR, et al. Strategy for cross-protection among Shigella flexneri serotypes. Infect Immun 1999;67:782–8.
24. Van de Verg LL, Herrington DA, Boslego J, et al. Age-specific prevalence of serum antibodies to the invasion plasmid and lipopolysaccharide antigens of Shigella species in Chilean and North American populations. J Infect Dis 1992;166:158–61.
25. Clemens JD, Stanton B, Stoll B, et al. Breast feeding as a determinant of severity in shigellosis. Evidence for protection throughout the first three years of life in Bangladeshi children. Am J Epidemiol 1986;123:710–20.
26. DuPont HL, Gangarosa EJ, Reller LB, et al. Shigellosis in custodial institutions. Am J Epidemiol 1970;92:172–9.
27. Cohen D, Green MS, Block C, et al. Serum antibodies to lipopolysaccharide and natural immunity to shigellosis in an Israeli military population. J Infect Dis 1988;157:1068–71.
28. Cohen D, Green MS, Block C, et al. Natural immunity to shigellosis in two groups with different previous risks of exposure to Shigella is only partly expressed by serum antibodies to lipopolysaccharide. J Infect Dis 1992;165: 785–7.
29. Foodborne Diseases Active Surveillance Network. Morb Mortal Wkly Rep 1997;46:258–61.
30. Preliminary FoodNet data on the incidence of foodborne illnesses-selected sites, United States. Morb Mortal Wkly Rep 2002;51:325–9.
31. Coker AO, Isokpehi RD, Thomas BN, et al. Human campylobacteriosis in developing countries. Emerg Infect Dis 2002;8:237–44.
32. Rao MR, Naficy AB, Savarino SJ, et al. Pathogenicity and convalescent excretion of Campylobacter in rural Egyptian children. Am J Epidemiol 2001;154:166–73.
33. Taylor DN, Perlman DM, Echeverria PD, et al. Campylobacter immunity and quantitative excretion rates in Thai children. J Infect Dis 1993;168:754–8.
34. Calva JJ, Ruiz-Palacios GM, Lopez-Vidal AB, et al. Cohort study of intestinal infection with campylobacter in Mexican children. Lancet 1988;1:503–6.
35. Taylor DN, Echeverria P, Pitarangsi C, et al. Influence of strain characteristics and immunity on the epidemiology of Campylobacter infections in Thailand. J Clin Microbiol 1988;26:863–8.
36. Torres O, Cruz JR. Protection against Campylobacter diarrhea: role of milk IgA antibodies against bacterial surface antigens. Acta Paediatr 1993;82:835–8.
37. Ruiz-Palacios GM, Calva JJ, Pickering LK, et al. Protection of breast-fed infants against Campylobacter diarrhea by antibodies in human milk. J Pediatr 1990;116:707–13.
38. Martin PM, Mathiot J, Ipero J, et al. Immune response to Campylobacter jejuni and Campylobacter coli in a cohort of children from birth to 2 years of age. Infect Immun 1989;57:2542–6.
39. Walz SE, Baqar S, Beecham HJ, et al. Pre-exposure anti-Campylobacter jejuni immunoglobulin a levels associated with reduced risk of Campylobacter diarrhea in adults traveling to Thailand. Am J Trop Med Hyg 2001;65:652–6.

CHAPTER 23

IMMUNOPROPHYLAXIS AND IMMUNOLOGIC CONTROL

MYRON M. LEVINE, MD, DTPH

ANN-MARI SVENNERHOLM, MD, PhD

When individuals from industrialized countries travel to less developed regions of the world, acute diarrhea is a common affliction that befalls them.[1] In general, the less developed the locale, the greater the chance of developing travelers' diarrhea and the risk is also generally increased in warm and wet seasons. Beginning in the late 1960s and continuing to the present time, an array of microorganisms have been incriminated as causative agents of travelers' diarrhea. Among the many bacterial pathogens incriminated, enterotoxigenic *Escherichia coli* (ETEC),[2–5] enteroaggregative *Escherichia coli (*EAggEC), and *Shigella* have been repeatedly incriminated in many geographic regions,[5–9] particularly in warm season (Table 1). In certain areas like Southeast Asia, *Campylobacter jejuni* has been shown to be an important warm season pathogen.[10] ETEC, the single most common cause of adult travelers' diarrhea in most studies, generally causes a moderate clinical illness that interferes with daily activity, although in occasional cases overt dehydration can ensue. Whereas overall *Shigella* is less common than diarrheagenic *E. coli,* it is capable of causing full blown bacillary dysentery, a more severe clinical form of diarrheal illness characterized by high fever, discomforting abdominal cramps, and overt blood in stools.[11] Another bacterial pathogen that uncommonly causes travelers' diarrhea but that is capable of causing copious watery diarrhea culminating in dehydration even in adults is *Vibrio cholerae* of serogroups O1 or O139 (see Table 1).[12,13] At a lesser frequency, three parasites have been incriminated as causes of travelers' diarrhea including *Giardia intestinalis, Cryptosporidium,* and *Entameba hisolytica* (see Table 1).[4,14] Of the many viruses associated with gastroenteritis, the noroviruses are the ones most often indicted as travelers' diarrhea pathogens.[15] In infant and young child travelers, rotavirus is an important etiologic agent that causes gastroenteritis (see Table 1).

Typhoid fever (caused by *Salmonella enterica* serovar Typhi) and paratyphoid fever (caused by *Salmonella enterica* serovar Paratyphi A and Paratyphi B), while representing clinical syndromes distinct from travelers' diarrhea, nevertheless manifest diarrhea in 20 to 40% of cases early in the course of illness. Enteric fevers are mentioned because the licensed oral (Ty21a) and parenteral (Vi polysaccharide) typhoid vaccines represent a paradigm for prevention of enteric pathogens,[16] because these organisms gain access to deeper tissues by targeting and entry through gut-associated lymphoid tissue.

The relative proportion of travelers' diarrhea that is attributable to this range of agents varies by geographic site, season, age, and local level of development (ie, quality of water supply, mechanisms for disposal of

Table 1 Prioritization of Vaccines for Prevention of Travelers' Diarrhea

Highest priority
Enterotoxigenic *E. coli*
Shigella
Rotavirus (for pediatric travelers)
Intermediate priority
Vibrio cholerae 01
Enteroaggregative *E. coli*
Campylobacter jejuni
Norovirus
Low priority
Cryptosporidium
Entameba histolytica
Giardia intestinalis
Vibrio cholerae 0139

E. = *Escherichia.*

human waste, adequacy of refrigeration for food preservation, and personal and food hygiene practices). It is evident that immunoprophylaxis of travelers' diarrhea (whether passively by oral administration of immunoglobulins or actively by vaccines) will require products active against several specific pathogens and multiple antigenic types or serotypes of certain pathogens. In the ensuing pages we review the few licensed vaccines that exist to prevent diarrhea caused by specific enteric pathogens and discuss progress made in development of vaccine candidates against many of the above-cited pathogens. We will emphasize vaccine candidates that are in clinical trials or for which clinical trials are imminent.

Vaccines against Enterotoxigenic *E. coli*

BACKGROUND

There are two fundamental steps in the pathogenesis by which ETEC causes diarrhea in humans or animals, namely: 1) attachment by fimbriae (protein adhesins) to specific receptors on enterocytes in the proximal small intestine (thereby overriding the powerful peristaltic defense that would otherwise remove the ETEC to the large intestine), followed by; 2) production of heat-stable (ST) or heat-labile (LT) enterotoxins that result in net intestinal secretion.[17–19] It is presumed that the main immunologic protection against ETEC diarrhea is mediated by secretory IgA (SIgA) antibodies that bind fimbrial antigens, thereby preventing attachment in the proximal small intestine. For some LT-producing ETEC strains, neutralizing anti-LT can also provide protection by preventing intestinal secretion.

Current dogma supposes that in order to provide broad-spectrum protection against ETEC, a vaccine will have to contain fimbrial antigens expressed by the most prevalent ETEC pathogens (Table 2). The most common fimbrial colonization factor antigens (CFAs) of human ETEC are colonization factor antigen I (CFA/I) and the adhesins found within the CFA/II and CFA/IV families of antigens.[20,21] Whereas CFA/I is a single antigenic moiety, coli surface antigen 1 (CS1), CS2, and CS3 collectively constitute the CFA/II "family" of fimbrial antigens; all CFA/II strains express CS3 fibrillae, either alone or in conjunction with CS1 or CS2. Similarly, CS4, CS5, and CS6 constitute the CFA/IV "family" and all CFA/IV strains express CS6, either alone or in conjunction with CS4 or CS5. Various other fimbrial antigens that are putative attachment factors for human intestinal cells, such as CS7, CS12, CS14, and CS17, are less frequent. The expression of CFAs by ETEC correlates with the O:H serotype and toxin phenotype.[20,21]

It has been shown that a substantial proportion of ETEC isolates from various studies of travelers' diarrhea in diverse geographic settings and from studies of endemic (mostly pediatric) diarrhea in developing countries express CFA/I and CS1-6. Approximately 60 to 90% of isolates that elaborate both LT and ST enterotoxins express these CFAs, whereas they are found on circa 40 to 70% of ST-only strains.[19,22–24] In striking contrast, only a small proportion of LT-only strains bear these CFAs.[19,24,25] Thus, if a multivalent ETEC vaccine contained CFA/I and CS1-6, it could theoretically protect against the majority of ETEC strains in most geographic areas (see Table 2). If an LT-derived immunogen is incorporated into the vaccine, it should be possible to achieve even broader protection. Finally, in the future, some of the less frequent fimbrial antigens such as CS7 and CS17 might be included in multivalent vaccines to augment the breadth of coverage.[19,26]

Several hallmark observations established the feasibility of immunoprophylaxis against ETEC and point the way for the type of vaccines that might be practical and effective. In an experimental challenge model of ETEC diarrhea in adult volunteers, Levine and colleagues demonstrated that an initial clinical diarrheal infection caused by a fimbriated LT/ST ETEC strain conferred ~ 80% protection against clinical illness upon subsequent rechallenge with the homologous ETEC strain.[27] In a proof-of-principle study, Levine and colleagues showed that immunization with a single 5×10^{10} colony forming unit (CFU) dose of a fimbriated ETEC strain (serotype O6:H16 expressing CS1 and CS3 fimbria) that had lost

Table 2 Epidemiologically Important Antigenic Types or Serotypes That an ETEC Vaccine and A *Shigella* Vaccine, Respectively, Will Need to Provide Broad Spectrum Protection

Enterotoxigenic *Escherichia coli*
Strains producing: LTh B subunit, colonization factor antigen I (CFA/I), coli surface antigens 1–6
Shigella
S. dysenteriae 1, all 14 classic *S. flexneri* serotypes and subtypes, *S. sonnei*

(Note: These 16 serotypes are the most important out of the total 45 classic types and subtypes of *Shigella*).

the genes encoding LT and ST conferred upon volunteers 75% protection against challenge with a heterologous ETEC serotype (O139:H28) expressing CS1 and CS3 fimbria and LT and ST.[17,28] Tacket and colleagues demonstrated that passive oral administration of cow milk-derived immunoglobulin from cows hyper immunized with a variety of fimbriated ETEC strains and LT conferred upon adult volunteers 90% protection against challenge with ETEC strain H10407 (serotype O78:H11) that expresses CFA/I fimbriae and LT and ST.[29] Finally, in a randomized controlled clinical trial in adult Finnish travelers going to Morocco, Peltola and colleagues showed that immunization with two doses of cholera toxin B-subunit/killed whole-cell cholera vaccine conferred 52% protection against ETEC diarrhea.[30] The assumption is that neutralizing SIgA antibodies stimulated by the cholera B subunit cross-neutralized LT, resulting in a moderate level of protection. Another randomized, double-blind, placebo-controlled trial of a two-dose regimen of cholera toxin B-subunit/killed whole-cell oral cholera vaccine was conducted in 502 US college students who went to study in Mexico.[31] Two doses (10 days apart) of vaccine or placebo were given immediately after arrival in Mexico. Rises in serum cholera antitoxin were demonstrated in 87% of vaccinees versus 8% of controls ($p < .001$). Vaccine efficacy against ETEC diarrhea was 50% (95% confidence interval, 14 to 71%), beginning 7 days after the second dose. However, three-quarters of the ETEC diarrhea cases occurred within 7 days of the second dose, when no efficacy was demonstrated. It is possible that administration of that vaccine prior to travel, rather than upon arrival, might have afforded greater overall protection.[31]

Collectively, the above-mentioned data demonstrate that stimulation of immune responses against ETEC fimbrial colonization factors and LT can significantly protect humans against ETEC diarrhea. These observations provide a rational basis for the expectation that efficacious ETEC vaccines can be developed to protect travelers from ETEC diarrhea.

Licensed Vaccines

Presently the only licensed vaccine that has an indication for prevention of (LT-producing) ETEC diarrhea is the oral inactivated cholera vaccine Dukoral (Table 3). Through its cholera toxin B-subunit component that confers cross protection against LT-producing ETEC, it is licensed in Canada and a number of other countries for protecting travelers against LT-producing ETEC, as well as against cholera. In European Union countries and Australia, Dukoral is licensed solely for the prevention of cholera.

Vaccines under Development

Inactivated Fimbriated ETEC Administered Orally in Combination with B Subunit of Cholera Toxin

The ETEC vaccine candidate that has had the most extensive testing in phase 1, 2, and 3 clinical trials consists of a mix of 1.0 mg of recombinant cholera toxin B subunit and $\sim 2 \times 10^{10}$ formalin-inactivated bacteria of ETEC strains SBL 101 (O78:H12, CFA/I, ST); SBL 104 (O25:H42, CS4); SBL 105 (O167:H5, CS5); SBL 106 (O6:H16, CS1); and SBL 107 (O rough:H6, CS2, CS3) (see Table 3).[22,23,32] Formalin treatment killed the ETEC without significant loss in antigenicity of the different colonization factors (CFs). Phase 1 and 2 trials of this CF-ETEC-rBS vaccine in Swedish, Bangladeshi, American, and Egyptian volunteers showed that the vaccine is well tolerated and in the majority of subjects elicits intestinal immune responses against the CFAs contained in the vaccine.[32–40] Pediatric clinical trials to assess the safety and immunogenicity of this inactivated ETEC vaccine were carried out in Bangladeshi toddlers and preschool children and in Egyptian preschool children (age 12 months to 5 years) who received two doses of vaccine or placebo (inactivated *E. coli* K-12) with 2 weeks between doses. There was no significant difference in the occurrence of adverse responses in vaccines versus controls, and the vaccine stimulated immune responses to B subunit and to vaccine CFAs in the majority of children. In Bangladeshi infants age 6 to 12 months, one-third of a full dose was well tolerated and immunogenic.[41] The safety and immunogenicity of this vaccine have also been documented in adult travelers.

There have been several controlled field trials undertaken to assess the efficacy of the CF-ETEC-rBS vaccine to prevent ETEC diarrhea in adults traveling from industrialized countries to developing countries in Latin America, Africa, and Asia. There has also been one trial that tested the efficacy of the vaccine in preventing endemic ETEC diarrhea in Egyptian children 6 to 18 months of age. Three vaccine efficacy trials, including one pilot study involving European travelers going to various developing countries, another involving European travelers going to Kenya, and a third in Israeli soldiers on training bases in areas where ETEC was prevalent, were unable to provide clear conclusions per protocol because an insufficient number of endpoint cases ensued.[42] However, the pilot study did show encouraging results by demonstrating 82% efficacy against ETEC diarrhea; regrettably, the number of cases fulfilling the study primary endpoint was low.[42,43] A placebo-controlled trial that enrolled ~ 700 US travelers going to Mexico and Guatemala did not show protection

Table 3 Licensed Vaccines (and Passive Immunoglobulin Preparations) against Forms of Travelers' Diarrhea and Candidates in Active Clinical Development

Type of Vaccine	Route of Immunization	Number of Doses	Name(s) of Licensed Product and Manufacturer	Developer of Experimental Vaccine
Cholera				
B subunit- inactivated whole vibrio combination	Oral	2	Dukoral, SBL (a Crucell Company)	
CVD 103-HgR recombinant live vaccine	Oral	1	Orochol, Mutacol, Berna Biotech (a Crucell Company)	
Enterotoxigenic *E. coli* *				
B subunit- inactivated whole vibrio combination +	Oral	2	Dukoral, SBL (a Crucell Company)	
B subunit- inactivated whole fimbriated ETEC combination	Oral	2		University of Goteborg and SBL (a Crucell Company)
Attenuated fimbriated non-toxigenic *E. coli* (derived from ETEC)	Oral	2 doses		Cambridge Biostability Ltd.
Attenuated *Shigella* strains expressing ETEC fimbrial colonization factors and LTh B subunit	Oral	2 doses		Center for Vaccine Development, University of Maryland School of Medicine
LTh alone or in combination with purified fimbrial colonization factors	Transcutaneous	2 doses		IOMAI Corporation
Shigella				
Attenuated *S. flexneri* 2a strain SC602	Oral	1–2 doses		Pasteur Institute, Paris
Attenuated *S. flexneri* 2a strain CVD 1208S	Oral	2 doses		Center for Vaccine Development, University of Maryland School of Medicine
Attenuated *S. sonnei* strain WRSS1	Oral	2 doses		Walter Reed Army Institute of Research
Attenuated *S. dysenteriae* 1 strain SC599	Oral	2 doses		Pasteur Institute, Paris
Shigella glycoconjugates (O polysaccharide covalently linked to carrier protein)	Intramuscular	2 doses		National Institute of Child Health and Human Development
Immunoglobulin preparation for passive prophylaxis against ETEC	Oral	1 caplet before every meal	Travelan, Anadis Ltd.	

*For brevity, several vaccine candidates that were tested in Phase 1 clinical trials but that do not appear to be in an active product development program are not listed

+ Cholera B subunit, which stimulates antitoxin that cross neutralizes LT of ETEC, provides short-term protection against LT-producing ETEC strains.

CVD = Center for Vaccine Development; *E.* = *Escherichia;* ETEC = enterotoxigenic *Escherichia coli*; *S.* = *Shigella.*

overall against ETEC diarrhea but did show 77% efficacy against more severe forms of ETEC diarrhea.[42,44] The ETEC-rBS did not protect Egyptian toddlers against ETEC diarrhea.[23,42,45] Based on the disappointing results from the pediatric efficacy trial in Egypt, work is in progress to try to improve vaccine efficacy by increasing the amounts of the CFs on the vaccine strains.

Live, Fimbriated, Nontoxigenic "ETEC" Administered Orally

A multivalent live oral ETEC vaccine under development is based on the administration of a mixture of fimbriated ETEC strains from which the genes encoding LT and ST are absent and other putative attenuating mutations have been introduced (see Table 3).[46–48] Three constructs clinically tested so far have not contained genes encoding the expression of LT B subunit or a mutant LTh to stimulate LT antitoxin, although such further modifications are planned. Strains PTL002 and PTL003 are further derivatives of strain E1392-75-2A, the O6:H16 prototype CFA/II vaccine strain that had spontaneously lost genes encoding LT and ST but retained genes for expression of CS1 and CS3 and had been shown in the 1980s to stimulate anti-CFA/II and to confer significant protection against experimental challenge with ETEC strain E24377A (O139:H28, LT/ST, CS1,CS3).[28] Both strains harbor a mutation in *aroC*; PTL002 has an additional mutation in *ompR*, while PTL003 has mutations in *ompC* and *ompF*.[46] In a Phase 1 clinical trial, both strains were well tolerated but significantly more recipients of PTL003 exhibited fecal shedding and mounted more robust serum antibody and IgA antibody secreting cell (ASC) responses to CFA/II.[46,49]

An initial experimental challenge study with virulent ETEC was carried out in North American volunteers immunized with two 2×10^9 CFU doses of PTL003 vaccine or placebo to assess preliminarily the ability of the strain to protect against ETEC diarrhea.[49] Subjects were challenged with 3×10^9 CFU of virulent LT/ST strain E24377A. Neither the attack rate for diarrhea nor total stool volume was significantly diminished in vaccines versus placebo recipients. It was hypothesized that the reason for the lack of protection compared to the positive results reported by Levine and colleagues[28] using the parent E1392-75-2A vaccine strain may have been the fact PTL003 was given at a 10-fold lower dose and a six-fold higher dose of challenge organisms. On the other hand, the parent E1392-75-2A prototype vaccine strain protected following administration of just a single dose.[28]

ACAM2010 is a similar vaccine candidate strain derived from wild type WS-1858B (O71:H$^-$, LT-/ST+, CFA/I, *astA*) by deleting STh (encoded by *estA*), EAST1 (EAggEC enterotoxin 1 encoded by *astA*), *aroC*, *ompC* and *ompF*.[48] In a small Phase 1 clinical trial, ACAM2010 was well tolerated and most recipients of a 10^9 CFU dose excreted the vaccine strain and had serum IgG and IgA ASC responses to CFA/I.[48]

Attenuated Shigella *Live Vector Strains Expressing ETEC Fimbrial Antigens and LTh B Subunit*

An ambitious public sector vaccine development project has been underway for several years in which five attenuated *Shigella* serotypes (*S. dysenteriae* 1, *S. flexneri* 2a, *S. flexneri* 3a, *S. flexneri* 6 and *S. sonnei*) have each been engineered to carry stable expression plasmids that encode various ETEC fimbriae and LTh B subunit (see Table 3). The five *Shigella* live vector strains in the final vaccine will collectively express CFA/I, CS1-6, and LTh B subunit.[50–54] Combinations of several attenuated *Shigella* strains expressing various ETEC fimbriae and LTh B subunit or a mutant LT (K63) have been shown in preclinical models (guinea pigs and Rhesus macaque nonhuman primates) to be well tolerated and to stimulate systemic immunoglobulin G (IgG) and mucosal immunoglobulin A (IgA) immune responses to both the ETEC and *Shigella* antigens.[50–54] In a preclinical model, the responses to the different fimbrial antigens are as robust when the strains are administered in combination as when they are administered as individual vaccines.[50,51] One of the five live vector strains, attenuated *Shigella flexneri* 2a strain CVD 1208S expressing CFA/I and LTh B subunit is currently under evaluation as a prototype in dose-escalating Phase 1 clinical trials to assess the live vector's clinical acceptability and immunogenicity in humans.

Purified ETEC Fimbriae and LT Administered by Transcutaneous Immunization

The skin is a highly active immunologic organ in which induction of immune responses can be initiated if antigens can penetrate the keratinized layer to reach the subepidermal region where Langerhans cells (a dendritic cell) are in abundance. Methods of penetrating the keratinized layer barrier include hydration,[55] electroporation, abrasives, and microneedles.[56] Proof-of-principle clinical trials were carried out in which adult North American volunteers received patches containing recombinant CS6 with LT or patches containing CS6 alone.[57] Three doses were given at 0, 1, and 3 months and serum antibodies and ASC responses were measured. The importance of the adjuvant effect of LT was clear, as there was no response to CS6 in the absence of LT.[57]

Since cholera toxin B subunit/whole cell cholera vaccine has been shown to confer ~ 50% protection for a few months against diarrhea caused by LT-producing ETEC in indigenous persons living in endemic developing countries and in travelers,[30,58] a group of 59 North American volunteers were randomized to be immunized transcutaneously with 50 μg of LT or placebo on days 0, 21 and 42. On day 56, 27 vaccinees and 20 controls were challenged with 6×10^8 CFU of wild type ETEC strain E24377A (O139:H28, LT/ST, CS1,CS3).[59] All vaccines had significant rises in serum IgG anti-LT. Following challenge, the attack rate for diarrhea was not significantly diminished in the vaccinees versus controls, but the vaccinees had a significantly longer time to onset of diarrhea, significantly fewer and smaller stools, and significantly fewer vaccinees needed for intravenous rehydration.[59] Collectively, these results demonstrate a biological effect of transcutaneous immunization with LT (see Table 3).

A randomized, controlled Phase 2 trial to assess the clinical acceptability, immunogenicity, and preliminary efficacy of two doses of LT administered via skin patch is underway among adult travelers to Central America (see Table 3). Notably, the two doses of vaccine are administered approximately 1 month before subjects commence their travel.

Some Other Prototype ETEC Vaccine Candidates Evaluated in Proof-of-Principle Clinical Trials

A number of nonliving and live oral vaccine prototypes have been evaluated for safety and immunogenicity in

Phase 1 clinical trials in recent years. These include transgenic plants (potato and corn) expressing LT B subunit,[60] attenuated *Salmonella* Typhi expressing LT B subunit, and polylactide/polyglycolide microspheres containing purified CS1 and CS3 fimbriae.[61] It is unclear if any of these is progressing to industrial product development.

Vaccines against *Shigella*

BACKGROUND

Because *Shigella* is an important pathogen incriminated in many studies of traveler's diarrhea and often causes clinically severe forms, including dysentery, protection against shigellosis is considered a high priority. However, a daunting problem to be overcome in *Shigella* vaccine development is achieving a practical strategy to confer broad spectrum protection because there are four species (*S. dysenteriae*, *S. flexneri*, *S. boydii*, and *S. sonnei*) and 49 classical serotypes and subtypes. *Shigella sonnei* (a single serotype) and *S. flexneri* (14 serotypes and subtypes) are the most common *Shigella* associated with traveler's diarrhea (see Table 2).[5] Nonhuman primate studies have convincingly shown that infection-derived immunity is species-specific and in many instances is likely to be serotype-specific.[62]

Licensed Vaccines

Presently there are no licensed vaccines to prevent shigellosis.

Vaccines under Development

Two generic types of *Shigella* vaccines, attenuated strains (employed as live oral vaccines) and parenteral conjugate vaccines (consisting of O polysaccharides covalently linked to carrier proteins) have provided proof that they can confer protection in randomized controlled field trials of efficacy. These vaccines are furthest along in development.

Streptomycin-Dependent and T32 Pioneer *Shigella* Vaccine Strains

In the 1960s and early 1970s, Mel and colleagues developed streptomycin-dependent (SmD) mutants of *Shigella* that were shown to be well tolerated and protective in randomized, controlled field trials.[63–70] Moreover, by administering combinations of attenuated SmD strains of several different *Shigella* serotypes, Mel and colleagues paved the way for future multivalent vaccines that might confer broad spectrum protection. However, these pioneering SmD vaccine strains suffered from some notable drawbacks that kept them from becoming licensed vaccines for widespread use. The drawbacks included an unknown (at the time) basis for attenuation, difficulty of large-scale manufacture and process control, and occasional lots that exhibited reversion to streptomycin independence (although the organisms remained attenuated and unable to invade epithelial cells).

During the same period as Mel's work, Istrati in Romania developed *S. flexneri* 2a vaccine strain T32, which was shown to be well tolerated; moreover, preliminary field use in nonrandomized trials suggested that the vaccine was efficacious.[71,72] Two decades later, in controlled field trials in China, Bingrui and colleagues demonstrated that T32 conferred significant protection against *S. flexneri* 2a disease.[73] Meanwhile, investigators at the Walter Reed Army Institute of Research (WRAIR) reported that the invasiveness plasmid in the T32 strain had a large deletion resulting in loss of three loci, (*ipaBCDA*, *invA* and *virG*) that crippled its ability to invade epithelial cells and resulted in attenuation.[74]

Building on Mel's pioneering observations, several different groups worldwide have applied recombinant deoxyribonucleic acid (DNA) technology and knowledge of molecular pathogenesis of shigellosis to create modern live oral *Shigella* vaccine candidates. For example, several different approaches have been taken to attenuate wild type *S. flexneri* 2a strain 2457T (shown to be virulent in volunteers),[75] resulting in live oral vaccine candidates that are well tolerated and immunogenic.

S. flexneri 2a Strain SC602

S. flexneri 2a strain SC602 harbors a deletion in *icsA* (also called *virG*), an invasiveness plasmid gene that encodes a protein involved in intracellular and intercellular spread of *Shigella*. SC602 also has a deletion in chromosomal *iuc* that encodes the iron sequestering protein aerobactin (see Table 3); this mutation diminishes virulence of *Shigella* in rabbit ileal loops.

In an initial dose response study, North American volunteers ingested 10^2, 10^4, 10^5, 10^6, 10^7, or 10^8 CFU of SC602.[76] At the highest dosage level (10^8 CFU), 2 of 3 subjects developed diarrhea, fever, abdominal cramps, and malaise.[76] An expanded dose selection trial was then undertaken wherein a dose of 10^6 CFU of SC602 was administered to 15 adult subjects, of whom 47% developed diarrhea, 33% fever, and 40% severe constitutional symptoms within 48 hours of vaccine ingestion.[76] Because of the substantial reactogenicity encountered at 10^6 CFU, another trial was carried out in which 12 volunteers were given 10^4 CFU of SC602. At the 10^4 CFU dosage level, none of the subjects developed fever, severe constitutional symptoms, or severe intestinal symptoms, and only one subject developed mild diarrhea;[76] 92% of the volunteers shed the vaccine organism.[76] Notably, the onset of fecal shedding was delayed in recipients of 10^4 CFU (72 h) compared to subjects who received 10^6 CFU (22 h). Significant IgA antibody secreting cell responses (ASC) to *S. flexneri* 2a O antigen were exhibited by 7 of the 12 recipients (58%) of 10^4 CFU and 4 of 12 (33%) developed seroconversions ($\geq$ four-fold) of serum IgG O antibody.

Eight weeks after ingesting the single 10^4 CFU dose of SC602, seven of the subjects participated in an experimental challenge study and ingested 10^3 CFU of fully virulent *S. flexneri* 2a strain 2457T, along with seven unvaccinated control subjects.[76] The challenge strain was excreted by 86% of both controls, and vaccinees and diarrhea was observed in 86% of controls and 43% of vaccinees.[76] However, the three vaccinees that developed diarrhea had significantly milder illness than the controls. For example, four of the seven controls (57%) developed dysentery, six had (86%) fever (mean temperature 102.7°F), and six (86%) manifested severe shigellosis; in contrast no vaccine had dysentery, fever, or severe illness.[76]

Two additional studies of SC602 were carried out in North American adults, including an inpatient study and a community study.[77] In the inpatient study, three volunteers ingested 10^3 CFU and nine ingested 10^4 CFU. One of nine who received 10^4 CFU developed fever and two manifested mild diarrhea.[77]

In the study in ambulatory community volunteers, 34 subjects ingested a single 10^4 CFU dose of SC602.[77] Five of 34 (15%) experienced fever, four of which occurred within 24 hours. Five subjects (15%) also experienced mild diarrhea that typically lasted for just 1 day. All but one subject excreted the vaccine strain, beginning on day 1 and continued to excrete for a mean of 11.6 days. One-half of the volunteers manifested a significant rise in serum IgA antibody to *S. flexneri* 2a O antigen. In summary, of 58 North American subjects who ingested 10^4 CFU of SC602 in the course of Phase 1 and 2 trials, 90% excreted the vaccine strain for at least 7 days and 19% manifested fever or diarrhea as adverse reactions.

Studies of SC602 were undertaken in adults and children in Bangladesh.[78] In an initial inpatient study, SC602 was well tolerated at dosage levels of 10^4, 10^5, and 10^6 CFU. In contrast with the prominent excretion of SC602 by North Americans, only a few Bangladeshis who received 10^6 CFU sporadically shed the vaccine strain. A trial was then carried out in 68 ambulatory Bangladeshi adults who similarly ingested 10^4, 10^5, and 10^6 CFU. No adverse reactions were recorded, nor did any vaccine excrete SC602 and immune responses were meager.

Descending in age, children 8 to 10 years of age were given doses of 10^4, 10^5, or 10^6 CFU, followed by children 12 to 36 months of age who were administered doses containing 10^3, 10^4, 10^5, or 10^6 CFU.[78] No child manifested adverse reactions nor did any child shed the vaccine strain or mount a significant immune response. Thus, subjects in a developing country manifested strikingly different clinical, bacteriologic, and immunologic responses to the SC602 vaccine strain compared to North Americans. Whereas in the Americans, SC602 in a low dose (10^4 CFU) was reactogenic in ~ 19% of the vaccinees, heavily excreted and moderately immunogenic, in the Bangladeshis it was virtually inert even in a 100-fold higher dose.[78]

S. flexneri 2a Vaccine Candidate Strains CVD 1203, CVD 1207, CVD 1208, and CVD 1208S Derived from Wild Type Strain 2457T

Prototype *S. flexneri* strain CVD 1203 harbors a deletion in *aroA* encoding an enzyme in the aromatic amino acid biosynthesis pathway that renders it nutritionally dependent on a substrate (para-aminobenzoic acid) that is insufficiently available in mammalian tissues to support extensive multiplication.[79] CVD 1203 also has a deletion in *virG*, thereby interfering with intracellular and intercellular spread.[79] In a Phase 1 clinical trial, North American adults were fed a single 10^6 CFU dose (N=10) or two doses of 10^8 CFU (N=11) or a dose of 10^9 CFU followed by a dose of 10^8 CFU (N=11), 14 days apart.[80] Whereas the 10^6 CFU dosage level was well tolerated, 18% of recipients of 10^8 CFU and 72% of subjects who ingested 10^9 CFU manifested adverse reactions (fever, diarrhea, or dysentery).[80] Ninety-one percent of vaccinees excreted the vaccine strain and 95% of the recipients of the two higher dosage levels developed strong responses of IgA ASC that recognize *S. flexneri* 2a O antigen. While the potent immune responses were encouraging, the reactogenicity dictated that alternative mutations should be evaluated to achieve a satisfactory degree of attenuation.

Strain CVD 1207 harbors a mutation in *guaBA* encoding enzymes involved in guanine nucleotide synthesis. In preclinical models, mutations in *guaBA* were more attenuating than mutations in *aroA*. CVD 1207 also has a deletion in *virG* that interferes with intra- and intercellular spread of *Shigella* and mutations in chromosomal *set* and plasmid *sen*, which respectively encode *Shigella* enterotoxins 1 and 2 (ShET1 and 2). ShET 2 is produced by all serotypes of *Shigella*,[81] while ShET1 production is limited almost exclusively to strains of *S. flexneri* 2a subtype.[82–84] These enterotoxins are believed to be responsible for the early watery diarrhea phase of shigellosis and to contribute to the diarrheal reactogenicity seen with certain live vaccine strains tested over the years.

Volunteers ingested single doses of 10^6, 10^7, 10^8, 10^9, or 10^{10} CFU of CVD 1207.[85] This live vaccine strain was remarkably well tolerated, as no subjects manifested adverse reactions through the 10^8 CFU dosage level.[85] Even at very high dosage levels of 10^9 and 10^{10} CFU, only one of 12 volunteers who ingested 10^9 and one of six who received 10^{10} CFU experienced mild diarrhea.[85] At dosage levels of 10^7, 10^8, 10^9, and 10^{10} CFU, 100%, 67%, 64%, and 100% of the vaccinees, respectively, exhibited significant IgA anti-O antigen ASC responses. The conclusion from the Phase 1 clinical trial of CVD 1207 was that the set of mutations in this strain may have resulted in hyper-attenuation.

CVD 1204 and CVD 1208 are isogenic derivatives of wild type strain 2457T that both carry deletions in *guaBA*.[86,87] However, in addition, CVD 1208 has deletions in *sen* and *set*. A randomized, double-blind clinical trial was carried out in which adult North American volunteers were given a single dose containing 10^7, 10^8, or 10^9 CFU of either CVD 1204 or CVD 1208.[87] This design allowed an assessment of the usefulness of inactivating the genes encoding ShET 1 and 2. Objective adverse reactions were observed in 8 of 23 recipients of CVD 1204 but in only 1 of 23 recipients of CVD 1208 ($p = .02$).[87] Immune responses to *S. flexneri* 2a O antigen (ASC, serum IgG, or fecal IgA) were seen in 86%, 43%, and 100% of recipients of CVD 1208. CVD 1208 was considered a highly attractive vaccine candidate that reflected the desired balance of clinical acceptability and good immunogenicity.

Because CVD 1208 had been constructed using culture media containing animal products, for regulatory purposes the strain was reconstructed using soy-based media, resulting in strain CVD 1208S (see Table 3). In a Phase 1 clinical trial, CVD 1208S exhibited the same clinical acceptability, excretion pattern, and immunogenicity as CVD 1208. Like CVD 1208, strain CVD 1208S has the characteristics of an ideal attenuated *Shigella* vaccine candidate, exhibiting an attractive balance of low reactogenicity and good immunogenicity. As such, it will constitute one of the five attenuated *Shigella* strains that comprise the CVD pentavalent *Shigella* vaccine and that serve as live vectors in the CVD multivalent *Shigella*/ETEC live vector combination vaccine.[26,51,88]

Shigella sonnei Vaccine Strain WRSS1

Investigators at WRAIR constructed vaccine strain WRSS1 by making a deletion in *virG* in the wild type Moseley strain.[89] In a Phase 1 trial in North American volunteers given a 10^3, 10^4, 10^5, or 10^6 CFU dose, the vaccine was well tolerated overall except that low-grade fever or mild diarrhea recorded in 6 of 27 vaccinees (22%).[90] IgA anti-LPS ASC responses were strong at all dosage levels.[90]

Safety/immunogenicity trials were next performed in ambulatory community adults in Israel who ingested 10^3, 10^4, or 10^5 CFU of WRSS1.[91] At the two lower dosage levels the vaccine was well tolerated with the exception of one of 30 subjects who developed moderate diarrhea and five who complained of mild diarrhea. In contrast, at the 10^5 CFU dosage level, 2 of 15 subjects developed fever and four experienced moderate diarrhea.[91] The 10^4 CFU dosage level provided the best balance of immunogenicity and clinical acceptability as all subjects manifested IgA anti-O antigen ASC responses and 73% of the vaccinees showed more than 50 IgA anti-O ASC/10^6 PBMC. WRSS1 colonized the vaccinees for a median of 5 days (and one individual excreted for 23 days).[91]

S. dysenteriae 1 Strain SC599

S. dysenteriae 1 candidate vaccine strain SC599 was engineered at the Pasteur Institute by making deletions in *icsA* (*virG*), *ent*, *fep*, and *stxA* (the gene encoding the enzymatically active A subunit of Shiga toxin).[78] In a Phase 1 trial in 28 British adults, groups of volunteers received 10^2, 10^3, 10^4, 10^5, 10^6, or 10^7 CFU under conditions of physical containment. The vaccine was well tolerated and no subjects developed fever or diarrhea.[78] Excretion of the vaccine was minimal, even at the highest dosage level, as only three of the 28 vaccinees had positive coprocultures and excretion persisted for only a single day. Only a limited proportion of subjects who ingested a dose of 10^5 CFU or higher exhibited modest ASC responses to *S. dysenteriae* 1 O antigen.

Salmonella enterica Typhi Strain Ty21a Expressing *Shigella* O Antigens

In the 1980s, Formal and colleagues at WRAIR developed a vaccine candidate consisting of licensed oral *Salmonella* Typhi live vaccine strain Ty21a engineered to express the O polysaccharide of *S. sonnei*. This live vector strain, 5076-1C, was very well tolerated but was highly variable in its immunogenicity and ability to protect in volunteer challenge studies where vaccinees and controls ingested wild type *S. sonnei* strain 53G.[92–94] The *S. sonnei* O polysaccharide was not firmly bound to the *S.* Typhi bacteria and it was subsequently hypothesized that this may have accounted for the variability in immune responses to different lots of vaccine.[95] Further development of 5076-1C was abandoned.

More recently, Kopecko and coworkers have succeeded in more reliably expressing the *S. sonnei* O antigen in Ty21a, as well as in expressing O polysaccharides of other important serotypes.[96] *Salmonella* has a LPS core that is chemically distinct from *Shigella*.[96] As a consequence, *S. sonnei* O polysaccharide in *S.* Typhi is expressed only as a non-core-linked surface-associated antigen.[96] These investigators are preparing a series of Ty21a-based live vector strains expressing *Shigella* O antigens.

Shigella/ETEC Live Vector

Investigators at the Center for Vaccine Development of the University of Maryland have prepared a multivalent *Shigella* vaccine that contains five attenuated strains of serotypes *S. dysenteriae* 1, *S. sonnei*, *S. flexneri* 2a, *S. flexneri* 3a, and *S. flexneri* 6.[26,51] *S. dysenteriae* 1 is included because that serotype causes epidemics and pandemics of severe Shiga dysentery and most strains of this serotype carry R factors encoding resistance to the majority of clinically useful antibiotics. *S. sonnei* is the single most important serotype causing traveler's shigellosis and remains a cause of pediatric diarrhea in certain subpopulations in industrialized countries, such as children attending day care. Finally, the *S. flexneri* serotypes collectively constitute the main *Shigella* associated with endemic disease in children in developing countries.[97] Epidemiologically, a global *Shigella* vaccine requires that protection be provided against all 14 *S. flexneri* serotypes and subtypes.[97] The *Shigella* vaccine development researchers at the Center for Vaccine Development include *S. flexneri* 2a, *S. flexneri* 3a, and *S. flexneri* 6 in their multivalent vaccine because these three serotypes have O antigen epitopes that are shared by the remaining 11 *S. flexneri* serotypes and subtypes.[88] They have demonstrated in an animal model that a multivalent vaccine containing serotypes *S. flexneri* 2a and *S. flexneri* 3a provides an impressive level of cross protection against other *S. flexneri* serotypes that share the common O epitopes.[88]

All five of the *Shigella* strains in the CVD multivalent vaccine harbor a deletion mutation in chromosomal *guaBA*,[86] and a deletion in *sen*, the plasmid gene that encodes *Shigella* enterotoxin 2 (ShET2).[81] In addition, the *S. flexneri* 2a strain (CVD 1208S) carries a deletion in *set*,[82–84] the chromosomal gene encoding ShET1, while the *S. dysenteriae* 1 strain is deleted of chromosomal *stxA*, which encodes the enzymatically active A subunit of Shiga toxin.[98] Each of these five attenuated *Shigella* strains carries a stable expression plasmid that encodes fimbrial colonization factors of ETEC or the B subunit of LTh;[50–54,99] collectively, the *Shigella* strains express CFA/I, CS1-6, and B subunit of LTh. A strong appeal of this multivalent *Shigella*-ETEC live vector vaccine is the potential for a single oral combination vaccine to protect against two of the most important pathogens associated with traveler's diarrhea and that cause endemic pediatric diarrhea in developing countries.

Shigella Conjugate Vaccines

Investigators at the National Institute of Child Health and Human Development, USA are developing a parenteral conjugate vaccine consisting of O polysaccharides derived from the LPS of relevant *Shigella* serotypes that are then each covalently linked to a carrier protein (*Pseudomona aeruginosa* exotoxin A) (see Table 3). Protection in this instance is hypothesized to be mediated by serum IgG, which is assumed to transude onto the surface of intestinal mucosa, thereby inactivating ingested *Shigella* early on before the bacteria have a chance to proliferate, interact with target cells of the intestinal mucosa (M cells, enterocytes and colonocytes), and initiate the pathogenesis of shigellosis.[100] A parenteral prototype vaccine consisting of *S. sonnei* O polysaccharide conjugated to *P. aeruginosa* exotoxin A was shown to be well tolerated and highly immunogenic in stimulating serum IgG O antibodies in young Israeli soldiers.[101,102] In a small, randomized, controlled, double blind Phase 3 efficacy trial involving several hundred Israeli soldiers, a single dose of the *S. sonnei* conjugate vaccine conferred 74% protection during an outbreak of *S. sonnei* diarrhea at an army base.[102]

Phase 2 trials assessed the clinical acceptability and immunogenicity of *S. sonnei* and *S. flexneri* 2a conjugate vaccines in Israeli children 4 to 7 years of age.[103] In these pediatric studies, a two-dose immunization schedule was used with doses spaced six weeks apart. The first injection of each vaccine stimulated a significant rise in homologous serum IgG antibodies. The second injection stimulated a booster response in the *S. flexneri* 2a vaccine recipients but not in those that got *S. sonnei* vaccine. By extrapolation, a Phase 3 trial of *S. sonnei* conjugate vaccine underway in pediatric subjects in Israel can hopefully address two important questions of relevance for protecting adult travelers. The questions include whether parenteral conjugate *Shigella* vaccines can elicit protection in immunologically naive subjects and whether protection will endure for many months.

Vaccines against EAggEC

EAggEC, a category of diarrheagenic *E. coli* characterized by strains that exhibit aggregated stacked brick attachment to Hep-2 cells, has come to be recognized as an important cause of traveler's diarrhea,[6,104,105] as well as a common cause of persistent diarrhea in children in developing countries and a common bacterial cause of acute pediatric diarrhea in industrialized countries.[106,107] The pathogenesis of diarrhea caused by EAggEC, which causes distinctive histopathological lesions evident in human intestinal specimens and in gnotobiotic piglets,[108] is being elucidated.[109] Most EAggEC strains express the fimbrial adhesins AAF/I, AAF/II, or AAF/III and elaborate enterotoxins, including either enteroaggregative *E. coli* heat-stable enterotoxin 1 (EAST) (which is also produced by some other pathovars of diarrheagenic *E. coli*) or plasmid encoded toxin (PET, found exclusively in EAggEC). These antigens are considered potential components of an EAggEC vaccine.

Vaccines against *Campylobacter jejuni*

In the 1990s, investigators at the Naval Medical Research Institute, USA developed a candidate oral vaccine against *C. jejuni* based on a combination of inactivated bacterial cells coadministered with mucosal adjuvant.[110] However, when the association between *C. jejuni* diarrheal infection and Guillain-Barré ascending paralysis came to be recognized based on mimicry between *C. jejuni* LPS epitopes and gangliosides,[111,112] safety concerns prudently led to abandonment of this approach. A more recent genomic approach based on the identification of common surface proteins as potential antigens has revived interest in *C. jejuni* vaccines.[113,114]

Vaccines against Cholera

BACKGROUND

The importance of cholera vaccines for travelers waxes and wanes in relation to increases or decreases in incidence and spread of cholera in the developing world. Nevertheless, certain geographic areas that remain highly endemic pose a risk for some categories of travelers, such as individuals with known risk factors. These include travelers with hypochlorhydria or those taking medication for peptic ulcer disease. It also includes individuals with cardiac disease for whom the fluid and electrolyte losses associated with severe forms of cholera can lead to arrythmias. In addition, it is prudent for travelers who expect to be many hours away from access to health care for days at a time to avail themselves of cholera vaccine. Should cholera gravis occur, severe dehydration culminating in hypovolemic shock, renal shutdown, and death can ensue within 8 hours of onset of diarrhea.

Although epidemic cholera caused by *V. cholerae* serogroup O139 appeared in South and Southeast Asia in the early 1990s, this serogroup is currently of only minor importance and has not become a problem in Africa. Accordingly, the currently licensed cholera vaccines only aim to confer protection against *V. cholerae* serogroup O1, the major cholera serogroup.

Licensed Vaccines

Two oral cholera vaccines are licensed in many countries (albeit not yet in the USA), including Dukoral, a nonliving antigen vaccine, and Orochol, an engineered attenuated strain (see Table 3).

Dukoral

The current commercial formulation of Dukoral contains $\sim 10^{11}$ heat-inactivated and formalin-inactivated *V. cholerae* O1, including a mix of classical and El Tor biotypes and Inaba and Ogawa serotypes, in combination with 1.0 mg of recombinant B subunit.[115] The vaccine is well tolerated by adults and children when administered as a two-dose immunization regimen, 10 to 14 days apart and is safe in young children (including infants as young as age 6 months), immunocompromised hosts, and human immunodeficiency virus (HIV)-positive subjects.[116–119] Whereas four-fold or greater rises in serum vibriocidal antibody in recipients of the commercial formulation are infrequent both in adults from industrialized countries and developing countries,[118,120] > 80% of subjects mount strong serum antitoxin responses.[118,120]

A three-dose regimen of a prototype B subunit-whole cell vaccine (that included B subunit purified from cholera toxin rather than produced by recombinant method) showed 85% efficacy in preventing cholera over 6 months in a large-scale field trial in Bangladesh and 50% efficacy over 3 years.[121,122] A post-hoc analysis of recipients of two doses of vaccine suggested that a two-dose regimen was also protective.[122]

The efficacy of a two-dose regimen (2 weeks apart) of the commercial Dukoral formulation derives from results of a randomized, double-blind, controlled trial in young adult Peruvian soldiers (710 vaccines, 714 placebo controls). During a 5-month follow-up, a high degree of protection (86% protective efficacy) against epidemic cholera was recorded in the course of exposure to a common source vehicle of transmission shortly after vaccination that resulted in a high rate of disease among placebo recipients.[116]

Dukoral, which is manufactured by SBL Vaccin AB, a Crucell Company located in Stockholm, Sweden, is licensed in more than 50 countries including the European Community, Canada, Australia, and different countries Latin America (see Table 3). The vaccine is given in a glass of water together with a bicarbonate buffer in two doses, 2 weeks apart; a booster dose is recommended after 1 or 2 years.

Orochol

Engineered single-dose recombinant live oral cholera vaccine CVD 103-HgR was derived from wild type *Vibrio cholerae* O1 classical Inaba strain 569B by deleting 94% of the gene encoding the enzymatically active (ADP ribosylating) A subunit of cholera toxin (leaving B subunit expression intact) and inserting a gene encoding resistance to mercury ions into the hemolysin A locus. CVD 103-HgR is licensed in a number of countries in Europe, Asia, and Australia and was available under the trade name Orochol; in Canada it is licensed under the name Mutacol (see Table 3). For a period of 2 years (2005 and 2006), supplies of CVD 103-HgR, manufactured by Berna Biotech, a Crucell Company, were exhausted and further manufacturing awaited completion of plant modifications. It is expected that CVD 103-HgR will be once again available in 2008.

The safety and immunogenicity of single-dose CVD 103-HgR oral vaccine has been documented in thousands of subjects as young as 3 months of age and as old as 65 years of age, including HIV+ subjects, through many randomized, placebo-controlled, double-blind clinical trials in Asia, Latin America, Africa, Europe, and North America.[123–133] The ability of CVD 103-HgR to protect against cholera caused by either biotype or serotype has been demonstrated in 10 experimental cholera challenge studies in adult North American volunteers. These clinical trials show that a single dose of CVD 103-HgR conferred on adult North American volunteers significant protection against experimental challenge with pathogenic *V. cholerae* O1 of either biotype or serotype.[134–137] Moreover, almost complete protection (> 95%) was conferred against moderate and severe diarrhea (total purge ≥ 3.0 liters) caused by either El Tor or classical biotype. In these experimental challenge studies, protection was evident as early as 8 days after vaccination and endured for at least 6 months (the shortest and longest intervals tested).[135,136] The single-dose efficacy and rapid onset of protection are attractive characteristics of CVD 103-HgR.

The formulation of CVD 103-HgR consists of two sachets, one containing lyophilized vaccine and the other buffer powder. The formulation for travelers, Orochol, contains ~ 10^8 CFU, while the formulation for populations in developing countries, Orochol E, contains ~ 10^9 CFU. A notable feature of vaccination with CVD 103-HgR is that high rates of seroconversion (> 90%) of vibriocidal antibody are recorded in groups of vaccinees who show low rates (~25%) of excretion of the vaccine strain.

Vaccines under Development

Peru 15

An attenuated El Tor Inaba strain, Peru 15, is being developed by Avant Immunotherapeutics. This strain has a deletion of the entire cholera toxin core element (that includes other virulence properties) and flanking segments *att*RS1 sequences that preclude reacquisition of the core element by site specific recombination. The *ctxB* gene that encodes the B subunit of cholera toxin was introduced into *recA*, which inactivates that locus making the strain unable to integrate exogenous DNA.[138,139] Peru 15 also manifests diminished motility.[139] Administered as a single oral dose containing 10^8 CFU to healthy adult North Americans, the vaccine was well tolerated and 98% showed a four-fold or greater rise in serum vibriocidal antibody.[140] Three months after vaccination, 24 vaccinees and 12 controls participated in an experimental challenge study. The vaccine provided 100% protection against moderate or severe cholera (total purge of ≥ 3.0 liters) (5 of 12 controls versus 0 of 24 vaccinees) and 93% protection against any severity of cholera.[140]

El Tor Ogawa Strain 638

Investigators at the Finlay Institute, Havana, Cuba have constructed an attenuated El Tor Ogawa vaccine strain by deleting the CTX/Phi prophage from a wild type parent and by inserting the gene encoding endoglucanase A of *Clostridium thermocellum* into the hemagglutinin/protease coding sequence of the vibrio. This oral vaccine was well tolerated and stimulated vibriocidal responses in 96% of the vaccinees.[141] In an experimental challenge study, 12 vaccinees (who received a single 10^9 CFU oral dose) and 9 placebo recipients 1 month later ingested 7 $\times 10^5$ CFU of virulent *V. cholerae* El Tor Ogawa (strain 3008). Seven of 12 controls but none of 12 vaccinees developed diarrhea; 2 controls manifested severe cholera (> 5.0 liters of diarrheal stool).[141]

Vaccines against Rotavirus

Rotavirus poses a risk for infants and toddlers everywhere in the world. Because rotavirus gastroenteritis can be severe and lead to dehydration, it is important that infant and young child travelers be protected by immunization with one of the new rotavirus vaccines. This is particularly critical if the pediatric subjects will be far from health care. A pentavalent rotavirus vaccine manufactured by Merck Vaccines (Rotateq) consisting of bovine rotavirus reassortants expressing the major human rotavirus G and P antigens is licensed in the USA and in many other countries. A monovalent human attenuated rotavirus strain (Rotarix) manufactured by GSK Vaccines is licensed in various countries in Europe, Latin America, and Asia. In large-scale, randomized, placebo-controlled safety and efficacy studies in infants, these vaccines proved to be well tolerated and highly protective.[142,143] Most importantly, these large safety studies demonstrated that the new vaccines were not associated with intussusception, a rare but serious adverse reaction that was triggered by immunization with an earlier tetravalent rhesus reassortant rotavirus vaccine.[144]

Vaccines against Norovirus

A candidate oral vaccine consisting of virus-like particles of Norwalk virus, a norovirus, was evaluated in Phase 1 clinical trials.[145,146] In two trials the vaccine was well tolerated and highly immunogenic.

Norwalk virus capsid protein expressed by transgenic by transgenic potatoes was also evaluated in a Phase 1 clinical trial.[146] The transgenic plant norovirus vaccine was well tolerated and 95% of subjects manifested immune responses to norovirus, albeit modest in magnitude.

Vaccines against *Entameba histolytica*

The amebic Gal/GalNAc lectin mediates adherence of *E. histolytica* to the mucosa of the colon and fecal anti-lectin IgA appears to protect against intestinal re-infection in children.[147,148] Miller-Sims and Petri and Houpt and colleagues showed that immunization with the *E. histolytica* native Gal/GalNAc lectin purified from the parasite or with a 64 kDa recombinant fragment ("LecA") can prevent cecal infection in a mouse model of amebic colitis.[147,148] It is not clear if this vaccine candidate will be further developed and will move into clinical trials.

Vaccines against *Cryptosporidium*

Elucidation of the full sequence of the genomes of *Cryptosporidium hominis* and *C. parvum* has led to the identification of several protein antigens that may serve as immunogens to elicit antibodies that can be used for passive prophylaxis or for use of the antigens to provide active immunity against cryptosporidiosis.[149,150]

Oral Immune Globulin Concentrates as Passive Protection against ETEC

The pioneering study of Tacket and colleagues demonstrated that volunteers could be protected against a potent challenge with wild type ETEC that caused diarrhea in 90% of control subjects by prior ingestion of milk immunoglobulin concentrate derived from cows hyperimmunized with ETEC expressing a variety of fimbrial and O antigens, LT, and cholera toxin.[29]

Anadis Ltd., an Australian Company, produces Travelan caplets containing cow immunoglobulin with ETEC antibodies (see Table 3). In an experimental challenge study carried out in Poland, Travelan prophylaxis conferred upon volunteers 91% protection compared to placebo controls when challenged with virulent ETEC.

Oral Immune Globulin Concentrates as Passive Protection against *Shigella*

Tacket and colleagues showed that bovine immunoglobulin concentrates that contained high titers of antibody directed against the O antigen of *S. flexneri* could protect volunteers against experimental challenge with *S. flexneri* 2a.[151]

Reference List

1. Steffen R, Tornieporth N, Clemens SA, et al. Epidemiology of travelers' diarrhea: details of a global survey. J Travel Med 2004;11:231–7.
2. Black RE. Pathogens that cause travelers' diarrhea in Latin America and Africa. Rev Infect Dis 1986;8S:S131–5.
3. Taylor DN, Echeverria P. Etiology and epidemiology of travelers' diarrhea in Asia. Rev Infect Dis 1986;8S:S136–41.
4. Black RE. Epidemiology of travelers' diarrhea and relative importance of various pathogens. Rev Infect Dis 1990; 12Suppl 1:S73–9.
5. Hyams KC, Bourgeois AL, Merrell BR, et al. Diarrheal disease during Operation Desert Shield. N Engl J Med 1991;325:1423–8.
6. Adachi JA, Jiang ZD, Mathewson JJ, et al. Enteroaggregative *Escherichia coli* as a Major Etiologic Agent in Traveler's Diarrhea in 3 Regions of the World. Clin Infect Dis 2001;32:1706–9.
7. Steffen R, Collard F, Tornieporth N, et al. Epidemiology, etiology, and impact of traveler's diarrhea in Jamaica. JAMA 1999;281:811–7.
8. Jiang ZD, Lowe B, Verenkar MP, et al. Prevalence of enteric pathogens among international travelers with diarrhea acquired in Kenya (Mombasa), India (Goa), or Jamaica (Montego Bay). J Infect Dis 2002;185:497–502.
9. Gascon J, Vargas M, Quinto L, et al. Enteroaggregative *Escherichia coli* strains as a cause of traveler's diarrhea: a case-control study. J Infect Dis 1998;177:1409–12.
10. Sanders JW, Isenbarger DW, Walz SE, et al. An observational clinic-based study of diarrheal illness in deployed United States military personnel in Thailand:

presentation and outcome of Campylobacter infection. Am J Trop Med Hyg 2002;67:533–8.

11. Levine MM. Bacillary dysentery: mechanisms and treatment. Med Clin North Am 1982;66:623–38.
12. Abrutyn E, Gangarosa E, Forrest J, et al. Cholera in a vaccinated American. Immunological response to vaccination and disease. Ann Intern Med 1971;74:228–31.
13. Taylor DN, Rizzo J, Meza R, et al. Cholera among Americans living in Peru. Clin Infect Dis 1996;22:1108–9.
14. Merson MH, Morris GK, Sack DA, et al. Travelers' diarrhea in Mexico. A prospective study of physicians and family members attending a congress. N Engl J Med 1976; 294:1299–1305.
15. Ko G, Garcia C, Jiang ZD, et al. Noroviruses as a cause of traveler's diarrhea among students from the United States visiting Mexico. J Clin Microbiol 2005;43:6126–9.
16. Levine MM, Taylor DN, Ferreccio C. Typhoid vaccines come of age. Pediatr Infect Dis J 1989;8:374–81.
17. Levine MM. *Escherichia coli* that cause diarrhea: enterotoxigenic, enteropathogenic, enteroinvasive, enterohemorrhagic, and enteroadherent. J Infect Dis; 1987;155: 377–89.
18. Kaper JB, Nataro JP, Mobley HL. Pathogenic *Escherichia coli.* Nat Rev Microbiol 2004;2:123–40.
19. Qadri F, Svennerholm AM, Faruque AS, et al. Enterotoxigenic *Escherichia coli* in developing countries: epidemiology, microbiology, clinical features, treatment, and prevention. Clin Microbiol Rev 2005;18:465–83.
20. Gaastra W, Svennerholm AM. Colonization factors of human enterotoxigenic *Escherichia coli* (ETEC). Trends Microbiol 1996;4:444–52.
21. Levine MM, Giron JA, Noriega F. Fimbrial vaccines. In: Klemm P, editor. Fimbriae: adhesion, biogenics, genetics and vaccines. Boca Raton: CRC Press; 1994. p. 255–70.
22. Walker RI, Steele D, Aguado T. Analysis of strategies to successfully vaccinate infants in developing countries against enterotoxigenic *E. coli* (ETEC) disease. Vaccine 2007.
23. Svennerholm AM, Steele D. Microbial-gut interactions in health and disease. Progress in enteric vaccine development. Best Pract Res Clin Gastroenterol 2004;18:421–45.
24. Levine MM, Ferreccio C, Prado V, et al. Epidemiologic studies of *Escherichia coli* infections in a low socioeconomic level Periurban community in Santiago, Chile. Am J Epidemiol 1993;138:849–69.
25. Qadri F, Das SK, Faruque ASG, et al. Prevalence of toxin types and colonization factors in enterotoxigenic *Escherichia coli* isolated during a 2-year period from diarrheal patients in Bangladesh. J Clin Microbiol 2000;38:27–31.
26. Levine MM. Immunization against bacterial diseases of the intestine. J Pediatr Gastroenterol Nutr 2000;31:336–55.
27. Levine MM, Nalin DR, Hoover DL, et al. Immunity to enterotoxigenic *Escherichia coli.* Infect Immun 1979;23: 729–36.
28. Levine MM, Morris JG, Losonsky G, et al. Fimbriae (pili) adhesins as vaccines. In: Lark DL, Normark S, Uhlin BE, Wolf-Watz H, editors. Protein-carbohydrate interactions in biological systems, The molecular biology of microbial pathogenicity. London: Academic Press; 1986. p. 143–5.
29. Tacket CO, Losonsky G, Link H, et al. Protection by milk immunoglobulin concentrate against oral challenge with enterotoxigenic *Escherichia coli.* N Engl J Med 1988;318: 1240–3.
30. Peltola H, Siitonen A, Kyrönseppä H, et al. Prevention of travellers' diarrhoea by oral B-subunit/whole-cell cholera vaccine. Lancet 1991;338:1285–9.
31. Scerpella EG, Sanchez JL, Mathewson III, et al. Safety, immunogenicity, and protective efficacy of the whole-cell/recombinant B subunit (WC/rBS) oral cholera vaccine against travelers' diarrhea. J Travel Med 1995;2:22–7.
32. Svennerholm A-M, Savarino SJ. Oral inactivated whole cell B subunit combination vaccine against enterotoxigenic *Escherichia coli.* In: Levine MM, Kaper JB, Rappuoli R, et al, editors. New generation vaccines. New York: Marcel Dekker; 2004. p. 737–50.
33. Svennerholm A-M, Ahren C, Jertborn M. Oral inactivated vaccine against enterotoxigenic *Escherichia coli.* In: Levine MM, Woodrow GC, Kaper JB, Cobon GS, editors. New generation vaccines. New York: Marcel Dekker; 1997. p. 865–74.
34. Ahren C, Jertborn M, Svennerholm AM. Intestinal immune responses to an inactivated oral enterotoxigenic Escherichia coli vaccine and associated immunoglobulin A responses in blood. Infect Immun 1998;66:3311–6.
35. Savarino SJ, Brown FM, Hall E, et al. Safety and immunogenicity of an oral, killed enterotoxigenic *Escherichia coli*-cholera toxin B subunit vaccine in Egyptian adults. J Infect Dis 1998;177:796–9.
36. Qadri F, Wenneras C, Ahmed F, et al. Safety and immunogenicity of an oral, inactivated enterotoxigenic *Escherichia coli* plus cholera toxin B subunit vaccine in Bangladeshi adults and children. Vaccine 2000;18:2704–12.
37. Qadri F, Ahmed T, Ahmed F, et al. Safety and immunogenicity of an oral, inactivated enterotoxigenic *Escherichia coli* plus cholera toxin B subunit vaccine in Bangladeshi children 18–36 months of age. Vaccine 2003; 21:2394–403.
38. Savarino SJ, Hall ER, Bassily S, et al. Introductory evaluation of an oral, killed whole cell enterotoxigenic *Escherichia coli* plus cholera toxin B subunit vaccine in Egyptian infants. Pediatr Infect Dis J 2002;21:322–30.
39. Savarino SJ, Hall ER, Bassily S, et al. Oral, inactivated, whole cell enterotoxigenic Escherichia coli plus cholera

toxin B subunit vaccine: results of the initial evaluation in children. PRIDE Study Group. J Infect Dis 1999;179:107–14.

40. Jertborn M, Ahren C, Svennerholm AM. Dose-dependent circulating immunoglobulin A antibody-secreting cell and serum antibody responses in Swedish volunteers to an oral inactivated enterotoxigenic *Escherichia coli* vaccine. Clin Diagn Lab Immunol 2001;8:424–8.

41. Qadri F, Ahmed T, Ahmed F, et al. Reduced doses of oral killed enterotoxigenic *Escherichia coli* plus cholera toxin B subunit vaccine is safe and immunogenic in Bangladeshi infants 6–17 months of age: dosing studies in different age groups. Vaccine 2006;24:1726–33.

42. World Health Organization. Future directions for research on enterotoxigenic *Escherichia coli* vaccines for developing countries. Wkly Epidemiol Rec 2006;81:97–104.

43. Wiedermann G, Kollaritsch H, Kundi M, et al. Double-blind, randomized, placebo controlled pilot study evaluating efficacy and reactogenicity of an oral ETEC B-subunit-inactivated whole cell vaccine against travelers' diarrhea (preliminary report). J Travel Med 2000;7:27–9.

44. Sack DA, Shimko J, Torres O. Randomized, double-blind, safety and efficacy trial of a killed oral vaccine for enterotoxigenic *E. coli* diarrhea of travelers to Guatemala and Mexico. Vaccine 2007.

45. Savarino SJ, Abu-Elyazeed R, Rao M, et al. Efficacy of an oral, inactivated whole-cell Enterotoxigenic *E. coli*/CholeraToxin B subunit vaccine in Egyptian infants. Arlington, VA: 6th Annual National Conference on Vaccine Research, National Foundation for Infectious Diseases; 2003.

46. McKenzie R, Bourgeois AL, Engstrom F, et al. Comparative safety and immunogenicity of two attenuated enterotoxigenic *Escherichia coli* vaccine strains in healthy adults. Infect Immun 2006;74:994–1000.

47. Turner AK, Terry TD, Sack DA, et al. Construction and characterization of genetically defined aro omp mutants of enterotoxigenic *Escherichia coli* and preliminary studies of safety and immunogenicity in humans. Infect Immun 2001;69:4969–79.

48. Turner AK, Beavis JC, Stephens JC, et al. Construction and phase I clinical evaluation of the safety and immunogenicity of a candidate enterotoxigenic *Escherichia coli* vaccine strain expressing colonization factor antigen CFA/I. Infect Immun 2006;74:1062–71.

49. Darsley M, Beavis J, Bourgeois AL, et al. Phase I safety, immunogenicity and challenge trials with components of a live attenuated vaccine for the prevention of ETEC diarrhoea. Montego Bay Jamaica: vaccines for enteric diseases; 2004.

50. Barry EM, Altboum Z, Losonsky G, et al. Immune responses elicited against multiple enterotoxigenic *Escherichia coli* fimbriae and mutant LT expressed in attenuated *Shigella* vaccine strains. Vaccine 2003;21:333–40.

51. Barry EM, Wang J, Wu T, et al. Immunogenicity of multivalent *Shigella*-ETEC candidate vaccine strains in a guinea pig model. Vaccine 2006;24:3727–34.

52. Altboum Z, Barry EM, Losonsky G, et al. Attenuated *Shigella flexneri* 2a)*guaBA* strain CVD 1204 expressing enterotoxigenic *Escherichia coli* (ETEC) CS2 and CS3 fimbriae as a live mucosal vaccine against *Shigella* and ETEC infection. Infect Immun 2001;69:3150–8.

53. Altboum Z, Levine MM, Galen JE, et al. Genetic characterization and immunogenicity of coli surface antigen 4 from enterotoxigenic *Escherichia coli* when it is expressed in a *Shigella* live-vector strain. Infect Immun 2003;71:1352–60.

54. Koprowski H II, Levine MM, Anderson RJ, et al. Attenuated *Shigella flexneri* 2a vaccine strain CVD 1204 expressing colonization factor antigen I and mutant heat-labile enterotoxin of enterotoxigenic *Escherichia coli.* Infect Immun 2000;68:4884–92.

55. Hammond SA, Guebre-Xabier M, Yu J, et al. Transcutaneous immunization: an emerging route of immunization and potent immunostimulation strategy. Crit Rev Ther Drug Carrier Syst 2001;18:503–26.

56. Levine MM. Can needle-free administration of vaccines become the norm in global immunization? Nat Med 2003; 9:99–103.

57. Guerena-Burgueno F, Hall ER, Taylor DN, et al. Safety and immunogenicity of a prototype enterotoxigenic *Escherichia coli* vaccine administered transcutaneously. Infect Immun 2002;70:1874–80.

58. Clemens JD, Sack DA, Harris JR, et al. Cross-protection by B subunit-whole cell cholera vaccine against diarrhea associated with heat-labile toxin-producing enterotoxigenic *Escherichia coli*: results of a large-scale field trial. J Infect Dis 1988;158:372–7.

59. McKenzie R, Bourgeois AL, Frech SA, et al. Transcutaneous immunization with the heat-labile toxin (LT) of enterotoxigenic *Escherichia coli* (ETEC): protective efficacy in a double-blind, placebo-controlled challenge study. Vaccine 2007.

60. Tacket CO, Mason HS, Losonsky G, et al. Immunogenicity in humans of a recombinant bacterial antigen delivered in a transgenic potato. Nat Med 1998;4: 607–9.

61. Tacket CO, Reid RH, Boedeker EC, et al. Enteral immunization and challenge of volunteers given enterotoxigenic E. coli CFA/II encapsulated in biodegradable microspheres. Vaccine 1994;12:1270–4.

62. Formal SB, Oaks EV, Olsen RE, et al. Effect of prior infection with virulent Shigella flexneri 2a on the

resistance of monkeys to subsequent infection with Shigella sonnei. J Infect Dis 1991;164:533–7.

63. Mel DM, Terzin AL, Vuksic L. Studies on vaccination against bacillary dysentery. 3. Effective oral immunization against *Shigella flexneri* 2a in a field trial. Bull WHO 1965; 32:647–55.

64. Mel DM, Arsic BL, Nikolic BD, et al. Studies on vaccination against bacillary dysentery. 4. Oral immunization with live monotypic and combined vaccines. Bull WHO 1968;39:375–80.

65. Mel DM, Gangarosa EJ, Radovanovic ML, et al. Studies on vaccination against bacillary dysentery. 6. Protection of children by oral immunization with streptomycin-dependent *Shigella* strains. Bull WHO 1971;45:457–64.

66. Mel DM, Arsic BL, Radovanovic ML, et al. Live oral *Shigella* vaccine: vaccination schedule and the effect of booster dose. Acta Microbiol Acad Sci Hung 1974;21:109–14.

67. Mel DM, Arsic BL, Radovanovic ML, et al. Safety tests in adults and children with live oral typhoid vaccine. Acta Microbiol Acad Sci Hung 1974;21:161–6.

68. Levine MM, Gangarosa EJ, Werner M, et al. Shigellosis in custodial institutions. III. Prospective clinical and bacteriologic surveillance of children vaccinated with oral attenuated Shigella vaccine. J Pediatr 1974;84:803–6.

69. Levine MM, Gangarosa EJ, Barrow WB, et al. Shigellosis in custodial institutions. IV. *In vivo* stability and transmissibility of oral attenuated streptomycin-dependent Shigella vaccines. J Infect Dis 1975;131:704–7.

70. Levine MM, Gangarosa EJ, Barrow WB, et al. Shigellosis in custodial institutions. V. Effect of intervention with streptomycin-dependent *Shigella sonnei* vaccine in an institution with endemic disease. Am J Epidemiol 1976; 104:88–92.

71. Meitert T, Istrati G, Sulea IT, et al. Prophylaxie de la dysenterie bacillaire par le vaccin vivant antidysentérique dans une collectivité d'enfants neuropsychiques. Arch Roum Path Exp Microbiol 1973;32:35–44.

72. Meitert T, Pencu E, Ciudin L, et al. Vaccine strain *Sh. flexneri* T32-Istrati. Studies in animals and in volunteers.Antidysentery immunoprophylaxis and immunotherapy by live vaccine Vadizen (*Sh. flexneri* T32-Istrati). Arch Roum Pathol Exp Microbiol 1984;43:251–78.

73. Bingrui W. Study on the effect of oral immunization of T32-Istrati strain against bacillary dysentery in field trials. Arch Roum Pathol Exp Microbiol 1984;43:285–9.

74. Venkatesan M, Fernandez Prada C, Buysse JM, et al. Virulence phenotype and genetic characteristics of the T32- ISTRATI Shigella flexneri 2a vaccine strain. Vaccine 1991;9:358–63.

75. Kotloff KL, Nataro JP, Losonsky GA, et al. A modified Shigella volunteer challenge model in which the inoculum is administered with bicarbonate buffer: clinical experience and implications for Shigella infectivity. Vaccine 1995;13:1488–94.

76. Coster TS, Hoge CW, VanDeVerg LL, et al. Vaccination against shigellosis with attenuated *Shigella flexneri* 2a strain SC602. Infect Immun 1999;67:3437–43.

77. Katz DE, Coster TS, Wolf MK, et al. Two studies evaluating the safety and immunogenicity of a live, attenuated *Shigella flexneri* 2a vaccine (SC602) and excretion of vaccine organisms in North American volunteers. Infect Immun 2004;72:923–30.

78. World Health Organization. Future needs and directions for *Shigella* vaccines. Weekly Epidemiological Record 2006;81:51–8.

79. Noriega FR, Wang JY, Losonsky G, et al. Construction and characterization of attenuated *)aroA)virG Shigella flexneri* 2a strain CVD 1203, a prototype live oral vaccine. Infect Immun 1994;65:5168–72.

80. Kotloff KL, Noriega F, Losonsky GA, et al. Safety, immunogenicity, and transmissibility in humans of CVD 1203, a live oral *Shigella flexneri* 2a vaccine candidate attenuated by deletions in aroA and virG. Infect Immun 1996;64:4542–8.

81. Nataro JP, Seriwatana J, Fasano A, et al. Identification and cloning of a novel plasmid-encoded enterotoxin of enteroinvasive Escherichia coli and Shigella strains. Infect Immun 1995;63:4721–8.

82. Fasano A, Noriega FR, Maneval DR Jr, et al. *Shigella* enterotoxin 1: an enterotoxin of Shigella flexneri 2a active in rabbit small intestine in vivo and in vitro. J Clin Invest 1995;95:2853–61.

83. Fasano A, Noriega FR, Liao FM, et al. Effect of Shigella enterotoxin 1 (ShET1) on rabbit intestine in vitro and in vivo. Gut 1997;40:505–11.

84. Noriega FR, Liao FM, Formal SB, et al. Prevalence of *Shigella* enterotoxin 1 among *Shigella* clinical isolates of diverse serotypes. J Infect Dis 1995;172:1408–10.

85. Kotloff KL, Noriega FR, Samandari T, et al. *Shigella flexneri* 2a Strain CVD 1207, with specific deletions in *virG, sen, set,* and *guaBA*, is highly attenuated in humans. Infect Immun 2000;68:1034–9.

86. Noriega FR, Losonsky G, Lauderbaugh C, et al. Engineered *DguaB-A, DvirG Shigella flexneri* 2a strain CVD 1205: construction, safety, immunogenicity and potential efficacy as a mucosal vaccine. Infect Immun 1996;64:3055–61.

87. Kotloff KL, Pasetti MF, Barry EM, et al. Deletion in the *Shigella* enterotoxin genes further attenuates *Shigella flexneri* 2a bearing guanine auxotrophy in a Phase 1 trial of CVD 1204 and CVD 1208. J Infect Dis 2004;190:1745–54.

88. Noriega FR, Liao FM, Maneval DR, et al. Strategy for cross-protection among *Shigella flexneri* serotypes. Infect Immun 1999;67:782–8.

89. Hartman AB, Venkatesan MM. Construction of a stable attenuated *Shigella sonnei* Delta*virG* vaccine strain, WRSS1, and protective efficacy and immunogenicity in the guinea pig keratoconjunctivitis model. Infect Immun 1998;66:4572–6.

90. Kotloff K, Taylor D, Sztein MB, et al. Phase 1 evaluation of a *vriG* deleted *Shigella sonnei* live, attenuated vaccine (strain WRSS1) in healthy adult volunteers. Infect Immun 2002;70:2016–21.

91. Orr N, Katz DE, Atsmon J, et al. Community-based safety, immunogenicity, and transmissibility study of the *Shigella sonnei* WRSS1 vaccine in Israeli volunteers. Infect Immun 2005;73:8027–32.

92. Tramont EC, Chung R, Berman S, et al. Safety and antigenicity of typhoid-Shigella sonnei vaccine (strain 5076-1C). J Infect Dis 1984;149:133–6.

93. Herrington DA, Van de Verg L, Formal SB, et al. Studies in volunteers to evaluate candidate Shigella vaccines: further experience with a bivalent *Salmonella typhi-Shigella sonnei* vaccine and protection conferred by previous *Shigella sonnei* disease. Vaccine 1990;8:353–7.

94. Van de Verg L, Herrington DA, Murphy JR, et al. Specific immunoglobulin A-secreting cells in peripheral blood of humans following oral immunization with a bivalent *Salmonella typhi-Shigella sonnei* vaccine or infection by pathogenic *S. sonnei.* Infect Immun 1990; 58:2002–4.

95. Seid RC, Kopecko DJ, Sadoff JC, et al. Unusual lipopolysaccharide antigens of a *Salmonella typhi* oral vaccine strain expressing the *Shigella sonnei* form I antigen. J Biol Chem 1984;259:9028–34.

96. Xu DQ, Cisar JO, Ambulos JN Jr, et al. Molecular cloning and characterization of genes for *Shigella sonnei* form I O polysaccharide: proposed biosynthetic pathway and stable expression in a live *Salmonella* vaccine vector. Infect Immun 2002;70:4414–23.

97. Kotloff KL, Winickoff JP, Ivanoff B, et al. Global burden of *Shigella* infections: implications for vaccine development and implementation of control strategies. Bull Wld Hlth Org 1999;77:651–66.

98. Greco KM, McDonough MA, Butterton JR. Variation in the Shiga toxin region of 20th-century epidemic and endemic *Shigella dysenteriae* 1 strains. J Infect Dis 2004; 190:330–4.

99. Levine MM, Galen J, Barry E, et al. Attenuated *Salmonella typhi* and *Shigella* as live oral vaccines and as live vectors. Behring Inst Mitt 1997. p. 120–3.

100. Robbins JB, Chu C, Schneerson R. Hypothesis for vaccine development: protective immunity to enteric diseases caused by non-typhoidal *Salmonellae* and *Shigellae* may be conferred by serum IgG antibodies to the O-specific polysaccharides of their lipopolysaccharides. Clin Infect Dis 1992;15:346–51.

101. Cohen D, Ashkenazi S, Green M, et al. Safety and immunogenicity of investigational Shigella conjugate vaccines in Israeli volunteers. Infect Immun 1996;64: 4074–7.

102. Cohen D, Ashkenazi S, Green MS, et al. Double-blind vaccine-controlled randomised efficacy trial of an investigational *Shigella sonnei* conjugate vaccine in young adults. Lancet 1997;349:155–9.

103. Ashkenazi S, Passwell JH, Harlev E, et al. Safety and immunogenicity of *Shigella sonnei* and *Shigella flexneri* 2a O-specific polysaccharide conjugates in children. J Infect Dis 1999;179:1565–8.

104. Adachi JA, Ericsson CD, Jiang ZD, et al. Natural history of enteroaggregative and enterotoxigenic *Escherichia coli* infection among US travelers to Guadalajara, Mexico. J Infect Dis 2002;185:1681–3.

105. Cohen MB, Hawkins JA, Weckbach LS, et al. Colonization by enteroaggregative *Escherichia coli* in travelers with and without diarrhea. J Clin Microbiol 1993;31:351–3.

106. Nataro JP, Mai V, Johnson J, et al. Diarrheagenic *Escherichia coli* infection in Baltimore, Maryland, and New Haven, Connecticut. Clin Infect Dis 2006;43:402–7.

107. Bhan MK, Raj P, Levine MM, et al. Enteroaggregative Escherichia coli associated with persistent diarrhea in a cohort of rural children in India. J Infect Dis 1989;159: 1061–4.

108. Tzipori S, Montanaro J, Robins-Browne RM, et al. Studies with enteroaggregative *Escherichia coli* in the gnotobiotic piglet gastroenteritis model. Infect Immun 1992;60:5302–6.

109. Nataro JP. Enteroaggregative *Escherichia coli* pathogenesis. Curr Opin Gastroenterol 2005;21:4–8.

110. Scott DA. Vaccines against *Campylobacter jejuni.* J Infect Dis 1997;176Suppl 2:S183–8.

111. Rees JH, Soudain SE, Gregson NA, et al. *Campylobacter jejuni* infection and Guillain-Barre syndrome. N Engl J Med 1995;333:1374–9.

112. Goodyear CS, O'Hanlon GM, Plomp JJ, et al. Monoclonal antibodies raised against Guillain-Barre syndrome-associated *Campylobacter jejuni* lipopolysaccharides react with neuronal gangliosides and paralyze muscle-nerve preparations. J Clin Invest 1999;104:697–708.

113. Sizemore DR, Warner B, Lawrence J, et al. Live, attenuated *Salmonella typhimurium* vectoring *Campylobacter* antigens. Vaccine 2006;24:3793–803.

114. Prokhorova TA, Nielsen PN, Petersen J, et al. Novel surface polypeptides of *Campylobacter jejuni* as traveller's diarrhoea vaccine candidates discovered by proteomics. Vaccine 2006;24:6446–55.

115. Holmgren J, Bergkvist C. Oral B subunit-killed whole cell cholera vaccine. In: Levine MM, Kaper JB, Rappuoli R,

et al, editors. New York: Marcel Dekker; 2004. p. 499–510.

116. Sanchez JL, Vasquez B, Begue RE, et al. Protective efficacy of oral whole-cell/recombinant-B-subunit cholera vaccine in Peruvian military recruits. Lancet 1994;344:1273–6.

117. Taylor DN, Cardenas V, Sanchez JL, et al. Two year study of the protective efficacy of the oral whole cell plus recombinant B subunit (WC/rBS) cholera vaccine in Peru. J Infect Dis 2000;181:1667–73.

118. Sanchez JL, Trofa AF, Taylor DN, et al. Safety and immunogenicity of the oral, whole cell/recombinant B subunit cholera vaccine in North American volunteers. J Infect Dis 1993;167:1446–9.

119. Ortigao-de-Sampaio MB, Shattock RJ, Hayes P, et al. Increase in plasma viral load after oral cholera immunization of HIV-infected subjects. AIDS 1998;12:F145–50.

120. Begue RE, Castellares G, Ruiz R, et al. Community-based assessment of safety and immunogenicity of the whole cell plus recombinant B subunit (WC/rBS) oral cholera vaccine in Peru. Vaccine 1995;13:691–4.

121. Clemens JD, Sack DA, Harris JR, et al. Field trial of oral cholera vaccines in Bangladesh. Lancet 1986;ii:124–7.

122. Clemens JD, Sack DA, Harris JR, et al. Field trial of cholera vaccines in Bangladesh: results from three year follow-up. Lancet 1990;335:270–3.

123. Kotloff KL, Wasserman SS, O'Donnell S, et al. Safety and immunogenicity in North Americans of a single dose of live oral cholera vaccine CVD 103-HgR: Results of a randomized, placebo-controlled, double-blind crossover trial. Infect Immun 1992;60:4430–2.

124. Cryz SJ, Levine MM, Kaper JB, et al. Randomized double-blind placebo controlled trial to evaluate the safety and immunogenicity of the live oral cholera vaccine strain CVD 103-HgR in Swiss adults. Vaccine 1990;8:577–80.

125. Suharyono, Simanjuntak C, Witham N, et al. Safety and immunogenicity of single-dose live oral cholera vaccine CVD 103-HgR in 5-9-year-old Indonesian children. Lancet 1992;340:689–94.

126. Simanjuntak CH, O'Hanley P, Punjabi NH, et al. The safety, immunogenicity, and transmissibility of single-dose live oral cholera vaccine CVD 103-HgR in 24 to 59 month old Indonesian children. J Infect Dis 1993;168: 1169–76.

127. Su-Arehawaratana P, Singharaj P, Taylor DN, et al. Safety and immunogenicity of different immunization regimens of CVD 103-HgR live oral cholera vaccine in soldiers and civilians in Thailand. J Infect Dis 1992;165: 1042–8.

128. Migasena S, Pitisuttitham P, Prayurahong P, et al. Preliminary assessment of the safety and immunogenicity of live oral cholera vaccine strain CVD 103-HgR in healthy Thai adults. Infect Immun 1989;57:3261–4.

129. Lagos R, Avendano A, Horwitz I, et al. Tolerancia e inmunogenicidad de una dosis oral de la cepa de *Vibrio cholerae* 01, viva-atenuada, CVD 103-HgR: estudio de doble ciego en adultos Chilenos. Rev Med Chile 1993;121: 857–63.

130. Lagos R, Avendano A, Prado V, et al. Attenuated live oral cholera vaccine strain CVD 103-HgR elicits significantly higher serum vibriocidal antibody titers in persons of blood group O. Infect Immun 1995;63:707–9.

131. Lagos R, Losonsky G, Abrego P, et al. Tolerancia, immunogenicidad, excresión y transmisión de la vacuna anti-colera oral viva-atenuada, CVD 103-HgR, estudio pareado de doble ciego en niños Chilenos de 24 a 59 meses. Bol Hosp Infant Mex 1996;53:214–20.

132. Lagos R, San Martin O, Wasserman SS, et al. Palatability, reactogenicity and immunogenicity of engineered live oral cholera vaccine CVD 103-HgR in Chilean infants and toddlers. Pediatr Infect Dis J 1999;18:624–30.

133. Perry RT, Plowe CV, Koumaré B, et al. A single dose of live oral cholera vaccine CVD 103-HgR is safe and immunogenic in HIV-infected and non-infected adults in Mali. Bull Wld Hlth Org 1998;76:63–71.

134. Levine MM, Kaper JB, Herrington D, et al. Safety, immunogenicity, and efficacy of recombinant live oral cholera vaccines, CVD 103 and CVD 103-HgR. Lancet 1988;2:467–70.

135. Tacket CO, Losonsky G, Nataro JP, et al. Onset and duration of protective immunity in challenged volunteers after vaccination with live oral cholera vaccine CVD 103-HgR. J Infect Dis 1992;166:837–41.

136. Levine MM, Tacket CO. Live oral vaccines against cholera. In: Ala'Aldeen DAA, Hormaeche CE, editors. Molecular and clinical aspects of bacterial vaccine development. Chichester: John Wiley & Sons; 1995. p. 233–58.

137. Tacket CO, Cohen MB, Wasserman SS, et al. Randomized, double-blind, placebo-controlled, multicentered trial of the efficacy of a single dose of live oral cholera vaccine CVD 103-HgR in preventing cholera following challenge with vibrio cholerae O1 El tor Inaba three months after vaccination. Infect Immun 1999;67: 6341–5.

138. Taylor DN, Killeen KP, Hack DC, et al. Development of a live, oral, attenuated vaccine against El Tor cholera. J Infect Dis 1994;170:1518–23.

139. Kenner JR, Coster TS, Taylor DN, et al. Peru-15, an improved live attenuated oral vaccine candidate for *Vibrio cholerae* O1. J Infect Dis 1995;172:1126–9.

140. Cohen MB, Giannella RA, Bean J, et al. Randomized, controlled human challenge study of the safety, immunogenicity, and protective efficacy of a single dose of Peru-15, a live attenuated oral cholera vaccine. Infect Immun 2002;70:1965–70.

141. Garcia L, Jidy MD, Garcia H, et al. The vaccine candidate *Vibrio cholerae* 638 is protective against cholera in healthy volunteers. Infect Immun 2005;73:3018–24.

142. Vesikari T, Matson DO, Dennehy P, et al. Safety and efficacy of a pentavalent human-bovine (WC3) reassortant rotavirus vaccine. N Engl J Med 2006;354:23–33.

143. Ruiz-Palacios GM, Perez-Schael I, Velazquez FR, et al. Safety and efficacy of an attenuated vaccine against severe rotavirus gastroenteritis. N Engl J Med 2006;354:11–22.

144. Murphy TV, Gargiullo PM, Massoudi MS, et al. Intussusception among infants given an oral rotavirus vaccine. N Engl J Med 2001;344:564–72.

145. Ball JM, Graham DY, Opekun AR, et al. Recombinant Norwalk virus-like particles given orally to volunteers: phase I study. Gastroenterol 1999;117:40–8.

146. Tacket CO, Sztein MB, Losonsky GA, et al. Humoral, mucosal, and cellular immune responses to oral Norwalk virus-like particles in volunteers. Clin Immunol 2003;108: 241–7.

147. Miller-Sims VC, Petri WA Jr. Opportunities and obstacles in developing a vaccine for *Entamoeba histolytica.* Curr Opin Immunol 2002;14:549–52.

148. Houpt E, Barroso L, Lockhart L, et al. Prevention of intestinal amebiasis by vaccination with the *Entamoeba histolytica* Gal/GalNac lectin. Vaccine 2004;22:611–7.

149. Xu P, Widmer G, Wang Y, et al. The genome of *Cryptosporidium hominis.* Nature 2004;431:1107–12.

150. Abrahamsen MS, Templeton TJ, Enomoto S, et al. Complete genome sequence of the apicomplexan, *Cryptosporidium parvum.* Science 2004;304:441–5.

151. Tacket CO, Binion SB, Bostwick E, et al. Efficacy of bovine milk immunoglobulin concentrate in preventing illness after *Shigella flexneri* challenge. Am J Trop Med Hyg 1992; 47:276–83.

Chapter 24

Pitfalls in Travelers' Diarrhea Management

Prativa Pandey, MD

Santanu Chatterjee, MBBS, DTM&H

Travelers' diarrhea is known to occur in 30 to 60%[1–7] of travelers to the developing world. Although it has been shown that improving health and food safety standards of hotels can reduce rates of travelers' diarrhea[9] in a country, the incidence and suffering from travelers' diarrhea is almost unchanged in the past 20 years.[4] One of the risk factors seems to be destination,[1-4,8] with certain destinations having very high risk compared to other destinations. Until basic hygiene and sanitation infrastructure improves in developing countries, we will continue to see high rates of travelers' diarrhea in travelers to these countries.

Travel medicine practitioners in the developing world who take care of a large number of travelers with travelers' diarrhea, come across myriads of problems faced by travelers in accessing and receiving care. Much of what is written in this chapter comes from the experience of authors as practitioners in the developing world in addition to what is available from scientific research.

Accessing Care

A traveler who is struck with an episode of travelers' diarrhea in the developing world may choose not to do anything about it and take the wait and see approach, may self-treat[3,4,10] depending on how well informed the traveler is and how comfortable the traveler feels with self treatment, or may seek care from a local physician.[3,4,10] Local medical care to some extent will depend on the destination and medical facilities that exist in that location. It will significantly depend on who the point of contact for the traveler is. Very often, guide books are consulted by travelers to find out information about doctors/clinics to be contacted should the traveler need to seek care locally. These guide books may point the traveler to seek the best locally available care because there is no financial reward involved in patient referrals. The point of contact for the traveler may also be the hotel doctor[3] or other doctors/clinics recommended by the hotel or the travel agent[4] where financial incentives may play a role in choosing where the traveler is referred to. It may be the Embassy that represents the traveler or friends of friends who are living in that country who are knowledgeable about existing local resources. For a traveler who is on a tight itinerary who runs the risk of ruining the trip due to illness,[4] significant amount of time may be lost trying to find the best locally available care that generates confidence and trust in the traveler.

Diagnostic Pitfalls

In many of the developing countries, the treating physician may have adequate knowledge of the microbial pathogens in the local population, but this may be different in travelers who have no immunity against many of these enteric pathogens. Even when pathogens are known, antimicrobial resistance patterns for the pathogens may not be known. Laboratory services may not exist or may not be reliable particularly where stool examinations are concerned[11] and fresh stool samples are rarely examined. Even when reliable services exist, it may not help the treating physician in immediate assessment and treatment of a person with travelers' diarrhea since laboratory results are often delayed for several days. What is seen very often is that certain diagnoses are missed and some are overdiagnosed. In Nepal, and probably true in several developing countries, many local laboratories will often report as *Escherichia (E.) histolytica* many different types of nonpathogenic ameba, resulting in overdiagnosis[12] and treatment for *E. histolytica*, which calls for prolonged therapy with metronidazole or tinidazole and a luminal agent. *E. histolytica* as a cause of traveler's diarrhea is of very low importance in published studies.[1,2,13–17] *Cyclospora cayatenensis*, which is a common pathogen in Nepal in the months of June and July to cause travelers' diarrhea, is never reported by most local laboratories, leading to missed diagnosis and prolonged suffering.

Treatment Issues

Because laboratory services are inadequate, polypharmacy is often the rule in developing countries, as is irrational fixed dose combinations and use of medications of uncertain efficacy.[18–21] What is a very simple problem may end up getting complicated due to polypharmacy.[18] A person with travelers' diarrhea often receives from the doctor up to 6 to 7 different combinations of medications eg, an antibacterial drug, an antiparasitic drug, a vitamin, an enzyme, an antiemetic, and an antimotility drug along with paracetmol/acetaminophen to reduce the fevers and rehydration powder sachets. With this approach, a person may get rid of the diarrhea but very often will suffer from side effects of some of these medications, such as dystonic reactions from excessive use of metoclopramide, severe nausea, vomiting, and loss of taste related to metronidazole, which may not have been needed in the first place.

In many developing countries, antibiotics can be purchased over the counter without a doctor's prescription.[29] Travelers will sometimes consult guide books that outline treatment for travelers' diarrhea and buy medication directly from a pharmacy. Antibiotics purchased over the counter could be substandard leading to ineffective therapy or a pharmacist may intervene and suggest additional remedies leading to polypharmacy. A certain brand of medication that has financial rewards to the pharmacist could be sold to the traveler. Substandard and counterfeit drugs are available[22] and are thriving businesses in some developing countries.[23,24]

Although waning in much of Asia, treatment with medication administration by injections when equally effective oral therapies exist is still a common practice in Latin America and Africa.[20,21] Patients in these countries are used to the doctor giving injections for treatment. This practice may cause increased risk of nosocomial hepatitis B, human immunodeficiency virus (HIV), and other infections.[25–27] This is not a problem of the developing world alone.[28] In rural health care settings, injections may be given by traditional and unlicensed practitioners where basic safety precautions may be ignored. For the treatment of travelers' diarrhea, injectable medications are rarely needed because oral therapy is highly effective.[3,30–32]

Severe Travelers' Diarrhea

An episode of travelers' diarrhea is often mild to moderate with few loose stools a day, but it could be severe and incapacitating[3,4,10,14] with several loose stools and any combination of symptoms of high fever, chills, abdominal cramps, nausea, vomiting, and prostration. These patients are often overwhelmed by the severe nature of their symptoms, which they are now facing in a foreign country away from their familiar environment. Some patients, especially the ones traveling alone, are usually too scared to be in a hotel room by themselves and prefer to be in a reassuring medical environment. Severe travelers' diarrhea, particularly if accompanied by vomiting and painful abdominal cramps, may be something that they have not experienced before and the experience could be a frightening one. At this point in time, the traveler with travelers' diarrhea is forced to seek care in the country that they are traveling in. In some clinics around the world, and this could be true in the developed world as well, a tourist patient is looked upon as a "cash cow" who gives a chance to the treating doctor to make good money. Some clinics/hospitals will give financial incentives to taxi drivers, hotels/lodges, or travel agents who bring foreign patients into their settings. As a result, patients do not always end up being in the best place that exists in that city that may not be giving out commissions. It is also financially rewarding to admit a patient with traveler's diarrhea to administer intravenous fluids for a day or two and often longer. There is another aspect to this. Patients often feel greatly improved after they receive intravenous fluids, and some patients will insist on receiving them. This can often be achieved during a day visit or with an overnight stay and should not necessitate a lengthy inpatient admission because recovery from severe travelers' diarrhea is usually rapid with treatment. In some instances, a patient who is insured and does not have to pay out of pocket will insist on being admitted, irrespective of the severity of illness, to undergo recuperation in a comfortable hospital bed that provides for rest in between days of rough and hectic backpacking low-budget travel.

Conclusion

Although medical care is improving in many of the developing countries, standards of care are not uniform, and there is much less accountability compared to the developed countries. Laboratory services are not always adequate and drug monitoring systems are not as effective as they should be, leading at times to production and sale of substandard and counterfeit drugs. Added to these problems is the financial incentive scheme for patient referrals practiced by some individuals and institutions that may not allow a traveler to seek the best local resource available. Specialty destination travel medicine clinics only exist in a handful of destinations that have brought about optimal care for travelers to some developing countries.

While we wait for basic sanitation infrastructure, personal hygiene, and restaurant hygiene to improve in developing countries, which will eventually decrease high rates of travelers' diarrhea, campaigns should be aimed at educating the traveler to seek pretravel consultation and to carry medication for self treatment of travelers' diarrhea. From the airport surveys of travelers regarding knowledge, attitudes, and practices, it is known that only 31 to 52% of travelers will seek pretravel health advice.[34–36] Pretravel advice alone with emphasis on dietary preventive measures have not been effective in preventing travelers' diarrhea.[3,4,33] Self treatment if used properly, works well[3,10] in treating travelers' diarrhea and is highly cost effective for the traveler. New preventive strategies[37] are now available that could also be discussed during the pre-travel visit. Providing a list of reliable health care facilities in the country of travel will be very reassuring to the naïve traveler. There are many resources available to identify competent clinics or health care facilities worldwide. International Society of Travel Medicine travel clinic directory that resides on the website <www.istm.org> is one such wonderful resource. It remains a challenge to educate the traveler who has not sought pretravel consultation. Very often, they are the ones who will consult travel guide books or the hotels or travel agents first and spend time and money seeking treatment for travelers' diarrhea.

References

1. DuPont HL, Khan FM. Travelers' diarrhea: epidemiology, microbiology, prevention, and therapy. J Travel Med 1994; 1:84–93.
2. von Sonnenburg F, Tornieporth N, Waiyaki P, et al. Risk and aetiology of diarrhoea at various tourist destinations. Lancet 2000;356:133–4.
3. Hill DR. Occurrence and self-treatment of diarrhea in a large cohort of Americans traveling to developing countries. Am J Trop Med Hyg 2000;62:585–9.
4. Steffen R, Tornieporth N, Clemens SA, et al. Epidemiology of travelers' diarrhea: details of a global survey. J Travel Med 2004;11:231–8.
5. Steffen R. Epidemiology of traveler's diarrhea. Clin Infect Dis 2005;41(Suppl 8):S536–40.
6. Ahlm C, Lundberg S, Fesse K, Wistrom J. Health problems and self-medication among Swedish travellers. Scand J Infect Dis 1994;26:711–7.
7. Cobelens FG, Leentvaar-Kuijpers A, Kleijnen J, Coutinho RA. Incidence and risk factors of diarrhoea in Dutch travellers: consequences for priorities in pre-travel health advice. Trop Med Int Health 1998;3:896–903.
8. Freedman DO, Weld LH, Kozarsky PE, et al. Spectrum of disease and relation to place of exposure among ill returned travelers. New Engl J Med 2006;354:119–30.
9. Ashley DV, Walters C, Dockery-Brown C, et al. Interventions to prevent and control food-borne diseases associated with a reduction in traveler's diarrhea in tourists to Jamaica. J Travel Med 2004;11:364–7.
10. Putnam SD, Sanders JW, Frenck RW, et al. Self reported description of diarrhea among military populations in operations Iraqi Freedom and Enduring Freedom. J Travel Med 2006;13:92–9.
11. Gill CJ, Lau J, Gorbach SL, Hamer DH. Diagnostic accuracy of stool assays for inflammatory bacterial gastroenteritis in developed and resource-poor countries. Clin Infect Dis 2003;37:365–75.
12. Leiva B, Lebbad M, Winiecka-Krusnell J, et al. Overdiagnosis of Entamoeba histolytica and Entamoeba dispar in Nicaragua: a microscopic, triage parasite panel and PCR study. Arch Med Res 2006;37:529–34.
13. Hoge CW, Shlim DR, Echeverria P, et al. Epidemiology of diarrhea among expatriate residents living in a highly endemic environment. JAMA 1996;275:533–8.
14. Riddle MS, Sanders JW, Putnam SD, Tribble DR. Incidence, etiology, and impact of diarrhea among long-term travelers (US military and similar populations): a systematic review. Am J Trop Med Hyg 2006;74:891–900.
15. Leena M. Clinical features and duration of traveler's diarrhea in relation to its etiology. Clin Infect Dis 1994; 19:728–34.
16. Hoge CW, Shlim DR, Rajah R, et al. Epidemiology of diarrhoeal illness associated with coccidian-like organism among travellers and foreign residents in Nepal. Lancet 1993;341:1175–9.
17. Jiang ZD, Lowe B, Verenkar MP, et al. Prevalence of enteric pathogens among international travelers with diarrhea acquired in Kenya (Mombasa), India (Goa), or Jamaica (Montego Bay). J Infect Dis 2002;185:497–502.
18. Cave W, Pandey P, Chatterjee S. Irrational prescribing in South Asia: a case of fluoroquinolone-associated phototoxicity. J Travel Med 2003;10:290–2.
19. Hazra A, Tripathi SK, Alam MS. Prescribing and dispensing activities at the health facilities of a non-governmental organization. Natl Med J India 2000;13:177–82.

20. Mallet HP, Njikam A, Scouflaire SM. Evaluation of prescription practices and of the rational use of medicines in Niger. Sante 2001;11:185–93.

21. Hogerzeil HV, Bimo, , Ross-Degnan D, et al. Field tests for rational drug use in twelve developing countries. Lancet 1993;342:1408–10.

22. WHO fact sheet. The safety of medicines. September 2005. Available at: http://www.who.int/mediacentre/factsheets/fs293/en/index.html (accessed October 27, 2006).

23. McGregor A. Counterfeit drugs flood developing world. Lancet 1997;350:1690.

24. Newton P, Green M, Fernandez F, et al. Counterfeit anti-infective drugs. Lancet infect dis 2006;6:602–13.

25. Rosenthal VD, Maki DG, Salomao R, et al. Device associated nosocomial infections in 55 intensive care units of 8 developing countries. Ann Intern Med 2006;145:582–91.

26. Imarengiaye CO, Enosolease ME, Iribhogbe PE, Ehigiegba AE. Risk of transfusion—transmitted hepatitis C virus in a tertiary hospital in Nigeria. Public Health 2006; 120:274–8.

27. Hauri AM, Armstrong GL, Hutin YJ. The global burden of disease attributable to contaminated injections given in health care settings. Int J STD AIDS 2004;15:7–16.

28. Samandari T, Malakmadze N, Balter S, et al. A large outbreak of hepatitis B virus infections associated with frequent injections at a physician's office. Infect Control Hosp Epidemiol 2005;26:745–50.

29. Ray K, Mukhopadhyay S, Dutt D, et al. Cross-sectional study of consumption, compliance and awareness about antibiotic utilisation amongst the urban community in Kolkata. J Indian Med Assoc 2003;101:79–10.

30. Ericsson CD, Johnson PC, Dupont HL, et al. Ciprofloxacin or trimethoprim-sulfamethoxazole as initial therapy for travelers' diarrhea: a placebo-controlled randomized trial. Ann Intern Med 1987;106:216–20.

31. Taylor DN, Sanchez JL, Candler W, et al. Treatment of travelers' diarrhea: ciprofloxacin plus loperamide compared with ciprofloxacin alone. A placebo-controlled, randomized trial. Ann Intern Med 1991;114:731–4.

32. Kuschner RA, Trofa AF, Thomas RJ, et al. Use of azithromycin for the treatment of Campylobacter enteritis in travelers to Thailand, an area where ciprofloxacin resistance is prevalent. Clin Infect Dis 1995;21:536–41.

33. Shlim DR. Looking for evidence that personal hygiene precautions prevent travelers' diarrhea. Clin Infect Dis 2005;41(Suppl 8):S531–5.

34. Hamer DH, Connor BA. Travel health knowledge, attitudes and practices among United States travelers. J Travel Med 2004;11:23–6.

35. Wilder-Smith A, Khairullah NS, Song JH, et al. Travel health knowledge, attitudes and practices among Australasian travelers. J Travel Med 2004;11:9–15.

36. Herck K, Castelli F, Zuckerman J, et al. Knowledge, attitudes and practices in travel related infectious diseases. The European airport survey. J Travel Med 2004;11:3–8.

37. Dupont HL, Jiang ZD, Okhuysen PC, et al. A randomized, double-blind, placebo-controlled trial of rifaximin to prevent travelers' diarrhea. Ann Intern Med 2005;142: 805–12.

Chapter 25

Nonspecific Treatment: Diet and Oral Rehydration Therapy

Juan-Pablo Caeiro, MD

William B. Greenough III, MD

Travelers' diarrhea occurs in approximately 40% of persons traveling from industrialized countries to low-income countries with decreased hygiene.[1] Food is considered the major source of infection, with water and ice being less commonly the culprit. Bacterial enteropathogens are the most important cause of travelers' diarrhea worldwide.[2] Diarrheagenic *Escherichia coli* (enterotoxigenic *Escherichia coli* [ETEC] and enteroaggregative *Escherichia coli* [EAEC]) are the principal organisms. *Salmonella, Shigella,* and *Campylobacter* spp. are the other significant group.

There are three general modalities for the therapy of travelers' diarrhea: diet and rehydration, symptomatic therapy, anti-inflammatory microbistatic agents (Pepto-Bismol, Bismuth Subsalicylate) antimotility agents like loperamide, and antimicrobial treatment.[3] They can be used alone or in combination.

In this chapter we will discuss diet and rehydration modalities.

Oral Rehydration Therapy

Oral rehydration therapy (ORT) has decreased diarrheal death world wide.[4] In 1968, the effectiveness of oral rehydration therapy was demonstrated in adult patients with cholera.[5] The oral route is the best way to treat dehydration in patients with acute diarrhea.

The small bowel absorbs sugars, amino acids, and oligopeptides via transporters that couple their absorption to the movement of sodium. The coupled transport of sodium and glucose is the basis for oral rehydration therapy in acute diarrhea.[6]

For treatment of acute travelers' diarrhea maintenance of water and electrolyte losses or balance is always desirable.

Travelers' diarrhea is often self-limited and not severe, but at the start of any episode the risk for dehydration is unknown and early use of oral rehydration is recommended. In certain vulnerable populations like children, pregnant women, elderly persons and immunocompromised patients, early and adequate use of oral rehydration solutions (ORS) can prevent hospitalizations and complications.

Evidence

The only study evaluating oral rehydration therapy in patients with travelers' diarrhea was done in Mexico.[7] It compared loperamide alone versus ORT plus loperamide. The study showed no difference decreasing dry mouth, dizziness, or thirst if persons were permitted to drink ad libitum. Persons were healthy young adults with minimal dehydration.

Oral rehydration solution is necessary in patients with important dehydration or with severe diarrhea. WHO and UNICEF recommend a low osmolarity oral rehydration solution for the treatment of dehydration due to diarrhea in children and adults.[8]

Recent data from the International Centre for Diarrhoeal Disease Research in Bangladesh showed that the risk of symptomatic hyponatremia in patients

Table 1

Available ORS in US

	Na MMOL/L	K MMOL/L	Osmolarity MOSM/L	Base MMOL/L	CHO G/L
CeraLyte	50	20	< 200	30	40
Pedialyte (also generic available)	50	20	250	30	100
Rehydralyte (close to WHO)	75	20	310	30	100
Homemade	50–70	---------	80	-------	50–80

CHO = carbohydrate; K = potassium; MMOL/L = millimoles/Liter; MOSM/L = miliosmoles/Liter; Na = sodium; WHO = World Health Organization.

receiving reduced osmolarity ORS was minimal.[9] There were 53,280 patients studied; 22,536 were children less than 60 months of age and 24,651 were persons > 15 years of age. The authors concluded that the reduced osmolarity ORS was safe and it may be utilized in the therapy of patients with diarrhea irrespective of the age and cause of diarrhea. Glucose-based ORS successfully hydrates patients but does not reduce the severity or duration of diarrhea. Rice-based ORS accomplishes both hydration and may reduce severity and duration of diarrhea.[10]

In the rare situation of persons with severe nausea, vomiting, and dehydration, the use of intravenous fluid may be necessary.

Recommendation

The majority of patients with travelers' diarrhea may drink fluids ad libitum with the acute event, but should avoid heavily sugared drinks, which are hyperosmolar and can increase fluid loss. Vulnerable persons should start an ORS early to avoid dehydration. For travelers desiring a rice-based ORS, CeraLyte is available (Table 1).

Intravenous solution is only necessary for the rare case of severe diarrhea associated with hypotension or the inability to drink.

Diet

The gastrointestinal tract depends on the intraluminal nutrients for repair, growth, and improvement. It is clear that early feeding is important in patients with acute diarrhea that can tolerate oral intake.[11]

Some authorities recommend the use of the "BRAT" diet (B, bananas; R, rice; A, applesauce; and T, toast) and refraining from dairy products for persons with acute diarrhea.[12]

Evidence

A recent pilot study compared the effects of a restricted physiologic diet with the effects of an unrestricted diet on the extent and symptoms of acute travelers' diarrhea among US healthy adults treated with an antibacterial drug in Mexico.[13] The restricted diet initially consisted of clear fluids like mineral water, consommé, jello, sherbet, or Manzanilla tea and food like salted crackers, tortillas, bread, and toast. Then, as diarrhea improved, bananas, rice, potatoes, and baked chicken, or fish were allowed. Food not permitted was red meat, milk, butter, ice cream, vegetables, fried foods, coffee, alcohol, cheese, and fruit other than bananas.

The duration of diarrhea and clinical symptoms were similar in both groups. The results indicate that the restriction of diet during therapy with antibacterial drug is not correlated with amelioration of clinical symptoms or diarrhea.

Patients with acute travelers' diarrhea can be advised to eat if they are hungry. Early feeding does not prolong or worsen the diarrhea and may hasten recovery.

Future studies may need to address the need of dietary restrictions or supplements in persons with travelers' diarrhea not receiving antibiotics.[14]

Recommendations

Patients with diarrhea should be allowed to eat if they are hungry. No specific food is indicated. Early feeding does not prolong diarrhea. If the patient is suffering significant nausea and vomiting, short-term fasting may be necessary.

References

1. DuPont HL. What's new in enteric infectious diseases at home and abroad. Curr Opin Infect Dis 2005;18:407–12.
2. DuPont HL. Travellers' diarrhoea: contemporary approaches to therapy and prevention. Drugs 2006;66:303–14.
3. DuPont HL. Travelers' diarrhea: antimicrobial therapy and chemoprevention. Nat Clin Pract Gastroenterol Hepatol 2005;2:191–8; quiz 1 p following 198.
4. Victora CG, Bryce J, Fontaine O, Monasch R. Reducing deaths from diarrhoea through oral rehydration therapy. Bull World Health Organ 2000;78:1246–55.
5. Nalin DR, Cash RA, Islam R, Molla M, Phillips RA. Oral maintenance therapy for cholera in adults. Lancet 1968;2:370–3.

6. Field M. Intestinal ion transport and the pathophysiology of diarrhea. J Clin Invest 2003;111:931–43.

7. Caeiro JP, DuPont HL, Albrecht H, Ericsson CD. Oral rehydration therapy plus loperamide versus loperamide alone in the treatment of traveler's diarrhea. Clin Infect Dis 1999;28:1286–9.

8. Duggan C, Fontaine O, Pierce NF, et al. Scientific rationale for a change in the composition of oral rehydration solution. JAMA 2004;291:2628–31.

9. Alam NH, Yunus M, Faruque AS, et al. Symptomatic hyponatremia during treatment of dehydrating diarrheal disease with reduced osmolarity oral rehydration solution. Jama 2006;296:567–73.

10. Fontaine O, Gore SM, Pierce NF. Rice-based oral rehydration solution for treating diarrhoea. The Cochrane Library. Issue No 1. 2005.

11. Duggan C, Nurko S. "Feeding the gut": the scientific basis for continued enteral nutrition during acute diarrhea. J Pediatr 1997;131:801–8.

12. Thielman NM, Guerrant RL. Clinical practice. Acute infectious diarrhea. N Engl J Med 2004;350:38–47.

13. Huang DB, Awasthi M, Le BM, et al. The role of diet in the treatment of travelers' diarrhea: a pilot study. Clin Infect Dis 2004;39:468–71.

14. Steffen R, Gyr K. Diet in the treatment of diarrhea: from tradition to evidence. Clin Infect Dis 2004;39:472–3.

CHAPTER 26

SYMPTOMATIC THERAPY

JAVIER A. ADACHI, MD

STEPHEN HANAUER, MD

The idea behind the use of symptomatic drugs is not to treat the microorganisms that cause the diarrheal syndrome in travelers, but to relieve symptoms, mainly the severity and frequency of loose stools passed, allowing the travelers to return more prompt to their planned schedule.[1–3] This chapter will concentrate on the medical literature pertaining specifically to diarrhea in travelers and will briefly review agents that have not been well studied but which might have value based on their mechanism of action. The use of probiotics for prevention of traveler's diarrhea and the role of diet and oral rehydration have been reviewed extensively in previous chapters (Chapter 21, "Probiotics in Traveler's Diarrhea" and Chapter 25, "Nonspecific Treatment: Diet and Oral Rehydration Therapy," respectively) and the use of antimicrobial agents will be reviewed in Chapter 27, "Antimicrobial Therapy."

Historically, symptomatic drugs have been used for the treatment of diarrhea in travelers for many decades. Symptomatically acting medications were the first treatments used to manage traveler's diarrhea, with different degrees of success.[1–6] They are especially useful for treatment of mild to moderate diarrhea, and they may be used to augment fluids therapy.

Three main intestinal mechanisms lead to acute diarrhea.[3–5] The most common pathophysiologic mechanism in acute infectious diarrhea is alteration of fluid and electrolyte movement from the serosal to the mucosal surface of the gut (secretory diarrhea). This alteration may occur as a result of cyclic nucleotide stimulation (as a second messenger) or by an inflammatory process that releases cytokines. The second mechanism, malabsorption or presence of nonabsorbed substances in the lumen of the bowel, and the third, acceleration of intestinal motility, are more important in prolonged or chronic forms of infectious and noninfectious diarrhea, such as tropical and nontropical sprue, Whipple's disease, scleroderma, malabsorption, irritable bowel syndrome, and inflammatory bowel disease. The best approach to classify the symptomatic agents for the treatment of traveler's diarrhea is based on their main effect on the above mentioned pathophysiologic mechanisms, as outlined in Table 1.

In the next lines we are going to describe the different symptomatic medications for the treatment of traveler's diarrhea. Some of them are proven and are widely used, while others have been tested and been shown not to be of clinical benefit in traveler's diarrhea or to have not been marketed by the pharmaceutical industry. Bismuth subsalicylate and loperamide will be reviewed separately at the end of this chapter because they have multiple mechanisms of action and therefore cannot be classified in a single group.

Antimotility Drugs

The most important antimotility symptomatic medication is loperamide. Other drugs included in this group are diphenoxylate, difenoxin (both combined with atropine), tincture of opium, and anticholinergic drugs such as Mepenzolate bromide.

Difenoxin is a drug closely related to diphenoxylate and has been studied in the treatment of acute and chronic diarrhea, including one early study in Germany in which travelers with diarrhea were treated.[7,8]

Diphenoxylate (the active ingredient in Lomotil) has shown to be effective in the treatment of nonspecific diarrhea,[9–12] but has not been studied in travelers with diarrhea. One early review[13] suggested that loperamide was preferred as an antidiarrheal agent to diphenoxylate. The main risks of diphenoxylate with atropine are atropine-mediated anticholinergic effects, central opiate effects in children taking an overdose, and as per all antimotility drugs, rare potentiation of dysenteric diarrhea not treated also with antibacterial drugs.[14]

Table 1 Symptomatic Drugs for the Treatment of Travelers' Diarrhea and its Mechanism of Action

Mechanism	Agent	Traveler's Diarrhea References	Nonspecific Diarrhea References
Antimotility			
	Loperamide (mainly an antimotility drug)	44,46–49,51	50
	Difenoxin/diphenoxylate plus atropine	7,8	9–12,14
	Mepenzolate bromide (anticholinergic)	15*	
	Tincture opium		17
Antisecretory			
	Loperamide (mainly an antimotility drug)	44,46–49,51	50
	Bismuth subsalicylate (mainly an antisecretory drug)	40–44	
	SP-303 or Crofelemer, (chloride channel blocker)	20†	
	Zaldaride (calmodulin inhibitor)	21–23†	
	Racecadotril (enkephaline inhibitor)		24–26
Adsorbents			
	Bismuth subsalicylate (mainly an antisecretory drug)	40–44	
	Activated charcoal	*‡	9,28
	Calcium polycarbophil		30,31
	Kaolin/pectin	*‡	9
	Hydrated aluminium-magnesium silicate (Attapulgite)	33†	32†
	Tannin albuminate plus ethacridine lactate	28†	
	Dioctahedral smectite (Clay-like compounds)		35†
Antimicrobial			
	Bismuth subsalicylate (mainly an antisecretory drug)	40–44	

* Negative results in clinical trials in travelers.
† No Food and Drug Administration approval. Not commercially available in the US.
‡ H. L. DuPont and C. D. Ericsson, personal communication.

Mepenzolate bromide is not recommended in the treatment of traveler's diarrhea based on ineffectiveness in a trial among college students visiting Mexico, with a higher incidence of anticholinergic side effects (51% compared to 14% in the placebo group).[15]

Deodorized tincture of opium showed a similar efficacy compared to diphenoxylate in early studies,[16,17] but it has not been used since the 1970s and has not been studied in travelers with diarrhea.

Antisecretory Drugs

SP 303 or crofelemer, zaldaride, and racecadotril have been shown to have antisecretory activity in clinical trials, but are not currently available commercially. The two available drugs with antisecretory activity (bismuth subsalycilate and loperamide) will be reviewed later in the chapter.

Crofelemer is an oligomeric proanthocyanidin extracted from the bark latex of the Croton tree, which is a potent inhibitor of chloride secretion.[18,19] In one placebo-controlled trial in Mexico or Jamaica, crofelemer was found to be effective in the treatment of travelers' diarrhea, reducing the duration of diarrhea by 21%.[20] The drug is currently being re-evaluated and in acute and persistent diarrhea but is as yet not approved by the US Food and Drug Administration.

Zaldaride, a calmodulin inhibitor, has shown to be similar to loperamide in two clinical trials (one in Mexico and the other in Egypt) for the treatment of traveler's diarrhea,[21–23] but the drug has not yet been marketed.

Racecadotril, an enkephalinase inhibitor, has been studied in patients with diarrhea but not in travelers. Racecadotril was shown to be comparable to loperamide in the clinical studies when used in a loading dose.[24] Racecadotril was not better than placebo in the treatment of cholera patients[25] and a recent review has suggested that further research is needed to determine the proper role of this drug in diarrhea treatment.[26,27] These data and the lack of studies in traveler's diarrhea disallow a recommendation for the treatment of diarrhea in travelers.

Adsorbents

In general, adsorbents are safe and may have benefit in the treatment of travelers' diarrhea by making stools more formed, but they are less effective than other symptomatic agents.

This class includes a great variety of substances, including activated charcoal, calcium polycarbophil, kaolin and pectin, hydrated aluminum-magnesium silicate, the combination of tannin albuminate and ethacridine lactate, and other clay-like compounds.

Activated charcoal and calcium polycarbophil have shown mixed results in cases with nonspecific diarrhea[9,28–31] but have not been effective in the treatment of travelers' diarrhea (DuPont HL and Ericsson CD, personal communication).

Kaolin/pectin was shown increase the form of stools in subjects with traveler's diarrhea (DuPont HL and Ericsson CD, personal communication) as well as nonspecific diarrhea.[9]

Attapulgite, a hydrated aluminium-magnesium silicate, has been studied in nonspecific diarrhea patients.[32] Also, it was safe but not better than loperamide in a study of traveler's diarrhea.[33]

Tannin albuminate plus ethacridine lactate was found to be superior to activated charcoal in alleviating symptoms of diarrhea illness in travelers visiting Turkey.[28]

Dioctahedral smectite (Smectite) and other natural clay compounds[34] are able to adsorb microorganisms in vitro. Smectite has been shown to be effective in the therapy of infectious diarrhea in children, mainly in developing countries,[35,36] but it has not been studied in the treatment of traveler's diarrhea.

Bismuth Subsalicylate

As mention above, bismuth subsalicylate (BSS) is one of the compounds that has multiple mechanisms of action. The salicylate shows antisecretory activity, and the bismuth moiety posses antimicrobial properties.[37–39] BSS has been available for near a century and it has a proven safety record. Its prophylactic activity is reviewed in Chapter 20, "Prophylactic Use of Drugs."

Several clinical trials have shown the benefit of BSS in traveler's diarrhea.[40–44] The sentinel placebo-controlled study[40] was done in US travelers to Mexico, showing a 16% reduction in passage of unformed stools in the group treated with the current recommended dose of 4.2 g (or 8 oz) of BSS over 4 hours, especially in those travelers infected with different strains of diarrheagenic *Escherichia coli*, the most common pathogen associated with traveler's diarrhea in this part of the world.[45] Also, it is important to mention that BSS did not prolong the infection by invasive microorganisms such as *Shigella* spp. The same modest but statistically significant result was confirmed later in a second study of travelers with diarrhea acquired while visiting West Africa or Mexico.[43]

A third study[44] compared BSS to loperamide in Mexico and other Latin America countries and demonstrated that loperamide afforded a 42% reduction of number of unformed stools passed compared with a lower 16 to 18% reduction for BSS.

In general, BSS is more effective than placebo and although it is not as effective as loperamide, it has a role in the treatment of mild to moderate episodes of travelers' diarrhea. Some important limitations of this drug are: it is not widely available in Europe and Oceania, it could produce salicylate toxicity in persons taking other salicylates as well as BSS, and it gives a black stain to the tongue and stools (harmless bismuth sulfide) in treated patients.[37,38]

Loperamide

The primary effect of loperamide is related to its antimotility effects. Loperamide also possess minor antisecretory activity.[13]

Loperamide has an excellent safety profile and is generally well tolerated. The University of Texas research program has evaluated the effectiveness of loperamide in traveler's diarrhea occurring in Mexico. This study confirmed the activity of loperamide along with additive effects when combined with trimethoprim-sulfamethoxazole.[46] In other studies of therapy among travelers to Mexico, loperamide was shown to more effectively control diarrhea than BSS.[41–44]

There has been an increased interest in combining loperamide with an antimicrobial agent, as outlined in Table 2. In early studies trimethoprim/sulfamethoxazole was combined with loperamide.[46,47] Most of the studies have shown that this combination could reduce the duration of diarrhea in travelers to a matter of few hours.[46–49] Loperamide plus quinolones (ciprofloxacin or ofloxacin)[46–49] or azithromycin in travelers to Mexico (Ericsson CD, personal communication), and loperamide plus ciprofloxacin in native population in Thailand[50] have demonstrated that the combination of both drugs was better than either drug alone. More recently, a new clinical trial combining loperamide with rifaximin, a novel nonabsorbed ($<$ 0.4%) antimicrobial agent, has also shown additive drug effects in the treatment of diarrhea among travelers to Mexico.[51]

Two studies carried out in Asia or Africa have not shown important additive effects by combing loperamide with ciprofloxacin in the treatment of travelers' diarrhea.[52,53]

Based on findings that loperamide offers rapid relief of symptoms while antibacterial drugs cure the infection

Table 2 Clinical Trials of the Combination of Loperamide with an Antimicrobial Agent

Loperamide plus	Study	Results	Reference
TMP/SMX	Randomized, double-blind, placebo controlled trial of: single dose of TMP/SMX (320/1,600 mg), or 3 days of loperamide alone, TMP/SMX (160/800 mg BID) alone, or the combination of both, for traveler's diarrhea in Mexico	Combination of loperamide and TMP/SMX showed the shortest duration of diarrhea	46
	Randomized, double-blind trial of 3 days loperamide PLUS 3 days of TMP/SMX (160/800 mg BID), or one single large dose of TMP/SMX (320/1,600 mg), or a large loading dose followed by 3 days of regular dose of TMP/SMX, for traveler's diarrhea in Mexico	Combination of loperamide and a large loading dose of TMP/SMX followed by 3 days standard doses was the most efficacious one	47
Ciprofloxacin	Randomized, double-blind, placebo-controlled trial of 3 days of ciprofloxacin (500 mg BID) PLUS loperamide or placebo, for adults with bacillary dysentery in Thailand	Combination of ciprofloxacin and loperamide showed the less median duration of diarrhea	50
	Randomized, double-blind, placebo-controlled trial of 3 days of ciprofloxacin (500 mg BID) PLUS loperamide or placebo, for military personnel with diarrhea in Egypt	Combination of loperamide and ciprofloxacin was not better than ciprofloxacin alone	52
	Randomized trial of single large dose of ciprofloxacin PLUS placebo, single large dose of ciprofloxacin (750 mg) with loperamide or 3 days of ciprofloxacin (500 mg BID) and placebo for military personnel with diarrhea in Thailand	The three treatment groups showed similar duration of diarrheal illness	53
Ofloxacin	Randomized, evaluator-blinded trial of single dose of ofloxacin (400 mg) alone or with 3 days of loperamide, or 3 days of ofloxacin (200 mg BID), for traveler's diarrhea in Mexico	Combination of single dose of loxacin plus loperamide showed less duration of diarrhea	48
	Randomized trial of loperamide PLUS single large dose of ofloxacin (400 mg) or loading dose of ofloxacin (400 mg) followed by 3 days of regular dose of ofloxacin (200 mg BID), for traveler's diarrhea in Mexico	The two treatment groups showed similar duration of diarrheal illness	49
Azithromycin	Trial of single dose of azithromycin (500 mg) with loperamide for traveler's diarrhea in Mexico	Combination of azithromycin and loperamide was more efficacious, showing less duration of diarrhea	*
Rifaximin	Randomized, double-blind trial of 3 days of rifaximin (200 mg TID), 2 days of loperamide, or the combination of both medications, for traveler's diarrhea in Mexico	Combination of rifaximin and loperamide was more efficacious, showing less duration of diarrhea and faster improvement	51

BID = twice a day; TID = three times a day; TMP/SMX = trimethoprim/sulfamethoxazole.
*C. D. Ericsson, personal communication.

and shorten the duration of diarrhea, many travel medicine experts recommend the combination of loperamide and antibacterial therapy in the treatment of most cases of traveler's diarrhea.

In conclusion, two nonantimicrobial agents are available and useful for treating traveler's diarrhea: BSS and loperamide. BSS has been shown to reduce the passage of loose stools by 16 to 18% and it should be reserved for the treatment of milder cases of watery, nonfebrile, nondysenteric traveler's diarrhea. Loperamide appears to represent the most effective symptomatic antidiarrheal drug showing an approximately 50% reduction in the passage of unformed stools, and has been especially useful in combination with antimicrobial agents. Additional study is needed with the more physiologic antisecretory drugs alone and in combination with antibacterial agents in the treatment of travelers' diarrhea.

Acknowledgment

I would like to thank my mentors and friends, Dr. H.L. DuPont and Dr. C. D. Ericsson.

References

1. Ericsson CD. Non antimicrobial agents in the prevention and treatment of traveler's diarrhea. Clin Infect Dis 2005; 41(Suppl 8):S557–63.
2. Ericsson CD, DuPont HL, Johnson PC. Non-antibiotic therapy for travelers' diarrhea. Rev Infect Dis 1986;8(Suppl 2):S202–6.
3. DuPont HL, Ericsson CD. Prevention and treatment of travelers' diarrhea. N Engl J Med 1993;328:1821–7.
4. Gorbach SL, Edelman R. Travelers' diarrhea: National Institutes of Health Consensus Development Conference. Rev Infect Dis 1986;8(Suppl 2):S109–S233.

5. Diemert DJ. Prevention and self-treatment of traveler's diarrhea. Clin Microb Rev 2006;19:583–94.
6. Kean BH. The diarrhea of travelers to Mexico: summary of five year study. Ann Intern Med 1963;59:605–14.
7. Stransky M, Schwarzenbach FH. Double-blind study of difenoxin hydrochloride among travelers to tropical countries. Ther Umsch 1979;36:267–70.
8. Steffen R. Special consideration of clinical and traveling medical criteria. Arzneimittelforschung 1979;29:685–8.
9. Alestig K, Trollfors B, K. S. Acute non-specific diarrhea, studies on the use of charcoal, kaolin-pectin and diphenoxylate. Practitioner 1979;222:859–62.
10. Cornett JWD, Aspeling RL, Mallegol D. A double-blind comparative evaluation of loperamide versus diphenoxylate with atropine in acute diarrhea. Curr Ther Res 1977;21: 629–37.
11. Palmer KR, Corbett CL, Holdsworth CD. Double-blind cross-over study comparing loperamide, codeine and diphenoxylate in the treatment of chronic diarrhea. Gastroenterology 1980;79:1272–5.
12. Lustman F, Walters EG, Shroff NE, Akber TA. Diphenoxylate hydrochloride (Lomotil) in the treatment of acute diarrhoea. Br J Clin Pract 1987;41:646–51.
13. Ericsson CD, Johnson PC. Safety and efficacy of loperamide. Am J Med 1990;88(Suppl 6A):S105–45.
14. DuPont HL, Hornick BB. Adverse effect of Lomotil therapy in shigellosis. JAMA 1973;226:1525–8.
15. Reves RR, Bass P, DuPont HL, et al. Failure to demonstrate effectiveness of an anticholinergic drug in the symptomatic treatment of acute travelers' diarrhea. J Clin Gastroenterol 1983;5:223–7.
16. Schoen AM. Tincture of opium. N Engl J Med 1984;310: 1124.
17. Kramer P. Effect of antidiarrheal and antimotility drugs in ileal excreta. Am J Dig Dis 1977;22:327–32.
18. Fischer H, Machen TE, Widdicombe JH, et al. A novel extract SB-300 from the stem bark latex of *Croton lechleri* inhibits CFTR-mediated chloride secretion in human colonic epithelial cells. J Ethnopharmacol 2004;93:351–7.
19. Gabriel SE, Davenport SE, Steagall RJ, et al. A novel plant-derived inhibitor of cAMP-mediated fluid and chloride secretion. Am J Physiol 1999;276:G58–63.
20. DiCesare D, DuPont HL, Mathewson JJ, et al. A double blind, randomized, placebo-controlled study of SP-303 (Provir) in the symptomatic treatment of acute diarrhea among travelers to Jamaica and Mexico. Am J Gastroenterol 2002;97:2585–8.
21. Okhuysen PC, DuPont HL, Ericsson CD, et al. Zaldaride malaete (a new calmodulin antagonist) versus loperamide in the treatment of travelers' diarrhea: randomized, placebo-controlled trial. Clin Infect Dis 1995;21:341–4.
22. DuPont HL, Ericsson CD, Mathewson JJ, et al. Zaldaride maleate, an intestinal calmodulin inhibitor, in the therapy of traveler's diarrhea. Gastroenterology 1993;104: 709–15.
23. Silberschmidt G, Schick MT, Steffen R, et al. Treatment of travelers' diarrhea: zaldaride compared with loperamide and placebo. Eur J Gastroenterol Hepatol 1995;7:871–5.
24. Prado D, Global Racecadotril Study Group. A multinational comparison of racecadotril and loperamide in the treatment of acute watery diarrhoea in adults. Scand J Gastroenterol 2002;37:656–61.
25. Alam NH, Ashraf H, Khan WA, et al. Efficacy and tolerability of racecadotril in the treatment of cholera in adults: a double blind, randomised, controlled clinical trial. Gut 2003;52:1419–23.
26. Huighebaert S, Awouters F, Tytgat GN. Racecadotril versus loperamide: antidiarrheal research revisited. Dig Dis Sci 2003;48:239–50.
27. Farthing MJ. Antisecretory drugs for diarrheal disease. Dig Dis 2006;24:47–58.
28. Ziegenhagen DJ, Raedsch R, Kruis W. Traveler's diarrhea in Turkey. Prospective randomized therapeutic comparison of charcoal versus tannin albuminate/ethacridine lactate. Med Klin (Munich) 1992;87:637–9.
29. Danhof IE. Pharmacology, toxicology, clinical efficacy, and adverse effects of Calcium polycarbophil, an enteral hydrosorptive agent. Pharmacotherapy 1982;2:18–28.
30. Toskes PP, Gonnery KL, Ritchey TW. Calcium polycarbophil compared with placebo in irritable bowel syndrome. Aliment Pharmacol Ther 1993;7:87–92.
31. Chiba T, Kudara N, Sato M, et al. Colonic transit, bowel movements, stool form, and abdominal pain in irritable bowel syndrome by treatment with calcium polycarbophil. Hepatogastroenterology 2005;52:1416–20.
32. Zaid MR, Hasen M, Khan AA. Attapulgite in the treatment of acute diarrhea: a double-blind placebo-controlled study. J Diarrhoeal Dis Res 1995;13:44–6.
33. DuPont HL, Ericsson CD, DuPont MW, et al. A randomized, open-label comparison of nonprescription loperamide and attapulgite in the symptomatic treatment of acute diarrhea. Am J Med 1990;88(Suppl 6A):20S–3S.
34. Vermeer DE, Ferrel RF Jr. Nigerian geophagical clay: a traditional antidiarrheal pharmaceutical. Science 1985;227: 634–6.
35. Gaurino A, Bisceglia M, Castellucci G, et al. Smectite in the treatment of acute diarrhea: a nationwide randomized controlled study of the Italian Society of Pediatric Gastroenterology and Hepatology (SIGEP) in collaboration with primary care pediatricians. SIGEP study group for smectite in acute diarrhea. J Pediatr Gastroenterol Nutr 2001;32:71–5.

36. Seajewska H, Dziechciarz P, Mrukowicz J. Meta-analysis: smective in the treatment of acute infectious diarrhoea in children. Aliment Pharmacol Ther 2006;23:217–27.

37. Ericsson CD. Bismuth subsalicylate in the treatment and chemoprophylaxis of travelers diarrhea in adults. Drug Therapy 1990;6:31–5.

38. Rao G, Aliwalas MG, Slaymaker E, Brown B. Bismuth revisited: an effective way to prevent travelers' diarrhea. J Travel Med 2004;11:239–41.

39. Ericsson CD, Tannenbaum C, Charles TT. Antisecretory and anti-inflammatory properties of bismuth subsalicylate. Rev Infect Dis 1990;12(Suppl 1):S16–20.

40. DuPont HL, Sullivan P, Pickering LK, et al. Symptomatic treatment of diarrhea with bismuth subsalicylate among students attending a Mexican university. Gastroenterology 1977;73:715–8.

41. DuPont HL, Sanchez JF, Ericsson CD, et al. Comparative efficacy of loperamide hydrochloride and bismuth subsalicylate in the management of acute diarrhea. Am J Med 1990;88(Suppl 6A):15S–9S.

42. Steffen R. Worldwide efficacy of bismuth subsalicylate in the treatment of travelers' diarrhea. Rev Infect Dis 1990;6: 153–7.

43. Steffen R, Mathewson JJ, Ericsson CD, et al. Travelers' diarrhea in tourists in West Africa and in students in Mexico: comparison of fecal transport systems and evaluation of liquid bismuth subsalicylate for therapy. J Infect Dis 1988;157:1008–13.

44. Johnson PC, Ericsson CD, DuPont HL, et al. Comparison of loperamide with bismuth subsalicylate for the treatment of acute travelers' diarrhea. JAMA 1986;255:757–60.

45. Adachi JA, Jiang ZD, Mathewson JJ, et al. Enteroaggregative *Escherichia coli* as a major etiologic agent in traveler's diarrhea in 3 regions of the world. Clin Infect Dis 2001;32:1706–9.

46. Ericsson CD, DuPont HL, Mathewson JJ, et al. Treatment of traveler's diarrhea with sulfamethoxazole and trimethoprim and loperamide JAMA, 1990;263:257–61.

47. Ericsson CD, Nicholls-Vasquez I, DuPont HL, et al. Optimal dosing of trimethoprim/sulfamethoxazole when used with loperamide to treat travelers' diarrhea. Antimicrol Agents Chemother 1992;36:2821–4.

48. Ericsson CD, DuPont HL, Mathewon JJ. Single dose ofloxacin plus loperamide compared with single dose or three days of ofloxacin in the treatment of traveler's diarrhea. J Trav Med 1997;4:3–7.

49. Ericsson CD, DuPont HL, Mathewson JJ. Optimal dosing of ofloxacin with loperamide in the treatment of non-dysenteric travelers' diarrhea. J Travel Med 2001;6:207–9.

50. Murphy GS, Bodhidatta L, Echeverria P, et al. Ciprofloxacin and loperamide in the treatment of bacillary dysentery. Ann Intern Med 1993;118:582–6.

51. DuPont HL, Jiang Z-D, Belkind-Gerson J, et al. Treatment of travelers' diarrhea: randomized trial comparing rifaximin, rifaximin plus loperamide, and loperamide alone. Clin Gastroenterol Hepatology 2007 [In press].

52. Taylor DN, Sanchez JL, Candler W, et al. Treatment of traveler's diarrhea: ciprofloxacin plus loperamide compared with ciprofloxacin alone. A placebo-controlled, randomized trial. Ann Intern Med 1991;114:731–4.

53. Petruccelli BP, Murphy GS, Sanchez JL, et al. Treatment of traveler's diarrhea with ciprofloxacin and loperamide. J Infect Dis 1992;165:557–60.

Chapter 27

Antimicrobial Therapy

David R. Tribble, MD, DrPH

Thomas Weinke, MD

The recognition of travelers' diarrhea as a distinct syndrome of primarily infectious bacterial etiology by Kean and colleagues set the stage for antimicrobial-based strategies of prevention and treatment.[1] Seminal investigations by Gorbach and colleagues documented the importance of enterotoxigenic *Escherichia coli* (ETEC) as the predominant pathogen leading to travelers' diarrhea.[2] Soon thereafter, numerous investigations demonstrated the impact antibiotics might have on prevention and treatment of this syndrome.[3–5] Based on therapeutic response to antibacterial therapy, it is estimated that approximately 80% of cases are due to bacterial enteropathogens.[6] Among bacterial etiologies, ETEC is commonly observed as the major cause on a global basis; however, important regional and seasonal differences exist.[6–11]

Antimicrobial Therapy Contribution to Overall Management

The management approach in acute bacterial diarrhea involves a primary clinical assessment, consideration and potential application of laboratory analysis, and a plan for assessing therapeutic response. Immediate assessment of fluid status with timely rehydration therapy is the cornerstone of diarrheal management. The decision to treat with medications, nonspecific antidiarrheal and/or an antimicrobial agent is based on illness severity assessment (often placed in the context of an individual's activities) or the results of screening or pathogen-specific lab tests. The nonspecific antidiarrheal medications fall into one of the three classes (adsorbents, antisecretory or antimotility) based on mechanism of action.[12] These agents are often all that is necessary for mild to moderate acute diarrhea. Further information is provided in Chapter 27, "Symptomatic Therapy."

Antibiotics have been demonstrated to reduce symptom duration in travelers' diarrhea from an average of 50 to 93 hours to 16 to 30 hours.[12–16] Antibiotic therapy has also been demonstrated to be efficacious in moderate to severe acute bacterial diarrhea in community-based studies in industrialized countries, shigellosis, and early treatment of campylobacteriosis (< 72 hours).[12,17–26] Antibiotic treatment is justified by more rapid abatement of symptoms during the acute process as well as potentially preventing postinfectious sequelae ranging from rare complications such as reactive arthritis or Guillain-Barré syndrome to more common postinfectious irritable bowel syndrome.[27–30] Empiric antibiotic therapy is the usual approach given the typical lack of a definitive etiologic agent at the time of primary assessment. Diarrhea management algorithms have been proposed to assist the clinician in targeting antibiotic therapy toward patients that would most benefit and limiting antibiotic-related risks and costs in patients with a brief self-limited mild illness.[13,14] Clinicians responsible for caring for patients with diarrhea should become familiar with the potential pathogen exposures in their target patient population, natural history of these enteropathogens with or without antibiotic therapy, availability and test performance characteristics of relevant lab tests, and antimicrobial resistance patterns of the primary enteropathogen threats. Special circumstances such as outbreaks and refugee medicine require an even greater structured approach to surveillance, triage, and attention to comorbid illnesses and resource allocation. In the field of travel medicine, the most common application of antimicrobial therapy for traveler's diarrhea is likely by self medication. Further discussion of approaches to empiric self treatment of acute traveler's diarrhea and post-travel management in the returning traveler are provided in Chapter 29,

"Approach to Prolonged Diarrhea in the Returning Traveler."

Evolution of Treatment Recommendations

Treatment recommendations have evolved related to availability of new agents; however, changes in management have frequently been driven by a continued need to seek alternative antibiotics following emergence of resistance. Antibiotic treatment trials in civilian and military travelers to developing regions fulfilling criteria for travelers' diarrhea have provided much of the current knowledge required to design empiric therapeutic regimens. An important observation when considering empiric travelers' diarrhea therapy is the self-limited placebo cure rates by 72 hours of approximately 50 to 60%.[31] Early trials were frequently performed using a placebo group in order to assure the active drug led to therapeutic benefit. This finding has now repeatedly demonstrated that antimicrobial therapy provides approximately a 34- to 63-hour reduction in duration of illness.

Not unlike many other infectious diseases, etiologic agents of travelers' diarrhea have demonstrated an ability to acquire resistance to antibiotics commonly used in empiric therapy. An extensive series of clinical trial investigations have been undertaken by DuPont, Ericsson, and colleagues in students traveling to Mexico,[3,32–46] Department of Defense investigators among military personnel on deployment to either Thailand or Egypt,[47–50] and other investigators[51,52] to establish efficacy for various antibiotics and regimens. Trials have also provided evidence of diminished efficacy of empiric regimens, such as ampicillin, as the bacteria develop resistance.[33] Initial studies documented efficacy of trimethoprim-sulfamethoxazole (TMP/SMX) in various regimens, both alone and in combination with loperamide, resulting in common use throughout the 1980s and early 1990s.[36,38,53,54] Increasing TMP/SMX antimicrobial resistance and the introduction of the fluoroquinolone antibiotics in the late 1980s led to several investigations to establish alternative regimens.[55] During the 1990s, increasing fluoroquinolone resistance among *Campylobacter* species prompted studies to evaluate the macrolide antibiotic azithromycin, which has now been demonstrated to have equal efficacy to fluoroquinolone antibiotics.[46,49] Early trials also demonstrated the efficacy of nonabsorbable antibiotics in treatment of travelers' diarrhea, including bicozamycin, aztreonam, and nifuroxazide, after initial lack of efficacy with oral neomycin in pediatric shigellosis.[32,39,56,57] Treatment and prevention strategies using nonabsorbed antibiotics have been revived with the rifamycin derivative, rifaximin.[43,45,56,58–61] This agent has been in use since 1987 in Europe for several gastrointestinal (GI)-related disorders including infectious diarrhea, *Clostridium difficile*-associated diarrhea, small intestinal bacterial overgrowth syndrome, and hepatic encephalopathy.[60]

Initial studies investigated empiric regimens with treatment duration of 5 days to establish efficacy.[20,37,53,54] Multiple daily doses or longer courses of therapy add to a regimen's inconvenience and increase likelihood of noncompliance. Given these concerns, studies have been undertaken to establish efficacy with shorter less cumbersome regimens.[36,38,42,44,52] Shorter duration of antibiotic therapy has been demonstrated to be equally effective for 3- versus 5-day regimens, as it has shown good results with single-dose therapy. [36,38,42,44,50,52]

Currently Recommended Antimicrobial Agents

FLUOROQUINOLONES

Fluoroquinolones remain active against most bacterial enteropathogens such as ETEC, *Shigella*, and *Salmonella*.[62,63] Fluoroquinolone-resistant travel-associated and domestic *Campylobacter* cases in industrialized countries have been increasingly reported and not restricted to countries such as Thailand and Spain.[64–66] *Campylobacter* species have also been well documented to develop in vivo resistance during therapy with fluoroquinolones.[67,68] In addition to antimicrobial resistance concerns with *Campylobacter*, nontyphoidal *Salmonella* isolates with reduced quinolone susceptibility have been documented in travelers returning from Southeast Asia (most commonly Thailand) with increasing nalidixic acid resistance in Thailand.[69–71] Ciprofloxacin resistance remains very low in *Salmonella* and *Shigella* isolates from Europe and Latin America; however, nalidixic acid resistance rates of 5 to 16% are concerning.[72] This is of concern given the association between nalidixic acid (NA) resistance and decreased FQ susceptibility.[73] NA resistance was also documented in 6% of ETEC isolates from traveler's diarrhea cases in India as well as rare fluoroquinolone resistance.[74]

The recommended standard empiric antibiotic therapy for travelers' diarrhea is a 1- to 3-day course with a fluoroquinolone.[12,14] As mentioned previously, several studies investigating fluoroquinolone antibiotics have demonstrated efficacy across 3- and 5-day regimen ranges.[35,37,42,44,75] Single-dose fluoroquinolone therapy has also been shown to have equal effectiveness in 3- or 5-day regimens for travelers' diarrhea, as well as specific therapy for shigellosis (not *Shigella dysenteriae*).[19–21,42,48,52] Important caveats when considering short-course or even single-dose fluoroquinolone therapy for travelers' diarrhea include the frequent finding of quinolone-resistant *Campylobacter jejuni* and the greatly reduced cure rates in *S. dysenteriae* using short-course therapy (although a very infrequent cause of travelers' diarrhea).[21] Ciprofloxacin was the first fluoroquinolone studied for travelers' diarrhea treatment[35,47,48] and was soon followed by other antibiotics in this class to include norfloxacin, ofloxacin, and levofloxacin with similar documented efficacy.[24,42,44,46,50,51,76,77]

There are many favorable features of fluoroquinolone pharmacokinetics leading to broad application for treatment of infectious GI syndromes. These include excellent oral bioavailability (70 to 96%) and fecal levels 100- to 1,000-fold greater than in serum.[78] In addition, once daily dosing is possible given the long half-life of these agents. Providers should be aware of the potential for reduced bioavailability of fluoroquinolones during coadministration with magnesium- or aluminum-containing antacids or ferrous sulfate.[79]

Fluoroquinolones are generally well tolerated, with most adverse effects being mild and transient GI (such as nausea, vomiting, or diarrhea) or central nervous system (such as headache, dizziness, or insomnia) side effects shared by all quinolones.[80–82] The incidence of GI symptoms ranges from 2 to 20% but most typically less than 5% and drug-related central nervous system (CNS) effects in approximately 1 to 2%.[82] *C. difficile*-associated diarrhea has also been reported with fluoroquinolone use.[83,84] Dermatologic side effects can also occur and are typically self-limited rash and/or pruritus in less than 3% and uncommon phototoxic reactions in less than 0.5%.[82] Musculoskeletal adverse events occur uncommonly and may include arthropathy or tendinopathy (including tendon rupture more often seen in association with renal disease and corticosteroid use).[85] Postmarketing surveillance, particularly observed with gatifloxacin in elderly patients, documented uncommon hypo- or hyperglycemic reactions more often in diabetic patients in the range of 6 to 13 per 1,000 persons, but also observed in nondiabetic patients at lower rates, 0.07 to .03 per 1,000 persons.[82] Prolongation of the QT interval has been rarely observed related to fluoroquinolone therapy and may lead to fatal dysryhthmias.[86,87] These side effects are much less common but have serious consequences. The adverse event profile should be factored into the decision to use these agents for travelers' diarrhea treatment. Also, consideration should be given to the potential for drug interactions in a given patient.[79]

AZITHROMYCIN

A recent multisite survey of azithromycin susceptibility in bacterial enteropathogens (predominantly ETEC, enteroaggregative E. coli, *Salmonella*, and *Shigella*) demonstrated minimum inhibitory concentration $(MIC)_{90}$ of 0.0625 μg/mL providing greater confidence for clinical use.[88] Surveys in Thailand in the 1990s documented azithromycin resistance in 4 to 15% of ETEC, 3 to 5% of *Salmonella*, and 2 to 8% of *Shigella* isolates, highlighting the importance of continued surveillance.[71,89] Azithromycin is more potent than other antibiotics against enteropathogenic *Campylobacter* species with MIC_{90} of 0.12 μg/mL.[72] *Campylobacter* species have maintained a relatively stable level of macrolide resistance around 5%; although, a higher rate of resistance is seen with the less common species *C. coli* as compared to *C. jejuni*.[72,90]

Azithromycin has been proposed as an alternative therapy for patients unable to take quinolones or travelers to areas with known high *Campylobacter* endemicity.[62,63] Azithromycin 500 mg daily was compared with ciprofloxacin 500 mg daily (each 3-day regimens) for diarrhea in US service personnel during Cobra Gold 1993 (military exercise in Thailand) and was found to have comparable efficacy.[49] There were only two clinical failures in the entire study group, both being ciprofloxacin-treated *Campylobacter* cases. Significant differences in improved microbiologic eradication of *Campylobacter* were demonstrated with azithromycin; however, this did not translate into statistically significant clinical differences. A trial in Bangladesh was conducted comparing azithromycin (500 mg initially then 250 mg daily over 5 days—total 1.5 gm) with ciprofloxacin 500 mg twice daily for 3 days in patients treated with shigellosis, and found the regimens comparable.[23] A single 1 gm dose of azithromycin was also compared with a 3-day course of ciprofloxacin in patients with shigellosis, and again the results were comparable.[91] A single-dose azithromycin regimen was efficacious in travelers to Mexico.[46] In this study, azithromycin recipients had ETEC recovered in 52%, *Shigella* in 5%, no *Campylobacter*, time to last unformed stool < 24 hours, no apparent increase in nausea/vomiting over levofloxacin comparator group, microbiologic eradication in 58%, and 9.5% treatment failures. In a follow-on trial in US military in Thailand, azithromycin was demonstrated to be the preferred antibiotic over levofloxacin for traveler's diarrhea empiric treatment in Thailand.[50] A single 1 g dose led to a 96% cure at 72 hours as compared to 85% with a 3-day regimen and 71% with levofloxacin. Single-dose azithromycin also had the shortest median time to last unformed stool (TLUS) at 35 hours.

Azithromycin, an azalide antibiotic, has favorable pharmacokinetics for single-dose use with an average half-life of 11 to 14 hours after a single 500 mg dose achieving high tissue concentrations.[92,93] Oral bioavailability of azithromycin (500 mg dose) is approximately 37%; however, on average 46% of active drug is nonabsorbed and passed in the feces.[94] The elimination dynamics provide theoretic advantage in the treatment of bacterial enteritis. Estimated GI luminal levels of azithromycin exceed 200 μg/mL in the 6-hour period after a 500 mg dose.[94] These levels far exceed the MIC_{90} of common enteric pathogens.[95]

Azithromycin is generally well tolerated, with minimal side effects consisting mainly of GI complaints.[95–100] In a study of 3,995 patients receiving azithromycin, 5-day regimen (total 1.5 gm) or single dose (1 gm), were less likely to report side-effects, 12% versus 14%, as compared to 3,108 patients receiving one of 12 other antibiotics (such as penicillin, amoxicillin, erythromycin, doxycycline, cephalexin, and cefaclor).[101] The most common symptoms were diarrhea (3.6%), abdominal pain (2.5%), nausea (2.6%), vomiting (0.8%), and headaches and dizziness (1.3%), all of which occurred less frequently than with the comparison antibiotics.[102] The only side effects occurring more commonly than the standard comparison antibiotics were vaginitis (0.4%) and rash (0.6%). The only laboratory abnormality noted was a mild, transient increase in the hepatic transaminases in 1.7% of patients. Only 0.7% of patients receiving the 5-day course discontinued the drug due to side effects. Single-dose azithromycin (1,250 mg weekly) for *Mycobacterium avium* complex prophylaxis in acquired immunodeficiency syndrome (AIDS) patients is discontinued in approximately 6% due to GI side effects.[103] Further suggestion of azithromycin dose-related GI side effect relationship is the 34% GI complaint rate observed in a study assessing gonorrhea therapy using a particularly large, single dose of 2 gm.[98] Assessment of GI side effects during a travelers' diarrhea treatment trial demonstrated new-onset nausea in 8 to 17% (higher in the 1-gm dose recipients) that was mild and of brief duration.[50] The GI side effects observed among azithromycin recipients in this study are higher than reported nausea rates for both 500 mg (3-day) and 1 gm single dose regimens in azithromycin treatment trials of non-GI infections, 3% and < 1%, respectively.[102,104,105] The higher rates are likely due to the exacerbating effect of the primary illness. Given the improved efficacy, likely improved compliance, and ease of dosing schedule, the mild side effects would seem to be outweighed toward selection of the single-dose regimen. Comparable efficacy may be achieved, with potentially lower GI side effect rates, using single doses less than 1,000 mg; however, this remains to be determined.

Rifaximin

Poorly absorbed antibiotics providing topical treatment and microbiological eradication have been studied for several mucosal infectious disease syndromes including acute infectious diarrhea. Oral bicozamycin and aztreonam, nonabsorbed antibiotics, have demonstrated treatment efficacy in travelers' diarrhea but were not further developed.[32,39] The rifamycin derivative, rifaximin, has been studied in several clinical trials documenting efficacy as an alternative agent for a patient with watery diarrhea and low risk of an invasive pathogen.[43,45,59,61,106] Rifaximin is almost completely nonabsorbed with measured blood levels less than 1% in both healthy patients and patients with ulcerative colitis.[107–109]

Promising data thus far, over several years of clinical use, have not documented induction of resistance that leads to lack of clinical efficacy. Rifaximin has moderately high MIC values as evidenced by MIC_{90} of 50 μg/mL for bacterial enteropathogens isolated in a study in travelers to Mexico.[110] In this study, the majority of the isolates were ETEC (83%) with lower proportion of *Shigella* (12%) and *Salmonella* (5.5%). Notably, the fecal levels of rifaximin achieved in these patients receiving a 400 mg twice daily (BID) regimen for 3 days was on average 7,961 μg/g of stool on the first day post treatment. Microbiological eradication for ETEC occurs at a lower rate, 77%, as compared to ciprofloxacin, 93%.[58] In addition, there is a relatively high rate, 53%, of ≥ fourfold rise in MIC post treatment in ETEC isolates, although the reduced susceptibility did not impact clinical response and traditional susceptibility breakpoints cannot be established. Induction of rifampin resistance in *Mycobacterium (M.) tuberculosis* is also a concern with this rifamycin derivative; however, in vitro experiments did not identify emergent rifampin resistance in *M. tuberculosis* strains.[111] Rifaximin has also not shown increases in antimicrobial resistant GI flora or enterococci during treatment.[112] Continued surveillance for clinically significant enteropathogen resistance will be needed as rifaximin has broader clinical use.

Rifaximin has recently been approved for use in *E. coli*-induced, noninvasive travelers' diarrhea.[56,113,114] Four randomized controlled trials employing both placebo and comparator treatments have definitively demonstrated rifaximin efficacy in the majority of cases of travelers' diarrhea with TLUS ranging from 22 to 32 hours from first antibiotic dose.[43,45,58,59] Superiority was observed against TMP/SMX in one trial[43] and equivalence with ciprofloxacin in two trials in varied locations.[45,58] Rifaximin efficacy has been documented in twice- and thrice-daily dosing regimens. Rifaximin does not adequately treat invasive pathogens, which account for approximately 20% of travelers' diarrhea cases, such as *Campylobacter*, *Salmonella*, and *Shigella*; therefore, it cannot be recommended for areas where these invasive pathogens have been shown to frequently cause diarrhea.[58,61,106] Rifaximin was ineffective in *Campylobacter* cases with only 23.5% clinical cures as detailed in the package insert making this a poor choice for an area such as Thailand. A recently published study demonstrated greater than 50% of patients with invasive pathogens failing to achieve wellness with rifaximin therapy.[58] This result is in contrast to earlier efficacy demonstrated against mild invasive infection and shigellosis with the nonabsorbed antibiotics bicozamycin and aztreonam.[32,39] Rifaximin did demonstrate efficacy in prevention of experimental shigellosis.[115]

The safety for this agent has been excellent as might be anticipated due the lack of systemic absorption. There is also no concern for drug interactions, unlike rifampin, given the lack of activation of cytochrome P_{450} (CYP_{450}) isoenzymes.[60] Rifaximin is contraindicated in patients with known hypersensitivity to rifamycin agents. Rifaximin had an equal frequency of adverse events observed as both placebo and ciprofloxacin in travelers' diarrhea trials.[58]

COMBINATION ANTIMICROBIAL AND LOPERAMIDE THERAPY

To minimize the impact of travelers' diarrhea, empiric treatment regimens consisting of an appropriate antibiotic and the antimotility agent loperamide have been recommended. Nonantibiotic antidiarrheal therapy with antimotility agents, such as loperamide, leads to more rapid clinical recovery when used as an adjunct to antibiotics. This observation has been demonstrated in ETEC-predominant areas with TMP/SMX and fluoroquinolone antibiotics.[36,38,42,44,47] These studies have documented the potential of combined antibiotic and loperamide to limit diarrhea duration to less than 12 hours. An earlier study in Thailand, a *Campylobacter*-predominant region, did not demonstrate added benefit with loperamide plus ciprofloxacin.[48] No studies have been performed with and without adjunctive loperamide to assess the potential impact with either azithromycin or rifaximin.

Special Considerations

Antibiotic therapy recommendations in children and during pregnancy are limited due to lack of data from randomized controlled trials. In general, oral rehydration should be aggressively provided. Due to concerns over the possibility of cartilage/articular damage with fluoroquinolones noted in animal studies, this class of antibiotics is currently not approved in children or in pregnancy. Rifaximin is not approved for use in pregnancy and has not been studied in children younger than 12 years. Azithromycin is generally considered safe in children and when taken during pregnancy. Given current azithromycin use in children and during pregnancy, these data in acute bacterial enteritis can reasonably be extrapolated for clinical application in these populations where concerns exist for fluoroquinolone and rifaximin use. Recommended pediatric dosing is 10 mg per kg daily for 3 days.[116] An alternative agent is nalidixic acid at a dosage of 55 mg per kg per day in four divided doses (maximum per day not greater than 1 g/24 hours)[116]

Antimicrobial Selection

Important considerations in the selection of an empiric antibiotic include likelihood of treatment efficacy and rapidity of response, probable target pathogens and antimicrobial resistance regional patterns, safety and tolerance profile of the antibiotic, considerations that may impact effectiveness of the dosing regimen such as patient compliance, and cost. Table 1 details dosing regimens for currently recommended antibiotics as well as several considerations in antibiotic selection. Treatment efficacy for watery noninvasive diarrhea appears to be equal between fluoroquinolones, azithromycin, and rifaximin. There is some evidence of a more rapid therapeutic response for fluoroquinolones in the first 24 hours as compared to the other two agents.[45,46,58] Clinical illness suggestive of an invasive pathogen should prompt use of a fluoroquinolone or azithromycin rather than rifaximin. The increasing incidence of fluoroquinolone-resistant *Campylobacter* and the propensity to cause an invasive clinical syndrome argues for azithromycin over a fluoroquinolone, particularly in areas such as Thailand.[50,117] Rifaximin is most advantageous from a safety standpoint over other first-line antibiotics.

Another important consideration is the alternate uses for the antibiotic and the possibility of promoting resistance in the community as an unintended consequence. Two key strategies to maintain fluoroquinolone class efficacy are to limit use to situations where benefit has been documented and use an antibiotic with optimal activity against likely pathogens.[118] This is a sound strategy that applies to most antibiotics; however, in the case of *Campylobacter* and *Salmonella* species, the complicating concern of antibiotic usage in animal husbandry must also be considered when developing public health and patient treatment strategies to limit emergence of antibiotic resistance.[90] Antibiotic therapy should be restricted to patients with moderate to severe

Table 1 Currently Recommended Oral Antimicrobial Therapies for Travelers' Diarrhea

	Recommended Dose and Regimen	Comments
Fluoroquinolone	Ciprofloxacin 500 mg BID × 1–3 days Ciprofloxacin 500 mg (single dose) Levofloxacin 500 mg QD × 1–3 days Levofloxacin 500 mg (single dose) Norfloxacin 400 mg BID × 1–3 days Ofloxacin 400 mg BID × 1–3 days Gatifloxacin 400 mg BID × 1–3 days	Most experience and direct trial evidence for ciprofloxacin, ofloxacin, and levofloxacin; adjunctive loperamide has been shown to speed recovery with these agents; should review patient's medical history and medication profile to avoid increase risk of side effects (eg, dysglycemic reactions in diabetics, higher risk of tendinopathy in patients with renal disease or steroid use), or drug interactions; not approved for use in children < 12 years old or during pregnancy
Azithromycin	500 mg BID × 3 days 1000 mg (single dose)	First-line agent in regions with high rates of fluoroquinolone-resistant *Campylobacter* (eg, Thailand); approved for use in children and during pregnancy
Rifaximin	200 mg TID × 3 days 400 mg BID × 3 days	Do not use if invasive diarrhea; not approved for use in children < 12 years old or during pregnancy

BID = twice daily; TID = three times daily; QD = once daily.

illness, individuals at risk for poor clinical outcomes based on comorbid illnesses, or high tempo settings with complicating issues such as risk of heat-associated illness (frequently the case in deployed military personnel). Azithromycin has become a widely used antibiotic particularly for empiric treatment of acute respiratory infections.[119] A concern for broadening azithromycin indications to include acute bacterial enteritis is the development of resistance as observed with fluoroquinolone antibiotics. *C. jejuni* macrolide resistance has been relatively stable worldwide with rates of 0 to 11% (typically higher rates with *C. coli*) in contrast to progressively rising fluoroquinolone-resistance observed in many countries.[90] Fluoroquinolone and azithromycin resistance potentially increasing in enteropathogenic *E. coli*, *Salmonella*, and *Shigella* requires ongoing surveillance as well as consideration of rifaximin use in cases with watery diarrhea.

The efficacy of single-dose regimens for both fluoroquinolones and azithromycin are favorable features supporting their acceptability and promoting effective application.[42,44,46,50,52] Fluoroquinolone antibiotics remain appropriate first-line therapy in much of the developing world and rifaximin is also a reasonable first-line agent for patients presenting with watery diarrhea. As previously discussed, azithromycin should be considered the first-line agent in areas with high rates of *Campylobacter*.[116,120,121] Additional traveler's diarrhea scenarios when azithromycin should be considered first-line include children, pregnancy, and fluoroquinolone or rifamycin drug allergy or prior intolerance. In cases where either fluoroquinolone or rifaximin is used as chemoprophylaxis or for treatment and fails, then azithromycin would be an appropriate next step. Cost of treatment will vary based on antibiotic selected, regimen chosen, and pharmacy source. Based on self-pay prices from an online mail-order delivery outlet <drugstore.com> and using commonly prescribed examples the costs are relatively similar: ciprofloxacin at 500 mg BID × 3 days ($29.80), levofloxacin at 500 mg QD × 3 day ($32.74), rifaximin at 200 mg TID ($35.72), azithromycin as 1,000 mg single dose ($29.20) and azithromycin as 500 mg QD × 3 days ($43.80).

In summary, an extensive series of traveler's diarrhea treatment trials highlight several key findings: 1) self-limited placebo cure rates by 72 hours are typically as high as 50 to 60%, 2) regional antimicrobial resistance can decrease cure rates (as evidenced by ETEC and *Shigella* ampicillin resistance leading to 49% cure rate in Mexico[33] or fluoroquinolone resistance in *Campylobacter* in Thailand demonstrating 71% cure rates[50]) leading to not recommending previous empiric therapy choices such as TMP/SMX, 3) shorter duration of antibiotic therapy often equally effective (as evidenced by 3- versus 5-day regimens, as well as, good results with single-dose therapy for fluoroquinolones and azithromycin), and 4) the currently recommended travelers' diarrhea antibiotic armamentarium includes systemic antibiotics, fluoroquinolones, and azithromycin, and the nonabsorbed antibiotic, rifaximin, which all have advantages and rationale supporting their use as first-line agents in particular circumstances. Continued research to optimize current regimens and evaluate alternative agents remains important.

References

1. Kean BH. The diarrhea of travelers to Mexico. Summary of five-year study. Ann Intern Med 1963;59:605–14.
2. Gorbach SL, Kean BH, Evans DG, et al. Travelers' diarrhea and toxigenic Escherichia coli. N Engl J Med 1975;292:933–6.
3. DuPont HL, Reves RR, Galindo E, et al. Treatment of travelers' diarrhea with trimethoprim/sulfamethoxazole

and with trimethoprim alone. N Engl J Med 1982;307: 841–4.

4. DuPont HL, Evans DG, Rios N, et al. Prevention of travelers' diarrhea with trimethoprim-sulfamethoxazole. Rev Infect Dis 1982;4:533–9.

5. Sack DA, Kaminsky DC, Sack RB, et al. Prophylactic doxycycline for travelers' diarrhea. Results of a prospective double-blind study of Peace Corps volunteers in Kenya. N Engl J Med 1978;298:758–63.

6. Black RE. Epidemiology of travelers' diarrhea and relative importance of various pathogens. Rev Infect Dis 1990; 12Suppl 1:S73–9.

7. Jiang ZD, Lowe B, Verenkar MP, et al. Prevalence of enteric pathogens among international travelers with diarrhea acquired in Kenya (Mombasa), India (Goa), or Jamaica (Montego Bay). J Infect Dis 2002;185:497–502.

8. Taylor DN, Echeverria P. Etiology and epidemiology of travelers' diarrhea in Asia. Rev Infect Dis 1986;8Suppl 2:S136–41.

9. Mattila L, Siitonen A, Kyronseppa H, et al. Seasonal variation in etiology of travelers' diarrhea. Finnish-Moroccan Study Group. J Infect Dis 1992;165:385–8.

10. Ericsson CD, DuPont HL, Mathewson IJ. Epidemiologic observations on diarrhea developing in US and Mexican students living in Guadalajara, Mexico. J Travel Med 1995;2:6–10.

11. Riddle MS, Sanders JW, Putnam SD, Tribble DR. Incidence, etiology, and impact of diarrhea among long-term travelers (US military and similar populations): a systematic review. Am J Trop Med Hyg 2006;74:891–900.

12. Scarpignato C, Rampal P. Prevention and treatment of traveler's diarrhea: a clinical pharmacological approach. Chemotherapy 1995;41Suppl 1:48–81.

13. Ericsson CD. Travelers' diarrhea. Epidemiology, prevention, and self-treatment. Infect Dis Clin North Am 1998; 12:285–303.

14. Ericsson CD, DuPont HL. Travelers' diarrhea: approaches to prevention and treatment. Clin Infect Dis 1993;16:616–24.

15. Katelaris PH, Farthing MJ. Traveler's diarrhea: clinical presentation and prognosis. Chemotherapy 1995;41Suppl 1:40–7.

16. De Bruyn G, Hahn S, Borwick A. Antibiotic treatment for travellers' diarrhoea. Cochrane Database Syst Rev 2000; (3):CD002242.

17. Pichler HE, Diridl G, Stickler K, Wolf D. Clinical efficacy of ciprofloxacin compared with placebo in bacterial diarrhea. Am J Med 1987;82:329–32.

18. Dryden MS, Gabb RJ, Wright SK. Empirical treatment of severe acute community-acquired gastroenteritis with ciprofloxacin. Clin Infect Dis 1996;22:1019–25.

19. Oldfield EC 3rd, Bourgeois AL, Omar AK, Pazzaglia GL. Empirical treatment of Shigella dysentery with trimethoprim: five-day course vs. single dose. Am J Trop Med Hyg 1987;37:616–23.

20. Gotuzzo E, Oberhelman RA, Maguina C, et al. Comparison of single-dose treatment with norfloxacin and standard 5-day treatment with trimethoprim-sulfamethoxazole for acute shigellosis in adults. Antimicrob Agents Chemother 1989;33:1101–4.

21. Bennish ML, Salam MA, Khan WA, Khan AM. Treatment of shigellosis: III. Comparison of one- or two-dose ciprofloxacin with standard 5-day therapy. A randomized, blinded trial. Ann Intern Med 1992;117:727–34.

22. Murphy GS, Bodhidatta L, Echeverria P, et al. Ciprofloxacin and loperamide in the treatment of bacillary dysentery. Ann Intern Med 1993;118:582–6.

23. Khan WA, Seas C, Dhar U, et al. Treatment of shigellosis: V. Comparison of azithromycin and ciprofloxacin. A double-blind, randomized, controlled trial. Ann Intern Med 1997;126:697–703.

24. Wistrom J, Jertborn M, Ekwall E, et al. Empiric treatment of acute diarrheal disease with norfloxacin. A randomized, placebo-controlled study. Swedish Study Group. Ann Intern Med 1992;117:202–8.

25. Salazar-Lindo E, Sack RB, Chea-Woo E, et al. Early treatment with erythromycin of Campylobacter jejuni-associated dysentery in children. J Pediatr 1986;109:355–60.

26. Goodman LJ, Trenholme GM, Kaplan RL, et al. Empiric antimicrobial therapy of domestically acquired acute diarrhea in urban adults. Arch Intern Med 1990;150:541–6.

27. Nachamkin I. Chronic effects of Campylobacter infection. Microbes Infect 2002;4:399–403.

28. McDowell RM, McElvaine MD. Long-term sequelae to foodborne disease. Rev Sci Tech 1997;16:337–41.

29. Connor BA. Sequelae of traveler's diarrhea: focus on postinfectious irritable bowel syndrome. Clin Infect Dis 2005;41Suppl 8:S577–86.

30. Halvorson HA, Schlett CD, Riddle MS. Postinfectious irritable bowel syndrome—a meta-analysis. Am J Gastroenterol 2006;101:1894–9; quiz 1942.

31. DuPont HL, Cooperstock M, Corrado ML, et al. Evaluation of new anti-infective drugs for the treatment of acute infectious diarrhea. Infectious Diseases Society of America and the Food and Drug Administration. Clin Infect Dis 1992;15Suppl 1:S228–35.

32. Ericsson CD, DuPont HL, Sullivan P, et al. Bicozamycin, a poorly absorbable antibiotic, effectively treats travelers' diarrhea. Ann Intern Med 1983;98:20–5.

33. DuPont HL, Ericsson CD, Galindo E, et al. Furazolidone versus ampicillin in the treatment of traveler's diarrhea. Antimicrob Agents Chemother 1984;26:160–3.

34. Johnson PC, Ericsson CD, DuPont HL, et al. Comparison of loperamide with bismuth subsalicylate for the treatment of acute travelers' diarrhea. JAMA 1986;255:757–60.

35. Ericsson CD, Johnson PC, Dupont HL, et al. Ciprofloxacin or trimethoprim-sulfamethoxazole as initial therapy for travelers' diarrhea. A placebo-controlled, randomized trial. Ann Intern Med 1987;106:216–20.

36. Ericsson CD, DuPont HL, Mathewson JJ, et al. Treatment of traveler's diarrhea with sulfamethoxazole and trimethoprim and loperamide. JAMA 1990;263:257–61.

37. DuPont HL, Ericsson CD, Mathewson JJ, DuPont MW. Five versus three days of ofloxacin therapy for traveler's diarrhea: a placebo-controlled study. Antimicrob Agents Chemother 1992;36:87–91.

38. Ericsson CD, Nicholls-Vasquez I, DuPont HL, Mathewson JJ. Optimal dosing of trimethoprim-sulfamethoxazole when used with loperamide to treat traveler's diarrhea. Antimicrob Agents Chemother 1992;36:2821–4.

39. DuPont HL, Ericsson CD, Mathewson JJ, et al. Oral aztreonam, a poorly absorbed yet effective therapy for bacterial diarrhea in US travelers to Mexico. JAMA 1992; 267:1932–5.

40. DuPont HL, Ericsson CD, Mathewson JJ, e al. Zaldaride maleate, an intestinal calmodulin inhibitor, in the therapy of travelers' diarrhea. Gastroenterology 1993;104:709–15.

41. Okhuysen PC, DuPont HL, Ericsson CD, et al. Zaldaride maleate (a new calmodulin antagonist) versus loperamide in the treatment of traveler's diarrhea: randomized, placebo-controlled trial. Clin Infect Dis 1995;21:341–4.

42. Ericsson CD, DuPont HL, Mathewson JJ. Single dose ofloxacin plus loperamide compared with single dose or three days of ofloxacin in the treatment of traveler's diarrhea. J Travel Med 1997;4:3–7.

43. DuPont HL, Ericsson CD, Mathewson JJ, et al. Rifaximin: a nonabsorbed antimicrobial in the therapy of travelers' diarrhea. Digestion 1998;59:708–14.

44. Ericsson CD, DuPont HL, Mathewson JJ. Optimal dosing of ofloxacin with loperamide in the treatment of non-dysenteric travelers' diarrhea. J Travel Med 2001;8:207–9.

45. DuPont HL, Jiang ZD, Ericsson CD, et al. Rifaximin versus ciprofloxacin for the treatment of traveler's diarrhea: a randomized, double-blind clinical trial. Clin Infect Dis 2001;33:1807–15.

46. Adachi JA, Ericsson CD, Jiang ZD, et al. Azithromycin found to be comparable to levofloxacin for the treatment of US travelers with acute diarrhea acquired in Mexico. Clin Infect Dis 2003;37:1165–71.

47. Taylor DN, Sanchez JL, Candler W, et al. Treatment of travelers' diarrhea: ciprofloxacin plus loperamide compared with ciprofloxacin alone. A placebo-controlled, randomized trial. Ann Intern Med 1991;114:731–4.

48. Petruccelli BP, Murphy GS, Sanchez JL, et al. Treatment of traveler's diarrhea with ciprofloxacin and loperamide. J Infect Dis 1992;165:557–60.

49. Kuschner RA, Trofa AF, Thomas RJ, et al. Use of azithromycin for the treatment of Campylobacter enteritis in travelers to Thailand, an area where ciprofloxacin resistance is prevalent. Clin Infect Dis 1995;21:536–41.

50. Tribble D, Sanders J, Pang L, et al. Travelers' diarrhea in Thailand: randomized, double-blind trial comparing azithromycin-based regimens (single dose and 3-day) versus levofloxacin (3-day). Clin Infect Dis 2006; accepted for publication.

51. Mattila L, Peltola H, Siitonen A, et al. Short-term treatment of traveler's diarrhea with norfloxacin: a double-blind, placebo-controlled study during two seasons. Clin Infect Dis 1993;17:779–82.

52. Salam I, Katelaris P, Leigh-Smith S, Farthing MJ. Randomised trial of single-dose ciprofloxacin for travellers' diarrhoea. Lancet 1994;344:1537–9.

53. DuPont HL, Ericsson CD, Reves RR, Galindo E. Antimicrobial therapy for travelers' diarrhea. Rev Infect Dis 1986;8Suppl 2:S217–22.

54. Ericsson CD, Johnson PC, DuPont HL, Morgan DR. Role of a novel antidiarrheal agent, BW942C, alone or in combination with trimethoprim-sulfamethoxazole in the treatment of traveler's diarrhea. Antimicrob Agents Chemother 1986;29:1040–6.

55. Sack RB, Rahman M, Yunus M, Khan EH. Antimicrobial resistance in organisms causing diarrheal disease. Clin Infect Dis 1997;24Suppl 1:S102–5.

56. Taylor DN. Poorly absorbed antibiotics for the treatment of traveler's diarrhea. Clin Infect Dis 2005;41Suppl 8:S564–70.

57. Haltalin KC, Nelson JD, Hinton LV, et al. Comparison of orally absorbable and nonabsorbable antibiotics in shigellosis. A double-blind study with ampicillin and neomycin. J Pediatr 1968;72:708–20.

58. Taylor DN, Bourgeois AL, Ericsson CD, et al. A randomized, double-blind, multicenter study of rifaximin compared with placebo and with ciprofloxacin in the treatment of travelers' diarrhea. Am J Trop Med Hyg 2006;74:1060–6.

59. Steffen R, Sack DA, Riopel L, et al. Therapy of travelers' diarrhea with rifaximin on various continents. Am J Gastroenterol 2003;98:1073–8.

60. Baker DE. Rifaximin: a nonabsorbed oral antibiotic. Rev Gastroenterol Disord 2005;5:19–30.

61. Adachi JA, DuPont HL. Rifaximin: a novel nonabsorbed rifamycin for gastrointestinal disorders. Clin Infect Dis 2006;42:541–7. Epub 2006 Jan 17.

62. Ansdell VE, Ericsson CD. Prevention and empiric treatment of traveler's diarrhea. Med Clin North Am 1999;83:945–73, vi.

63. Juckett G. Prevention and treatment of traveler's diarrhea. Am Fam Physician 1999;60:119–24, 135–6.

64. Hakanen A, Jousimies-Somer H, Siitonen A, et al. Fluoroquinolone resistance in Campylobacter jejuni isolates in travelers returning to Finland: association of ciprofloxacin resistance to travel destination. Emerg Infect Dis 2003;9:267–70.

65. Nachamkin I, Ung H, Li M. Increasing fluoroquinolone resistance in Campylobacter jejuni, Pennsylvania, USA, 1982–2001. Emerg Infect Dis 2002;8:1501–3.

66. Prevention. CfDCa. National antimicrobial resistance monitoring system: enteric bacteria 2000 annual report. Atlanta: The Centers 2000.

67. Segreti J, Gootz TD, Goodman LJ, et al. High-level quinolone resistance in clinical isolates of Campylobacter jejuni. J Infect Dis 1992;165:667–70.

68. Adler Mosca H, Luthy Hottenstein J, Martinetti Lucchini G, et al. Development of resistance to quinolones in five patients with campylobacteriosis treated with norfloxacin or ciprofloxacin. Eur J Clin Microbiol Infect Dis 1991;10:953–7.

69. Hakanen A, Kotilainen P, Huovinen P, et al. Reduced fluoroquinolone susceptibility in Salmonella enterica serotypes in travelers returning from Southeast Asia. Emerg Infect Dis 2001;7:996–1003.

70. Molbak K, Gerner-Smidt P, Wegener HC. Increasing quinolone resistance in Salmonella enterica serotype Enteritidis. Emerg Infect Dis 2002;8:514–5.

71. Hoge CW, Gambel JM, Srijan A, et al. Trends in antibiotic resistance among diarrheal pathogens isolated in Thailand over 15 years. Clin Infect Dis 1998;26:341–5.

72. Streit JM, Jones RN, Toleman MA, et al. Prevalence and antimicrobial susceptibility patterns among gastroenteritis-causing pathogens recovered in Europe and Latin America and Salmonella isolates recovered from bloodstream infections in North America and Latin America: report from the SENTRY Antimicrobial Surveillance Program (2003). Int J Antimicrob Agents 2006;27:367–75.

73. Hakanen A, Kotilainen P, Jalava J, et al. Detection of decreased fluoroquinolone susceptibility in Salmonellas and validation of nalidixic acid screening test. J Clin Microbiol 1999;37:3572–7.

74. Vila J, Vargas M, Ruiz J, et al. Quinolone resistance in enterotoxigenic Escherichia coli causing diarrhea in travelers to India in comparison with other geographical areas. Antimicrob Agents Chemother 2000;44:1731–3.

75. Steffen R, Jori R, DuPont HL, et al. Efficacy and toxicity of fleroxacin in the treatment of travelers ' diarrhea. Am J Med 1993;94:182s–6s.

76. Wistrom J, Jertborn M, Hedstrom SA, et al. Short-term self-treatment of travellers' diarrhoea with norfloxacin: a placebo-controlled study. J Antimicrob Chemother 1989; 23:905–13.

77. Thornton SA, Wignall SF, Kilpatrick ME, et al. Norfloxacin compared to trimethoprim/sulfamethoxazole for the treatment of travelers' diarrhea among US military personnel deployed to South America and West Africa. Mil Med 1992;157:55–8.

78. Hooper DC. Quinolones. In: Mandell GL, Bennett JE, Dolin R, editors. Principles and practices of infectious diseases, Vol 1. 6th ed. Philadelphia, PA: Elsevier Inc.; 2005. p. 451–73.

79. Oliphant CM, Green GM. Quinolones: a comprehensive review. Am Fam Physician 2002;65:455–64.

80. Dembry LM, Farrington JM, Andriole VT. Fluoroquinolone antibiotics: adverse effects and safety profiles. Infect Dis Clin Pract 1999;8:421–8.

81. Lipsky BA, Baker CA. Fluoroquinolone toxicity profiles: a review focusing on newer agents. Clin Infect Dis 1999;28: 352–64.

82. Sprandel KA, Rodvold KA. Safety and tolerability of fluoroquinolones. Clin Cornerstone 2003;Suppl 3:S29–36.

83. Oldfield EC 3rd. Clostridium difficile-associated diarrhea: resurgence with a vengeance. Rev Gastroenterol Disord 2006;6:79–96.

84. McDonald LC, Killgore GE, Thompson A, et al. An epidemic, toxin gene-variant strain of Clostridium difficile. N Engl J Med 2005;353:2433–41.

85. Melhus A. Fluoroquinolones and tendon disorders. Expert Opin Drug Saf 2005;4:299–309.

86. Owens RC Jr, Ambrose PG. Torsades de pointes associated with fluoroquinolones. Pharmacotherapy 2002;22:663–8; discussion 668–72.

87. Noel GJ, Natarajan J, Chien S, et al. Effects of three fluoroquinolones on QT interval in healthy adults after single doses. Clin Pharmacol Ther 2003;73:292–303.

88. Gomi H, Jiang ZD, Adachi JA, et al. In vitro antimicrobial susceptibility testing of bacterial enteropathogens causing traveler's diarrhea in four geographic regions. Antimicrob Agents Chemother 2001;45:212–6.

89. Isenbarger DW, Hoge CW, Srijan A, et al. Comparative antibiotic resistance of diarrheal pathogens from Vietnam and Thailand, 1996–1999. Emerg Infect Dis 2002;8:175–80.

90. Engberg J, Aarestrup FM, Taylor DE, et al. Quinolone and macrolide resistance in Campylobacter jejuni and C. coli: resistance mechanisms and trends in human isolates. Emerg Infect Dis 2001;7:24–34.

91. Shanks GD, Smoak BL, Aleman GM, et al. Single dose of azithromycin or three-day course of ciprofloxacin as therapy for epidemic dysentery in Kenya. Acute Dysentery Study Group. Clin Infect Dis 1999;29:942–3.

92. Foulds G, Shepard RM, Johnson RB. The pharmacokinetics of azithromycin in human serum and tissues. J Antimicrob Chemother 1990;25 Suppl A:73–82.

93. Lalak NJ, Morris DL. Azithromycin clinical pharmacokinetics. Clin Pharmacokinet 1993;25:370–4.

94. Luke DR, Foulds G. Disposition of oral azithromycin in humans. Clin Pharmacol Ther 1997;61:641–8.

95. Rakita RM, Jacques-Palaz K, Murray BE. Intracellular activity of azithromycin against bacterial enteric pathogens. Antimicrob Agents Chemother 1994;38:1915–21.

96. Alvarez Elcoro S, Enzler MJ. The macrolides: erythromycin, clarithromycin, and azithromycin. Mayo Clin Proc 1999;74:613–34.

97. Charles L, Segreti J. Choosing the right macrolide antibiotic. A guide to selection. Drugs 1997;53:349–57.

98. Drew RH, Gallis HA. Azithromycin—spectrum of activity, pharmacokinetics, and clinical applications. Pharmacotherapy 1992;12:161–73.

99. Jones K, Felmingham D, Ridgway G. In vitro activity of azithromycin (CP-62,993), a novel macrolide, against enteric pathogens. Drugs Exp Clin Res 1988;14:613–5.

100. Barza M, Eisenberg E. Clarithromycin and Azithromycin. Infect Dis Clin Pract 1996;5:291–302.

101. Hopkins S. Clinical toleration and safety of azithromycin. Am J Med 1991;91:40S–5S.

102. Treadway G, Pontani D, Reisman A. The safety of azithromycin in the treatment of adults with community-acquired respiratory tract infections. Int J Antimicrob Agents 2002;19:189–94.

103. Bartlett JG. Medical management of HIV infection: Johns Hopkins University, Department of Infectious Diseases; 1998.

104. Lister PJ, Balechandran T, Ridgway GL, Robinson AJ. Comparison of azithromycin and doxycycline in the treatment of non-gonococcal urethritis in men. J Antimicrob Chemother 1993;31 Suppl E:185–92.

105. Waugh MA. Open study of the safety and efficacy of a single oral dose of azithromycin for the treatment of uncomplicated gonorrhoea in men and women. J Antimicrob Chemother 1993;31 Suppl E:193–8.

106. Taylor DN, Bourgeois AL, Ericsson CD, et al. A randomized, double-blind, multicenter study of rifaximin compared with placebo and with ciprofloxacin in the treatment of travelers' diarrhea. Am J Trop Med Hyg 2006;74:1060–6.

107. Descombe JJ, Dubourg D, Picard M, Palazzini E. Pharmacokinetic study of rifaximin after oral administration in healthy volunteers. Int J Clin Pharmacol Res 1994; 14:51–6.

108. Rizzello F, Gionchetti P, Venturi A, et al. Rifaximin systemic absorption in patients with ulcerative colitis. Eur J Clin Pharmacol 1998;54:91–3.

109. Gionchetti P, Rizzello F, Ferrieri A, et al. Rifaximin in patients with moderate or severe ulcerative colitis refractory to steroid-treatment: a double-blind, placebo-controlled trial. Dig Dis Sci 1999;44:1220–1.

110. Jiang ZD, Ke S, Palazzini E, et al. In vitro activity and fecal concentration of rifaximin after oral administration. Antimicrob Agents Chemother 2000;44:2205–6.

111. Soro O, Pesce A, Raggi M, et al. Selection of rifampicin-resistant Mycobacterium tuberculosis does not occur in the presence of low concentrations of rifaximin. Clin Microbiol Infect 1997;3:147–51.

112. DuPont HL, Jiang ZD. Influence of rifaximin treatment on the susceptibility of intestinal Gram-negative flora and enterococci. Clin Microbiol Infect 2004;10:1009–11.

113. Diemert DJ. Prevention and self-treatment of traveler's diarrhea. Clin Microbiol Rev 2006;19:583–94.

114. DuPont HL. Travellers' diarrhoea: contemporary approaches to therapy and prevention. Drugs 2006;66: 303–14.

115. Taylor DN, McKenzie R, Durbin A, et al. Rifaximin, a nonabsorbed oral antibiotic, prevents shigellosis after experimental challenge. Clin Infect Dis 2006;42:1283–8.

116. Yates J. Traveler's diarrhea. Am Fam Physician 2005;71: 2095–100.

117. Sanders JW, Isenbarger DW, Walz SE, et al. An observational clinic-based study of diarrheal illness in deployed United States military personnel in Thailand: presentation and outcome of Campylobacter infection. Am J Trop Med Hyg 2002;67:533–8.

118. Scheld WM. Maintaining fluoroquinolone class efficacy: review of influencing factors. Emerg Infect Dis 2003;9:1–9.

119. Sanchez F, Mensa J, Martinez JA, et al. Is azithromycin the first-choice macrolide for treatment of community-acquired pneumonia? Clin Infect Dis 2003;36:1239–45.

120. Adachi JA, Ostrosky-Zeichner L, DuPont HL, Ericsson CD. Empirical antimicrobial therapy for traveler's diarrhea. Clin Infect Dis 2000;31:1079–83.

121. Shlim DR. Update in traveler's diarrhea. Infect Dis Clin North Am 2005;19:137–49.

CHAPTER 28

EMPIRIC MANAGEMENT OF ACUTE TRAVELERS' DIARRHEA ABROAD AND IN THE RECENTLY RETURNED TRAVELER

BRADLEY A. CONNOR, MD

JOSEPH TORRESI, MBBS, BMedSci, FRACP, PhD

Commencing an effective treatment for acute travelers' diarrhea should help to reduce the immediate and possibly the long-term impact of this condition for travelers. Most cases of travelers' diarrhea are not dehydrating particularly when effective therapy is expeditiously begun; therefore, the classic role of oral rehydration solutions is much less relevant in the usual management of travelers and will not be dealt with further here. Details about Oral rehydration solutions (ORS) can be found in Chapter 26, "Symptomatic Therapy." The high prevalence of bacterial microorganisms as the underlying etiological agents of acute travelers' diarrhea has made antibiotic therapy the mainstay of the treatment of travelers' diarrhea. The principles that guide our treatment of the returned traveler with acute travelers' diarrhea apply as well to enlightened self treatment by the traveler acutely ill with travelers' diarrhea in the field. The benefits of antibiotic treatment of travelers' diarrhea are clear with treated travelers experiencing both faster resolution and less severe diarrhea. A recent Cochrane analysis demonstrated that travelers receiving antibiotics were almost six times more likely to have more rapid resolution of diarrhea compared to untreated travelers.[1] This may also ultimately translate to a lower likelihood of developing chronic diarrhea and irritable bowel syndrome, although clinical trials to confirm this are still lacking.

The earliest antibiotics used to treat travelers' diarrhea were tetracycline and ampicillin. Resistance to these drugs led to the use of trimethoprim/sulfamethoxazole (TMP/SMX) in the early 1980s.[2] By the end of that decade, many bacterial enteropathogens had become resistant to this combination, which led to the use of fluoroquinolones, initially nalidixic acid, and then norfloxacin and ciprofloxacin. The fluoroquinolones were extremely effective in promptly eradicating the bacterial pathogens and restoring a sense of well being to the traveler sometimes in a matter of hours. This was true across virtually any destination worldwide until sometime in the early 1990s when the emergence of ciprofloxacin-resistant *Campylobacter* in Thailand led to the empiric use of azithromycin for the treatment of travelers' diarrhea in this region.[3] With antimicrobial resistance becoming far more widespread among the common bacterial pathogens associated with travelers' diarrhea, choice of currently available antimicrobials will in time become more restricted.

With the growing recognition of resistance patterns, the choice of antibiotic for empiric treatment needs to be matched as best as possible to the destination. There is no clear threshold as to when antibiotic resistance mandates a change in empiric treatment. It is known that for certain destinations in Asia, such as Thailand and Nepal, *Campylobacter* isolates comprise approximately 25% of the bacterial pathogens. Considering

70 to 90% resistance to fluoroquinolones in these regions, one would expect a failure rate of up to 23% in travelers receiving this class of antibiotics for travelers' diarrhea.

Azithromycin has been shown to have antibacterial activity that is at least comparable to fluoroquinolones but is superior for the treatment of campylobacter infections.[4] Consequently azithromycin has become more widely accepted as an effective antibiotic for acute travelers' diarrhea, and for several travel destinations this antibiotic is the drug of choice for treatment of acute travelers' diarrhea. A newer antibiotic proposed for the treatment of travelers' diarrhea is rifaximin. Rifaximin is poorly absorbed and its actions are limited to the lumen of the intestinal tract. Although studies across several countries seemed to indicate that rifaximin was as effective as ciprofloxacin in empiric treatment of travelers' diarrhea,[5] the fact that the drug is not absorbed renders it ineffective in treating invasive pathogens such as *Shigella* spp. or *Campylobacter* spp.

So now instead of a "one drug fits all" strategy, we are forced to consider factors such as the resistance of specific pathogens, geographic regions, and invasive versus noninvasive organisms. Thus, the empiric treatment of travelers' diarrhea is not as simple as it was just a few years ago, requiring a more thoughtful strategy.

Self-Diagnosis and Self-Treatment of Travelers' Diarrhea

Allowing the traveler to recognize acute bacterial diarrhea and be able to distinguish it from less common causes of travelers' diarrhea (eg, parasitic) made standardization of pretravel advice possible. Viral gastroenteritis often cannot be distinguished clinically from bacterial diarrhea at the outset, but fortunate for the concept of empiric self therapy, studies have shown that viruses account for only 5 to 8% of travelers' diarrhea Likewise, toxic gastroenteritis, caused by ingestion of a preformed toxin, and not by a bacterial enteric infection, does not appear to be a common cause of travelers' diarrhea. Giardia is the most common protozoal pathogen in travelers, accounting for up to 10% of travelers' diarrhea at a destination travel medicine clinic in Nepal.[6] With an incubation period of 1 to 2 weeks, Giardia is not usually the cause of diarrhea during travel among short-term travelers. Travelers who prove to have a bacterial pathogen in their stool usually present for evaluation within 3 days of the onset of their illness, whereas those with protozoal pathogens do not present for evaluation until 2 weeks after the onset of their illness.[6] Diarrhea due to *Entamoeba histolytica* is much less common in travelers, accounting for 1 to 5% of cases in longer-term travelers and expatriates. *Cryptosporidium parvum* is another protozoan that not infrequently causes diarrhea in travelers. The illness is usually self-limiting with resolution over a week, and in travelers not responding to empiric antibiotic therapy, treatment with nitazoxanide could be considered.[7] *Cyclospora cayetanensis* causes an initial illness indistinguishable from bacterial diarrhea. However, after 2 to 3 days, the severe symptoms subside and a prolonged illness ensues.[8] Whereas TMP/SMX could be given for Cyclospora diarrhea, the drug is not effective enough against the majority of much more common bacterial pathogens to be used for initial empiric therapy.

Management of Travelers' Diarrhea

ANTIBIOTICS

As bacterial causes of travelers' diarrhea far outnumber other microbial etiologies, empiric treatment with an antibiotic directed at enteric bacterial pathogens remains the best and most definitive therapy for travelers' diarrhea. However, adjunctive agents like loperamide used for symptomatic control may also be recommended. The standard treatment regimens consist of 3 days of antibiotic, although when treatment is initiated promptly shorter courses, including single-dose therapy, may reduce the duration of the illness to a few hours (Table 1).

The benefit of treatment of travelers' diarrhea with antibiotics has been proven in a number of studies. The effectiveness of a particular antimicrobial agent depends on the etiologic agent and its antibiotic sensitivity. Both as empiric therapy or for treatment of a specific bacterial pathogen, first-line antibiotics include those of the fluoroquinolone class, such as ciprofloxacin or levofloxacin and the macrolide antibiotic, azithromycin.

FLUOROQUINOLONES

Fluoroquinolones have been the mainstay of antimicrobial treatment for travelers' diarrhea for the past two decades. The combination of fluoroquinolones and loperamide has proven not only to be especially effective in resolving diarrhea, but also to be safe, even in patients with *Shigella* dysentery.[9] However, in patients with fever and severe bloody diarrhea, it may be prudent to adopt a more cautious approach and initiate treatment with antibiotics alone.

All of the fluoroquinolones are well absorbed and have excellent oral bioavailability, making them suitable for the treatment of enteroinvasive bacteria. They are contraindicated in pregnancy and should be used with caution in young children, although a short course

Table 1 Antimicrobial Agents for the Treatment of Acute Travelers' Diarrhea

Antibiotic	Adult Dosing Regimens
Fluoroquinolone	
Norfloxacin	800 mg stat followed, if needed, by 400 mg BID for 1–3 days
Ciprofloxacin	1,000 mg followed, if needed, by 500 mg BID for 1–3 days
Levofloxacin	500 mg orally daily for 1–3 days
Azithromycin	1 g orally as a single dose or 500 mg daily for 3 days
Rifaximin	200 mg orally TID for 3 days

BID = twice daily; TID = three times daily.

fluoroquinolones as used for travelers' diarrhea is considered safe.[10]

Increasing microbial resistance to the fluoroquinolones, especially among Campylobacter isolates, may limit their usefulness in some destinations such as Thailand and Nepal. However, until good epidemiologic data are available from a larger number of regions throughout Asia, the impact of the growing antimicrobial resistance on the efficacy of fluoroquinolones for travelers' diarrhea is uncertain. Despite this gap in our knowledge, it appears that fluoroquinolones still work well in most destinations where travelers' diarrhea is a risk and remain first line agents for most travelers.

AZITHROMYCIN

Azithromycin has good activity against a wide range of enteric organisms and appears to be as effective as fluoroquinolones for the treatment of travelers' diarrhea acquired in Mexico and Thailand.[4,11] Azithromycin is active against *Campylobacter* species, providing it with a significant advantage over fluoroquinolones in regions where *Campylobacter* are prevalent. For travelers' diarrhea acquired in Thailand and Nepal, azithromycin is now the drug of choice for the treatment of travelers' diarrhea .[11]

RIFAXIMIN

Rifaximin is a nonabsorbable antibiotic that has recently become more widely available as another option for the treatment of travelers' diarrhea , especially diarrhea caused by enterotoxigenic or enteroaggregative E. coli. , Rifaximin has proven to be less effective than ciprofloxacin for the treatment of invasive enteric bacterial pathogens like Shigella and Campylobacter.[12] For travelers who use rifaximin empirically, an improvement in symptoms may not be seen if they are infected with an invasive pathogen; consequently, an alternate drug, effective against these pathogens, would need to be taken. Until further information is available about the efficacy of rifaximin for invasive intestinal pathogens it cannot be recommended as an empiric therapeutic option in these patients or in travelers to regions where invasive pathogens are especially prevalent, such as South East Asia.

If the use of the selected antibiotic fails to result in improvement in 48 hours, this could mean that the diagnosis is wrong (the patient may have a parasitic or viral infection), the bacteria could be resistant to that antibiotic, or (in the case of rifaximin) the patient has an invasive bacterium. In addition co-infection is a possibility. In this circumstance, the traveler would need to consider the possibility of an intestinal parasite as the underlying cause for their symptoms.

Symptomatic Treatment (see Chapter 27, "Antimicrobial Therapy")

ANTIMOTILITY AGENTS

Antimotility agents provide symptomatic relief and serve as useful adjuncts to antibiotic therapy in travelers' diarrhea .[13] Synthetic opiates, such as loperamide and diphenoxylate, can reduce bowel movement frequency and enable travelers to resume their activities while awaiting the effects of antibiotics. Loperamide also has antisecretory properties and has become the preferred agent of the two because it avoids the anticholinergic side effects of the atropine contained in diphenoxylate preparations.[14] Although earlier studies suggest these agents should not be used in diarrheal illness associated with high fever or blood in the stool, more recent studies suggest these medications may be used in such instances as long as antibiotics are administered concurrently. The combination of loperamide with antibiotic results in more rapid relief than either antibiotics or loperamide alone.[15] The recommendations for the use of antimotility agents in children also vary widely. In the US, loperamide and diphenoxylate are not recommended for children < 2 years of age while in the UK they are not recommended below 4 years of age and in Australia they are contraindicated in children under the age of 12 years.

ANTIEMETIC AGENTS

Additional symptomatic treatment may be offered with antiemetics. Most travelers probably do not need antiemetics for empiric therapy in their travel kit because nausea and vomiting are generally self-limiting in travelers' diarrhea. Antiemetics are available in oral, injectable, or suppository form. Suppositories are a practical way for a traveler to self-treat vomiting, but their usefulness may be limited by the concomitant presence of diarrhea. Orally disintegrating tablets of ondansetron may be effective because they do not require

Table 2 Algorithmic Approach to Self Treatment Abroad or Treatment of the Recently Returned Traveler with Acute Diarrhea

Presenting Symptoms of Acute Diarrhea	Empiric Therapeutic Intervention
Mild (tolerable)	Loperamide, or bismuth subsalicylate, if symptomatic relief is desired*
Moderate to severe (distressing)	Loperamide (especially if rapid control of symptoms is indicated) PLUS Invasive pathogen not expected: Rifaximin A fluoroquinolone Azithromycin Invasive pathogen expected: A fluoroquinolone Azithromycin Travel to regions like South and South East Asia** where fluoroquinolone-resistant *Camplyobacter* can be anticipated: Azithromycin
Severe (incapacitating)	An antimicrobial agent (invasive pathogens are more predictable) A fluoroquinolone Azithromycin (preferred for South and South East Asia) PLUS Loperamide when rapid control of symptoms is indicated

* Some authorities suggest no antibiotic for mild disease, especially in long-term travelers or expatriates, to help the traveler develop some immunity; others are proponents of early antibiotic treatment of mild disease.

** While the prevalence of fluoroquinolone-resistance enteropathogens varies within the region, we prefer to simplify the recommendation and suggest azithromycin for the entire region.

ingestion with fluids. These medications are most effective at the point at which the vomiting is waning and nausea is still prominent. By decreasing the nausea, and preventing further vomiting, the patient can pursue oral rehydration more vigorously; however, in our experience travelers can also be instructed to continue efforts at rehydration despite occasional vomiting, and they are usually successful in avoiding dehydration and in taking medication between waves of nausea without antiemetics.

NONSPECIFIC AGENTS

Bismuth subsalicylate (BSS or Pepto-Bismol) has been shown to decrease stool frequency and shorten the duration of illness in several placebo-controlled studies.[16] This agent is associated with a 16 to 18% reduction in unformed stooling compared to over 50% for loperamide. Side effects include black tongue, black stools, and tinnitus. BSS should be used with caution in travelers on aspirin therapy or anticoagulants and should be avoided in those who have significant renal insufficiency. In addition, BSS should be avoided in children with viral infections, such as *Varicella* or influenza, because of the risk of Reye syndrome. BSS is not available in many parts of the world such as Europe, Australia, and New Zealand. Other nonspecific agents, such as kaolin pectin, activated charcoal, and probiotics such as Lactobacillus GG and *Saccharomyces boulardii*, have had a limited role in the treatment of travelers' diarrhea.

Algorithmic Approach

Table 2 shows an algorithmic approach to the use of antimicrobial agents and the nonspecific agent, loperamide, in the treatment of acute travelers' diarrhea. While the use of loperamide in severe disease is somewhat controversial, it is reassuring that the combination of antibiotic and loperamide has been efficacious and safe even in dysentery. Travelers should remember that there are many species and strains causing travelers' diarrhea. Having one episode of diarrhea will not confer adequate protection against the syndrome and should not make the traveler complaisant about continuing to exercise good food and beverage choices.

References

1. Al-Abri SS, Beeching NJ, Nye FJ. Traveller's diarrhoea. Lancet Infect Dis 2005;5:349–60.
2. Black R. Epidemiology of travelers' diarrhea and relative importance of various pathogens. Rev Infect Dis 1990; 12(Suppl 1):S73–9.
3. Kuschner RA, Trofa AF, Thomas RJ, et al. Use of azithromycin for the treatment of *Campylobacter* enteritis in travelers to Thailand, an area where ciprofloxacin resistance is prevalent. Clin Infect Dis 1995;21:536–41.
4. Adachi JA, Ericsson CD, Jiang ZD, et al. Azithromycin found to be comparable to levofloxacin for the treatment of

US travelers with acute diarrhea acquired in Mexico. Clin Infect Dis 2003;37:1165–71.

5. Steffen R, Sack DA, Riopel L, et al. Therapy of travelers' diarrhea with rifaximin on various continents. Am J Gastroenterol 2003;98:1073–8.
6. Shlim DR. Update in traveler's diarrhea. Infectious disease clinics of North America 2005;19:137–49.
7. Rossignol JF, Ayoub A, Ayers MS. Treatment of diarrhea caused by *C. parvum*: a prospective randomized, double-blind, placebo-controlled study of nitazoxanide. J Infect Dis 2001;184:103–6.
8. Shlim DR, Cohen MT, Eaton M, et al. An alga-like organism associated with an outbreak of prolonged diarrhea among foreigners in Nepal. Am J Trop Med Hyg 1991;45:383–9.
9. Steffen R, Jori J, DuPont H, et al. Treatment of travelers diarrhea with fleroxacin: a case study. J Antimicrob Chemother 1993;31:767–76.
10. Adachi J, Ostrosky-Zeichner L, DuPont HL, Ericsson CD. Empirical antimicrobial therapy for traveler's diarrhea. Clin Infect Dis 2000;31:1079–83.
11. Tribble DR, Sanders JW, Pang LW, et al. Traveler's diarrhea in Thailand: randomized double-blind trial comparing single-dose and 3-day azithromycin-based regimens with a 3-day levofloxacin regimen. Clin Infect Dis 2007;44:338–46.
12. Taylor D, Bourgeois A, Ericsson C, et al. A randomized, double-blind, multicenter study of rifaximin compared with placebo and with ciprofloxacin in the treatment of travelers' diarrhea. Am J Trop Med Hyg 2006;74:1060–6.
13. Schiller LR, Santa Ana CA, Morawski SG, et al. Mechanism of the antidiarrheal effect of loperamide. Gastroenterology 1984;86:1475–14.
14. Ericsson CD, Johnson PC. Safety and efficacy of loperamide. Am J Med 1990;88(suppl 6A):10S–4S.
15. Murphy GS, Bedhidatta L, Echeverria P, et al. Ciprofloxacin and loperamide in the treatment of bacillary dysentery. Ann Intern Med 1993;118:582–6.
16. Ericsson CD. Non antimicrobial agents in treatment and prevention of travelers' diarrhea. Clin Infec Dis 2005;41: S557–63.

CHAPTER 29

APPROACH TO PROLONGED DIARRHEA IN THE RETURNING TRAVELER

BRADLEY A. CONNOR, MD

JOSEPH TORRESI, MBBS, BMedSci, FRACP, PhD

Although travelers' diarrhea is typically a self-limiting illness, some patients may experience a more prolonged clinical course. By convention, acute diarrhea is an illness that has lasted less than 2 weeks. Evaluation of persistent or prolonged symptoms in returned travelers requires an understanding of the epidemiology and potential causes of persistent travelers' diarrhea. Some cases of persistent travelers' diarrhea are those in which the diarrhea itself is actually a small complaint but associated gastrointestinal (GI) symptoms such as cramping, bloating, gaseousness, and rectal urgency may predominate. The etiology of prolonged symptoms is often related to persistent infection, co-infection, temporary postinfectious phenomena, malabsorptive syndromes, or underlying GI disease.[1–8] Recently, postinfectious irritable bowel syndrome (see Chapter 18, "Postinfectious Irritable Bowel Syndrome") has gained increased recognition as another potential cause of persistent diarrhea in returned travelers.[9]

Epidemiology of Prolonged Travelers' Diarrhea

Although the majority of cases of travelers' diarrhea are self-limiting, several published studies suggest that a minority of individuals will experience persistent symptoms.[10–12] One of these studies evaluated the health problems that occurred among 7,886 Swiss international tourists after travel to developing countries for ≤ 3 months.[10] Approximately 1% of patients reported chronic diarrhea, which was defined as persisting illness with at least three unformed stools per day that resulted in at least five medical consultations, hospitalization of at least 5 days, inability to work for at least 15 days, or no cure by 4 to 7 months after return. A second study estimated the incidence of chronic diarrhea among 4,607 US Peace Corps volunteers stationed in 43 countries.[11] During the previous 2 years, an estimated 78 volunteers (1.7%) experienced chronic diarrhea, which was defined as the presence of ≥ 3 loose stools per day that usually persisted for ≥ 3 months, marked fecal urgency, the absence of systemic symptoms, and no known etiology. In a third study, persistent diarrhea (ie, persisting for ≥ 2 weeks) occurred in 1 of 35 students (2.9%) who had traveled to Latin America.[12] Collectively, these three studies demonstrate that persistent diarrheal illnesses in travelers are not uncommon, with up to 3% of individuals experiencing symptoms for at least 2 weeks and up to several months.

Etiology of Prolonged Diarrhea in Travelers (Table 1)

PERSISTENT INFECTION

An infecting pathogen should be considered in the evaluation of individuals with persistent travelers' diarrhea. In general, the usual approach is to rule out a persistent bacterial or protozoan infection. Although carriage of bacteria such as *Salmonella* may persist, these pathogens are rarely associated with persistent symptoms.[2] Conversely, protozoa are more likely to cause

Table 1 Etiologies of Prolonged Travelers' Diarrhea

Conditions	Considerations
Persistent infection	• Persistent bacterial infection • Persistent protozoal infection
Co-infection	• Undocumented additional pathogen • *Clostridium difficile* after antibiotic therapy
Temporary postinfectious phenomena	• Intestinal disaccharidase deficiency • Small intestinal bacterial overgrowth
Malabsorption	• Tropical sprue • Celiac sprue
Underlying GI disease	• Inflammatory bowel disease • Colon cancer
Postinfectious irritable bowel syndrome	• GI consultation for management

GI = gastrointestinal.

protracted illness in travelers,[1,2] particularly in patients who describe an insidious onset of symptoms.[2] Parasitic infections probably represent the most common causes of persistent diarrhea in returning travelers. With symptoms continuing for more than 14 days, parasitic causes increase in likelihood. In travelers to Nepal, protozoans were detected in 10% of travelers with symptoms for less than 14 days and in 27% of those with symptoms for more than 14 days.[13,14] The most common protozoan pathogen isolated in travelers with persistent diarrheal symptoms is *Giardia lamblia.* [1] Other protozoan pathogens that commonly cause prolonged illness include *Cyclospora* and *Cryptosporidium.*[1,2] For some patients with persistent diarrhea, a stool analysis by microscopy may only identify "nonpathogenic" protozoa such as *Entamoeba coli*, *Endolimax nana*, and *Iodamoeba buetschlii.*[15]

CO-INFECTION

Persistent diarrhea may be due to co-infection with an untreated second infection (eg, *Giardia*) in patients effectively treated for another pathogen.[2] *Clostridium (C.) difficile* infections may be a cause of persistent diarrhea in returned travelers.[3] There is usually a history of prior treatment of diarrheal episodes with antibiotics. In some cases, diarrhea from *C. difficile* may result from the use of antimalarial chemoprophylactic agents. A careful history of prior antibiotic use and medications used during travel is important in suggesting this diagnosis. An examination of stool for *C. difficile* toxin should be included as part of the workup.

TEMPORARY POSTINFECTIOUS PHENOMENA

Temporary postinfectious phenomena may cause persistent symptoms in returned travelers as a result of GI damage or compromise.[2] or for example, an attack of acute infectious diarrhea may precipitate intestinal disaccharidase deficiency (eg, lactase or sucrase deficiency).[2,4,5] Patients typically report symptoms of chronic diarrhea, abdominal pain, and gaseous distention.[2] These symptoms usually resolve within a few weeks, although certain individuals with a genetic predisposition may have permanent lactose intolerance unmasked by an acute episode of infectious diarrhea.[2]

Another temporary postinfectious phenomenon that may lead to persistent symptoms is small intestinal bacterial overgrowth.[2] An acute enteric infection can cause changes in small bowel motility and lead to stasis and secondary bacterial overgrowth.

MALABSORPTION

Persistent diarrhea, especially when accompanied by weight loss, may be related to malabsorption.[2] Tropical sprue is a clinical entity of unknown etiology that is associated with chronic diarrheal illness and malabsorption in travelers and expatriates in developing countries.[16] Tropical sprue is, however, relatively uncommon.[17] More commonly, celiac sprue may be unmasked by an acute episode of infectious diarrhea and present as persistent travelers' diarrhea.[6] Celiac sprue, an autoimmune inflammatory condition of the bowel, is generally responsive to a gluten-free diet.

UNDERLYING GI DISEASE

Travelers' diarrhea may also uncover an underlying chronic GI disease. A review of the case notes of 129 returned travelers with bloody diarrhea admitted to the Hospital for Tropical Diseases in London from 1978 to 1984 found that one-quarter of the patients (32/129) had inflammatory bowel disease, and an additional 2 patients (2%) had colon cancer.[7] Other clinicians have described the detection of colon cancer in a patient who developed fever and diarrhea during international travel.[8]

POSTINFECTIOUS IRRITABLE BOWEL SYNDROME

A diagnosis of postinfectious irritable bowel syndrome (PI-IBS) should be considered in returned travelers with chronic symptoms for which no specific etiology is identified. PI-IBS is associated with an onset of IBS symptoms after an acute episode of an enteric infection in patients with previously normal bowel function.[9] Increasing evidence supports PI-IBS as a specific diagnosis.[2,9] Acknowledgement of PI-IBS represents a paradigm shift that assumes that a peripheral event (ie, infection) leads to prolonged, permanent changes in GI function.[2]

Although not conclusive, epidemiologic studies suggest that PI-IBS may be a relatively common complication of travelers' diarrhea. Increasing etiologic and pathologic data highlight the importance of effective prevention and treatment of acute bacterial illness as a strategy to reduce the risk of PI-IBS. Quantitative histology data indicating persistent low-grade inflammation following an acute enteric infection support additional studies to investigate the potential benefits of anti-inflammatory agents and antibiotics in the treatment of PI-IBS.

The increasing recognition of PI-IBS as a specific diagnosis also provides opportunities for additional areas of research. For example, a case definition of PI-IBS in the travelers' diarrhea population and the extent of workup necessary to establish a diagnosis of PI-IBS have yet to be clearly defined. In addition, retrospective analyses of biopsy and electron microscopy data from patients with PI-IBS may provide further information about the pathophysiology of this illness. Controlled trials are also needed to evaluate the potential benefit of anti-inflammatory and antibiotic therapies in the treatment of PI-IBS. In order to obtain clinically meaningful results from these studies, the optimal duration of therapy and appropriate endpoints need to be defined. These research activities will promote a more thorough understanding of PI-IBS, which may lead to improvements in the management of this illness.

Management

Management is beyond the scope of this chapter and depends on the underlying cause of the prolonged illness. If a workup for persisting or previously unrecognized enteropathogens is negative, some experts recommend an empiric trial of an antibiotic directed at possible persisting pathogens like enteroaggregative *Escherichia coli* that might not be detected in a routine microbiology laboratory. If symptoms suggest *Giardia* infection and empiric metronidazole, tinidazole or nitazoxanide might be tried. Simple dietary changes or bulking agents can be tried especially if PI-IBS is suspected. Antispasmodics and antidiarrheals may play in role in treatment as well. However, if the cause of persistent diarrhea is not clear and symptoms continue despite empiric interventions, consultation with a gastroenterologist is recommended for consideration of endoscopic evaluation in selected patients.

References

1. Taylor DN, Connor BA, Shlim DR. Chronic diarrhea in the returned traveler. Med Clin North Am 1999;83:1033–52.
2. Connor BA. Sequelae of traveler's diarrhea: focus on postinfectious irritable bowel syndrome. Clin Infect Dis 2005;41(suppl 8):S577–86.
3. Golledge CL, Riley TV. Clostridium difficile-associated diarrhoea after doxycycline malaria prophylaxis. Lancet 1995;345:1377–8.
4. Matthews SB, Waud JP, Roberts AG, Campbell AK. Systemic lactose intolerance: a new perspective on an old problem. Postgrad Med J 2005;81:167–73.
5. Muldoon C, Maguire P, Gleeson F. Onset of sucrase-isomaltase deficiency in late adulthood. Am J Gastroenterol 1999;94:2298–9.
6. Landzberg BR, Connor BA. Persistent diarrhea in the returning traveler: think beyond persistent infection. Scand J Gastroenterol 2005;40:112–4.
7. Harries AD, Myers B, Cook GC. Inflammatory bowel disease: a common cause of bloody diarrhoea in visitors to the tropics. Br Med J (Clin Res Ed) 1985;291:1686–7.
8. Scully RE, Mark EJ, McNeely WF, McNeely BU. Case records of the Massachusetts General Hospital. Weekly clinicopathological exercises. Case 33–1993. N Engl J Med 1993;329:561–8.
9. Spiller RC. Postinfectious irritable bowel syndrome. Gastroenterology 2003;124:1662–71.
10. Steffen R, Rickenbach M, Wilhelm U, et al. Health problems after travel to developing countries. J Infect Dis 1987;156:84–91.
11. Addiss DG, Tauxe RV, Bernard KW. Chronic diarrhoeal illness in US Peace Corps volunteers. Int J Epidemiol 1990; 19:217–8.
12. Guerrant RL, Rouse JD, Hughes JM, Rowe B. Turista among members of the Yale glee club in Latin America. Am J Trop Med Hyg 1980;29:895–900.
13. Hoge CW, Shlim DR, Echeverria P, et al. Epidemiology of diarrhea among expatriate residents living in a highly endemic environment. JAMA 1996;275:533–8.
14. Taylor DN, Houston R, Shlim DR, et al. Etiology of diarrhea among travelers and foreign residents in Nepal. JAMA 1988;260:1245–8.
15. Lee MB, Keystone JS, Kain KC. Cost implications of reporting nonpathogenic protozoa. Clin Infect Dis 2000;30:401–2.
16. Walker MM. What is tropical sprue? J Gastroenterol Hepatol 2003;18:887–90.
17. Shlim DR. Tropical sprue as a cause of traveler's diarrhea [response to letter to the editor]. Wilderness Environ Med 2000;11:140–1.

CHAPTER 30

A COST-EFFECTIVE APPROACH TO TRAVELERS' DIARRHEA

SANTIAGO PÉREZ CACHAFEIRO, MD, MSc

THOMAS D. SZUCS, MD, MPH, MBA, LLM

RON H. BEHRENS, BSc, MBChB, MD

Just consider how many people are traveling abroad every year. The United Nations World Tourist Organization (UNWTO) reported 806 million tourist arrivals worldwide in 2005, 275 million if Europe and North America are excluded, most of them visiting high-risk countries for travelers' diarrhea.[1] Now, think of those travelers in terms of policy making. Travelers' diarrhea attack rates are between 10 and 50%—a good estimate would be a 30%.[2–15] Thus, the global burden of travelers' diarrhea approaches 82 million episodes per year. In terms of quality of life, some studies found that the perceived quality of life decreased during a travelers' diarrhea episode by 14%[16] and travelers' diarrhea average duration without treatment is 3 to 4 days (Table 1).[(2–4,6,7,10,13,17–26)] Roughly, these numbers mean that one episode of travelers' diarrhea without treatment produces a loss of 0.0016 QALYs ([quality adjusted life years], equivalent to 0.6 days per episode), which is a small number. Nevertheless, this represents a annual global loss of 126,800 QALYs worldwide.

Travelers will not perceive this as a loss, but as a lost leisure opportunity consequent to their travelers' diarrhea. If an average vacation lasts 7 to 14 days, and costs around $850 US,[1] a lost day is equivalent to more than $60 to $120 US; because some visits can not be repeated, and leisure can not be replaced, many travelers obtain travel health insurance to financially compensate for ill health.

Overall, 82 million episodes of travelers' diarrhea per year represent a global cost of $69.7 billion (days of travel lost) and 82 million lost leisure activities in a host country, which has both a monetary and reputation value. Lost activity has a real economic burden for the host country. A traveler in bed does not use local services (apart from health services if that is the case) and does not benefit the local economy. No studies have been conducted pertaining host countries' perspective. In addition, recent trends show that travelers are more willing to visit high-risk areas than in the past.[45]

Thus, any economic evaluation of travelers' diarrhea should consider the most appropriate point of view, reflecting the disease impact most relevantly. This chapter will try to clarify some economic concepts and offer a brief explanation of different cost-effective approaches to travelers' diarrhea.

Some Economic Concepts

The most common methods employed by health economists are classical research designs such as cost-benefit-, cost-effectiveness- and cost-utility-analyses.

COST-BENEFIT ANALYSES

As applied to health care, cost-benefit analysis (CBA) measures all costs and benefits of competing therapies in terms of monetary units. For individual therapies, net benefits can be calculated by simply subtracting the costs form the benefits. If net benefits are positive, the intervention is worth undertaking from the economic perspective. Differences in net benefits of competing therapies or programs (eg, intensive care unit versus new diagnostic equipment or preventive measures) can in theory be readily compared for an efficient allocation of resources. However, CBA requires assigning monetary values to life and to health improvements measured in a variety of dimensions including quality of life. This

Table 1 Duration of Travelers' Diarrhea by Treatment Option. A Literature Review

Treatment option	References	Dose	Duration (hours)
No seek treatment*	[27]		74
Current treatment*	[28-32]		48-96
Pre-treatment*	[27, 33-37]		24-32
Placebo	[34, 36-39]		53 - 81
Azythromicin	[40]	1000mg single dose	22
	[41]	500mg 3 days	37
Levofloxacin	[40]	500mg single dose	22
Ofloxacin	[34]	300mg 3 days	39
		300mg 5 days	28
Ciprofloxacin	[41-43]	500mg bid 3 days	25 -44
	[38, 39]	500mg bid 5 days	29
	[36, 43]	single dose	25-36
Rifaximin	[35, 39]	200mg tid	32-37
	[35, 42]	400mg bid	26-39
	[35, 37]	600mg/day	33-53
	[37]	1200mg/day	33
Trimethoprim-sulfamethoxazole	[38][35]	160/800mg	20-56
Antibiotic with loperamide	[27, 43]		26-34
Probiotics	[44]		30

* No treatment shows duration of TD when it runs its course without any treatment; current treatment refers to duration of TD when it was treated following actual clinical practice; pretreatment is duration of TD before visiting any health professional, thus the real duration of TD with any intervention would be the sum of durations before (pretreatment) and after beginning treatment.

presents equal benefit issues (are benefits equal to everyone?) as well as substantial measurement problems. For these reasons, CBAs have not been widely used for evaluating drug therapies and the optimal allocation of resources. [46]

COST-EFFECTIVENESS ANALYSES

Cost-effectiveness studies measure changes in the cost of all relevant treatment alternatives, but they measure the differences in outcomes in some natural unit such as actual lives saved, years of lives saved, events prevented, or children immunized. Cost-effectiveness analyses (CEA) can also be applied equally to cases where the outcome is in terms of quality of life. CEA is useful in comparing alternative therapies that have the same outcome units, such as increase of life expectancy, but the treatments do not have the same effectiveness, that is one drug may lead to greater gains in life expectancy than another. The measure compared is the cost of therapy divided by the units of effectiveness and, hence, a lower number signifies a more cost-effective outcome.

This type of study has the advantage that it does not require the conversion of health outcomes to monetary units and thereby avoids equal benefit and other difficult issues of the valuing benefits. It is therefore among the most frequently used tools to identify the most efficient strategy to reach a specific health target (production efficiency). It has the disadvantage of not permitting comparisons across programs (see CBA). In other words, the cost-effectiveness of a drug that aims to reduce infant mortality cannot be compared with a drug designed to improve quality of life of senior citizens.[47] The value for money of an intervention is most usefully measured as what a the decision maker is willing to pay for a health gain. Moreover, it cannot compare outcomes measured in clinical units with quality of life measures.

COST-UTILITY ANALYSES

Cost-utility analysis (CUA) compares the added costs of therapy with the number of QALY gained. The quality adjustment weight is a utility value that can be measured as part of clinical trials or independently. The advantage of CUA is that therapies that produce improvement in different or multiple health outcomes can be more readily compared. The QALY measure is calculated by multiplying the length of time in a specific health state by the perceived utility of that health status (on a scale from 0 to 1). Many analysts are more comfortable with QALYs as a measure of the consequence of medical care than with the monetary units.

CUA is an improvement over CEA because it can measure the effects of multiple outcomes (such as the impact of vaccines on both morbidity and mortality or the impact on both pain and physical functional). Cost per QALY can be computed and compared across alternative treatment scenarios. This is especially useful when only a limited and fixed budget is available and allocation among competing programs/therapies has to be optimized. A comprehensive overview of QALY estimates has been published by Tengs and Wallace.[48]

As it is stated above, CBAs, CEAs, and CUAs compare two or more interventions. The result of a CEA is a cost-effectiveness ratio: average cost-effectiveness ratio (ACER), marginal cost-effectiveness ratio (MCER) or incremental cost-effectiveness ratio (ICER). It would be worth trying to explain the differences between them in few words. First, ACER represents the average cost per one unit of outcome (eg, average cost per day of diarrhea reduced) in each intervention. Second, MCER is the cost of increasing outcome (cost of increasing the intervention in order to avert a day of diarrhea) in each intervention. And finally, ICER shows how much cost units have to be invested to get one unit more of outcome with one intervention when it is compared to another (increase of cost needed to prevent 1 further day of diarrhea when using an intervention rather than the current intervention).[49,50]

ICER is the commonest measure employed when publishing CEA. It used to compare a new intervention with common practice, and its interpretation is linear when the result is positive. However, a negative ICER can be misleading.[51]

In addition, there is a specific CEA that compares the new intervention or interventions with the status quo or doing nothing. It is called generalized cost-effectiveness analysis (GCEA).[52] The World Health Organization (WHO), through WHO-CHOICE guidelines, recommends performing GCEA in order to improve allocative efficiency. When comparing different measures with doing nothing, the practice with smallest ICER would be to use resources most efficiently compared with the other(s).[a,46,47,49-53] If one of the others is the common practice, this implies that common practice is not cost effective.[49,52]

When talking about travelers' diarrhea, undertaking a GCEA is possible; maintaining the status quo or doing nothing is a possible intervention and should therefore be included in any cost-effective approach to travelers' diarrhea.

[a]This is a simplification of the interpretation of CEA and GCEA analysis. Further explanations may be obtained from WHO-CHOICE guidelines and the referenced economic evaluation guidelines at the end of the chapter.

Different Perspectives on Travelers' Diarrhea Economic Evaluations

Societal perspective is often the first perspective considered when analyzing the impact of any disease. WHO recommends disability adjusted life years (DALYs)/ quality adjusted life years (QALYs) when undertaking a CEA from a societal perspective,[49] allowing those measures that most benefit the society to be recognized. This stance becomes difficult with a disease such as travelers' diarrhea which produces a small decrease on QALYs for policy makers. The Institute of Medicine in the United States evaluated some possible vaccines against pathogens involved in travelers' diarrhea (enterotoxigenic *Escherichia (E.) coli, shigella*). They discovered that vaccines against these pathogens were not cost effective from a societal perspective (costing more than $100,000 per QALY gained).[54,55] However, it could be cost effective from other perspectives in some settings.[56]

Thoren and colleagues[57] evaluated the economic impact of acute diarrhea (including travelers' diarrhea) on the community. In this study, an episode of acute diarrhea generates a mean of 2 days sick leave; and the economic effects were higher in ages 20 to 30 years. They did not evaluate cost of different intervention strategies.

Thomson and colleagues[58] performed a cost-benefit analysis of travelers' diarrhea, demonstrating that benefit-cost ratios favor treatment strategies rather than prophylaxis. Previously, Reves and colleagues[59] conducted a CEA of antimicrobial agents and concluded that chemoprophylaxis with doxycycline or co-trimoxazole were more cost-effective than treatment strategies. However, Reves and colleagues used data from a Delphi survey pertaining to incapacitation produced by travelers' diarrhea that suggested higher incapacitation rates than actual data taken from the global survey of Steffen and colleagues[16] These higher incapacitation rates could skew the perspective towards using prophylaxis.

A second point of view is based from the perspective of the individual. When routine prophylaxis was not yet established as a useful intervention, microbiologists were using chemoprophylaxis when traveling abroad.[60] The questions this raises are (a) how much do travelers know about the disease and the different intervention strategies?; (b) how much are individuals willing to pay to avoid one day of diarrhea?; and (c) how much are they willing to pay to avoid a whole episode of illness? Normal travelers (package, sporting, and honeymoon) consider lost leisure and duration of sickness (incapacitation time) as an important factor. Whereas society considers society's costs (burden of disease), the traveler considers their personal costs as the most important economic factor when choosing measures. Steffen and colleagues calculated an average travelers' diarrhea episode per trip cost of $116.50 per patient or $27.5 per traveler.[13]

Risk perception, measured by those who seek pretravel advice or who use effective compliance with prophylactic measures,[9,16,61] or an individual's willingness to pay (WTP)[62] become important factors for a cost-effective approach to travelers' diarrhea from a traveler's perspective. Risk perception may also be influenced by other factors, including age. Younger individuals have the highest diarrhea attack rates,[14,63] and are not usually willing to pay for prevention.[62]

A third approach relates to business travelers, in whom lost time is of high economic value; thus, incapacitation has significant financial implications. Reves and colleagues demonstrated that the most important contributory component in the cost of travelers' diarrhea, was the time an individual was incapacitated and unable to undertake any activity.[59] Recent studies on a rifaximin prophylaxis as a strategy, described a more favorable benefit-cost ratio for the short-term business travelers than the current intervention reducing incapacitation.[64]

Incapacitation is also important in the military context. Since Napoleon, military leaders discovered that gastrointestinal disturbances in their troops are an important cause of morbidity during military campaigns.[12,65] Recent research during military exercises including operations Desert Shield, Iraqi Freedom, Enduring Freedom, Bright Star, and Restore Hope have described the impact of travelers' diarrhea on military performance.[3,7, 12] A future vaccine against the main aetiological agents leading to travelers' diarrhea may be the most cost-effective approach from the military and other long-term travelers perspective.[56]

The remainder of the chapter will examine the cost-effectiveness of travelers' diarrhea from the travelers' perspective, noting discrepancies as they occur compared to other perspectives.

Intervention Strategies

Apart form the baseline strategy in a GCEA (the status quo), there are two main ways to deal with travelers' diarrhea: prevention and treatment, either as self treatment and/or through medical care (Figure 1).[66-69] Prevention measures that could be evaluated include pretravel advice, chemoprophylaxis with antibiotics[70–72] or drugs without antibacterial effect,[73,74] and vaccination. Although there is still no vaccine against travelers' diarrhea, a number are being developed.[75–78] Current treatment strategies include oral rehydration therapy and intravenous rehydration, the use of antimotility agents such as loperamide, antibiotic therapy, and rarely hospitalization. Probiotics have been used for many decades for both the treatment and prevention of travelers' diarrhea, but their value is unclear.[68,74, 79-85] Bismuth subsalycylate has been similarly used and is licensed in some countries.[74,81,86]

There are two important determinants in CEA: coverage and compliance.[87] For example, If 40% of travelers seek pretravel advice and only 65% of these are compliant to the advice, the expected benefit falls from 60 to 15.6%. The same effect occurs with any chemoprophylaxis. Barriers to accessing prophylactic measures could also bias the effectiveness of such measures.[88] The analysis of vaccine effectiveness is more complex because it may confer protection against disease but may not necessarily reduce infection. Thus, the risks

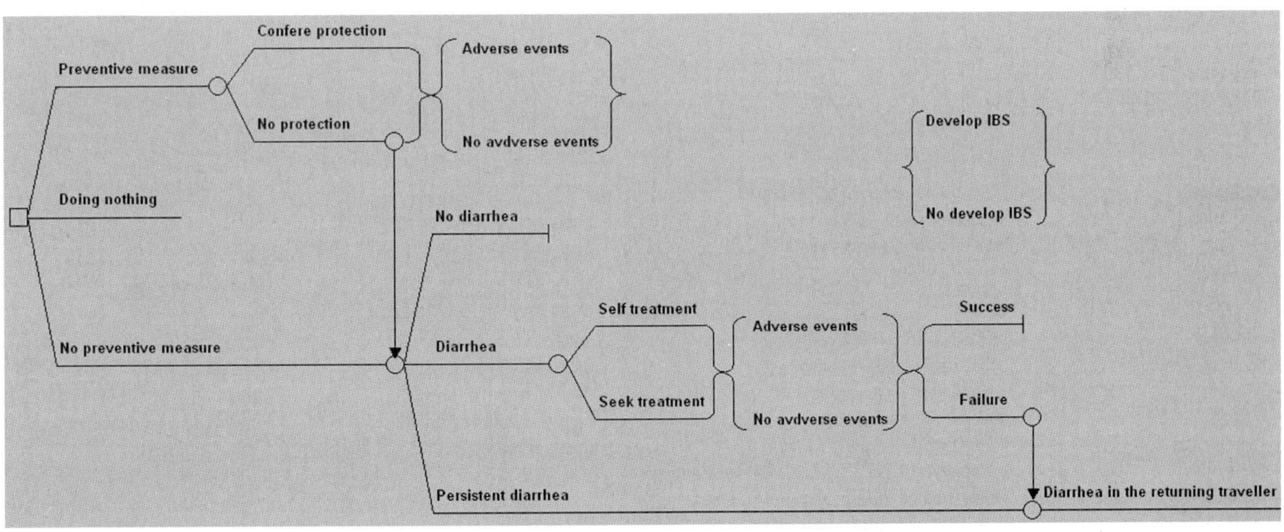

Figure 1 Model describing possible interventions on Travelers' Diarrhea and short and long-term effects to consider in a cost-effectiveness analysis.

of long-term sequelae, such as Guillain-Barré or irritable bowel syndrome (IBS) may still remain after a subclinical infection.[4, 8] Some studies of prophylactic interventions, such as the use of probiotics, report higher attack rates in intervention groups.[71–73] This has also been described in groups receiving pretravel advice and other measures such as a *E. Coli* vaccine.[9,78,84] One possible explanation of this paradox is that protected travelers may take more risks than unprotected individuals, a phenomenon called *moral hazard.* Preventative measures may reduce diarrhea attack rates but also reduce the perceived threat of diarrhea by travelers.

The major treatment options available include: (a) oral rehydration, (b) antibiotics, (c) nonantibiotic drugs such as loperamide and bismuth subsalycilate, (d) intravenous rehydration, and (e) hospitalization. Loperamide is the most widely used drug measure to manage travelers' diarrhea and ciprofloxacin the most widely used antibiotic.[67–69,92]

In Figure 1, prevention and treatment are clearly complementary; when the prevention is effective there is no need for treatment, and treatment (or status quo) are the only option(s) during an episode of travelers' diarrhea.

For both strategies, adverse events need to be evaluated in any economic analysis. Any event that increases cost or decreases quality of life needs consideration. Long-term sequelae should also be included in all models. In the case of travelers' diarrhea, progression to IBS is the most obvious association.[4,8,89-91] Others could be Guillian-Barré Syndrome or postinfective polyarthritis following Campylobacter infection.[93]

Baseline Assumptions

Some variables that need to be included in a CEA of travelers' diarrhea are shown in Table 2. Cost and probabilities are shown alongside travelers' diarrhea intervention strategies. It is important to note that travelers' diarrhea incidence among other variables are important during a travelers' diarrhea-CEA, and these assume different values affected by country of origin of travelers, destination, reason, and duration of travel.[3,4,10,12,13,15,16,94] To select appropriate values for these variables in CEA, a literature review was undertaken and the results summarized in Table 3. Where no information was available in the literature, consensus conferences and Delphi studies may be used as a data source.[4,58]

The time-frame for a CEA might be the average short trip: 7 to 14 days and several months in long-term travelers. This biases the analysis by excluding long-term sequelae that occur years after infection. Some strategies like vaccination or establishing travel clinics are costly in the beginning while their benefits last for years. Thus the analytical horizon has to consider these costs and be long enough to dilute their impact on the CEA (decades).

Table 2 Variables to consider when undertaking a cost-effective analysis of Travelers' Diarrhea

	Variables	Costs	Disease outcomes
Travelers' Diarrhea • Classic TD • Moderate TD • Mild TD • Persistent TD • Chronic TD	• Origin and host countries • Number of travelers • Type of travel • Incidence of TD • Days of travel • Probability of incapacitation • Probability of IBS if not having TD • Probability of IBS after having TD	• Travel costs • Cost of incapacitation • Cost of long-term sequelae (IBS, Guillian-Barre, post-infectious polyarthritis)	• Duration of TD if runs its course • Duration of incapacitation
Prophylaxis • Probiotics • Bismuth • Antibiotics • Vaccine	• Coverage of prophylactic measures • Efficacy of prophylaxys • Probability of adverse events	• Instruction of traveler • Delivery of prevention • Cost of health visit • Cost of drug / vaccine • Costs of adverse events	
Treatment • No drug treatment • Probiotics • Bismuth • Loperamide • Antibiotics • iv fluids • hopitalisation	• Probability of no treatment • Probability of self treatment • Probability of choosing each of treatment options if self-treatment • Probability of seeking treatment • Probability of selecting each treatment option where treated by a health proffesional • Probability of treatment failure • Probability of adverse events	• Cost of visit abroad • Cost of each treatment option • Cost of adverse events • Cost of treatment failure • Costs of returning ill	• Duration of TD pre-treatment • Duration of TD per treatment option • Duration of hospitalisation

Table 3 Probabilities and values of variables related to cost and efficacy of TD intervention strategies.

	Probability (%)		References
PREVENTION			
Probability of seeking pre-travel advice	16.7-83.8		[95,96]
Protection confered by prevention measure	0-50	Lactobacilli GG	[96–101]
	80-100	Fluoroquinolones	
	79-94	TMP / SMX	
	72-77	Rifaximin	
	40-65	Bismuth	
Probability of adverse events due to prevention	0.06	Rifaximin	[100]
TREATMENT			
Probability of no treatment	38.3		[96]
Self-treatment			
Probability of self-treatment	20-36		[96,102]
Probability of probiotics if self-treated	61		[103]
Probability of Antibiotic if self-treated	7.6-28.6		[102,103]
Probability of loperamide if self-treated	15.4-51.6		[102,103]
Probability of bismuth	15.6		[102]
Probability of self-treatment lead to "cure"	79.9		[102]
Seek for health care			
Probability of seeking treatment	6.6-40.2		[96,102,104–109]
Probability of being treated (drugs) after visiting a health facility	<35-38.7		[104,110]
Probability of Antibiotic (alone)	26.8-78.7		[102,111]
Probability of loperamide	33.1-62		[102,104,111]
Probability of bismuth	13		[102]
Probability of iv treatment	0-16.5		[102,106,111]
Probability of hopitalisation	0-13		[96,102,104,106,108,109]
Probability of treatment failure	2.8-8.9	Overall	[106,111–116]
		Stratified by drug:	
	1.2-4.1	Loperamide	
	5.1-17.6	TMP/SMX	
	9.7-16.7	Rifaximin	
	4.9-10.6	Ofloxacin	
	1.2-6.7	Ciprofloxacin	
Probability of adverse events due to treatment	0-0.05	Severe adverse events	[106,113,117,118]
INCAPACITATION			
Probability of developing incapacitation due to Travelers' Diarrhea	2.8-56		[104,106,108,109]

Point of reference value for CEA might be the US dollars at the year 2000 ($Y2000) and its equivalencies with other currencies, which are freely available from WHO.[125] In order to generalize results, it is suggested to use this $Y2000 and to adjust any monetary value to this year using past observed inflation (ie, observe inflation rates for medical goods and services in the US Bureau of Labor Statistics).[126] Following the lead of the WHO-CHOICE, a 3% real discount rate is recommended to discount future cost to the current value, but a sensitivity analysis needs to be done.[49]

Measuring Costs

Use of health resources and cost savings may be divided into different components: (a) patient costs are those directly related with treatment, bed-day, transportation, etc. (b) program costs include delivery of care, education of personnel, mass media costs. And such like.[49-51] Cost of antibacterials may include the cost of clinical trials; because agents develop resistance to antimicrobials, clinical trials have to be periodically repeated in order to identify the most appropriate drug.[127,128]

Costs saved by an intervention include cost of subsequent IBS, cost of being incapacitated, or changes to routine daily activity and cost of leisure days lost. Persistent diarrhea, treatment failure, and late onset diarrhea in "returned" travelers generate costs because they require a number of visits to a health facility and a number of laboratory investigations in their native country.[94,128–130]

To improve the generalization of results, the WHO designed tables of health-related costs per country in 2000.[125] When costs are not in these tables, local values can be used. For drug costs there is an international guide;[131] nevertheless, drugs and other health resources can normally be obtained cheaper at the host country than before traveling,[132] and the lowest cost should be considered in CEA.

Measuring Effectiveness

The use of systematic reviews is the most reliable source of accurate values. But there are problems with these reviews because published literature often uses different outcome measures. Randomized, controlled trials do not always report duration of disease as an outcome or measure quality of life. The duration of disease may not always have the same endpoint measure. Duration may be expressed as a mean, a median, or a range of hours or days, and the endpoint may be time to last symptom or time to last unformed stool (TLUS).[133] To standardize outcomes in future travelers' diarrhea studies, it is suggested to use the median TLUS as a standardized variable. It may also be expressed as a mean with standard deviation because the duration of disease is a biological event and therefore should follow a normal distribution.[50,51]

An alternative endpoint would be time of incapacitation, which is reported in a small number of studies but is valuable when performing a travelers' diarrhea CEA from all perspectives.[16]

An important consideration are that many of these outcomes are country dependent: dependent on the origin and the destination of travelers.[3–5,10,13,15,16] Outcomes are also influenced by behavior, gender, age, and reason for travel.[134] The impact of travelers' diarrhea is increased in men and in younger people and decreased in business travelers.[10,16,45] Aetiological agents of TD also differ between countries and influence intervention to select.[4,13,15,45,49,76,79,88–93]

Another aspect to consider is when a combination of strategies is implemented. Treatments are commonly combined,[67,81] although there are only a few studies examining combination therapy (usually an antibiotic with loperamide).[4,6,25] In addition, antimicrobial randomized control trials (RCT) do not declare or control for confounders, such as the use of probiotics commonly used by travelers.[79]

Uncertainty and Sensitivity Analysis

Because of the biological basis of travelers' diarrhea, a Markov model is not absolutely necessary when analyzing travelers' diarrhea in a CEA. The lack of homogeneity of costs and outcomes and variability in incidence makes the use of a tool that deals with uncertainty of published data necessary. The MonteCarlo simulations are accepted as a way of analyzing uncertainty, and there are several software packages available for this purpose.[49,51,52]

A mathematical model of travelers' diarrhea pertaining to US travelers to Mexico from the travelers' perspective was created specifically for use based on published data (see Tables 1 and 3).[2–4,6–13,15–26,73,79,83,90,128,130,140–146] Any prophylactic measure appears to be more cost effective than treatment alone when efficacy is measured as days of incapacitation averted; however, there are no reliable data on incapacity averted by treatment because several studies report data on duration of travelers' diarrhea only. Self-treatment options become more cost effective when the outcome is measured as days of diarrhea averted (Table 4); nevertheless, preventative measures appear to be more effective (but more expensive). The break-even point from a societal perspective will differ between regions of travel.[147] The break-even point from an individuals perspective needs to be decided by the reader because the most useful measure is willingness to pay (WTP), which is not normally available.[62]

The sensitivity of each option allows uncertainty to be linked to each variable, which then reflects changes on both axis, as shown in Table 5. All prevention measures are influenced (sensitive) to coverage, incidence, and duration of travelers' diarrhea as well as costs of the intervention and the cost of sequelae (mainly IBS and "returning ill"). The treatment options (either self treatment or seeking treatment strategies) are not very

Table 4 MonteCarlo simulation. ICER of a GCEA from the traveler perspective expressed as $ per day of TD averted and mean days of TD averted per person in each intervention strategy. The source data are described in tables 1 and 3

	PREVENTION				TREATMENT	
	Advice	Probiotics	Ciprofloxacin	Rifaximin	Health Prof.	Self
Mean	$46	$59	$120	$125	$67	$39
Median	$43	$55	$109	$111	$60	$34
Range	$19-133	$14-193	$59-436	$57-665	$17-277	$12-110
Days ill averted per traveler	1.14	0.71	0.86	0.87	0.17	0.35

Table 5 Comparison of impact of variables on the three interventions. Analogic scale showing how much Cost-Effectiveness Ratios of three intervention strategies vary according to equivalent changes of different variables (influence of each variable on the intervention)

	Prevention	Self-treatment	Seek-treatment
Incidence of TD	++	-	-
Duration of TD	++	+	+
Probability of choosing the strategy (coverage)	+++	+++	+++
Cost of intervention	+++	++	++
Cost of sequalae	+	++	+++

-: little/no impact; +: the variable has some influence on the intervention; the variable has relevant influence on the intervention +++: the variable has significant influence on the intervention.

sensitive to the incidence of travelers' diarrhea, but are to duration of travelers' diarrhea and the likelihood and cost of receiving treatment. The increasing costs of sequelae make prophylaxis more cost effective; however, there is an inverse and much smaller effect on treatment (Figures 2 through 4).

Conclusion

The biggest limitation of this and other models in the analysis of travelers' diarrhea is lack of data where there are combinations of several interventions. The results in Table 4 points how the combination of pretravel advice and self treatment would provide the most cost-effective strategy if the ideal outcome was days of travelers' diarrhea averted. However, limitations in data relating to the treatment, because there are no measures of travelers' diarrhea days averted, makes it difficult to do an analysis (comparison with prophylaxis). Without an adequate comparison to treatment, prevention strategies that include pretravel advice and chemoprophylaxis appear to be the best combination for reducing days of incapacitation from travelers' diarrhea.

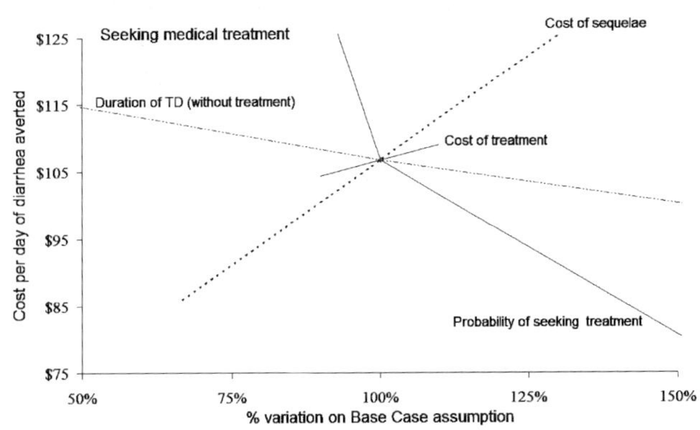

Figure 3 Sensitivity analysis of seek for care strategies showing the impact of modifying certain parameters on the incremental cost-effectiveness ratio expressed as cost per day diarrhea averted following medical treatment (compared with doing nothing). The Base case is calculated from the data described in tables 1 and 3.

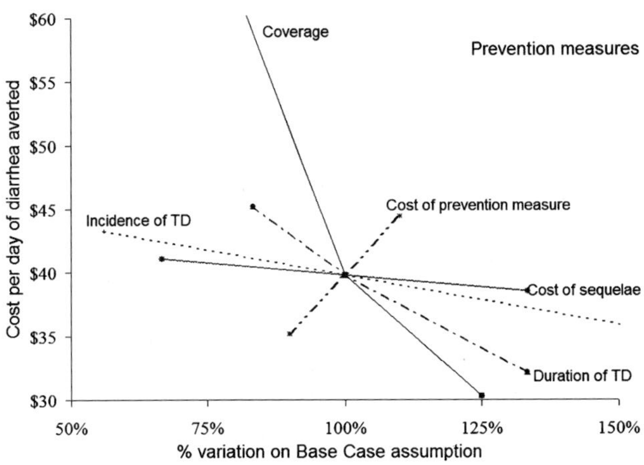

Figure 2 Sensitivity analysis of preventive measures shows the impact of modifying certain parameters on the incremental cost-effectiveness ratio expressed as cost per day diarrhea averted by preventative measures (compared with doing nothing). The Base case is calculated from the data described in tables 1 and 3.

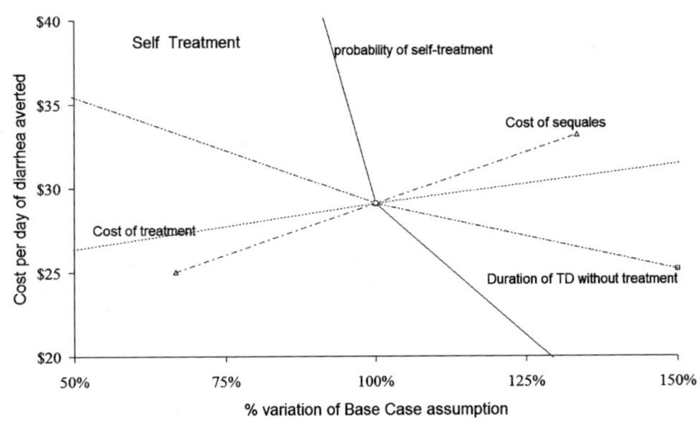

Figure 4 Sensitivity analysis of the self-treatment intervention showing the impact of modifying certain parameters on the incremental cost-effectiveness ratio expressed as cost per day diarrhea averted by self-treatment (compared with doing nothing). The Base case is calculated from the data described in tables 1 and 3.

Where the traveler is not willing to pay the cost of avoiding one day incapacitation, this strategy cannot be considered cost effective. Commonly, travelers pay more for treatment (and lost leisure) than they would pay for a preventative strategy; however, from their perspective, this looks cost effective even though it is more costly. Risk perception influences not just behavior, but likely benefits and potential costs of different interventions for travelers' diarrhea. Risk perception ultimately impacts what individuals are willing to pay.[88,128,142,148,149]

Where a National Health Service functions as free-of-charge provider, policy makers have to decide on the break-even point (WTP per traveler) for their service. Nevertheless, they should consider that from a societal point of view (QALYs), all interventions are probably not cost effective.

From a military perspective, the WTP may be higher because just one casualty has implications during a military campaign, and costs of treatment and evacuation may be significant. Prophylaxis becomes the main option and oral vaccines may in the future be the ideal intervention.

In conclusion, preventative measures reduce more days of disease than treatment, while treatment is the cheaper measure (particularly self-treatment). Willingness to pay becomes the objective for future research in order to measure the real cost-effectiveness ratio of each intervention from the travelers' perspective. Then, country and etiological-specific ratio need to be understood, stratified by age and income to produce a meaningful analysis.

References

1. UNWTO. Tourism highlights. 2006 Available at: http://www.unwto.org (accessed November 15, 2006).
2. Salam I, Katelaris P, Leigh-Smith S, Farthing MJ. Randomised trial of single-dose ciprofloxacin for travellers' diarrhoea. Lancet 1994;344:1537–9.
3. Rudland S, Little M, Kemp P. The enemy within: diarrheal rates among British and Australian troops in Iraq. Military Med 1996;161:728–31.
4. Riddle M, Sanders J, Putnam S, Tribble D. Incidence, etiology and impact of diarrhea among long-term travelers (US military and similar populations): a systematic review. Am J Trop Med Hyg 2006;75:762–7.
5. Redman C, MacLennan A, Wilson E, Walker E. Diarrhea and respiratory symptoms among travelers to Asia, Africa, South America and Central America from Scotland. J Travel Med 2006;13:203–11.
6. Petruccelli BP, Murphy GS, Sanchez JL, et al. Treatment of traveler's diarrhea with ciprofloxacin and loperamide. J Infect Dis 1992;165:557–60.
7. Putnam S, Sanders J, Frenck R, et al. Self-reported description of diarrhea among military populations in operations Iraqi Freedom and Enduring Freedom. J Travel Med 2006;13:92–9.
8. Okhuysen P, Jiang ZD, Carlin L, et al. Post-diarrhea chronic intestinal symptoms and irritable bowel syndrome in North American travelers to Mexico. Am J Gastroenterol 2004;99:1774–8.
9. McIntosh IB, Reed JM, Power KG, Swanson V. Travellers' diarrhoea and the effect of pre-travel health advice in general practice. Br J Gen Pract 1997;47:71–5.
10. Cavalcanti A, Costa Clemens SA, Von Sonnenburg F, et al. Traveler's diarrhea: epidemiology and impact on visitors to Fortaleza, Brazil. Revista Panamericana de Salud Publica/Pan American Journal of Public Health 2002;11: 245–52.
11. DuPont H, Jiang Z, Okhuysen P, et al. A randomized, double-blind, placebo-controlled trial of rifaximin to prevent travelers' diarrhea. Ann Intern Med 2005;142:805.
12. Sanchez JL, Gelnett J, Petruccelli BP, et al. Diarrheal disease incidence and morbidity among United States military personnel during short-term missions overseas. Am J Trop Med Hyg 1998;58:299–304.
13. Steffen R, Collard F, Tornieporth N, et al. Epidemiology, etiology, and impact of traveler's diarrhea in Jamaica. JAMA 1999;281:811–7.
14. Meuris B. Observational study of travelers diarrhea. J Travel Med 1995;2:11–5.
15. von Sonnenburg F, Tornieporth N, Waiyak P, et al. Risk and aetiology of diarrhoea at various tourist destinations. Lancet 2000;356:133–4.
16. Steffen R, Tornieporth N, Costa Clemens SA, et al. Epiemiology of travelers' diarrhea: details of a global survey. J Travel Med 2004;11:231–8.
17. DuPont HL, Ericsson C, Mathewson JJ, DuPont M. Five versus three days of ofloxacin therapy for traveler's diarrhea: a placebo-controlled study. Antimicrob Ag Chemo 1992;36:87–91.
18. Ericsson CD, Johnson PC, Dupont HL, et al. Ciprofloxacin or trimethoprim-sulfamethoxazole as initial therapy for travelers' diarrhea. A placebo-controlled, randomized trial. Ann Intern Med 1987;106:216–20.
19. Steffen R, Sack DA, Riopel L, et al. Therapy of travelers' diarrhea with rifaximin on various continents. Am J Gastroenterol 2003;98:1073–8.
20. Taylor DN, Bourgeois AL, Ericsson CD, et al. A randomized, double-blind, multicenter study of rifaximin compared with placebo and with ciprofloxacin in the treatment of travelers' diarrhea. Am J Trop Med Hyg 2006;74:1060–6.
21. Adachi JA, Ericsson CD, Jiang Z-D, et al. Azithromycin found to be comparable to levofloxacin for the treatment

of US travelers with acute diarrhea acquired in Mexico. Clin Infect Dis 2003;37:1165–71.

22. Kuschner RA, Trofa AF, Thomas RJ, et al. Use of azithromycin for the treatment of Campylobacter enteritis in travelers to Thailand, an area where ciprofloxacin resistance is prevalent. Clin Infect Dis 1995;21:536–41.
23. DuPont HL, Jiang Z-D, Ericsson CD, et al. Rifaximin versus ciprofloxacin for the treatment of traveler's diarrhea: a randomized, double-blind clinical trial. Clin Infect Dis 2001;33:1807–15.
24. DuPont HL, Ericsson CD, Mathewson JJ, et al. Rifaximin: a nonabsorbed antimicrobial in the therapy of travelers' diarrhea. Digestion 1998;59:708–14.
25. Caeiro J, Dupont H, Albrecht H, Ericsson C. Oral rehydratation therapy plus loperamide versus loperamide alone in the treatment of traveler's Diarrhea. Clin Infect Dis 1999;28:1286–9.
26. Herwaldt B, de Arrorayre K, Roberts J, Juranek D. A multiyear prospective study of the risk factors for and incidence of diarrheal illness in a cohort of peace corps volunteers in Guatemala. Ann Intern Med 2000;132:982–8.
27. Riddle M, et al. Incidence, etiology and impact of diarrhea among long-term travelers (US military and similar populations): a systematic review. Am J Trop Med Hyg 2006.
28. Cavalcanti A, et al. Traveler's diarrhea: Epidemiology and impact on visitors to Fortaleza, Brazil. Revista Panamericana de Salud Publica/Pan American Journal of Public Health 2002;11(4):245–252.
29. Herwaldt B, et al. A Multiyear Prospective Study of the Risk Factors for and Incidence of Diarrheal Illness in a Cohort of Peace Corps Volunteers in Guatemala. Ann Intern Med 2000;132:982–988.
30. Putnam S, et al. Self-reported description of diarrhea among military populations in operations Iraqi Fredom and Enduring Freedom. J Travel Med 2006;13(2):92–99.
31. Rudland S, Little M, Kemp P. The enemy within: diarrheal rates among British and Australian troops in Iraq. Military Med 1996;161:728–731.
32. Steffen R, et al. Epidemiology, etiology, and impact of traveler's diarrhea in Jamaica. Jama 1999;281(9):811–7.
33. Caeiro J, et al. Oral Rehydratation Therapy plus Loperamide versus Loperamide alone in the Treatment of Traveler's Diarrhea. Clin Infect Dis 1999;28:1286–1289.
34. DuPont HL, et al. Five versus three days of ofloxacin therapy for traveler's diarrhea: a placebo-controlled study. Antimicrob Ag Chemo 1992;36:87–91.
35. DuPont HL, et al. Rifaximin: a nonabsorbed antimicrobial in the therapy of travelers' diarrhea. Digestion 1998; 59(6):708–14.
36. Salam I, et al. Randomised trial of single-dose ciprofloxacin for travellers' diarrhoea. Lancet 1994;344(8936): 1537–9.
37. Steffen R, et al. Therapy of travelers' diarrhea with rifaximin on various continents. American Journal of Gastroenterology 2003;98(5):1073–1078.
38. Ericsson CD, et al. Ciprofloxacin or trimethoprim-sulfamethoxazole as initial therapy for travelers' diarrhea. A placebo-controlled, randomized trial. Ann Intern Med 1987;106(2):216–20.
39. Taylor DN, et al. A randomized, double-blind, multicenter study of rifaximin compared with placebo and with ciprofloxacin in the treatment of travelers' diarrhea. Am J Trop Med Hyg 2006;74(6):1060–6.
40. Adachi JA, et al. Azithromycin Found to Be Comparable to Levofloxacin for the Treatment of US Travelers with Acute Diarrhea Acquired in Mexico. Clinical Infectious Diseases 2003;37(9):1165–1171.
41. Kuschner RA, et al. Use of azithromycin for the treatment of Campylobacter enteritis in travelers to Thailand, an area where ciprofloxacin resistance is prevalent. Clin Infect Dis 1995;21(3):536–41.
42. DuPont HL, et al. Rifaximin versus ciprofloxacin for the treatment of traveler's diarrhea: A randomized, double-blind clinical trial. Clinical Infectious Diseases 2001; 33(11):1807–1815.
43. Petruccelli BP, et al. Treatment of traveler's diarrhea with ciprofloxacin and loperamide. J Infect Dis 1992; 165(3):557–60.
44. Allen S, et al. Probióticos para el tratamiento de la diarrea infecciosa (revisión cochrane traducida). The Cochrane Library 2006;(3).
45. Valerio L, Martínez O, Sabrià M, et al. High-risk travel abroad overtook low-risk travel from 1999 to 2004: characterization and trends in 2622 Spanish travelers. J Travel Med 2005;12:327–31.
46. Drummond M, O'Brien B, Stoddart G, Torrance G. Methods for the economic evaluation of health care programmes. 2nd ed. Oxford: Oxford University Press; 1997.
47. Gold M, Siegel J, Russel L, Weinstein M. Cost-effectiveness in health and medicine. New York: Oxford University Press; 1996.
48. Tengs T, Wallace A. One thousand quality-of-life estimates. Med Care 2000;38:592–637.
49. Edejer TT, Baltussen R, Adam T, et al. Making choices in health: WHO guide to cost-effectiveness analysis. Geneva: WHO; 2003.
50. Haddix A, Teusch S, Corso P. Prevention effectiveness: a guide to decision analysis and economic evaluation. 2nd ed. New York: Oxford University Press; 2003.
51. Fox-RubyCairns. Economic evaluation: Open University Press; 2005.

52. Murray C, Evans D, Acharya A, Baltussen R. Development of WHO guidelines on generalized cost-effectiveness analysis. Health Economics 2000;9:235–51.

53. Alban A, Gyldmark M, Pedersen A, Sogaard J. The Danish approach to standards for economic evaluation methodologies. Pharmaco Economics 1997;12:627–36.

54. Stratton K, Durch J, Lawrence R. Vaccines for the 21st century: a tool for decision making. Washington DC: Institute of Medicine. National Academy Press; 1999.

55. New vaccine development establishing priorities. Washington DC: National Academy Press; 1986.

56. Perez Cachafeiro S. Cost-effectiveness of developing a new vaccine against traveller's diarrhoea. London: London School of Hygiene and Tropical Medicine; 2006.

57. Thoren A, Lundberg O, Bergdahl U. Socioeconomic effects of acute diarrhoea in adults. Scan J Infect Dis 1988;20:317–22.

58. Thomson MA, Booth IW. Treatment of traveller's diarrhoea. Economic aspects. Pharmacoeconomics 1996; 9:382–91.

59. Reves RR, Johnson PC, Ericsson CD, DuPont HL. A cost-effectiveness comparison of the use of antimicrobial agents for treatment or prophylaxis of travelers' diarrhea. Arch Intern Med 1988 Nov;148:2421–7.

60. Ala'Aldeen D. A microbiologist's guide to travellers abroad: do as I say not as I do. J Hosp Infect 1997;35: 255–7.

61. Laverone E, Boccalini S, Bechini A, et al. Travelers' compliance to prophylactic measures and behaviour during stay abroad: results of a retrospective study of subjects returning to a travel medicine center in Italy. J Travel Med 2006;13:338–44.

62. Yeung R, Abdullah A, McGhee S, Hedley A. Willingness to pay for preventive travel health measures among Hong Kong Chinese residents. J Travel Med 2005;12:66–71.

63. Steffen R, van der Linde F, Gyr K, Schär M. Epidemiology of diarrhea in travelers. JAMA 1983;249:1176–80.

64. Cichon B. Cost-benefit analysis of Rifaximin prophylaxis. London: London School of Hygiene and Tropical Medicine; 2006.

65. Kilpatrick M. Diarrhoeal disease: current concepts and future challenges. Transactions Royal Soc Trop Med Hyg 1993;87(Suppl 3):S47–8.

66. deBruyn G, Hahn S, Borwick A. Antibiotic treatment for traveller's diarrhoea. The Cochrane Library. Chichester, UK: John Wiley & Sons, Ltd; 2006;3.

67. Adachi J, Ostrosky-Zeichner L, Dupont H, Ericsson C. Empirical antimicrobial therapy for traveler's diarrhea. Clin Infect Dis 2000;31:1079–83.

68. DuPont HL, Ericsson CD. Prevention and treatment of traveler's diarrhea. New England J Med 1993;328:1821–7.

69. Diemert DJ. Prevention and self-treatment of traveller's diarrhea. Clin Microbiol Rev 2006;19:583–94.

70. Sack R. Prophylactic antimicrobials for travelers' diarrhea: an early history. Clin Infect Dis 2005;41(Suppl 8):S553–6.

71. Taylor DN. Poorly absorbed antibiotics for the treatment of travelers' diarrhea. Clin Infect Dis 2005;41(Suppl 8): S564–70.

72. DuPont HL, Jiang Z, Okhuysen P, et al. Antibacterial chemoprophylaxis in the prevention of travelers' diarrhea: evaluation of poorly absorbed oral rifaximin. Clin Infect Dis 2005;41(Suppl 8):S571–6.

73. Rendi-Wagner P, Kollaritsch H. Drug prophylaxis for travelers' diarrhea. Clin Infect Dis 2002;34:628–33.

74. Ericsson CD. Nonantimicrobial agents in the prevention and treatment of travelers' diarrhea. Clin Infect Dis 2005; 41(Suppl 8):S557–63.

75. Walker RI. Considerations for development of whole cell bacterial vaccines to prevent diarrheal diseases in children in developing countries. Vaccine 2005;23:3369–85.

76. Levine MM. Enteric infections and the vaccines to counter them: future directions. Vaccine 2006;24:3865–73.

77. Girard MP, Steele D, Chaignat CL, Kieny MP. A review of vaccine research and development: human enteric infections. Vaccine 2006;24:2732–50.

78. Steffen R, Castelli F, Nothdurft H, et al. Vaccination against enterotoxigenic escherechia coli, a cause of travelers' diarrhea. J Travel Med 2005;12:102–7.

79. Reinthaler FE, Feierl G, Beubler E, et al. Treatment of travelers' diarrhea among Austrian tourists. J Travel Med 2004;11:66–8.

80. Guerrant R, Gilder T, Steiner T. Practice guidelines for the management of infectious diarrhea. Clin Infect Dis 2001; 32:331–50.

81. DuPont H. Travellers' diarrhoea: contemporary approaches to therapy and prevention. Drugs 2006;66:303.

82. Sharma AK, Mohan P, Nayak BB. Probiotics: making a comeback. Indian J Pharmacol 2005;37:358–65.

83. Allen S, Okoko B, Martinez E, et al. Probióticos para el tratamiento de la diarrea infecciosa (revisión cochrane traducida). The Cochrane Library. Oxford: Update Software Ltd. Spanish; 2006. p. 3.

84. Sazawal S, Hiremath G, Dhingra U, et al. Efficacy of probiotics in prevention of acute diarrhoea: a meta-analysis of masked, randomised, placebo-controlled trials. Lancet Infect Dis 2006;6:374–82.

85. Alvarez-Olmos M, Oberhelman R. Probiotic agents and infectious diseases: a modern perspective on a traditional therapy. Clin Infect Dis 2001;32:1567–76.

86. Rao G, Aliwalas M, Slaymaker E, Brown B. Bismuth revisited: an effective way to prevent travelers' diarrhea. J Travel Med 2004;11:239–42.

87. Hillel O, Potasman I. Correlation between adherence to precautions issued by WHO and diarrhea among long-term travelers to India. J Travel Med 2005;12:243–7.

88. Angell S, Cetron M. Health disparities among travelers visiting friends and relatives abroad. Ann Intern Med 2005;142:67–72.

89. Wang L, Fang X, Pan G. Bacillary disentery as a causative factor of irritable bowel syndrome and its pathogenesis. Gut 2004;53:1096–101.

90. Stermer E, Lubezky A, Potasman I, et al. Is traveler's diarrhea a significant risk factor for the development of irritable bowel syndrome? A prospective study. Clin Infect Dis 2006;43:898–901.

91. Connor B. Sequelae of travelers' diarrhea: focus on postinfectious irritable bowel syndrome. Clin Infect Dis 2005;41(Suppl 8):S577–86.

92. Heymann DL. Control of communicable diseases manual. 18th ed. Washington DC: American Public Health Association; 2004.

93. Crushell E, Harty S, Sharif F, Bourke B. Enteric campylobacter: purging its secrets. Pediatr Res 2004;55: 3–12.

94. Reinthaler FE, Feierl G, Stunzner D, Marth E. Diarrhea in returning Austrian tourists: epidemiology, etiology, and cost-analyses. J Travel Med 1998;5:65–72.

95. Steffen R, et al. Epiemiology of travelers' diarrhea: details of a global survey. J Travel Med 2004;11:231–238.

96. McIntosh IB, et al. Travellers' diarrhoea and the effect of pre-travel health advice in general practice. British Journal of General Practice 1997;47(415):71–75.

97. Rendi-Wagner P, Kollaritsch H. Drug prophylaxis for Travelers' Diarrhea. Clin Infect Dis 2002;34:628–633.

98. DuPont HL. Travelers' diarrhea: antimicrobial therapy and chemoprevention. Nature Clinical Practice 2005.

99. Sack D, et al. Prophylactic doxycicline for traveler's diarrhea. Results of a prospective double blind study of Peace Corps volunteers in Kenya. N Engl J Med 1978;298: 758–763.

100. DuPont H, et al. A randomized, double-blind, placebo-controlled trial of rifaximin to prevent travelers' diarrhea. Annals of Internal Medicine 2005;142(10):805.

101. DuPont HL, et al. Antibacterial chemoprophylaxis in the prevention of Travelers' Diarhea: evaluation of poorly absorbed oral rifaximin. Clin Infect Dis 2005;41(Suppl 8): S571–S576.

102. Putnam S, et al. Self-reported description of diarrhea among military populations in operations Iraqi Fredom and Enduring Freedom. J Travel Med 2006;13(2):92–99.

103. Reinthaler FE, et al. Treatment of travelersdiarrhea among Austrian tourists. J Travel Med 2004;11:66–68.

104. Cavalcanti A, et al. Traveler's diarrhea: Epidemiology and impact on visitors to Fortaleza, Brazil. Revista Panamericana de Salud Publica/Pan American Journal of Public Health 2002;11(4):245–252.

105. Okhuysen P, et al. Post-diarrhea chronic intestinal symptoms and irritable bowel syndrome in North American travelers to Mexico. Am J Gastroenterol 2004; 99:1774–1778.

106. Riddle M, et al. Incidence, etiology and impact of diarrhea among long-term travelers (US military and similar populations): a systematic review. Am J Trop Med Hyg 2006.

107. Sanchez JL, et al. Diarrheal disease incidence and morbidity among United States military personnel during short-term missions overseas. Am J Trop Med Hyg 1998; 58(3):299–304.

108. Steffen R, et al. Epidemiology, etiology, and impact of traveler's diarrhea in Jamaica. Jama 1999;281(9):811–7.

109. von Sonnenburg F, et al. Risk and aetiology of diarrhoea at various tourist destinations. Lancet 2000;356:133–134.

110. Riddle M, et al. Knowledge, attitudes and practices regarding epidemiology and management of traveler's diarrhea: a survey of front-line providers in Iraq and Afghanistan. Military Med 2005;170:492–495.

111. Sanders J, et al. An observational clinic-based study of diarrheal illness in deployed United States military personnel in Thailand: presentation and outcome of Campylobacter infection. Am J Trop Med Hyg 2002; 67(5):533–538.

112. Adachi JA, DuPont HL. Rifaximin: A novel nonabsorbed rifamycin for gastrointestinal disorders. Clinical Infectious Diseases 2006;42(4):541–547.

113. DuPont HL, et al. Five versus three days of ofloxacin therapy for traveler's diarrhea: a placebo-controlled study. Antimicrob Ag Chemo 1992;36:87–91.

114. Ericsson CD, et al. Ciprofloxacin or trimethoprim-sulfamethoxazole as initial therapy for travelers' diarrhea. A placebo-controlled, randomized trial. Ann Intern Med 1987;106(2):216–20.

115. Petruccelli BP, et al. Treatment of traveler's diarrhea with ciprofloxacin and loperamide. J Infect Dis 1992;165(3): 557–60.

116. Steffen R, et al. Therapy of travelers' diarrhea with rifaximin on various continents. American Journal of Gastroenterology 2003;98(5):1073–1078.

117. DuPont HL, et al. Rifaximin versus ciprofloxacin for the treatment of traveler's diarrhea: A randomized, double-blind clinical trial. Clinical Infectious Diseases 2001; 33(11):1807–1815.

118. Rifaximin is a safe effective antibacterial for treating noninvasive traveller's diarrhoea Drugs & Therapy Perspectives 2006;22(7):1–5.

119. Rudland S, Little M, Kemp P. The enemy within: diarrheal rates among British and Australian troops in Iraq. Military Med 1996;161:728–731.

120. Halvorson H, Schlett C, Riddle M. Postinfectious irritable bowel syndrome - a meta-analysis. Am J Gastroenterol 2006;101:1–6.

121. Ansart S, et al. Illnesses in travelers returning from the tropics: a prospective study of 622 patients. J Travel Med 2005;12:312–318.

122. Stermer E, et al. Is traveler's diarrhea a significant risk factor for the development of irritable bowel syndrome? A prospective study. Clin Infect Dis 2006;43:898–901.

123. Freedman D, et al. Spectrum of disease and relation to place of exposure among ill returned travelers. N Engl J Med 2006;354(2):119–130.

124. Estimates of unit costs for patients services. Available at: http://www.who.int/choice/country (accessed August 11, 2006).

125. Consumer price index (CPI). Available at: http:/ www.bls.gov/cpi/#data (accessed August 11, 2006).

126. Nelson J, Smith K, Vugia D, et al. Prolonged diarrhea due to ciprofloxacin-resistant Campylobacter infection. J Infect Dis 2004;190:1150–7.

127. Travers K, Barza M. Morbidity of infections caused by antimicrobial-resistant bacteria. Clin Infect Dis 2002; 43(Suppl 3):S131–4.

128. Freedman D, Weld L, Kozarsky P, et al. Spectrum of disease and relation to place of exposure among ill returned travelers. N Engl J Med 2006;354:119–30.

129. Spira A. Assessment of travellers who return home ill. Lancet 2003;361:1459–69.

130. Ansart S, Perez L, Vergely O, et al. Illnesses in travelers returning from the tropics: a prospective study of 622 patients. J Travel Med 2005;12:312–8.

131. International drug price indicator guide 2005. Cambridge: WHO; 2006.

132. Goldberg J. Cost of treating travelers' diarrhea. Ann Intern Med 1991;115:331.

133. Huang DB, Awasthi M, Le B-M, et al. The role of diet in the treatment of travelers' diarrhea: a pilot study. Clin Infect Dis 2004;39:468–71.

134. Moreira Lima A. Tropical diarrhoea: new developments in traveller's diarrhoea. Curr Opin Infect Dis 2001;14:547–52.

135. Cohen MB, Hawkins JA, Weckbach LS, et al. Colonization by enteroaggregative Escherichia coli in travelers with and without diarrhea. J Clin Microbiol 1993;31:351–3.

136. Jiang Z, Mathewson JJ, Ericsson CD, Svennerholm A, et al. Characterization of Enterotoxigenic Escherechia coli strains in patients with travelers' diarrhea acquired in Guadalajara, Mexico, 1992–1997. J Infect Dis 2000;181: 779–82.

137. DuPont HL, Jiang ZD. Influence of rifaximin treatment on the susceptibility of intestinal Gram-negative flora and enterococci. Clin Microbiol Infect 2004;10:1009–11.

138. Mattila L. Clinical features and duration of travelers' diarrhea in relation to its etiology. Clin Infect Dis 1994;19: 728–34.

139. Taylor DN, Houston R, Shlim D, et al. Etiology of diarrhea among travelers and foreign residents in Nepal. JAMA 1988;260:1245–8.

140. DuPont HL. Travelers' diarrhea: antimicrobial therapy and chemoprevention. Nat Clin Pract Gastroenterol Hepatol 2005;2:191–8.

141. Sack D, Kaminsky D, Sack R, et al. Prophylactic doxycicline for traveler's diarrhea. Results of a prospective double blind study of Peace Corps volunteers in Kenya. N Engl J Med 1978;298:758–63.

142. Riddle M, Tribble D, Jobanputra N, et al. Knowledge, attitudes and practices regarding epidemiology and management of traveler's diarrhea: a survey of front-line providers in Iraq and Afghanistan. Military Med 2005;170: 492–5.

143. Sanders J, Isenbarger D, Walz S, et al. An observational clinic-based study of diarrheal illness in deployed United States military personnel in Thailand: presentation and outcome of Campylobacter infection. Am J Trop Med Hyg 2002;67:533–8.

144. Adachi JA, DuPont HL. Rifaximin: a novel nonabsorbed rifamycin for gastrointestinal disorders. Clin Infect Dis 2006;42:541–7.

145. Rifaximin is a safe effective antibacterial for treating noninvasive traveller's diarrhoea Drugs Ther Perspect 2006;22:1–5.

146. Halvorson H, Schlett C, Riddle M. Postinfectious irritable bowel syndrome—a meta-analysis. Am J Gastroenterol 2006;101:1–6.

147. WHO. Treshold values for intervention cost-effectiveness by region. Available at: http://www.who.int/choice/costs/CER_levels/en/print.html (accessed August 11, 2006).

148. Mattila L, Siitonen A, Kyronseppa H, et al. Risk behaviour for travelers' diarrhea among Finnish travelers. J Travel Med 1995;2:77–84.

149. Johnson J, McMullen L, Hasselback P, et al. Travelers' knowledge of prevention and treatment of travelers' diarrhea. J Travel Med 2006;13:351–5.

CHAPTER 31

PAST PROGRESS AND FUTURE DIRECTIONS FOR TRAVELERS' DIARRHEA

SHERWOOD L. GORBACH, MD

When considering the prospects for future advancements in travelers' diarrhea, it is necessary to reflect on the progress over the past 50 years that we have recognized this condition and it has been subjected to systematic scrutiny. By examining the pace of progress over this era of scientific discovery, we can gain insight into the prospects for future developments. The overall conclusion is that there has been virtually no change in the incidence of travelers' diarrhea, and only modest, but not breakthrough, advances in etiology, prevention, and treatment.

Incidence of Travelers' Diarrhea

According to recent surveys, > 60% of travelers to resource-deprived countries will develop travelers' diarrhea during a 2-week trip. The figures vary from country to country, from 20 to 90% in high-risk countries. Yet a look at the incidence over the past 50 years in Mexico, for example, where 21 studies have been reported since 1957, shows remarkably little change. The conclusion: not much improvement in the incidence of travelers' diarrhea over the past 50 years of observation.

Etiology of Travelers' Diarrhea

While significant improvements have been made over the past half century in defining the etiology of travelers' diarrhea, serious gaps in our knowledge remain and continue to confound a full understanding of this condition. Traditional folklore of travelers' diarrhea has spawned such etiologic theories as change in the water, too much noonday sun, spicy foods, and the general vicissitudes of travel. As improved laboratory methods became available, particularly testing for enterotoxigenic *Escherichia coli* (ETEC), it became apparent that travelers' diarrhea is caused in the main by infectious microorganisms that are acquired in food and drink. Several studies have isolated specific microbial pathogens from the feces of sick tourists. The causal link between infection and clinical disease has been solidified by field trials that have demonstrated the efficacy of antibacterial drugs in preventing and treating travelers' diarrhea. Indeed, prevention rates of 80% or more, achieved with a variety of antimicrobial drugs, strongly implicate bacterial pathogens, and probably gram-negative enteric organisms, as the cause of most travelers' diarrhea cases.

Microbiological studies of travelers' diarrhea have been carried out in many parts of the world. An array of pathogens has been found, but it is apparent that the leading culprits are various forms of *Escherichia (E.) coli*, particularly ETEC and enteroaggregative *E. coli*. Some geographic differences have become apparent in the isolation rates of ETEC in travelers. In Latin America, for example, the median isolation rate of ETEC in travelers' diarrhea cases has been 42% (range 26 to 72%), compared with a median of 16% in Asia (range 0 to 37%).

Several studies have reported more than one pathogen in travelers' diarrhea cases, up to 15% in Mexico and 33% in Thailand. To confuse the issue further, no pathogens have been identified despite careful laboratory methodology—up to 40% or more in some studies from several parts of the world. The high incidence of mixed infections, along with the inability to isolate pathogens in many cases, casts some doubt on the veracity of etiologic studies altogether. It is disappointing that that the multitude of studies over the past 50 years have failed to elucidate the cause of this disease in the mixed infections and the "undiagnosed" cases, which in many studies number nearly one-half of persons with travelers' diarrhea. Nevertheless, the striking efficacy of prophylaxis and treatment directed against bacterial pathogens suggests that travelers' diarrhea is indeed a bacterial infection in most cases, but we have made this surmise for several decades.

Prevention of Travelers' Diarrhea

It is certainly beneficial to prevent an attack of diarrhea, especially one that can interfere with an overseas journey. Having stated the obvious, such prevention is not easy to accomplish unless one travels with sterile, hermetically sealed containers of food and drink. Four approaches to preventing travelers' diarrhea can be conceived: avoiding unsafe foods and beverages, use of anti-infective drugs, use of other medications, and immunization.

Although there seems to be a direct relationship between dietary indiscretions and the incidence of travelers' diarrhea, some studies have failed to show any benefit from dietary restriction, probably because this advice is followed more in theory than in practice. Despite recommendations about safe consumption of food and drink, it is apparent that most travelers are unable to maintain perfect vigilance during a pleasure trip. Thus, this approach, although universally recommended, does not in reality provide complete protection.

Drug prophylaxis of travelers' diarrhea can be dated to before World War II, when iodochlorohydroxyquin, commonly known as Entervioform, was used to prevent what was felt to be the principle pathogen, *Entamoeba histolytica.* This practice continued unabated for several decades and was unquestioned until Ben Kean, whom many revere as the "scientific father of travelers' diarrhea," published in 1959 what is clearly the first blinded, placebo-controlled clinical trial of prophylactic drugs to 610 US students going to Mexico for the summer. Since the classic study by Kean and colleagues, many placebo-controlled trials have been conducted. Significant protection compared with placebo was noted in all but three studies, two of which involved neomycin and the third doxycycline in twice weekly doses rather than the usual daily doses. Protection rates have varied from 28 to 100%; the lower rates have been seen with what would now be recognized as poorly effective antimicrobial drugs, such as sulfonamides and streptomycin, or when a high level of resistance to the drug is found in ETEC isolated in the area.

Resistance to antimicrobial drugs is a universal occurrence and the bacteria causing travelers' diarrhea are involved in this trend. The enteric pathogens, especially *Shigella, Salmonella, Campylobacter and* ETEC, have developed a high degree of resistance to several antimicrobial agents in many developing countries. Resistance has been increasing to trimethoprim/sulfamethoxazole (TMP-SMX) and tetracycline, which were widely used in the past for travelers' diarrhea, and a great increase in resistance among coliforms, including diarrhea pathogens, has been witnessed in recent years to fluoroquinolones. It appears that many of the favored drugs for prevention have been compromised by these developments in antimicrobial resistance. Although no resistance was observed in the initial rifaximin trials with small numbers of participants, there is a concern that this drug, which is related to rifampin, an agent that is known to readily induce antimicrobial resistance, might be associated through widespread use with a similar problem.

So what progress has been made over the past 50 years in prophylaxis of travelers' diarrhea? The earlier drugs such as iodochlorohydroxyquin, neomycin, and sulfa compounds have all been discarded for prophylaxis due to lack of efficacy or side effects or both. As newer agents came into service, first tetracyclines, then TMP-SMX, and finally the quinolones, each has been seriously compromised by the spread of antimicrobial resistance, which is even more pervasive in countries with high incidences of travelers' diarrhea. The high level of resistance is promoted in these countries by uncontrolled dispensing of antimicrobial drugs at pharmacies and by the overzealous use of antimicrobial drugs in animal feed. Particularly concerning in this latter regard is the widespread use of fluoroquinolones in poultry, which induces widespread resistance in *Campylobacter* and *Salmonella.* Thus far, rifaximin has not been cursed with development of resistance, but it is in its early days for use in the developing world. If it follows the course of indiscriminate usage seen with other antimicrobial drugs, we can expect resistance to develop to rifaximin as well.

Universal prophylaxis to 50 million travelers who travel each year to resource-restrained countries is not, however, a rational or even feasible solution to travelers' diarrhea. Such an approach will surely invite the induction of antimicrobial resistance not only in potential pathogens but in components of the normal flora, and it might be associated with side effects for what is usually a mild illness in an otherwise healthy population. Surely, some few individuals should receive antibiotic prophylaxis for travelers' diarrhea, but not all of the 50 million travelers at risk.

Various commercial preparations of Lactobacillus, Sacchromyces, and *Streptococcus faecium* (SF 68) have been used prophylactically for travelers' diarrhea, and the effects have generally been inconsistent or, frankly, negative.

For immunological approaches, several investigators have employed passive antibody to ETEC with decidedly mixed results. In recent studies, colostrum-derived antibody to ETEC failed in clinical trials and in volunteer studies despite some earlier, largely unsubstantiated claims for success.

Although several avenues appear promising, there is no current vaccine that can be recommended for preventing travelers' diarrhea. Most vaccine work is focused on controlling ETEC because it is the major pathogen. Another approach employs cholera vaccine or the toxin B subunit, which induces protection against ETEC. These various approaches are being pursued vigorously in several laboratories, and active vaccine or passive antibodies may become available in the future for use in travelers' diarrhea as well as the important problem of diarrhea in developing countries. In prevention of travelers' diarrhea, however, it is not clear that an ETEC-directed immunologic strategy will ultimately prove successful in this condition. As noted above, travelers' diarrhea is associated with many pathogens, from bacterial, surely the most common, to protozoa, and more recently to viruses, particularly Norovirus. In addition, the vaccine approach may be confounded by the lack of identification of a specific pathogen, or the converse, the finding of at least two or more pathogens isolated in many cases.

Even if a successful vaccine could be produced—and this is a major assumption—there remains the imposing challenge of administering it to the approximately 50 million persons who travel each year from industrialized countries to resource-constrained countries.

Treatment of Travelers' Diarrhea

The shelves of all pharmacies and apothecaries around the globe are filled with various proprietary anti-diarrhea medicines or herbals. Starches, talcs, chalks, and absorbent compounds have been prescribed for diarrheal diseases for as long as recorded history. Kaolin and pectin, for example, are included in several over-the-counter formulations, yet there is no substantive evidence that these products can alter the volume or electrolyte content of diarrhea stool. Despite widespread prescribing and self-medicating, these products have not proven useful in travelers' diarrhea. Such knowledge, even if negative, can be judged as a sign of progress over the past few decades.

We have also learned by careful field trials that some cases of travelers' diarrhea are mild enough that specific treatment can be withheld without adverse consequences. Several antibiotics have been used successfully in treatment of moderate-to-severe travelers' diarrhea. In reviewing previous studies of these various agents, it is important to recognize that the playing field is constantly shifting as antimicrobial resistance becomes increasingly a major segment of the epidemiologic landscape. In the past, it was shown that TMP-SMX or TMP alone, ciprofloxacin, fleroxacin, norfloxacin, and aztreonam have been used successfully for treatment of travelers' diarrhea. However, all of these drugs have been compromised as effective therapeutic agents in many countries. Of the drugs that currently enjoy some currency due to continuing sensitivity of the pathogens, rifaximin and azithromycin have gained support for treatment of travelers' diarrhea.

Antimotility drugs have engendered considerable favor among tourists for providing relief from the intestinal indignities of travel, and their approbation is supported by good scientific studies. The most effective relief from symptoms of travelers' diarrhea has been provided by a combination of an antimicrobial drug and an antimotility drug.

Treatment is an area where it can be said beyond peradventure that we have gained in knowledge over the past 50 years. We have learned which products have limited efficacy, which antimicrobial drugs have lost their activity due to rising incidences of resistance, and which antimicrobial drugs can still be used for treatment. In addition, it does seem that the combination of antimotility drugs and antimicrobial agents can offer rapid and substantial relief from the agonies of travelers' diarrhea.

Future Directions

Because international travel has expanded, particularly to exotic and eco-travel destinations as well as to the resource-limited countries, where the adventures are both challenging as well as financially feasible, travelers' diarrhea continues to be the uninvited and unwelcome travel companion. It is estimated now that 50 million travelers sojourn each year to areas of significant travelers' diarrhea risk. This brief review has provided what is a disappointing report card on scientific progress in travelers' diarrhea over the past 50 years, and looking ahead does not provide any exciting prospects for improvement. On the other hand, it is known that at the turn of the 20th Century diarrhea morbidity and mortality in North America was very high, comparable to the figures now seen in resource-deprived countries. Over the first half of the past century, diarrhea rates fell dramatically in the industrialized countries related to improvements in food production and infrastructure, sewage handling, and nearly universal availability of potable water.

The future of improvements in reducing the incidence of travelers' diarrhea lies not in further developments in treatment nor even in prevention modalities, particularly given the uncertain and thus far disappointing results with vaccines or immunological products. The future in reductions of travelers' diarrhea is rooted in public health measures in resource-deprived countries in food handling, sewage handling, and water supplies—proven measures to lift up the health status of the local population that will incidentally have a salutary effect on travelers' diarrhea rates. This is the only approach that could offer protection from travelers' diarrhea to nearly all travelers without inviting the potentially unpleasant compromises associated with universal drug prophylaxis, an option that is unlikely to be applied successfully to all travelers at risk. In addition, any sensible prevention measure for so many individuals at risk must take the responsibility for daily self administration out their hands and transfer it to a universal and generalizable approach. Some countries are developing these public health capacities but, alas, many regions, including some of the most popular tourist attractions, have made very little progress. The continuing high incidence of travelers' diarrhea serves as a canary in the mine, reminding us of the woeful condition of public health infrastructure in many of the economically deprived areas of our world.

INDEX